Hartman's Complete Guide for the Patient Care Technician

Hartman Publishing, Inc.

hartmanonline.com

Hartman

Credits

Managing Editor
Susan Alvare Hedman

Developmental Editor
Kristin Calderon

Designer
Kirsten Browne

Production
Anika Steppe

Photography
Matt Pence, Pat Berrett, Art Clifton, and Dick Ruddy

Proofreaders
Sapna Desai, Danielle Lescure, and Zella Mansson

Editorial Assistant
Angela Storey

Sales Manager
Kendra Robertson

Sales/Marketing
Deborah Rinker-Wildey, Erika Walker, Col Foley, Erin Kleymann, and Caroyl Scott

Operations Manager
Fran Desmond

Customer Service
Thomas Noble, Hank Bullis, Della Torres, Kate Plath, and Brian Fejer

Information Technology
Eliza Martin

Warehouse Coordinator
Eric Cruz

Copyright Information

1313 Iron Avenue SW
Albuquerque, New Mexico 87102
(505) 291-1274
web: hartmanonline.com
email: orders@hartmanonline.com

ISBN 978-1-60425-162-3

PRINTED IN CANADA

Notice to Readers

Though the guidelines and procedures contained in this text are based on consultations with healthcare professionals, they should not be considered absolute recommendations. The instructor and readers should follow employer, local, state, and federal guidelines concerning healthcare practices. These guidelines change, and it is each reader's responsibility to be aware of these changes and of the policies and procedures of their healthcare facility.

The publisher, authors, editors, and reviewers cannot accept any responsibility for errors or omissions or for any consequences from application of the information in this book and make no warranty, express or implied, with respect to the contents of the book. The publisher does not warrant or guarantee any of the products described herein or perform any analysis in connection with any of the product information contained herein.

Gender Usage

This textbook uses gender pronouns interchangeably to denote healthcare team members and patients.

Special Thanks

A heartfelt thank you goes to our insightful and wonderful reviewers, listed in alphabetical order:

Sylvia Beste, MEd, MT (ASCP)
El Paso, TX

Mary M. Bradley, MSN, RN, CEN
Baltimore, MD

Gale Chambers Cabe, RN, CPCT
Schertz, TX

Janet M. Cadeau, MSEL, BS, CMA (AAMA)
Farmington Hills, MI

Jennifer L. James, DNP, APRN
Carpenter, WY

Michele Knorpp, LVN
Palestine, TX

We are very appreciative of the many sources who shared their informative photos with us:

3M

American Hospital Association

Baxter International Inc.

B. Braun Medical Inc.

Becton, Dickinson and Company

Benchmark Scientific

CleanLife Products

Detecto

Dreamstime

Encompass Group, LLC

Exergen Corporation

Globe Scientific, Inc.

Greiner Bio-One

Harrisburg Area Community College

Hollister Incorporated

The International Dysphagia Diet Standardisation Initiative

Invacare Corporation

Dr. Jere Mammino, DO

Magnetic Concepts

March of Dimes

Marketlab, Inc.

McKesson Medical-Surgical

The Medcom Group, Ltd.

Medline Industries, LP

National Pressure Injury Advisory Panel

North Coast Medical, Inc.

Nova Biomedical

Nova Medical Products

Occupational Safety and Health Administration (OSHA)

Philips RS North America LLC.

Royal Philips

Skil-Care Corporation

Statewide Program for Infection Control and Epidemiology (SPICE)

Teleflex Incorporated

Vancare, Inc.

Verathon, Inc.

Zoll Medical Corporation

Contents

Learning Objective — *Page*

Procedures

Procedure	*Page*

Using a Hartman Textbook

Understanding how this book is organized and what its special features are will help you make the most of this resource!

We have assigned each chapter its own colored tab. Located on the side of every page, each colored tab contains the chapter number and title.

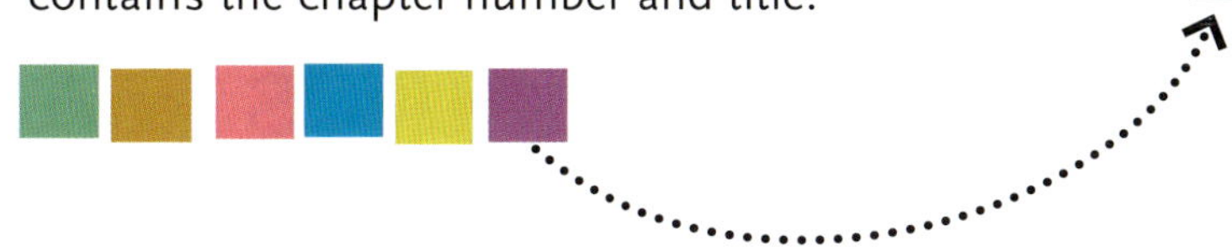

1. Discuss common legal concepts and responsibilities in health care

Everything in this book, the student workbook, and the instructor's teaching material is organized around learning objectives. A learning objective is a very specific piece of knowledge or a very specific skill. After reading the text, if you can do what the learning objective says, you know you have mastered the material.

---

bloodborne pathogens

Bold key terms are located throughout the text, followed by their definitions. They are also listed in the glossary at the back of this book.

Making an occupied bed

All care procedures are highlighted by a black bar for easy recognition.

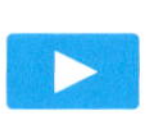

This icon indicates that Hartman Publishing offers a corresponding video for this skill.

Guidelines: Legal and Ethical Behavior

Guidelines and Observing and Reporting lists are colored green for easy reference.

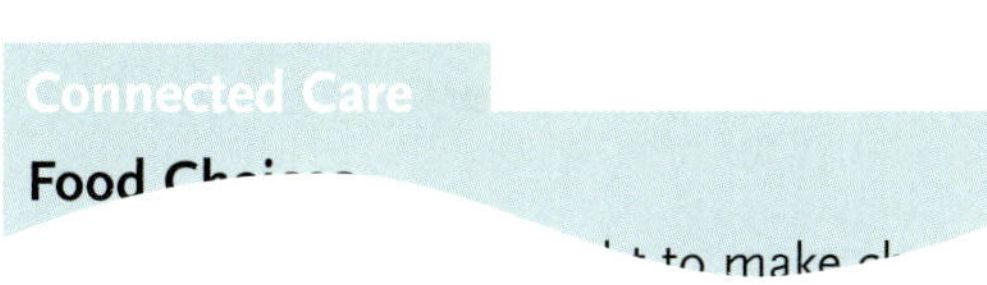

Blue Connected Care boxes relate to providing care that promotes patient dignity and protects patient rights.

Chapter Review

Chapter-ending questions test your knowledge of the information found in the chapter. If you have trouble answering a question, you can return to the text and reread the material.

Beginning and ending steps in care procedures

For most care procedures, these beginning and ending steps should be performed. Understanding why they are important will help you remember to perform each step every time care is provided.

Beginning Steps

Identify yourself by name. Identify the patient according to facility policy.	Before any procedure, knock and wait for permission to enter the patient's room. Upon entering his room, identify yourself and state your title. Patients have the right to know who is providing their care. Identify and greet the patient. This shows courtesy and respect. It also establishes correct identification. This prevents care from being performed on the wrong person.
Wash your hands.	Handwashing provides for infection prevention. Nothing fights infection in facilities like performing consistent, proper hand hygiene. Handwashing may need to be done more than once during a procedure. Practice Standard Precautions with every patient.
Explain the procedure to the patient. Speak clearly, slowly, and directly. Maintain face-to-face contact whenever possible.	Patients have a legal right to be involved in their care, which includes knowing what care you will provide.
Provide for the patient's privacy with a curtain, screen, or door.	Doing this maintains patients' rights to privacy and dignity. Providing for privacy in a facility is not simply a courtesy; privacy is a legal right.
Adjust the bed to a safe level, usually waist high. Lock the bed wheels.	Locking the bed wheels is an important safety measure. It ensures that the bed will not move as you are performing care. Raising the bed helps you to remember to use proper body mechanics. This helps prevent injury to you and to patients.

Ending Steps	
Make the patient comfortable.	Make sure the sheets are wrinkle-free and lie flat under the patient's body. This helps prevent pressure injuries. Replace bedding and pillows. Check that the patient's body is in proper alignment. This promotes comfort and health after you leave the room.
Return the bed to its lowest position. Remove privacy measures.	Lowering the bed provides for the patient's safety. Remove extra privacy measures added during the procedure. This includes anything you may have draped over and around the patient, as well as privacy screens.
Place the call light within the patient's reach.	A call light allows the patient to communicate with staff as necessary. It must always be left within reach of the patient's hand. You must respond to call lights promptly.
Wash your hands.	Handwashing is the most important thing you can do to prevent the spread of infection.
Report any changes in the patient to the nurse. Document the procedure using facility guidelines.	You will spend a lot of time with patients, so you are in the best position to note any changes in a patient's condition. Every time you provide care, observe the patient's physical and mental capabilities, as well as the condition of the patient's body. For example, a change in a patient's ability to get out of bed may signal a greater problem. After you have finished giving care, document the care using facility guidelines. Do not record care before it is given. If you do not document the care you gave, legally it did not happen.

In addition to the beginning and ending steps listed above, remember to follow infection prevention guidelines. Even if a procedure in this book does not tell you to wear gloves or other PPE, there may be times when it is appropriate.

For example, the procedure for measuring blood pressure does not include gloves. Gloves are usually not required for this. However, if the patient has open sores or cuts on his arm, gloves are necessary.

1

The Role of the Patient Care Technician

1. Explain the patient care technician's role

Patient care technicians (PCTs) are skilled healthcare workers who perform assigned tasks such as measuring vital signs and providing or assisting with personal care. PCTs may also draw blood and perform simple tests at a patient's bedside. They may conduct electrocardiograms (EKGs), a test of heart activity. PCTs work under the supervision of a licensed healthcare professional, usually a registered nurse.

The patient care technician role is similar to the roles of nursing assistants (NAs) and medical assistants (MAs), but there are several differences. One key difference is the workplace, or setting. NAs usually work in **long-term care** (**LTC**) facilities. (The term *nursing homes* was once widely used to refer to these facilities.) MAs usually work in doctors' offices, clinics, or urgent care centers. PCTs may work in long-term care or in a medical office, but more often they work in hospitals and other inpatient settings (Fig. 1-1). The next learning objective has more information about these settings.

A PCT's duties include some that nursing assistants do not usually perform. NAs do not draw blood or conduct EKGs unless they receive special training. Other skills that relate to inpatient care, such as removing an IV, are not common for NAs. In addition to having clinical duties, many medical assistants are trained in administrative tasks. They may assist with payment collection, insurance claims, and managing patient records. Most PCTs only have direct patient care duties.

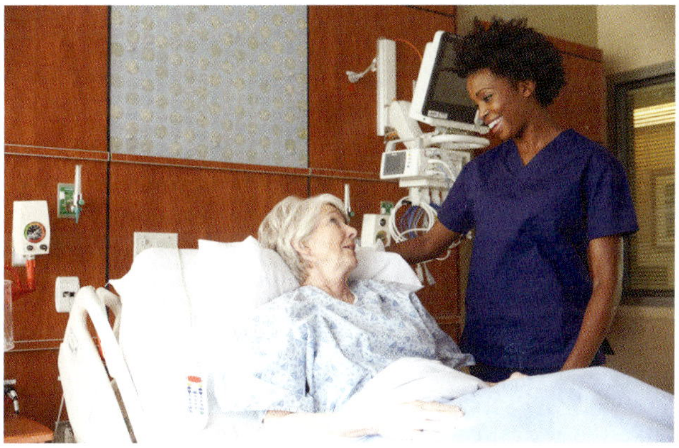

***Fig. 1-1.** More than half of PCTs work in hospitals, according to industry surveys.*

Each state sets its own rules about which tasks PCTs can perform. The following is a list of common PCT tasks:

- Assisting with admitting new patients to units and preparing the room prior to their arrival
- Assisting patients with bathing, grooming, and elimination
- Measuring vital signs (temperature, pulse rate, respiratory rate, and blood pressure)
- Transferring patients, for example from a bed to a gurney (stretcher) or from a gurney back to a bed

- Assisting with range of motion exercises and ambulation
- Assisting with timed tests and specimen collections, such as 24-hour urine tests
- Drawing blood
- Conducting **point-of-care tests** (tests performed at the patient's bedside) such as fingerstick glucose tests (Fig. 1-2)

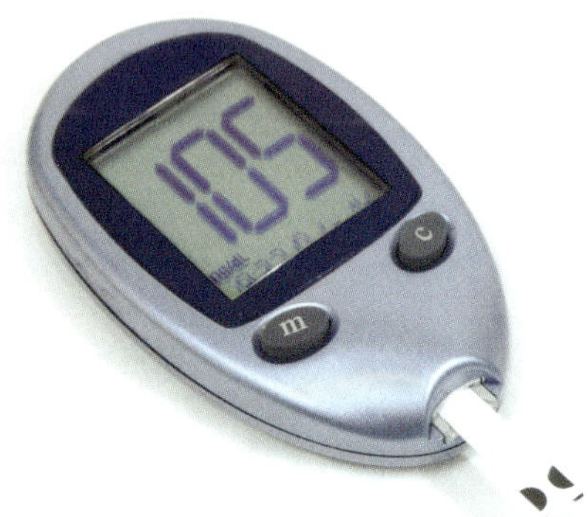

***Fig. 1-2.** Point-of-care tests are performed at the patient's bedside. Blood sugar (glucose) levels are often tested this way.*

- Conducting EKGs and setting up other types of cardiac monitoring
- Helping to prepare patients for surgery and caring for patients after surgery
- Making beds and changing linens on beds
- Caring for supplies and equipment

PCTs spend most of their time working directly with patients. Observing changes in a patient's condition and reporting them is a very important duty of the PCT. Patients' care can be revised or updated as conditions change. Another duty of the PCT is noting and recording important information about the patient; this is called **charting**, or documenting.

PCTs are part of a healthcare team. The team includes providers, nurses, social workers, therapists, dietitians, and specialists. The patient and patient's family are part of the team. Everyone, including the patient, works closely together to meet recovery goals.

2. Describe healthcare settings where patient care technicians work

Health care can take place in either an inpatient or outpatient setting. Because PCTs most often work in hospitals, this book emphasizes the skills needed in an inpatient setting. Inpatient facilities are facilities where patients spend at least 1 night while receiving care. They include traditional hospitals and the following facilities:

- Specialty hospitals such as heart care hospitals and cancer centers
- Skilled nursing facilities (SNFs), rehabilitation centers, or other long-term care facilities (LTCFs) where patients may receive extended care after a hospital stay
- Inpatient mental health facilities

Medical offices, urgent care clinics, specialty clinics, and same-day surgery centers are examples of outpatient settings. In these settings, patients arrive, receive care, and leave on the same day. PCTs who work in these settings may measure vital signs, assist providers with examinations, help prepare patients for procedures, draw blood, and conduct EKGs (Fig. 1-3).

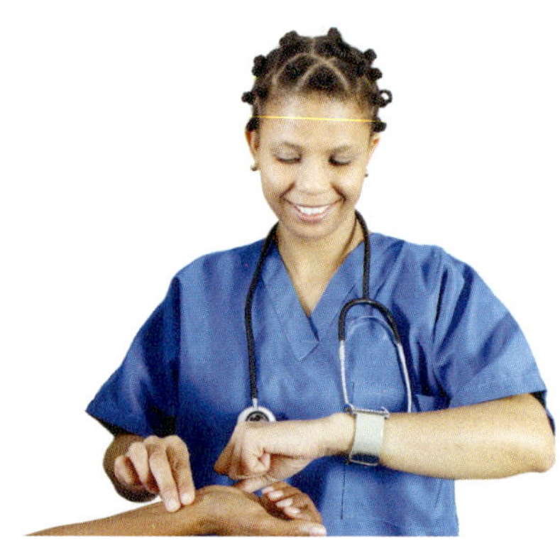

***Fig. 1-3.** In outpatient settings, PCTs measure patient vital signs and assist healthcare providers.*

Assisted living facilities and home health care agencies may also hire PCTs. **Assisted living facilities** are residences for people who need some help with daily care, such as showering, meals, and dressing. People who live in these facilities do not need 24-hour skilled care. Some assisted living facilities have memory care units for people who have mild dementia. These people are unable to live alone but are still fairly independent. **Dementia** is defined as the serious loss of mental abilities, such as thinking, remembering, reasoning, and communicating.

Home health care, or home care, is provided in a person's home. This type of care is often given to people who are older and are chronically ill but who are able to and wish to remain at home. Home health care may also be needed when a person needs assistance after a recent hospital stay. PCTs who work in home care help with personal care, measure vital signs, help with mobility, and may also help with housekeeping tasks.

3. Identify members of the healthcare team

Patients have different needs and conditions. Healthcare professionals with a wide range of education and experience help care for them together (sometimes referred to as an *interdisciplinary approach*). This group is known as the *care team*. Members of the care team include the following:

Patient care technician (PCT): The PCT is an unlicensed healthcare worker who performs assigned tasks, such as measuring vital signs, and provides or assists with personal care, such as bathing patients and helping with elimination needs. PCTs spend much of their time working with patients. That is why they act as the "eyes and ears" of the team. Observing and reporting changes in the patient's condition or abilities is a very important duty of the PCT. There is no national standard for training of PCTs. States may set standards and facilities may also have requirements for PCT training and certification.

Registered nurse (RN): In hospitals and long-term care facilities, a registered nurse is a licensed healthcare professional who coordinates, manages, and provides skilled nursing care. This includes administering special treatments and giving medication as prescribed by a physician. A registered nurse also assigns tasks and supervises daily care of patients by PCTs. A registered nurse has graduated from a 2- to 4-year nursing program. RNs have diplomas or college degrees and have passed a national licensure examination. Registered nurses may have additional academic degrees or education in specialty areas.

Licensed practical nurse (LPN) or **licensed vocational nurse (LVN)**: A licensed practical nurse or licensed vocational nurse is a licensed healthcare professional who administers medications and gives treatments. A licensed practical nurse or vocational nurse has completed 1 to 2 years of education and has passed a national licensure examination.

Advanced practice registered nurse (APRN): An advanced practice registered nurse (sometimes called an *advanced practice nurse*, or *APN*) is a registered nurse who has completed training at the postgraduate level (master's or doctoral). There are 4 types of APRNs: nurse practitioner (NP), nurse anesthetist (CRNA), nurse midwife (CNM), and clinical nurse specialist (CNS). APRNs can make diagnoses and prescribe treatment. Nurse practitioners and clinical nurse specialists may receive additional certification in many areas, including acute care, cardiac care, gerontology, neonatal care, and psychiatric/mental health care.

Physician or **doctor (MD** or **DO [doctor of osteopathy])**: A doctor is a licensed healthcare professional who diagnoses disease or disability and prescribes treatment and medication (Fig. 1-4). A doctor has graduated from a 4-year medical school, which they attended after first receiving a bachelor's degree. Many doctors also attend specialized training programs after medical school.

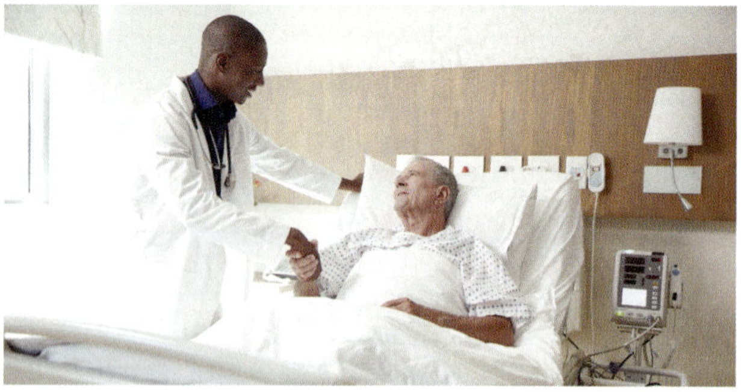

Fig. 1-4. A doctor makes a diagnosis and prescribes treatment.

Physician assistant (PA): A physician assistant is a licensed healthcare professional who diagnoses disease or disability and develops treatment plans, as well as prescribes medication. PAs work together with doctors to provide care. PAs have received master's degrees and have to pass a national licensure examination before they can practice.

Pharmacist (RPh): A pharmacist is a licensed healthcare professional who prepares and dispenses prescribed medications. Pharmacists help manage medications to ensure safety and prevent potential problems. They also educate patients and healthcare providers. A pharmacist has graduated from a doctoral degree program and must pass national and state licensure examinations before they can practice.

Physical therapist (PT or DPT): A physical therapist is a licensed healthcare professional who evaluates a person and develops a treatment plan to increase movement, improve circulation, promote healing, reduce pain, prevent disability, and regain or maintain mobility (Fig. 1-5).

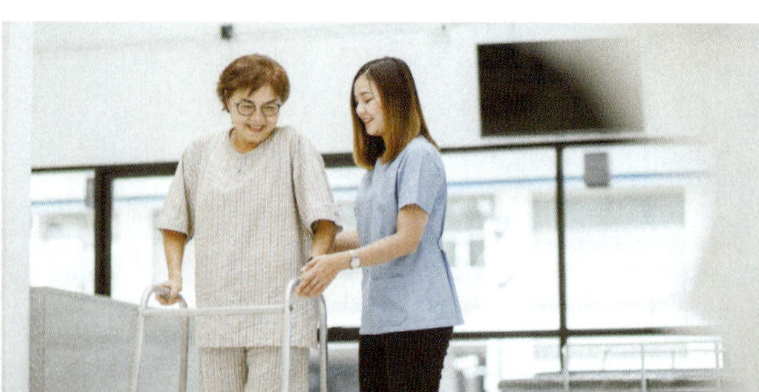

Fig. 1-5. A physical therapist helps exercise muscles, bones, and joints to improve strength or restore abilities.

A PT or DPT (doctor of physical therapy) administers therapy in the form of heat, cold, massage, ultrasound, electrical stimulation, and exercise to muscles, bones, and joints. A physical therapist has graduated from a doctoral degree program after receiving an undergraduate degree. PTs have to pass national licensure examinations before they can practice.

Occupational therapist (OT): An occupational therapist is a licensed healthcare professional who helps patients learn to adapt to disabilities. An OT may help train patients to perform activities of daily living (ADLs), such as bathing, dressing, and eating. This often involves the use of special equipment called *assistive devices* (Fig. 1-6). The OT evaluates the patient's needs and develops a treatment program. Occupational therapists have earned a master's or doctoral degree and must pass a national licensure examination before they can practice. (As of July 2027, the Accreditation Council for Occupational Therapy Education [ACOTE] will require occupational therapists to have a doctoral degree.)

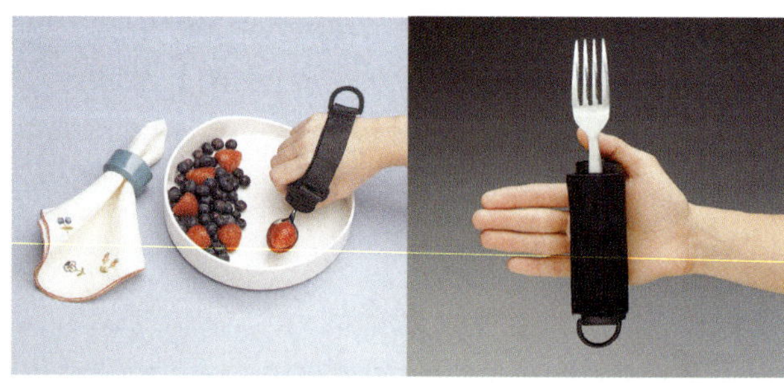

Fig. 1-6. An occupational therapist will help patients learn to use assistive devices, such as this special fork and plate. (PHOTOS COURTESY OF NORTH COAST MEDICAL, INC., WWW.NCMEDICAL.COM)

Speech-language pathologist (SLP): A speech-language pathologist, or speech therapist, is a licensed healthcare professional who identifies communication disorders, addresses factors involved in recovery, and develops a plan of care to meet improvement or recovery goals. An SLP teaches exercises to help the patient improve or overcome speech problems. An SLP also evaluates a person's ability to swallow food and drink. Speech-language pathologists have earned a master's degree in speech-language pathology. They must pass a national certification exam before they can practice.

Registered dietitian (**RD**) or **registered dietitian nutritionist** (**RDN**): A registered dietitian or registered dietitian nutritionist assesses a patient's nutritional status and develops a treatment plan to improve health and manage illness. An RD/RDN creates diets to meet patients' special needs and may also supervise the preparation of food and educate people about nutrition. RDs/RDNs have completed a bachelor's degree or master's degree, and in most states they must be licensed to practice. (As of 2024, the Commission on Dietetic Registration [CDR] will require RDNs to have a master's degree.)

Medical social worker (**MSW**): A medical social worker is a licensed healthcare professional who determines patients' needs and helps get them support services, such as counseling and financial assistance. An MSW may help patients obtain clothing and personal items they would not otherwise have after discharge from the facility. An MSW may help patients book appointments and transportation for follow-up care. MSWs have earned a master's degree in social work and must be licensed to work.

Patient and patient's family: The patient is an important member of the care team. Providing **person-centered care** means placing the patient's well-being first, and giving her the right to make decisions about her care. The patient helps plan care, and the patient's family may also be involved in these decisions. The care team revolves around the patient and her condition, goals, priorities, treatment, and progress. Without the patient, there is no care team.

4. Understand delegation and scope of practice

A PCT carries out instructions given to her by a nurse. The nurse is acting on the instructions of a doctor or other member of the care team. This is called the **chain of command**. It describes the line of authority and helps to make sure that patients get proper health care. The chain of command also protects employees and employers from liability. **Liability** is a legal term that means someone can be held responsible for harming someone else. An example is a situation in which a task that a PCT performs for a patient harms that patient. However, the task was in the care plan and was done correctly. In this case, the PCT may not be liable, or responsible, for hurting the patient. However, if the PCT does something that is not in the care plan that harms a patient, she could be held responsible. That is why it is important to follow instructions in the care plan and for the facility to have a chain of command (Fig. 1-7).

In addition to respecting their facility's chain of command, PCTs must understand what they can and cannot do. This is important so that they do not harm patients or involve themselves or their employers in lawsuits. **Scope of practice** refers to the roles, responsibilities, and procedures that are within the knowledge, training, and legal definition of a profession. Scope of practice for the PCT varies by state and facility. Some states have laws for PCTs' scope of practice, overseen by boards of nursing or medicine. In states without legal guidelines, scope of practice is guided by the facility in which the PCT works.

Everything PCTs do in their job must be assigned to them by a licensed healthcare professional. When planning care, nurses decide which tasks to delegate to others, including PCTs. **Delegation** means transferring responsibility to a person for a specific task. PCTs do not delegate tasks; they have tasks delegated to them. Licensed nurses are accountable for care, including all delegated tasks.

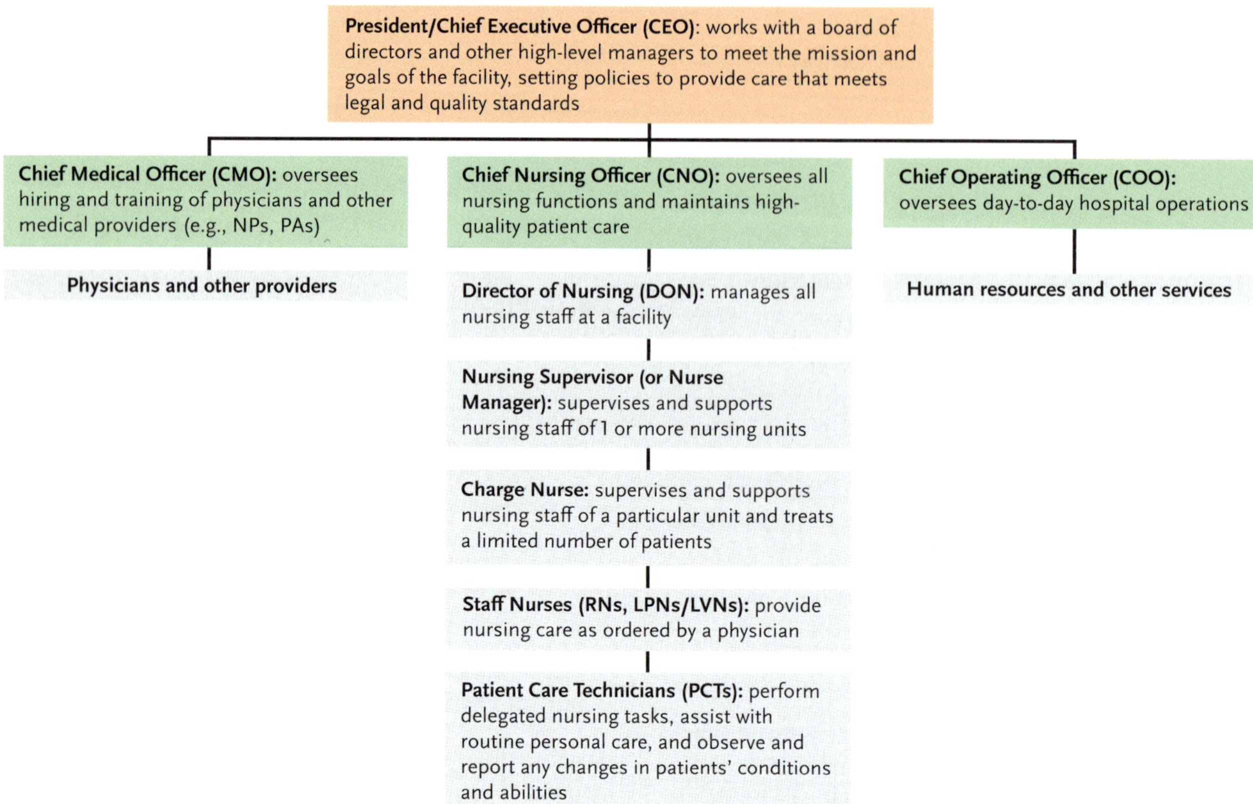

Fig. 1-7. *The chain of command describes the line of authority in a facility and helps ensure that the patient receives proper care.*

The National Council of State Boards of Nursing (NCSBN, ncsbn.org) has identified the Five Rights of Delegation. This can be used as a mental checklist to help nurses in the decision-making process. The Five Rights of Delegation are the Right Task, Right Circumstance, Right Person, Right Direction/Communication, and Right Supervision/Evaluation. Before delegating tasks, nurses consider these questions:

- Is there a match between the patient's needs and the PCT's skills, abilities, and experience?
- What is the level of patient stability?
- Is the patient care technician the right person to do the job?
- Can the nurse give appropriate direction and communication?
- Is the nurse available to give the supervision, support, and help that the patient care technician needs?

These are questions PCTs may want to consider before accepting a task:

- Do I have all the information I need to do this job? Are there questions I should ask?
- Do I believe that I can do this task? Do I have the necessary skills?
- Do I have the needed supplies, equipment, and other support?
- Do I know who my supervisor is and how to reach that person?
- Have I told my supervisor of any special needs for help and support?
- Do we both understand who is doing what?

A PCT should never be afraid to ask for help. They should always ask if they need more information or are unsure about something. If a PCT feels that they do not have the skills for a task or that the task is not within their scope of practice, they should talk to the nurse. Requests that are outside the PCT's scope of practice must always be refused. Refusing to do something that the PCT cannot legally do is the PCT's right and responsibility.

5. Define *professionalism* and list examples of professional behavior

Professional means having to do with work or a job. **Personal** refers to life outside a job, such as family, friends, and home life. **Professionalism** is behaving properly when on the job. It includes dressing appropriately and speaking well. It also includes being on time, completing tasks, and reporting to the nurse. For a PCT, professionalism means following the care plan, making careful observations, and reporting accurately.

Following policies and procedures is an important part of professionalism. A **policy** is a course of action that should be taken every time a certain situation occurs. For example, a common policy is that healthcare information must remain **confidential** (private). A **procedure** is a method, or way, of doing something. For example, a facility will have a procedure for reporting information about patients. The procedure explains what, when, and how often to document patient information. Most facilities have published policies and procedures that can be accessed at any time by employees.

Patients, coworkers, and supervisors respect employees who behave professionally. Professionalism helps people keep their jobs and may also help them earn promotions and raises.

A professional relationship with patients includes the following:

- Providing person-centered care, or care that promotes each patient's individual preferences, choices, and dignity
- Keeping a positive attitude
- Doing only the assigned tasks that are in the care plan and that the PCT is trained to do
- Keeping all patients' information confidential
- Always being polite (Fig. 1-8)

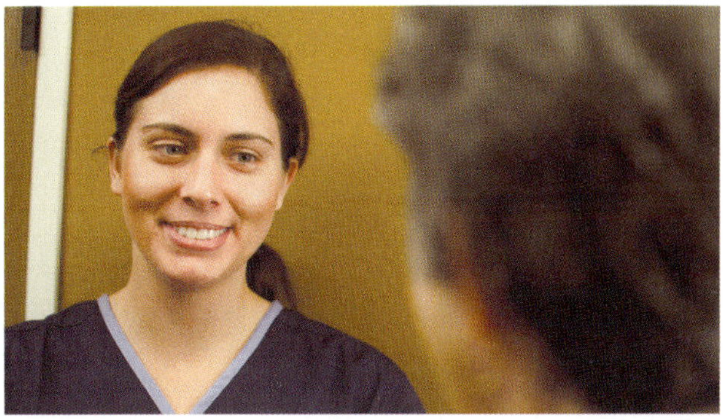

Fig. 1-8. *PCTs are expected to be polite and professional in all circumstances.*

- Not discussing personal subjects with patients or with coworkers when providing care
- Not using personal phones in patients' rooms or in any patient care area
- Not using profanity, even if a patient does
- Listening to the patient
- Calling a patient Mr., Mrs., Ms., or Miss, and their last name, or by the name the patient prefers; terms such as sweetie, honey, and dearie are disrespectful and should not be used
- Using the pronouns a patient prefers (she/her, he/him, they/them)
- Never giving or accepting gifts
- Always explaining care before providing it
- Following practices, such as handwashing, to protect oneself and patients

A professional relationship with an employer includes the following:

- Completing tasks efficiently
- Always following policies and procedures
- Documenting and reporting carefully and correctly

- Reporting problems with patients or tasks
- Reporting anything that keeps a patient care technician from completing duties
- Asking questions when the patient care technician does not know or understand something
- Taking directions or feedback without getting upset
- Being clean, neatly dressed, and groomed
- Always being on time
- Telling the employer if the patient care technician cannot report for work
- Following the chain of command
- Participating in education programs
- Being a positive role model for the facility

PCTs must be

Compassionate: Being **compassionate** means being caring, concerned, considerate, empathetic, and understanding. Demonstrating **empathy** means identifying with the feelings of others. People who are compassionate understand other people's problems. They care about them. Compassionate people are also sympathetic. Showing **sympathy** means sharing in the feelings and difficulties of others.

Honest: An honest person tells the truth and can be trusted. Patients need to feel that they can trust the people who care for them. The care team depends on honesty in planning care. Employers count on truthful records of the care provided and the observations made.

Tactful: Being **tactful** means showing sensitivity and having a sense of what is appropriate when dealing with others. It is the ability to speak and act without offending others.

Conscientious: People who are **conscientious** try to do their best. They are guided by a sense of right and wrong. They are alert, observant, accurate, and responsible. Giving conscientious care means making accurate observations and reports, following the care plan, and taking responsibility for one's actions (Fig. 1-9).

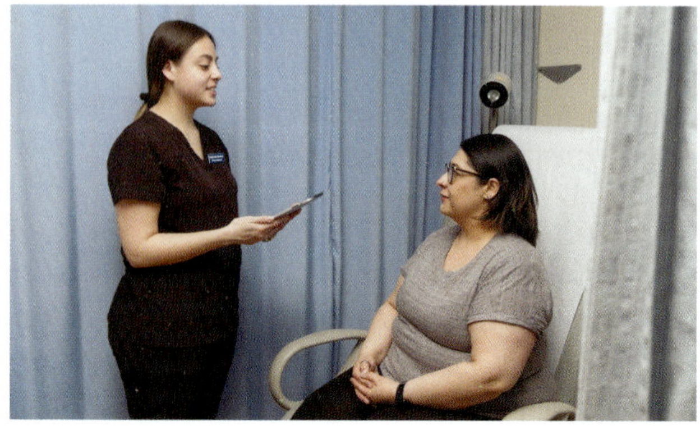

Fig. 1-9. *Observing carefully and documenting accurately are a part of providing conscientious care.*

For example, accurately measuring vital signs, such as temperature or pulse rate, is important. Other members of the care team will make treatment decisions based on the documented measurements. Without conscientious care, a patient's health and well-being are in danger.

Dependable: PCTs must be able to make and keep commitments. They must report to work on time. They must skillfully do assigned tasks, avoid absences, and help their peers when needed.

Organized: PCTs must manage their time well while taking care of patients. There are many tasks that must be done during their shifts. Planning ahead, prioritizing (doing the most important tasks first), and making a schedule are ways PCTs can be organized in their work.

Patient: People who are patient do not lose their tempers easily. They do not act irritated or complain when things are hard. Patients may be sick or in pain. They may become upset. PCTs must be patient. They must not rush patients or act annoyed.

Respectful: Being respectful means valuing other people's individuality, including their age, religion, culture, feelings, practices, and beliefs. People who are respectful treat others politely and kindly. They care about other people's self-esteem and do not gossip about them. PCTs may not like or agree with all patients or their families. However, their job is to care for each patient as assigned, not to judge them. PCTs should respect each patient as an individual.

Unprejudiced: PCTs work with people from many different backgrounds. They must give each patient the same quality care regardless of age, gender, sexual orientation, gender identity, religion, race, ethnicity, body size, or condition.

Proactive: Being proactive means anticipating potential problems and needs before they occur. PCTs who pay close attention to patients and their environments are more likely to anticipate needs and prevent problems, rather than simply reacting after something occurs. Observing and reporting carefully are key ways to be proactive.

Personal appearance is also part of professionalism. Professional dress inspires trust. Proper hygiene and careful grooming are essential qualities of healthcare workers (Fig. 1-10).

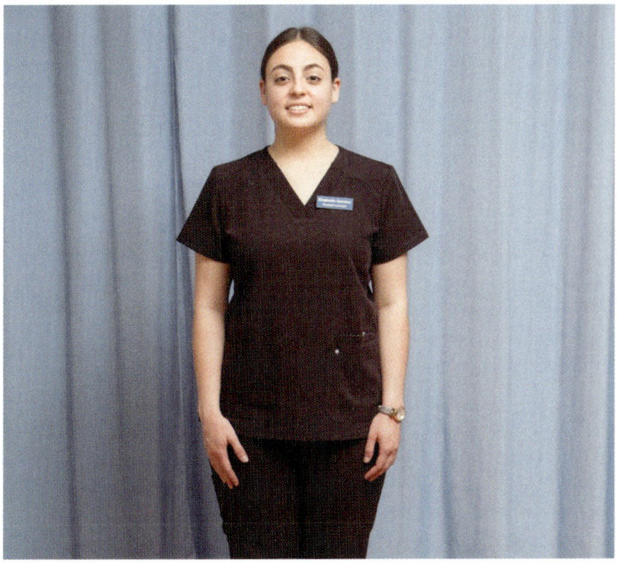

Fig. 1-10. *A PCT should look professional.*

Guidelines: Grooming and Appearance

- **G** Bathe or shower daily.
- **G** Brush and floss your teeth regularly, at least twice a day.
- **G** Wear deodorant and do not use scented sprays, body washes, perfumes, or lotions. Patients may not like scents or may have allergies.
- **G** Comb or brush your hair, pulling long hair back and securing it into a ponytail or bun.
- **G** Groom facial hair regularly and keep it clean and neat.
- **G** Wear little or no makeup.
- **G** Keep fingernails short, smooth, and clean.
- **G** Do not wear artificial nails, nail polish, or nail wraps. Artificial nails and wraps can harbor bacteria, no matter how well you wash your hands.
- **G** Wear a clean, wrinkle-free uniform that fits properly.
- **G** Wear an identification badge that is clearly visible.
- **G** Limit jewelry to small earrings and a simple watch that can count seconds.
- **G** Wear comfortable, clean, high-quality shoes. They must have closed toes and soles that do not slip easily.
- **G** Do not wear earbuds or headphones while working.

6. Describe the certification process

PCTs are eligible for national certification after they complete a qualifying patient care technician program. Not all states require PCTs to be certified. Some may require that PCTs be certified as nursing assistants before they can become certified as PCTs. Certification (if available) is valued by employers. It is a sign of professionalism. Certification proves that the PCT has achieved a certain level of knowledge.

Many agencies offer certification, and requirements vary. They usually include providing proof of course completion and passing a test given by the certification agency (Fig. 1-11). Some agencies allow people who have received on-the-job training in a healthcare setting or in the military to apply for certification. Applicants still must pass a certification exam. A high school diploma or GED certificate (general educational development tests showing knowledge equivalent for a high school diploma) is required for PCT certification. Once certified, the PCT must maintain certification through annual training called **continuing education** (**CE**).

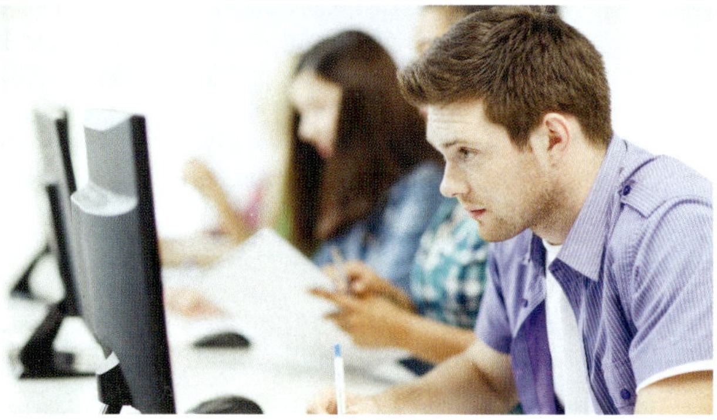

Fig. 1-11. PCTs must pass an exam as part of the certification process.

The National Healthcareer Association (NHA, nhanow.com) and the National Center for Competency Testing (NCCT, ncctinc.com) both offer widely recognized and respected PCT certifications. The agency used may depend on the PCT's training program or employer. If a PCT is able to choose, it is best to use an agency that is accredited by an outside organization such as the National Commission for Certifying Agencies (NCCA). An accredited certification program is confirmed to meet quality standards.

Certified PCTs are in high demand in inpatient and outpatient settings. PCTs can also choose to earn additional certifications in phlebotomy, electrocardiography (EKG), or other areas. Additional training and education can improve employment opportunities and benefits. PCTs can also return to school and pursue careers in nursing, medicine, and many other healthcare fields.

Chapter Review

1. In what settings do PCTs typically work?
2. List 4 common PCT tasks.
3. Explain the difference between an outpatient and an inpatient facility and give an example of each.
4. What type of care do residents of an assisted living facility typically need?
5. Which care team members can diagnose diseases/disorders and prescribe treatment?
6. Explain why the patient is considered an important part of the care team.
7. List 3 questions a PCT should ask himself before accepting an assignment.
8. What should the PCT do if asked to do something they are not legally allowed to do or do not feel they have the skills to do?
9. What is person-centered care? Give 2 examples of things a PCT can do to provide person-centered care.
10. Choose 3 of the words listed in Learning Objective 5 that describe qualities important in PCTs (compassionate, honest, etc.). Give an example of how a PCT can show that quality at work.
11. How is a professional certification different from continuing education?
12. What is 1 benefit of being nationally certified as a PCT?

2 Legal and Ethical Issues

1. Define the terms *law* and *ethics* and list examples of legal and ethical behavior

Ethics and laws guide behavior. **Ethics** are the knowledge of right and wrong. An ethical person has a sense of duty and responsibility toward others. He tries to do what is right. If ethics tell people what they *should* do, **laws** tell them what they *must* do. Laws are usually based on ethics. Governments establish laws to help people live peacefully together and to ensure order and safety. When someone breaks the law, they may be punished by having to pay a fine or spend time in prison.

Ethics and laws are extremely important in health care (Fig. 2-1). They protect people receiving care and guide people giving care. Patient care technicians and other healthcare workers should be guided by a code of ethics. They must also know the laws that apply to their jobs. Legal and ethical behavior is key to professionalism in health care.

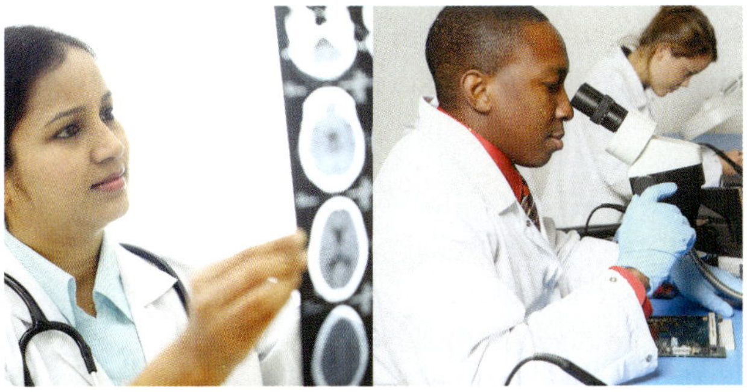

Fig. 2-1. *All healthcare providers must behave ethically and follow the law.*

Guidelines: Legal and Ethical Behavior

- **G** Be honest at all times. Stealing and lying about the care you provided are examples of dishonesty. Communicate honestly with all team members.
- **G** Protect patients' privacy. Do not discuss their cases except with other members of the care team. All team members must keep patient information confidential. It is the law, and it is one of the rights protected in the Patient Care Partnership (covered in the next learning objective).
- **G** Keep staff information confidential. You should not share information about your coworkers at home or anywhere else.
- **G** Report abuse or suspected abuse of patients. Help patients report abuse if they wish to make a complaint of abuse.
- **G** Follow the care plan and your assignments. Report any mistakes you make promptly. This helps prevent any further problems. Reporting mistakes promotes the safety and well-being of all patients.
- **G** Do not perform any task outside your scope of practice.
- **G** Report all patient incidents according to facility policy. An incident is any unexpected event during the course of care (e.g., a patient falls). Learning Objective 7 has more information on incident reports.

- Document accurately and promptly.
- Follow rules for safety and infection prevention (Chapters 5 and 6).
- Do not accept gifts or tips.
- Do not get personally or sexually involved with patients or their family members or friends. Keep interactions professional. Do not share or exchange personal information.

Many organizations and companies have created a code of ethics for their members or employees to follow. These vary, but generally they focus on promoting proper conduct and high standards of practice. If a facility has its own code of ethics, all staff members will be given a copy and expected to follow it.

2. Explain patients' rights and why they are important

Patients' rights specify how patients must be treated as they receive medical care. They provide an ethical code of conduct for healthcare workers. In 1973 the American Hospital Association introduced the *Statement on a Patient's Bill of Rights.* All healthcare facilities were encouraged to use it. This document described 15 rights to which all patients are entitled when receiving care. The document was updated over the years and was eventually replaced by the *Patient Care Partnership* (Fig. 2-2). Although the Patient Care Partnership relates to hospital care, it can be applied to any healthcare setting. The Patient Care Partnership includes the following rights:

High-quality hospital care. This includes the patient's right to know the title and identity of any person providing care. The patient also has a right to know if that person is a student, medical resident, or trainee.

A clean and safe environment. This addresses infection prevention and control (covered in Chapter 5). It also emphasizes communicating with the patient about any incident that might have an impact on her care.

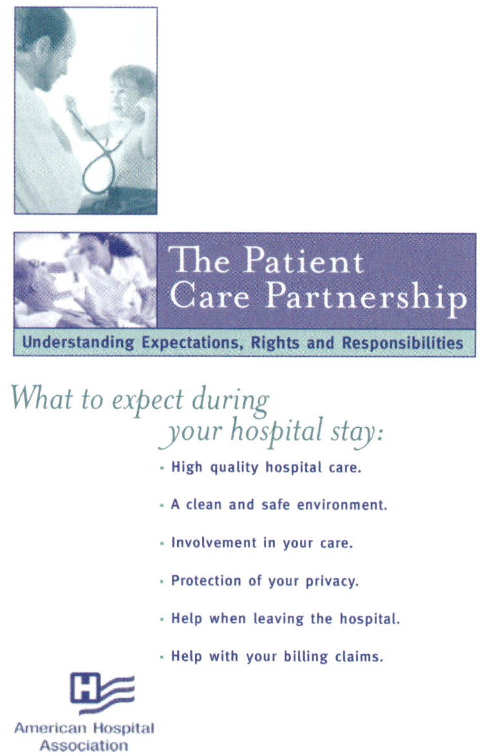

***Fig. 2-2.** The Patient Care Partnership describes rights patients are entitled to when in the hospital.*

Involvement in your care. Doctors and other healthcare providers must explain care, including risks and benefits. This process is called *informed consent.* Doctors must also tell patients if a treatment is experimental or part of a research study. Patients must agree to participate in these studies based on a detailed explanation. Patients have a right to know what may happen if they refuse a treatment or type of care. They also have the right to be informed about the cost of care. All of this information must be given in a language the patient understands. Patients have responsibilities related to their care as well. They must provide accurate information about their condition, symptoms, history, and insurance coverage.

Patients have the right to have—and the responsibility to communicate—**advance directives**. Advance directives are legal documents that allow people to decide what kind of medical care they wish to have in the event they are unable to make those decisions themselves. The **Patient Self-Determination Act** (**PSDA**), which came into effect in 1991, requires that facilities provide patients with information about advance directives.

Uniform Anatomical Gift Act

The Uniform Anatomical Gift Act was first passed in 1968 and was updated in 1987 and again in 2006. This act creates a framework for decisions about organ donation upon death. Patients can express their consent to organ donation in different ways. Most states have online donor registries and an option to indicate donor status on driver's licenses. Wishes about organ donation may also be outlined in advance directives. It is a patient's right to decide whether or not to donate organs.

One type of advance directive is a **living will**, also known as *directive to physicians* and *healthcare directive*. This document outlines specific medical care a person wants or does not want to receive.

A **do not resuscitate** (**DNR**) order is an advance directive that says the patient does not want cardiopulmonary resuscitation (CPR) performed in case of cardiac or respiratory arrest. A **do not intubate** (**DNI**) order means that no breathing tube will be placed in the person, even though some CPR measures and medications may be used. An advance directive can also name a person other than the patient to make medical decisions if the patient becomes ill or disabled. This is called **durable power of attorney for health care**.

Patients who are seriously ill may work with a doctor to complete a document known as **Physician Orders for Life-Sustaining Treatment** (**POLST**). This medical order is part of a patient's record and must be honored. It describes the care a patient wishes to receive during a health emergency. It is more specific than advance directives.

Protection of your privacy. Healthcare providers must follow federal, state, and local laws about patient privacy. They also must let patients know about their privacy policies. Patients are required to sign documents confirming that they have received this material. If a patient wishes for their health information to be shared with someone outside the facility, they must sign a release allowing it.

Help when leaving the hospital. When a patient leaves a medical facility after treatment, the facility must provide information about any follow-up care needed. This may include training about particular care procedures or about the use of prescribed medications.

Help with your billing claims. Hospital staff file claims with a patient's insurer or with programs such as Medicare or Medicaid. If a patient does not have insurance, the hospital may direct him to possible sources of assistance. Hospitals employ medical social workers who are available to help with financial issues and other assistance a patient may need.

Guidelines: Protecting Patients' Rights

- **G** Never abuse a patient. Abuse includes rough handling of a patient. It can also be verbal. Speaking abusively to a patient is a violation of her rights.
- **G** Call the patient by the name the patient prefers. Use pronouns the patient prefers (he/him, she/her, or they/them).
- **G** Allow the patient to make as many choices as possible about how care is performed.
- **G** Always keep a patient informed about what they can expect. Explain a procedure to a patient before performing it.
- **G** Follow all facility procedures regarding infection prevention.
- **G** Respect a patient's refusal of care. Patients have a legal right to refuse treatment and care. Inform patients about the provider's reasons for suggesting specific care. As appropriate, ask respectfully about the patient's reasons for refusal. Never perform refused care. Report the refusal to a supervisor immediately.

- G Tell your supervisor if a patient has questions, concerns, or complaints about a procedure.
- G Be truthful when documenting care.
- G Do not talk or gossip about patients.
- G Keep all patient information confidential.

3. Explain HIPAA and discuss ways to protect patients' privacy

To respect confidentiality means to keep private things private. PCTs learn confidential (private) information about patients. They learn about a patient's health and see information such as address, date of birth, and phone number. Ethically and legally, they must protect this information. This means that PCTs should not share information about patients with anyone other than the patients themselves, the care team, or the patients' legal representatives (such as parents or guardians of children under 18).

Congress passed the **Health Insurance Portability and Accountability Act** (**HIPAA**, hhs.gov/hipaa) in 1996. It has been further defined and revised since then. The US Department of Health and Human Services (HHS) is in charge of enforcing this law. One reason HIPAA was passed was to help keep health information private and secure. All healthcare organizations must take special steps to protect health information. They and their employees can be fined and/or imprisoned if they do not protect patient privacy.

Protected health information (**PHI**) is information that can be used to identify a person and that relates to the patient's physical or mental condition, any health care the person has had, and payment for that health care. Examples of PHI include a person's name, address, telephone number, social security number, email address, and medical record number. Only people who must have information to provide care or to process records should know a person's private health information. They must make sure they protect the information so that it does not become known or used by anyone else. It must be kept confidential. In 2008, the **Genetic Information Nondiscrimination Act** (**GINA**) was passed, adding to the privacy protections of HIPAA. It bans discrimination in employment and healthcare coverage based on genetic information.

The Health Information Technology for Economic and Clinical Health (HITECH) Act became law at the end of 2009. HITECH was passed to protect consumers' **electronic health records** (**EHR**). It increases the penalties for sharing or accessing PHI and makes it easier to enforce these penalties. HITECH also gives providers and organizations incentives for using EHR.

HIPAA applies to all healthcare workers, including doctors, nurses, PCTs, and any other members of the care team. PCTs cannot give out any information about a patient to anyone who is not directly involved in the patient's care unless the patient gives formal consent or unless the law requires it.

Guidelines: Protecting Privacy

- G Make sure you are in a private area when you are listening to or reading your messages.
- G Know with whom you are speaking on the phone. If you are not sure, get a name and number to call back after you find out it is all right to share information with this person.
- G Do not talk about patients in public (Fig. 2-3). Public areas include elevators, grocery stores, lounges, waiting rooms, parking garages, schools, restaurants, etc.
- G Do not take photos or videos at work.
- G Do not share any patient information on social media sites. This includes photos and videos, even if the patient is not named in your post. Do not share patient information via text messages.

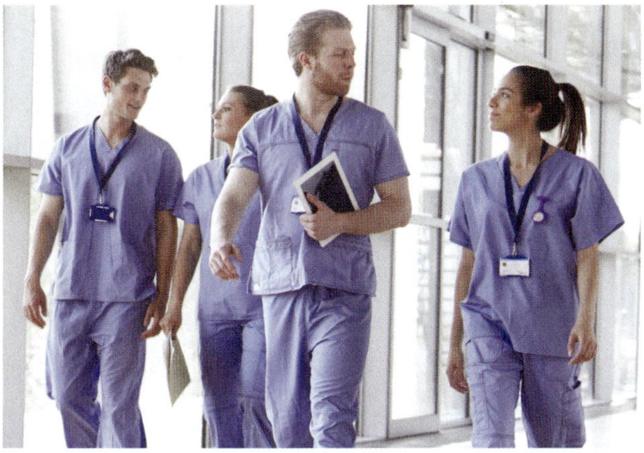

Fig. 2-3. *Patient care should only be discussed in private settings and not in lobbies or other areas open to the public.*

- **G** Ensure privacy when discussing patient information with other care team members. Keep your voice low when discussing patient information with other care team members.
- **G** Make sure nobody can see private and protected health or personal information on your computer screen while you are working. Log out and/or exit the program when you are finished with any computer work.
- **G** Do not give confidential information in emails; you do not know who has access to your messages.
- **G** Make sure fax numbers are correct before faxing healthcare information. Use a cover sheet with a confidentiality statement.
- **G** Do not leave confidential documents where others may see them.

All healthcare workers must comply with HIPAA regulations, no matter where they are or what they are doing. There are serious penalties for violating these regulations, including the following:

- Fines ranging from $100 to $1.5 million
- Prison sentences of up to 10 years

Maintaining confidentiality is a legal and ethical obligation. It is part of respecting patients and their rights. Discussing a patient's care or personal affairs with anyone other than members of the care team violates the law.

4. List other laws and organizations that affect hospitals

The laws described in Learning Objective 3 relate closely to a PCT's job. Many other laws also apply to PCTs and other healthcare workers, as well as to healthcare facilities. Several different government and nonprofit agencies help regulate the care given in these facilities.

The **Centers for Medicare & Medicaid Services** (**CMS**, cms.gov) is a federal agency within HHS. CMS runs 2 national healthcare programs: Medicare and Medicaid. They both help pay for health care and health insurance for millions of Americans. CMS has many other responsibilities as well. **Medicare** (medicare.gov) is a federal health insurance program that was established in 1965 for people aged 65 or older. It also covers people of any age with permanent kidney failure or certain disabilities. **Medicaid** (medicaid.gov) is a medical assistance program for people who have a low income, as well as for people with disabilities.

Individual states generally certify healthcare facilities to receive Medicaid payments. To receive these payments, the facilities must meet certain standards. The standards relate to the patient's experience at a facility. CMS also makes sure that facilities meet the requirements of the **Clinical Laboratory Improvement Amendments** (**CLIA**). This law applies to medical laboratories and testing. The goal is to make sure tests are done by qualified workers who use the correct methods.

State survey agencies certify that facilities meet CMS standards. States often have contracts with independent, nongovernment agencies to conduct surveys. The **Joint Commission** is an independent, not-for-profit organization that evaluates and accredits healthcare organizations.

It is the most common way hospitals in the US are accredited. In many states, facilities that are surveyed by the Joint Commission are not required to have surveys done by state inspectors. Whether a survey is done by the Joint Commission, another organization, or a state agency, all parts of patient care and facility operations are inspected. It guarantees that a facility is meeting all state and federal requirements.

The **Clinical and Laboratory Standards Institute** (**CLSI**) is another not-for-profit organization related to quality of care at healthcare facilities. CLSI develops standards for medical testing. They do not survey or accredit facilities, but meeting CLSI standards is one way facilities can show their testing procedures are done correctly.

Laws also apply to specific areas of a facility's operations. The **Americans with Disabilities Act** (**ADA**, dol.gov/general/topic/disability/ada) is a federal law passed in 1990 that prohibits discrimination because of a disability. People with disabilities must be able to get into and around buildings and use the bathrooms, drinking fountains, and other areas. The law requires new buildings to be accessible and older buildings to be updated. This law applies to healthcare facilities. In addition, the ADA requires that people with disabilities have equal access to education, employment, and all the services offered to the public. Healthcare facilities must make reasonable accommodations to provide this access.

The **Emergency Medical Treatment and Labor Act** (**EMTALA**) is another law that affects hospitals. It requires hospitals to provide necessary emergency medical treatment to patients even if they cannot pay. A patient who arrives at a hospital's emergency department must be checked by a medical professional. Examination and treatment cannot be delayed due to a patient's inability to pay. If the patient has an emergency medical condition, the patient must receive treatment to stabilize the condition. If the facility is not able to provide the needed treatment, the patient must be transferred to a facility that can provide it. EMTALA covers patients who arrive at an emergency department in labor (preparing to give birth).

The Occupational Safety and Health Administration (OSHA, osha.gov) and the Centers for Disease Control and Prevention (CDC, cdc.gov) are federal agencies. OSHA makes rules to protect workers from hazards on the job. The CDC issues guidelines to protect and improve the health of individuals and communities. More information about these laws and guidelines is found in Chapters 5 and 6.

HCAHPS

The Agency for Healthcare Research and Quality (AHRQ, ahrq.gov), like CMS, is part of the federal Department of Health and Human Services. CMS and AHRQ worked together to develop a survey to gather information about patients' experiences in hospitals. Many hospitals had their own surveys, but because they were all different, they could not be compared to each other. The **Hospital Consumer Assessment of Healthcare Providers and Systems** (**HCAHPS**, hcahpsonline.org) was first used in 2006. HCAHPS (pronounced H-caps) asks patients to report how often they experienced certain important parts of hospital care. Hospitals send HCAHPS surveys to patients. These patients are selected at random. Hospitals that receive Medicare payments must submit at least 300 HCAHPS survey results each year.

HCAHPS has 3 stated goals: to allow for comparisons between hospitals; to encourage hospitals to improve quality of care; and to increase accountability for hospitals that receive public funds. An accountable organization takes responsibility for its work and is transparent, or clear, about how it functions.

5. Discuss common legal concepts and responsibilities in health care

There are 2 types of law that deal with wrongdoing. **Criminal law** deals with offenses considered to harm all of society. Even though the victims may be individuals, the public is thought to be harmed by acts that violate criminal law. These acts are called *crimes*. **Civil law** deals with disputes between individuals, and violations of civil law are called *torts*. Failing to keep a patient's protected health information confidential can violate both criminal and civil law.

Civil offenses (torts) deal with wrongdoing between individuals. Torts may be intentional or they may occur as a result of negligence. They can result in lawsuits against a healthcare worker or facility. For example, a PCT who speaks or writes defamatory (insulting) or untrue comments about a patient or coworker may be guilty of slander or libel. Slander is a civil offense related to spoken words that are untrue or defamatory. Libel relates to written words. Such comments should never be documented in a patient's chart or spoken to coworkers, patients, or family members. They should never be posted on social media. Healthcare workers can be taken to court for such actions.

Negligence and abuse are other possible causes of legal action against healthcare workers. **Negligence** is a civil offense describing actions, or the failure to act, that result in injury to a patient. An example is a PCT forgetting to lock a patient's wheelchair before transferring her and the patient falls. *Malpractice* is also a type of negligence. An example of malpractice is a doctor using nonsterile instruments during surgery. Many healthcare workers have professional liability/malpractice insurance to protect themselves against claims of liability and the expense of a lawsuit.

Abuse is purposeful mistreatment that causes physical, mental, or emotional pain or injury to someone. Assault and battery are legal terms that describe behavior that is abusive. **Assault** is the use of words or actions to cause another person to feel fearful of being harmed. **Battery** is the intentional touching of a person without permission. Rough handling of a patient is a form of battery and is considered abuse. PCTs must never abuse patients and must follow all policies and procedures to avoid possible harm to patients, as well as to protect against charges of negligence. All healthcare workers are **mandated reporters**, which means they are legally required to report suspected or observed abuse or neglect. There is more information about reporting abuse and neglect in the next learning objective.

Connected Care

Consent

The concept of consent is a very important legal issue for healthcare workers. Before a patient gets medical treatment of any kind, she must provide consent. This means she must agree to be treated. In most cases, a facility requires that a patient sign a general consent form. This general consent is considered valid for routine care, including examinations, laboratory tests, and blood draws. This way, a hospitalized patient will not need to sign a new consent form for each routine service provided. Patients need to sign a separate form for care that is not routine, such as a surgical procedure. The provider must explain the care and risks both of receiving and refusing the care. This type of consent is known as *informed consent*.

In most cases, a parent or guardian must provide consent for a patient under 18 years old. Some adults may also require the consent of a guardian or caretaker. Adults may be considered legally incompetent (unable) to give consent if they have intellectual disabilities or illnesses that affect their cognitive ability (ability to think and process information). An adult who is considered unable to provide consent will have a legal representative who can do so.

In emergency situations it can be difficult to get informed consent. The patient may be unconscious or in shock. A child's parent may not be available. In these cases, patients may be treated with *implied consent*. Laws vary from state to state, but when a person is temporarily unable to provide informed consent, healthcare workers can generally provide care that a "reasonable person" would consent to in order to protect his life and well-being.

6. Discuss abuse and neglect and explain how to report abuse and neglect

PCTs, like all healthcare workers, are mandated reporters and are legally required to report suspected or observed abuse, neglect, or exploitation. There are many forms of abuse, including physical abuse, psychological abuse, verbal abuse, and sexual abuse. Neglect is different from negligence, which was described in the last learning objective. **Neglect** is the failure to provide needed care that results in physical, mental, or emotional harm to a person. **Exploitation** is the act of taking advantage of a person for personal gain. A caregiver for a developmentally disabled person who takes that person's money for her own benefit, for example, is committing exploitation.

PCTs are in an excellent position to observe and report abuse, neglect, and exploitation. Children, elderly people, and people whose condition requires that others be closely involved with their care are especially vulnerable.

Observe and Report: Abuse, Neglect, and Exploitation

The following injuries are considered suspicious and should be documented and reported to the nurse:

- O/R Poisoning or traumatic injury
- O/R Teeth marks
- O/R Belt buckle or strap marks
- O/R Unexplained bruises, contusions, welts, scars, fractures, or dislocations
- O/R Burns of unusual shape or in unusual locations, cigarette burns
- O/R Scalding burns
- O/R Unexplained scratches or puncture wounds
- O/R Scalp tenderness or patches of missing hair
- O/R Swelling in the face, broken teeth, nasal discharge
- O/R Bruises, bleeding, or discharge from the vaginal or anal area

The following signs could be associated with abuse:

- O/R Yelling obscenities
- O/R Fear, apprehension, fear of being alone
- O/R Poor self-control
- O/R Constant pain
- O/R Threatening to hurt others
- O/R Withdrawal or apathy (Fig. 2-4)

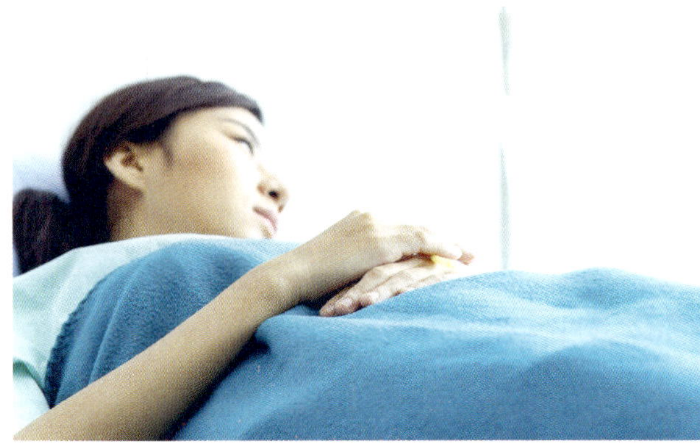

Fig. 2-4. *When a patient seems to have withdrawn from others, this is an important sign to report.*

- O/R Alcohol or drug abuse
- O/R Agitation or anxiety, signs of stress
- O/R Low self-esteem
- O/R Mood changes, confusion, disorientation
- O/R A family member/caregiver is present during all conversations and does not allow private conversations

The following signs could indicate neglect:

- O/R Pressure injuries
- O/R Unclean body
- O/R Body lice
- O/R Poorly fitting clothing
- O/R Unmet needs relating to hearing aids, eyeglasses, etc.
- O/R Weight loss, poor appetite
- O/R Dehydration

The following signs could indicate exploitation:

- O/R A family member/caregiver is present during all conversations and does not allow private conversations

- O/R Insulting remarks from the caregiver toward the patient
- O/R The caregiver is hostile toward the patient and/or healthcare providers
- O/R The caregiver gives inconsistent explanations for the patient's condition
- O/R The patient's condition shows the possibility of nonconsensual sexual activity

The PCT has an important role in protecting patients and keeping the healthcare environment safe. Signs of abuse, neglect, and exploitation should be reported immediately. Facility policy and chain of command should be followed.

In some cases a PCT may find it necessary to report directly to an outside authority. If reports of abuse are being ignored within the chain of command or if the PCT suspects a provider or coworker of abuse, the PCT has a duty to report this. Laws exist to protect people who make reports against coworkers or employers. They are often called *whistleblower laws*. They protect employees from being fired or treated badly for reporting legal concerns about their workplace.

7. Describe incident reporting

An **incident** is an accident, problem, or unexpected event during the course of care. It is something that is not part of the normal routine. A mistake in care, such as collecting a specimen from the wrong patient, is an incident. A patient falling or being injured in a medical facility is another type of incident. Accusations made by patients against staff, as well as employee injuries, are other types of incidents.

State and federal guidelines require that incidents be recorded in an incident report. An incident report (also called an *occurrence*, *accident*, *accident/incident*, or *event report*) is a report that documents the incident and the response to it. The report is a factual, objective account of what happened. The information in an incident report is confidential. It is intended for internal use to help prevent future incidents.

Incident reports are also used to document unsafe activities that could cause injury to patients and/or staff. Healthcare workers must observe for unsafe practices or conditions. Incident reports are not *punitive*, or intended for punishment. They are meant to improve quality of care and patient safety. Incident reports should be filed when any of the following occurs:

- A patient falls (all falls must be reported, even if the patient says they are fine)
- A staff member or a patient breaks or damages something
- A PCT (or any healthcare worker) makes a mistake in care
- A patient makes sexual advances or remarks
- Anything happens that makes a PCT feel uncomfortable, threatened, or unsafe
- A PCT is injured on the job
- A PCT is exposed to blood or other body fluids

When an employee is injured on the job, there may be federal reports to complete in addition to any facility reports. Reporting and documenting incidents protects everyone involved. This includes the patient, the employer, and the PCT. When documenting incidents, PCTs should complete reports as soon as possible. This is important so they do not forget any details. PCTs should write brief and accurate descriptions of the events as they happened. They should not place blame or liability within the report.

Guidelines: Incident Reporting

- G Tell what happened. State the time and the mental and physical condition of the person.
- G Describe the person's reaction to the incident, including information about the person's mental and physical condition.

- **G** State the facts; do not give opinions.
- **G** Do not write anything in the incident report on the medical record. Referring to an incident report in the patient's medical record makes it a part of the record. Medical records are subject to subpoena, which means they can be ordered to be used as evidence in a lawsuit.
- **G** Describe the action taken to give care.

A **sentinel event** is an unexpected occurrence that results in death or in serious physical or psychological injury. A *sentinel* is a soldier who stands guard. Sentinel events are called *sentinel* because they signal the need for an immediate investigation and response. The sentinel events most often reviewed by the Joint Commission in 2022 were as follows:

1. Falls
2. Delay in treatment (e.g., a patient not getting needed medications on time)
3. Unintended retention of a foreign object (e.g., a sponge left inside a patient during surgery)
4. Wrong surgery (e.g., surgery on the wrong side of the body or on the wrong patient)
5. Suicide

A sentinel event must be reported to the proper agency.

Chapter Review

1. What is the difference between ethics and laws?
2. List 8 examples of legal and ethical behavior for a PCT.
3. Define *advance directives* and briefly describe 2 examples.
4. What is an important reason that HIPAA was passed?
5. List 5 examples of a person's protected health information (PHI).
6. Which patients are covered under Medicare? What is the purpose of Medicaid?
7. Give 2 examples of public building modifications that meet requirements of the Americans with Disabilities Act (ADA).
8. What are the 3 goals of the Hospital Consumer Assessment of Healthcare Providers and Systems (HCAHPS)?
9. What is the difference between criminal law and civil law?
10. Explain why it would be illegal for a health-care worker to post something about a patient on social media.
11. Explain the difference between abuse and neglect. Give an example of each.
12. What is a mandated reporter?
13. What are 3 types of consent in health care and when/how are they applied?
14. Give an example of an action that can be considered exploitation.
15. What is a whistleblower law?
16. What is the purpose of an incident report and when should it be completed?
17. Give an example of a sentinel event.

3 Communication and Diversity

1. Define *communication*

Communication is the process of exchanging information with others. It is a process of sending and receiving messages. People communicate by using signs and symbols, such as words, drawings, and pictures. They also communicate through their behavior.

The simplest form of communication is a 3-step process that takes place between 2 people (Fig. 3-1). In the first step, the sender (the person who communicates first) sends a message. In the second step, the receiver receives the message. Receiver and sender constantly switch roles as they communicate. The third step involves providing feedback. The receiver repeats the message or responds to it in some way. This lets the sender know that the message was received and understood. Feedback is especially important when working in health care. PCTs must take time to make sure patients understand messages and that they understand what patients are communicating.

All 3 steps must occur before the communication process is complete. During a conversation, this process is repeated over and over.

Closed-Loop Communication

A tool that is often used in healthcare settings is closed-loop communication. This builds on the concept of providing feedback as part of the communication process. With closed-loop communication, the receiver repeats the message to make sure it was understood and the sender confirms to "close the loop." Doing this helps avoid errors and misunderstandings and promotes safety.

Effective communication is a critical part of a PCT's job. PCTs must communicate with nurses, other members of the care team, patients, and family members. A patient's health depends on how well a PCT communicates observations and concerns to the nurse. The PCT will also need to communicate clearly and respectfully in stressful or confusing situations. Some patients may need help in communicating clearly with the care team.

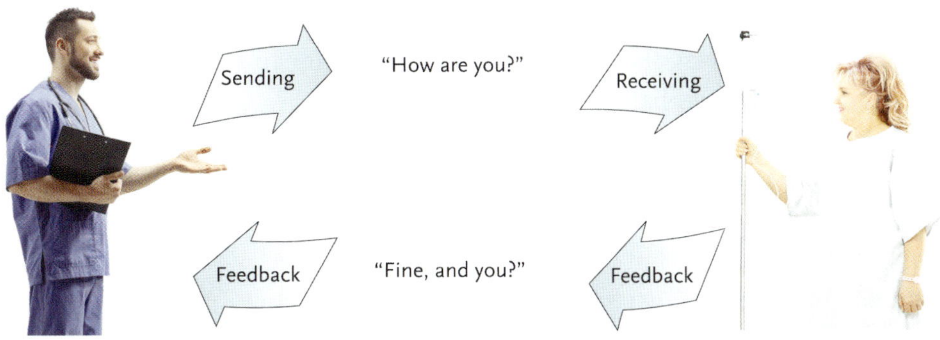

Fig. 3-1. The communication process consists of sending a message, receiving a message, and providing feedback.

Communication is either verbal or nonverbal. **Verbal communication** involves the use of words, spoken or written. A PCT telling a nurse about his observations is an example of verbal communication. When communicating verbally, it is important to use words that have the same meaning to both the sender and the receiver. Misunderstandings may occur if each person interprets the same words differently. For example, if a PCT asks a patient to "use the light" when she needs help, the patient may not understand that the PCT meant for her to push the call button.

Nonverbal communication is communicating without using words. It also includes how a person says something. For example, a PCT says kindly, "I'll be right with you, Mrs. Gonzales." This communicates that the PCT is ready and willing to help. But saying the same phrase in a different tone or emphasizing different words can communicate frustration and annoyance: *"I'll be right with you, Mrs. Gonzales!"*

Body language is another form of nonverbal communication. Movements, facial expressions, and posture can express different attitudes or emotions. Body language sends messages, just as speaking does. Other people receive and interpret these messages. For example, slouching in a chair and sitting up straight send 2 different messages (Fig. 3-2). Slouching says that a person is bored, tired, or hostile. Sitting up straight says that the person is interested and respectful. Other examples of positive nonverbal communication include smiling, nodding one's head, and looking at the person who is speaking.

Sometimes people send one message verbally and a very different message nonverbally. Nonverbal communication often shows how someone is feeling. This message may be quite different from what he is saying. For example, a patient who says, "I'm feeling fine," but is moving slowly and wincing is sending 2 very different messages. Paying attention to nonverbal communication helps PCTs give better care. In this example, the PCT should tell the nurse that the patient is moving slowly and appears to be wincing in pain, despite what he says.

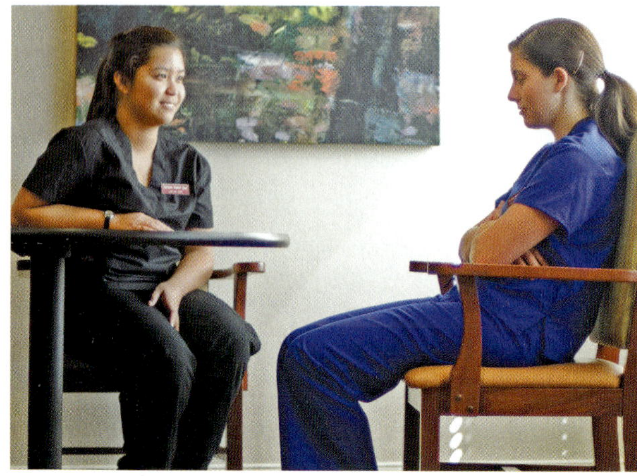

Fig. 3-2. *Body language sends messages just as words do. Which of these people seems more interested in their conversation—the person on the right who is looking down with her arms crossed or the person on the left who is sitting up straight and smiling?*

PCTs must also be aware of their own verbal and nonverbal messages. If a PCT says, "It's nice to see you today, Mr. Lee," but does not smile or look him in the eye, Mr. Lee may feel that the PCT is not really happy to see him.

When communication is confusing, the PCT should try to clarify by asking for an explanation. The PCT can say, "Mrs. Jones, you've just told me something that I don't understand. Would you explain it to me?" Or she can state what she has observed and ask if the observation is correct. For example, "Mrs. Jones, I see that you're smiling, but I also see that you are holding your stomach. Are you having stomach pains or nausea?" Taking time to clarify communication can make care more effective.

2. Define *diversity* and understand the importance of responding to diversity without bias

PCTs work with people from varied backgrounds and with different life experiences. The word

diversity is often used to refer to the variety among people. People who respond to diversity with judgment (negative or positive) or with assumptions based on personal beliefs are responding with **bias**. Bias, whether it is negative or positive, prevents a PCT from treating a patient as an individual. Any kind of bias can have a negative impact on patient care.

Diversity can refer to these differences:

Race or ethnicity: **Race** typically refers to physical characteristics shared by people with common ancestry. **Ethnicity** may involve a combination of race, culture, nationality, language, and other factors. A person who identifies as Latino or Latina, for instance, may be Black, white, Indigenous, Asian, or of mixed race.

Culture: The learned beliefs and behaviors practiced by a group of people influence how they behave. This is that group's **culture**. Culture may be tied to race, ethnicity, or nationality, but it may also relate to other factors, such as where people live or the beliefs people share. People may be influenced by many different cultures. For example, a Mexican American person may be an evangelical Christian and a US Marine. All of those groups may have a cultural influence on that person.

Religion: Patients' religious beliefs will vary. PCTs do not always know what a person's beliefs are, but those beliefs may be very important to patients' views on health care. Some patients may consider themselves deeply religious, while others may think of themselves as spiritual but not religious. Other patients may not consider themselves spiritual or religious at all.

Age: People of all ages need medical care. Some hospitals specialize in caring for children. Most facilities, however, have a wide range of ages among their patients.

Body shape and size: PCTs care for people of all heights, weights, and body shapes. Genetics (the influence of genes from a person's parents) play a strong role in determining a person's physical attributes, including height, weight, and body shape.

Connected Care

Weight-Inclusive Care

A tendency to treat people with larger bodies as unhealthy or undesirable (sometimes called *weight bias*, *anti-fat bias*, or *fatphobia*) can cause poorer health outcomes for patients of all sizes. The assumption that a larger body means a person is unhealthy is not correct. Poor health in a person who is overweight or obese may result from unequal care or stigma. People with larger bodies may not seek care because they often receive treatment that is dismissive or shaming. Healthcare providers may emphasize weight loss for health problems that are not, in fact, related to a patient's weight. They may make incorrect assumptions about a person's habits based on cultural or personal bias. Behaving as if having a large body is a moral failure increases the risk of disordered eating and exercise. *Weight-inclusive care* seeks to prevent weight bias in health care. It emphasizes creating environments where patients of all sizes are accommodated (e.g., comfortable seating is available in a variety of sizes and hallways allow easy passage for all). Eating and exercise are addressed as they relate to wellness, not size. Research indicates this approach can improve health.

Gender identity: A person's **gender identity** is a deeply felt sense of one's gender. A person may have the gender identity of a man or a woman or may not fit into either of those categories (terms related to these gender identities include *nonbinary*, *genderqueer*, and *genderfluid*). A person's gender identity may or may not be the same as their sex assigned at birth due to anatomy.

Sexual orientation: **Sexual orientation** refers to a person's physical, emotional, and/or romantic attraction to another person. It is different from gender identity. People may be attracted to people of the same gender (**gay** or **lesbian**), a different gender (**straight**), or to either their own or other genders (**bisexual** or **pansexual**). People may also relate to emotional or romantic partners—of any gender—in a nonsexual way (**asexual**).

Health status: A range of situations can lead to hospitalization (Fig. 3-3). Some patients may be having scheduled nonurgent surgery. Some may have been in accidents or experienced violence. Others may be receiving treatment for an acute situation such as a stroke, or for a chronic condition that has gotten worse.

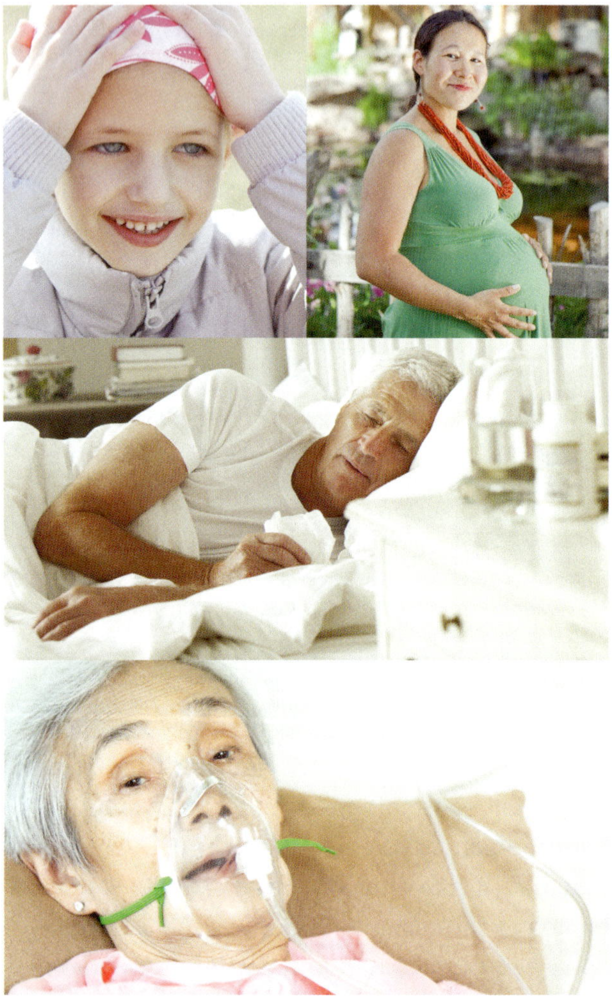

Fig. 3-3. *PCTs work with patients in many different states of health.*

Ability/disability: Patients with physical, developmental, and intellectual disabilities, as well as patients with no disabilities, require medical care. People with disabilities are not all the same. Many types of disability can exist in a range from mild to severe.

PCTs should respond to diversity of all kinds without bias. The best care is given when healthcare workers treat patients as individuals and do not make assumptions or judgments. This is easier in theory than it is in practice. Even people who do not intend to be biased may act with unconscious bias (sometimes called *implicit bias*). Recognizing this type of bias helps to reduce its impact.

Guidelines: Unbiased Behavior with Patients

- **G** Do not make assumptions about a patient's race, ethnicity, or gender identity. Do not question how a patient identifies.
- **G** Treat each person as an individual who deserves high-quality medical care. Your personal beliefs should not influence your approach to care. For example, some people have strong religious beliefs related to sexual orientation and gender identity. PCTs who believe that certain forms of sexual or gender expression are wrong must not allow these beliefs to affect how they treat patients.
- **G** Do not dismiss patients' input based on the patient's education level, income, age, condition, disability, or any other factor.
- **G** Understand that patients who are disabled or have a chronic illness are not defined by their condition. They may have health concerns not related to their condition (Fig. 3-4).

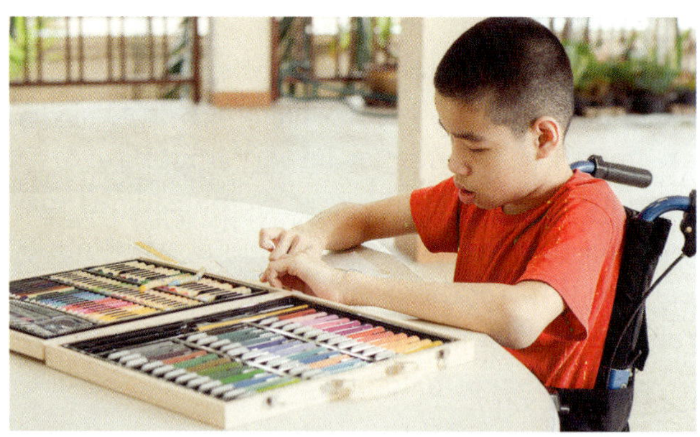

Fig. 3-4. *People with disabilities and people who have chronic medical conditions have interests, ambitions, and concerns that are not related to their disability or condition.*

- **G** Be aware of your own bias and realize that it may be unconscious. People may be more likely to respond sympathetically to people like them. They may be less likely to view people different from them as having the same needs or feelings. Being aware of this will help prevent it. Empathize with patients. Believe what they say about their own health.

G Approach a patient's symptoms, conditions, and social/medical history without judgment. Behaving as if a patient's medical situation or history is shameful or their fault does not improve their health. Patients who feel safe and accepted are more likely to be honest and open with the care team. This leads to better care.

3. Describe therapeutic communication

Effective communication between healthcare workers and patients is very important to patient health. This communication can be challenging. All of the factors listed in the last learning objective can affect how a patient sends and receives messages, both verbal and nonverbal. There are also differences between individuals. Each person has their own communication style and preferences. Being in a hospital, even if the patient's health is not in danger, is difficult. Hospitals are noisy. People do not have the privacy they have at home, even in a private room. They often receive care from many different healthcare workers.

All of this makes clear communication both more difficult and more important. *Therapeutic communication* describes communication techniques that build trust between a patient and a healthcare worker. Therapeutic communication is clear and professional. It promotes the patient's health and well-being. The following promote appropriate therapeutic communication:

Be a good listener. The PCT should allow the patient to express her ideas completely. He should concentrate on what the patient is saying and not interrupt. The PCT should not finish the patient's sentences even if he knows what she is going to say. When the patient is finished, the PCT should restate the message in his own words to make sure he has understood.

Provide feedback. Active listening means focusing on the person sending the message and giving feedback. Feedback might be an acknowledgment, a question, or repeating the sender's message. The PCT should offer general but leading responses, such as "Oh?" or "Go on," or "Hmm." By doing this, he is actively listening, providing feedback, and encouraging the sender to expand the message.

Bring up topics of concern. If the PCT knows of a topic that might concern a patient, he can raise the issue in a general, nonthreatening way. This lets the patient decide whether or not to discuss it. For example, if the PCT observes that a patient is unusually quiet, he could say, "Mrs. Jones, you seem so quiet today." Or he may notice a certain emotion. He might say, "Mrs. Jones, you seemed upset earlier. Would you like to talk about it?"

Let some pauses happen. Using silence for a few moments at a time encourages the patient to gather her thoughts and compose messages.

Do not engage in religious discussions. Religious differences can affect communication. Religion can be very important in some people's lives, particularly when they are facing health challenges. Other people are not religious and may feel strongly about that. A PCT should allow patients to express religious thoughts if they wish to express them. The PCT should not question the patients' beliefs or discuss his beliefs with them.

Understand the importance of touch. Softly touching patients' hands or shoulders or holding their hands may communicate caring. Some people's backgrounds may make them less comfortable being touched. The PCT should ask permission before touching patients and should be sensitive to their feelings. PCTs must touch patients in order to do their jobs. However, they should recognize that some patients feel more comfortable when there is little physical contact. The PCT should adjust care to patients' needs.

Ask for more. When patients report symptoms, events, or feelings, the PCT should have them repeat what they have said and ask them for more information.

Avoid changing the subject when a patient is discussing something. This is true even if the subject makes the PCT feel uncomfortable or helpless. For example, a patient might say, "I'm so scared to get my test results." The PCT should not avoid the topic by asking an unrelated question or responding with a cliché (such as "I know everything will be fine.") This makes the patient feel that the PCT is not interested in him or what he is talking about.

Do not ignore a patient's request. A patient may request that a particular test be done, for example, or that the doctor consider a specific diagnosis. These requests must be communicated to the nurse or provider, even if the PCT does not think the patient is correct. Ignoring a request is negligent behavior. It is the nurse's or provider's job to decide how best to respond to the patient.

Do not talk down to patients. A PCT should talk to patients and their families as she would talk to any person.

Connected Care

Communication Styles

Communication styles may be categorized as *passive*, *aggressive*, or *assertive*. Passive communication emphasizes the needs and desires of others, excluding one's own needs and desires. It interferes with professional communication because it does not allow all needs to be considered. It can lead to a feeling of being taken advantage of or to resentment. Aggressive communication emphasizes one's own needs and desires, excluding the needs of others. It leaves people feeling ignored, dismissed, or bullied. Assertive communication considers the needs and desires of everyone involved. A person who is communicating assertively expresses her own thoughts clearly and also shows concern for the thoughts of others. Assertive communication is more professional. It is likely to be more successful than passive or aggressive communication.

Therapeutic communication can be blocked or disrupted in many ways (Fig 3-5). When this happens, patient care can suffer. PCTs should be aware of the following barriers to communication and know how to avoid them:

Patient does not hear PCT, does not hear correctly, or does not understand. The PCT should stand directly facing the patient. He should speak slowly and clearly. He should not shout, whisper, or mumble. The PCT should speak in a normal voice, using a pleasant tone. If the patient wears a hearing aid, the PCT should make sure it is turned on.

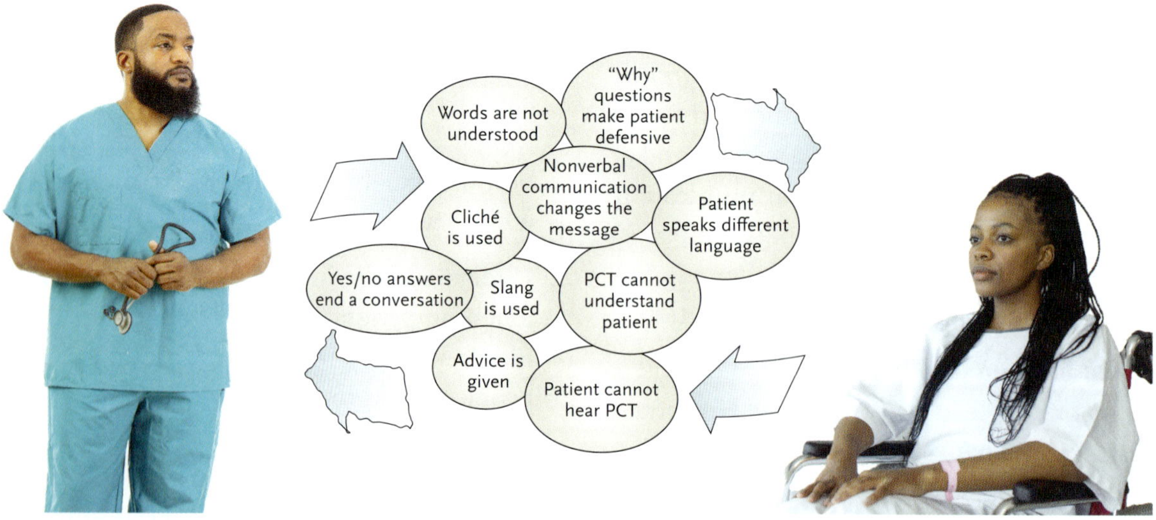

Fig. 3-5. *Barriers to communication.*

Patient is difficult to understand. The PCT should be patient and take time to listen. He can ask the patient to repeat or explain the message, and then state the message in his own words to make sure he has understood.

PCT, patient, or others use words that are not understood. The PCT should not use medical terminology with patients or their family members. He should speak in simple, everyday words and ask what a word means if he is not sure.

PCT uses slang or profanity. The PCT should avoid using slang words and expressions. They are unprofessional and may not be understood. He should not use profanity, even if the patient does.

PCT uses clichés. Clichés are phrases that are used over and over again and do not really mean anything. For example, "Everything will be fine" is a cliché. Instead of using a cliché, the PCT should respond with a meaningful message. For example, if a pediatric patient is afraid that a blood draw will be painful, the PCT can say "I know this is scary. It might hurt a little bit, but I will do my best to be quick" instead of saying "Oh, it'll be over before you know it."

Connected Care

Validating Patients' Concerns

When a patient expresses doubt, worry, or fear, responding with a cliché can make the patient feel ignored or dismissed. Telling a patient they should not feel a certain way is also dismissive. Patients have a right to have their feelings and opinions taken seriously. Even if a PCT does not share a patient's concern or believes the patient is mistaken, she can still validate the patient's feelings. This means expressing an understanding of the patient's concerns. In the example of the pediatric patient having blood drawn, when the PCT acknowledges that blood draws can be scary and may hurt, the patient knows they have been heard. A patient is more likely to trust and respect a PCT who listens and validates them.

PCT responds with "Why?" The PCT should avoid asking "Why?" when a patient makes a statement. "Why" questions make people feel defensive. For example, a patient may say she does not want to do range of motion exercises. If the PCT asks "Why not?" he may receive an angry response. Instead, he can ask "Are you having pain right now?" The patient may be willing to talk about it.

PCT gives advice. The PCT should not offer his opinion or give advice. Giving medical advice is not within a PCT's scope of practice. It could be dangerous.

PCT asks questions that only require yes/no answers. The PCT should ask open-ended questions that need more than a "yes" or "no" answer. "Yes" and "no" answers end conversation. For example, if a PCT wants to hear how a patient's night went, he should not ask, "Did you have a good night?" Instead, he should ask, "Can you tell me about your night?"

Patient speaks a different language. If a patient speaks a different language than the PCT does, the PCT should speak slowly and clearly, without exaggerating his words. He should keep his messages short and simple. He should be alert for words the patient understands and also be alert for signs that the patient is only pretending to understand. The PCT should be patient and calm. He may need to use a medical interpreter or an interpretation service. If an interpreter is used, the PCT should still address the patient and not the interpreter. Family members or friends should not be used as interpreters.

PCT or patient uses nonverbal communication. Nonverbal communication can change a message. The PCT should be aware of his body language and gestures. He can look for nonverbal messages from patients and clarify them. For example, "Mr. Feldman, you say you're feeling fine but you seem to be in pain. Can you tell me more about how you're feeling?"

4. Explain the difference between facts and opinions

A fact is something that is definitely true. "Mr. Garcia's temperature is 99.7°F," for example, is a fact. This fact has evidence to back it up: using a thermometer to measure Mr. Garcia's body temperature. An opinion is something someone believes to be true, but is not definitely true or cannot be proven. "Mr. Garcia looks feverish" is an opinion. This statement might be true, but it cannot be backed up with evidence. It is important to be able to separate facts from opinions.

Using facts instead of opinions is a more professional and effective way to communicate. When communicating with the care team, distinguishing between facts and opinions is important. For example, "Mr. Morgan is acting like he had a stroke" is an opinion and could very well be wrong. Instead, the facts should be reported: "Mr. Morgan has lost strength on his right side, and his speech is slurred." When reporting opinions, the PCT can introduce them with "I think...". Then it is clear that she is offering her opinion and not a fact she has observed.

5. Explain objective and subjective information and describe how to observe and report accurately

When making any kind of report, the right kind of information must be collected before documenting it. Facts, not opinions, are most useful to the care team. Two kinds of factual information are needed in reporting. **Objective information** is based on what a person sees, hears, touches, or smells. Objective information is collected by using the senses. It is also called *signs*. **Subjective information** is something a person cannot or did not observe. It is based on something that the patient reported that may or may not be true. It is also called *symptoms*.

An example of objective information is, "Mr. Hartman is holding his head and rubbing his temples." A subjective report of the same situation might be, "Mr. Hartman says he has a headache." The care team needs factual information in order to make decisions about care and treatment. Both objective and subjective reports are valuable.

In any report, what is observed (signs) and what the patient reports (symptoms) need to be clearly noted. "Ms. Scott reports pain in her left shoulder" is an example of clear reporting. PCTs are not expected to make diagnoses based on signs and symptoms observed. This is beyond their scope of practice. Their observations, however, can alert the care team to possible problems.

In order to report accurately, a PCT must observe patients accurately. To observe accurately, as many senses as possible should be used to gather information (Fig. 3-6).

Sight: The PCT should look for changes in the patient's appearance. These may include rashes, redness, paleness, swelling, discharge, weakness, sunken eyes, and posture or gait (walking) changes.

Hearing: The PCT should listen to what the patient says about his condition and needs. Is the patient speaking clearly and making sense? Does he show emotions, such as anger, frustration, or sadness? Is his breathing normal? Does he wheeze, gasp, or cough?

Touch: Does the patient's skin feel hot or cool, moist or dry? Is the pulse rate normal? (Chapter 10 includes information on counting pulse rate.)

Smell: Are there any odors coming from the patient's body? Odors could suggest infection, incontinence, or a need for bathing. **Incontinence** is the inability to control the bladder or bowels. Breath odor could suggest the use of alcohol or tobacco, indigestion, or poor mouth care.

Using all the senses allows a PCT to make the most complete report of a patient's situation.

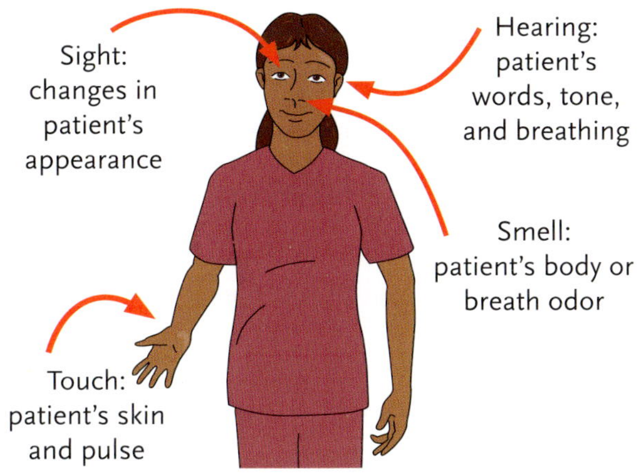

Fig. 3-6. *Reporting observations accurately requires using more than one sense.*

6. Describe basic medical terminology and abbreviations

Throughout a PCT's training, he will learn medical terms for specific conditions. For example, the medical term for fainting is *syncope*; skin that is blue or gray is called **cyanotic**. Using medical terminology makes medical communication more precise.

PCTs use medical terminology so that they can communicate clearly with other team members. These terms should not be used with patients, their family members, or anyone who is not trained to understand them. Facilities may have medical references (books or electronic options) available for PCTs to check terms.

Medical terms are often made up of roots, prefixes, and suffixes. A root is a part of a word that contains its basic meaning or definition. The prefix is the word part that comes before the root to help form a new word. The suffix is the word part added to the end of a root that helps form a new word. Prefixes and suffixes are called *affixes* because they are attached, or affixed, to a root. Here are some examples:

- The root *derm* or *derma* means skin. The suffix *itis* means inflammation. *Dermatitis* is an inflammation of the skin.
- The prefix *brady* means slow. The root *cardia* means heart. *Bradycardia* is slow heartbeat or pulse.
- The suffix *pathy* means disease. The root *neuro* means of the nerve or nervous system. *Neuropathy* is a nerve disease or disease of the nervous system.

Abbreviations are another way to communicate more efficiently with care team members. For example, the abbreviation *prn* means *as necessary*. *BP* means *blood pressure*. *CBC* means *complete blood count*, a common blood test. A patient who has been ordered to not consume any food or liquids is *NPO*. This is an abbreviation for *nil per os*, which is Latin for *nothing by mouth*.

PCTs should learn the standard medical abbreviations their facility uses. They can use them to report information briefly and accurately. They may also need to know these abbreviations to read assignments or to understand some parts of a patient's record. A brief list of abbreviations follows, and more are located at the end of this textbook and in the instructor's guide. There may be other terms in use at a facility, so it is important for PCTs to know the correct abbreviations. Misunderstanding can result in patient injury or death. The Joint Commission has an official "do not use" list, which appears as an appendix to this book. It includes abbreviations that could be easily misunderstood and cause problems in care.

Common Abbreviations	
$\bar{a}$	before
abd	abdomen
ac, a.c.	before meals
ad lib	as desired
ADLs	activities of daily living
amb	ambulate, ambulatory
AP	apical pulse
b.i.d., bid	2 times a day

BM	bowel movement
BP, B/P	blood pressure
$\overline{c}$	with
C	Celsius
CHF	congestive heart failure
c/o	complains of
CPR	cardiopulmonary resuscitation
DNR	do not resuscitate
DX, dx	diagnosis
F	Fahrenheit
FBS	fasting blood sugar
f/u, F/U	follow-up
FWB	full weight-bearing
GI	gastrointestinal
H_2O	water
h, hr, hr.	hour
Hx	history
inc	incontinent
I&O	intake and output
NKDA	no known drug allergies
NPO	nothing by mouth
NWB	non-weight-bearing
O_2	oxygen
OOB	out of bed
$\overline{p}$	after
pc, p.c.	after meals
PO	by mouth
prn, PRN	as necessary
PWB	partial weight-bearing
$\overline{q}$	every
ROM	range of motion
$\overline{s}$	without
SOB	shortness of breath
stat, STAT	at once, immediately
t.i.d., tid	3 times a day
TPR	temperature, pulse, respiration
URI	upper respiratory infection
UTI	urinary tract infection
v.s., VS	vital signs
w/c, W/C	wheelchair

7. Explain how to communicate patient information during shift changes

PCTs must be able to communicate information about patients to their supervisors and to other members of the care team. This communication may be oral or written, and it must be brief but accurate. Communicating careful observations is very important to the health and well-being of all patients. Signs and symptoms that should be reported will be discussed throughout this textbook. Some observations will need to be reported immediately to the nurse. Deciding what to report immediately involves critical thinking. Anything that endangers patients should be reported immediately, including the following:

- Falls
- Chest pain
- Severe headache
- Difficulty breathing
- Abnormal pulse, respiration, or blood pressure
- Change in mental status
- Sudden weakness or loss of mobility
- Fever
- Loss of consciousness
- Change in level of consciousness
- Bleeding
- Swelling of a body part
- Change in patient's condition

- Bruises, abrasions, or other possible signs of abuse (see Chapter 2)

PCTs may use oral reports to discuss experiences with patients. These may be shared with the PCT's supervisor and/or with the PCT who will be caring for the patient on the next shift. Facts, not opinions, should be used for oral reports. It is a good idea for PCTs to make notes so that important details are not forgotten (Fig. 3-7). When needing to give an oral report, unless the situation is urgent, the PCT should approach the care team member and wait for her to complete the task she is doing. Once the person has acknowledged the PCT, she can briefly state the message. Waiting until the person is ready to listen helps reduce the risk of error.

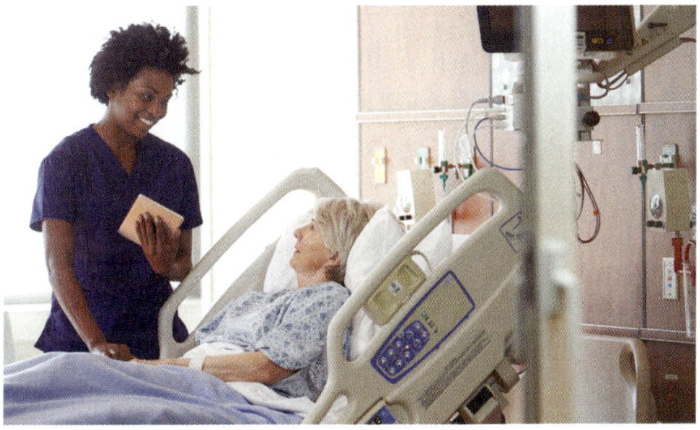

Fig. 3-7. *Taking notes helps PCTs to remember facts and report accurately.*

Following an oral report, PCTs must document when, why, about what, and to whom an oral report was given. EHRs may include a checkbox style shift change report. Documentation should always occur after the information is communicated, not before.

Sometimes the nurse or another member of the care team will give a PCT a brief oral report about a patient. The PCT should listen carefully and take notes. Information shared may include the following:

- Whether a patient has a strict intake and output (I&O) order (I&O is the fluid a person consumes and eliminates; a strict I&O order emphasizes the importance of monitoring everything consumed and eliminated.)
- Whether urine is being collected for a 24-hour urine specimen
- Any changes to the vital sign measurement schedule (e.g., for pre- or postoperative patients)
- Whether the patient is considered to be at an increased risk of falls and any safety measures needed

PCTs should ask about anything they do not understand. At the end of the conversation, the PCT can restate what they have been told to make sure they understand.

When communicating about patients, PCTs must remember that all patient information is confidential. Information should only be shared with members of the care team.

SBAR and I PASS the BATON

Accurate communication between members of the care team is very important to patient safety and well-being. This can be challenging in all healthcare settings. In a hospital, patients may be critically ill. Their care may be shared between several departments and providers. This makes communication even more challenging. It makes accurate and timely communication even more important.

There are several different systems that may be used to promote accurate communication about patient care. Hospitals may use special communication systems. Two of these systems are SBAR and I PASS the BATON. SBAR stands for *situation, background, assessment, recommendation*. This framework was established by the military in the 1940s to communicate important safety information. In health care it may be used during handoffs, or transfers of authority between shifts or departments.

I PASS the BATON was developed by the AHRQ (Agency for Healthcare Research and Quality) and the US Department of Defense. It is specifically designed for handoffs between healthcare professionals and departments. Each letter stands for an important part of the handoff:

- I = Introduction
- P = Patient
- A = Assessment
- S = Situation
- S = Safety

the

- B = Background
- A = Actions
- T = Timing
- O = Ownership
- N = Next

It is beyond the scope of practice for PCTs to assess patients or plan care. It is helpful, though, for PCTs to understand the information that is communicated to provide the best, safest patient care. PCT observations are a very important part of this process.

8. Describe a standard patient record and patient record systems

Patient records include the following information:

- Demographic information, such as name, birthdate, address, email address, and contact number(s)
- Administrative records, including insurance information, billing records, appointment scheduling, referrals, release of information requests, and letters
- Medical history, including illnesses, injuries, diseases, and surgeries
- Social history, including education, living conditions, health habits, and tobacco/alcohol use
- Family health history, including diseases and conditions in close relatives such as siblings and parents
- Known allergies to medications, foods, or other substances (e.g., latex)
- Current health conditions, diagnoses, treatments (including medications), and procedures
- Consent forms, both general and for procedures and surgeries
- Provider notes describing assessments, diagnoses, and treatment plans
- Test results

Healthcare providers depend on up-to-date records to care for their patients. Accurate records are necessary to provide high-quality care.

Medical records can be stored electronically in software systems or manually in paper charts. Most healthcare facilities have adopted the use of **electronic medical records** (**EMR**) or electronic health records (EHR) for documenting patient care. An *EMR* is a system that can only be accessed by a single healthcare facility. Information in the *EHR* can be shared between healthcare organizations.

Electronic record systems are expensive and require special training to operate. Healthcare facilities must choose systems that are HIPAA compliant to protect health information.

Electronic Medical Records

Electronic medical records are digital records of a patient's medical information. One benefit of the EMR is that, unlike a paper chart, it can be used by multiple people in a healthcare organization at the same time. EMRs also reduce the risk of errors due to unclear handwriting, a common problem with paper charts. These records can also be easily stored and maintained. However, EMRs are limited to a single healthcare facility. They cannot be accessed by providers outside that system.

Electronic Health Records

Electronic health records are also digital records of a patient's medical information. The EHR can be used by more than one person at a time. Unlike the EMR, the EHR can be accessed across many healthcare facilities and systems. This makes it the most accessible patient medical record available.

Paper Charts

Paper charting is the traditional way to keep patient medical records. Paper charts are only available to one person at a time. They require a large amount of space for storage. Steps must be taken to keep them secure and confidential. Paper medical records are inexpensive to use, but charts can be misfiled or lost. Important information can also be overlooked more easily. Almost all hospitals use electronic systems.

Medical records may be organized in several ways. Paper records are often organized according to source or category. For example, test results are in one location and provider progress notes in another. In an electronic record, there may be tabs or menu items for these categories.

Because medical records contain protected health information (PHI), there are laws about how the records are managed. All medical records must be stored securely. Electronic records must be secured on password-protected computer systems. They must have security measures such as firewalls and data encryption. A *firewall* is a security feature that protects computer files from being accessed by or sent to unauthorized users. Information in medical records should also be *encrypted*, or converted into codes to prevent unauthorized access.

HIPAA requires that electronic records also have a backup system. This means that if an equipment failure, power outage, fire, or other disaster occurs, the data is not lost. Backup methods vary, but the records must be stored outside the healthcare facility. EHR software systems often include HIPAA-compliant backup.

In many electronic systems, users have a unique username and password login. Other systems use badges for access. The person uses their badge to tap in on a workstation and later tap out to end the session. PCTs and other care team members should access the needed record(s) and then log out or tap out before stepping away from the screen. Usernames and passwords should never be shared. Healthcare workers must always use their own credentials to log in. Monitor screens must be placed so that protected health information cannot be viewed by people who are not part of the care team (Fig. 3-8).

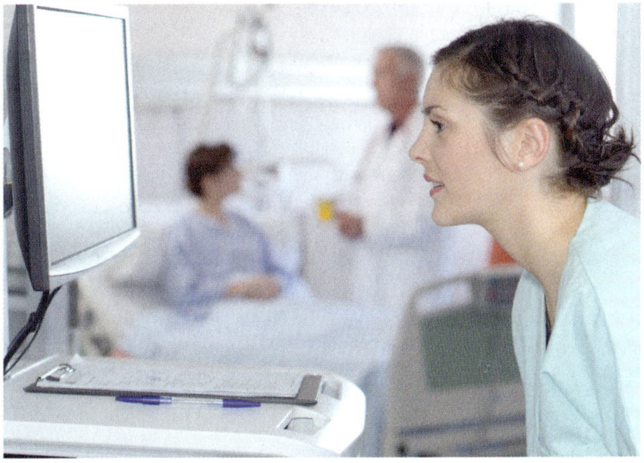

Fig. 3-8. *Computer screens should be oriented so that only healthcare team members can view them.*

Paper medical records must also be stored securely. File cabinets must lock and should be fire-resistant. Record rooms should be located in areas not accessible to the public.

Chapter Review

1. Briefly describe 3 steps in the communication process.
2. What type of communication involves repeating a message to be sure it was understood and receiving confirmation from the sender?

3. Define *nonverbal communication* and give one example that is not listed in the textbook.
4. What does the word *culture* mean?
5. How can a healthcare worker provide unbiased care?
6. Why should "why" questions be avoided when talking with patients?
7. If a patient speaks a different language than the PCT does, how can the PCT communicate?
8. What is one way to provide feedback while listening?
9. What does it mean to validate a patient's concerns?
10. What are 3 examples of therapeutic communication?
11. What is the difference between facts and opinions? What is the difference between objective and subjective information?
12. With whom should PCTs use medical terminology—care team members or patients and their families?
13. When communicating information about a patient, should the PCT use facts or opinions?
14. List 10 patient observations that are considered urgent and should be reported immediately.
15. What is one thing the PCT can do to let the supervisor know that he has understood a verbal instruction at shift change?
16. Explain the difference between an electronic health record (EHR) and an electronic medical record (EMR).
17. What is one way to protect patients' protected health information (PHI) while using a computer in a healthcare facility?

4

Human Needs and Human Development

1. Identify basic human needs

People have different genes, physical appearances, cultural backgrounds, ages, and social and financial positions. But all human beings have the same basic physiological needs. **Physiological needs** relate to the processes and activities that keep living things alive:

- Food and water
- Protection and shelter
- Activity
- Sleep and rest
- Comfort, especially freedom from pain

Activities of daily living, such as eating, eliminating, bathing, and grooming, are the ways people meet their most basic physiological needs. By assisting with ADLs or helping patients perform them independently, PCTs help patients meet their basic needs.

Human beings also have **psychosocial needs**, which involve social interaction, emotions, intellect, and spirituality. Although they are not as easy to define as physiological needs, psychosocial needs include the following:

- Love and affection
- Acceptance by others
- Safety and security
- Self-reliance and independence in daily living
- Contact with others (Fig. 4-1)
- Success and self-esteem

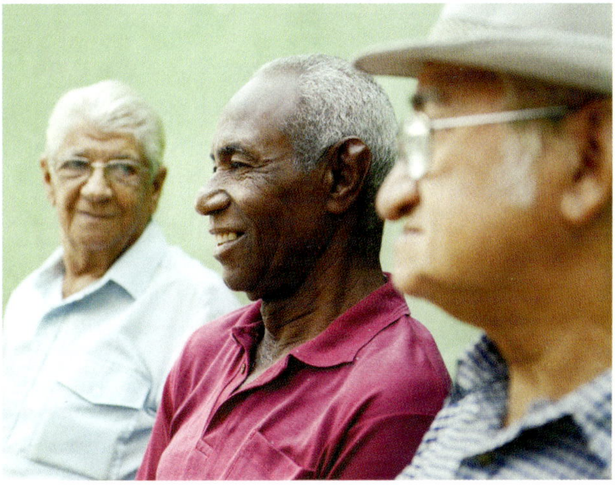

Fig. 4-1. *Interaction with other people is a basic psychosocial need. Social contact is important.*

Health and well-being affect how well psychosocial needs are met. Stress and frustration occur when basic needs are not met. This can lead to fear, anxiety, anger, aggression, withdrawal, indifference, and depression. Stress can also cause physical problems that may eventually lead to illness.

Abraham Maslow, a researcher of human behavior, wrote about human physiological and psychosocial needs. He arranged these needs by order of importance. He thought that physiological needs must be met before psychosocial needs can be met. His theory is called *Maslow's Hierarchy of Needs* (Fig. 4-2).

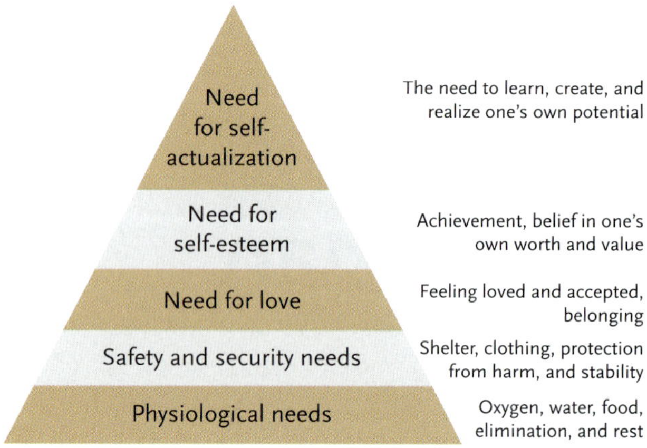

Fig. 4-2. *Maslow's Hierarchy of Needs is a model developed by Abraham Maslow to show how physiological and psychosocial needs are arranged in order of importance. Maslow believed that physiological needs must be met before psychosocial needs can be met.*

After meeting physiological needs, safety and security needs must be met. Feeling safe means not feeling afraid or unstable. Many things can cause a person to feel unsafe. An illness or disability can be frightening and make a person feel fearful and insecure.

After physiological and safety needs are met, the need for love and belonging is important. This level involves feeling accepted, needed, and cared for. The need for self-esteem is the next level. This need involves respecting and valuing oneself, which comes from within, as well as from other people. Achievements that make a person feel valued are important.

Self-actualization is the highest level. It means that a person tries to be the best person they can be; they try to reach their full potential. This may mean different things for each person. The quest to meet this need continues and changes throughout a person's life.

PCTs provide care that is focused mostly on physiological needs. However, meeting these needs provides a foundation for meeting psychosocial needs. It is in meeting those needs that people gain a sense of fulfillment in life. It is important to remember that medical care affects more than just a person's physical health.

2. Discuss holistic care and person-centered care

Holistic means considering a whole system, such as a whole person, rather than dividing the system up into parts. **Holistic care** means caring for the whole person—the mind as well as the body. Holistic care takes into account a person's physiological, psychological, social, and spiritual needs. Caring for a person holistically is part of providing person-centered care. Person-centered care is a type of care that revolves around the patient and promotes their individuality, preferences, choices, dignity, and interests.

A simple example of holistic care is taking time to talk with a patient in between vital signs measurements. The PCT is getting to know the patient as a person, which allows for better, more individualized care. Another way of practicing holistic care is considering psychosocial factors in illness, as well as physiological factors. For example, if there is a change in a patient's desire to get out of bed or care for himself, the cause may be depression rather than worsening physical health. The PCT does not make diagnoses. However, by talking with him she can learn things that help the provider. For example, she may learn that the patient is worried he will never recover and will not be able to work. She should document this information and share it with the nurse.

3. Describe the stages of human growth and development

Throughout their lives, people change physically and psychologically. Physical changes occur in the body. Psychological changes occur in the mind and also in the person's behavior. These changes are called human growth and development.

Everyone will go through the same stages of development during their lives. However, no 2 people will follow the exact same pattern or rate of development. The age ranges given in this learning objective provide a general idea of developmental stages, not an exact description. Each patient must be treated as an individual and as a whole person who is growing and developing, rather than someone who is merely ill or receiving a particular medical treatment.

Infancy (Birth to 12 Months)

Infants grow and develop very quickly. In 1 year, a baby moves from total dependence to the relative independence of moving around, communicating basic needs, and feeding herself. Physical development in infancy moves from the head down. For example, infants gain control over the muscles of the neck before they are able to control the muscles in their shoulders. Control over muscles in the trunk area, such as the shoulders, develops before control of the arms and legs (Fig. 4-3).

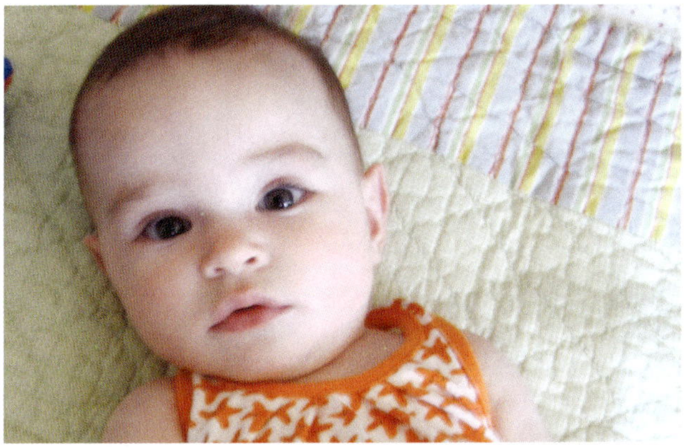

Fig. 4-3. *An infant's physical development moves from the head down.*

This head-to-toe sequence should be respected when caring for infants. For example, newborns must be supported at the shoulders, head, and neck. Babies who cannot sit or crawl should not be encouraged to stand or walk.

Toddler (Ages 1 to 3)

During the toddler years, children gain independence. One part of this independence is new control over their bodies. Toddlers learn to speak, gain coordination of their limbs, and to control their bladders and bowels (Fig. 4-4). Toddlers assert their new independence by exploring. Poisons and other hazards, such as sharp objects, must be locked away. Psychologically, toddlers learn that they are individuals, separate from their parents. Children at this age may try to control their parents. They may try to get what they want by throwing tantrums, whining, or refusing to cooperate. This is a key time for parents to set rules and standards.

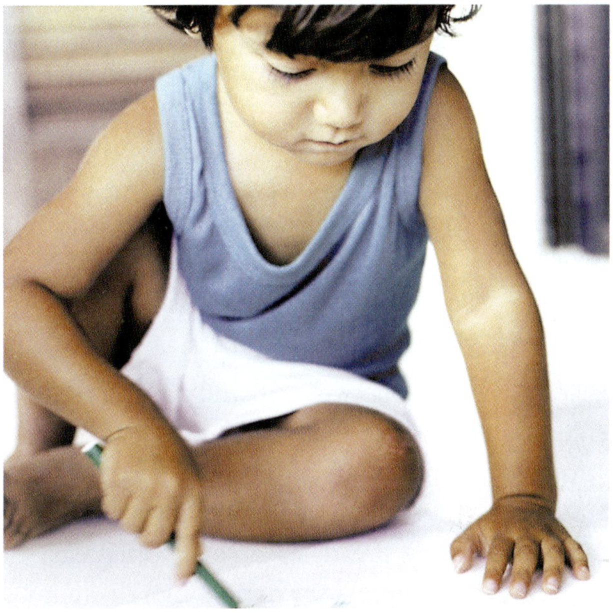

Fig. 4-4. *Toddlers gain coordination of their limbs.*

Preschool (Ages 3 to 5)

Children in their preschool years develop skills that help them become more independent and have social relationships (Fig. 4-5). They develop a vocabulary and language skills. They learn to play in groups. They become more physically coordinated and learn to care for themselves. Preschoolers also develop ways of relating to family members. They begin to learn right from wrong.

School Age (Ages 5 to 10)

School-age children's development is centered on **cognitive** (related to thinking and learning) and social development. As children enter school, they also explore the world around them. They relate to other children through games, peer groups, and classroom activities. In these years, children learn to get along with each other. They also begin to develop a conscience, morals, and self-esteem.

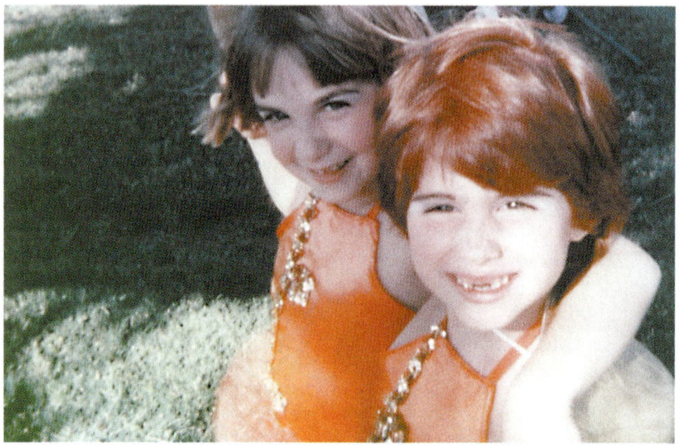

Fig. 4-5. *Children in their preschool years develop social relationships.*

Preadolescence (Ages 10 to 12)

During the years between 10 and 12, children enjoy a growing sense of self-identity and a strong sense of identity with their peers. They tend to be very social. This is usually a relatively calm period, and preadolescents are often easy to get along with and able to handle more responsibility at home and school. Childhood fears of ghosts or monsters will give way to fears based in the real world. It is important that preadolescents feel able to trust in the attention and care of parents or other adults.

Children generally begin puberty during this stage, although this varies based on factors such as genetics and health status. Girls start puberty, on average, 1 year earlier than boys. During puberty, a person develops secondary sex characteristics. In females, these characteristics include growth of body hair and development of breasts and hips. In males, they include growth of body hair, growth of the testes and penis, broadening of the shoulders, and a lower voice.

Adolescence (Ages 12 to 18)

During adolescence, children become sexually mature. If they did not reach puberty during the previous stage, it will start here. Many teenagers have a hard time adapting to the rapid changes that occur in their bodies after puberty. Peer acceptance is important to them. Adolescents may be afraid that they are unattractive or abnormal. This concern for body image and peer acceptance, combined with changing hormones that influence moods, can cause rapid mood swings. Conflicting pressures develop as they remain dependent on their parents and yet need to express themselves socially and sexually (Fig. 4-6). This can cause conflict and stress.

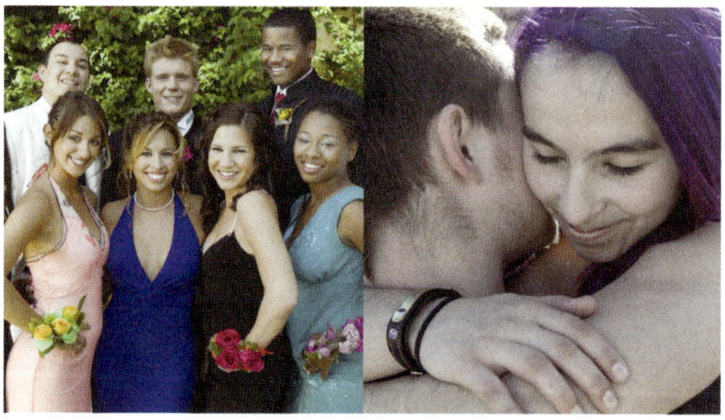

Fig. 4-6. *Adolescence is a time of adapting to change.*

Young Adulthood (Ages 18 to 40)

Physical growth has usually been completed by this time. Adopting a healthy lifestyle in these years can make life better now and prevent health problems in later adulthood. Psychological and social development continues, however. The tasks of these years include the following:

- Selecting an appropriate education
- Selecting an occupation or career
- Selecting a mate (Fig. 4-7)
- Learning to live with a mate or others
- Raising children
- Developing a satisfying sex life

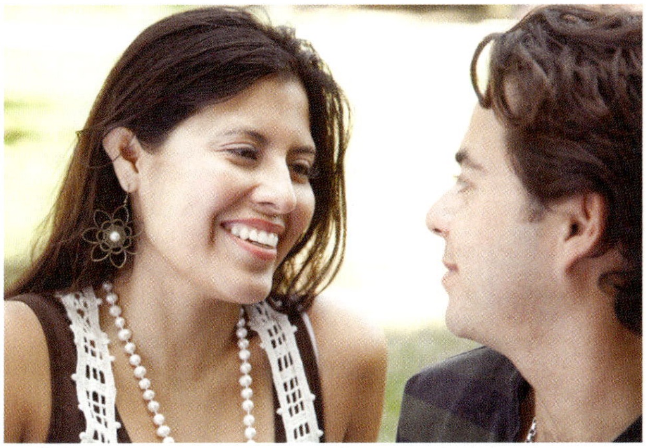

Fig. 4-7. Young adulthood often involves finding a mate.

Middle Adulthood (Ages 40 to 65)

In general, people in middle adulthood are more comfortable and stable than they were in previous stages. Many of their major life decisions have already been made. In the early years of middle adulthood people sometimes experience a "midlife crisis." This is a period of unrest centered on a subconscious desire for change and fulfillment of unmet goals.

Physical changes related to aging also occur in middle adulthood. Adults in this age group may notice that they have difficulty maintaining their weight or notice a decrease in strength and energy. Metabolism and other body functions slow down. Wrinkles and gray hair appear. Vision and hearing loss may begin. Women experience **menopause**, the end of menstruation (occurs when a woman has not had a menstrual period for 12 months). This occurs when the ovaries stop secreting hormones. Many diseases and illnesses can develop in these years. These disorders can become chronic and life-threatening.

Late Adulthood (65 years and older)

Persons in late adulthood must adjust to the effects of aging. These changes can include the loss of strength and health, the death of loved ones, retirement, and preparation for their own death. Although the developmental tasks of this age appear to deal entirely with loss, solutions often involve new relationships, friendships, and interests.

Developmental Disabilities

Developmental disabilities are disabilities that are present at birth or emerge during childhood, up to age 22. A developmental disability is a chronic condition. It restricts physical and/or mental ability. These disabilities prevent a child from developing at a normal rate. Language, mobility, learning, and the ability to perform self-care may be affected. The care patients need will depend on the type and the extent of their disability.

Intellectual disability (formerly called *mental retardation*) is the most common developmental disability. It is neither a disease nor a mental health disorder (see next learning objective). People with an intellectual disability develop at a below-average rate. They have below-average mental functioning. They have difficulty with learning, communicating, and moving, and may have problems adjusting socially. Their ability to care for themselves may be affected.

Patients who have an intellectual disability have the same emotional and physical needs that others have. They experience the same emotions, such as anger, sadness, love, and joy, as others do, but their ability to express their emotions may be limited.

4. Discuss mental health and mental health disorders

Mental health is the normal functioning of emotional and intellectual abilities. A person who is mentally healthy is able to

- Get along with others (Fig. 4-8)
- Adapt to change
- Care for herself and others
- Give and accept love
- Deal with situations that cause anxiety, disappointment, and frustration
- Take responsibility for decisions, feelings, and actions
- Control and fulfill desires and impulses appropriately

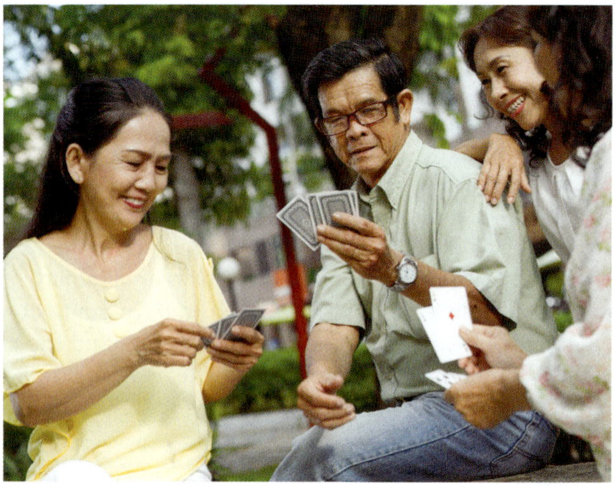

Fig. 4-8. The ability to interact well with other people is a characteristic of mental health.

Although it involves the emotions and mental functions, a **mental health disorder** is like a physical disorder in many ways. It may have physical causes, such as differences in a person's brain structure or the way the brain works. It produces signs and symptoms and affects the body's ability to function. It responds to proper treatment and care. A mental health disorder disrupts a person's ability to function in the family, home, or community. It often causes inappropriate behavior. Some signs and symptoms of mental health disorders include confusion, disorientation, agitation, and anxiety.

Physical factors related to the brain may cause a mental health disorder or make one more likely to develop. Illness, disability, or aging can cause stress that may lead to a mental health disorder. Substance abuse or a chemical imbalance and traumatic brain injury can also cause mental health disorders.

There are many degrees and types of mental health disorders, from mild to severe. A person with a severe mental health disorder may lose touch with reality and become unable to communicate or make decisions. Some people with a mild type, however, function normally. They may sometimes become overwhelmed by stress or be highly emotional. Many signs of mental health disorders are simply extreme behaviors most people occasionally experience. Being able to recognize such behaviors may make it easier to understand patients with these disorders.

Anxiety Disorders: **Anxiety** is uneasiness, worry, or fear, often about a situation or condition. When a person who is mentally healthy feels anxiety, he can usually identify the cause. The anxiety fades once the cause is removed. A person who has an anxiety disorder may feel anxious all the time and not know why. Anxiety causes physical symptoms, such as shaking, muscle aches, sweating, cold and clammy hands, dizziness, chest pain, rapid heartbeat, cold or hot flashes, a choking or smothering sensation, and a dry mouth. Some types of anxiety disorders include the following:

Generalized anxiety disorder (**GAD**) is characterized by chronic anxiety and worry, even when there is no reason for concern. A person with GAD may be excessively worried about health, finances, work, or other issues.

Panic disorder is characterized by panic attacks. A panic attack is an episode of intense fear that occurs along with physical symptoms, such as rapid heartbeat, chest pain, dizziness, and shortness of breath. A person having a panic attack may think he is having a heart attack or dying. When a person has panic disorder, he has regular panic attacks or lives with chronic anxiety about having another attack.

When a person has **social anxiety disorder** (social phobia), she has intense anxiety and extreme discomfort in social situations. A **phobia** is an intense, irrational fear of or anxiety about an object, place, or situation, such as a fear of dogs or a fear of flying. Having social anxiety disorder is not the same as being shy. A person with this disorder is very self-conscious and may feel she is being judged or criticized by others to the point where she actively avoids social functions.

Obsessive-Compulsive and Related Disorders: **Obsessive-compulsive disorder (OCD)** is a disorder characterized by recurring intrusive behavior or thoughts that cause anxiety or stress. For example, a person may repeatedly check to make sure the door is locked. A person with OCD is unable to stop these thoughts and feels compelled (forced) to perform these actions.

Trauma and Stressor-Related Disorders: **Post-traumatic stress disorder (PTSD)** is a disorder caused by experiencing or witnessing a traumatic experience, such as being a victim of violence (e.g., sexual or physical assault, other violent crimes), being involved in combat while in the military, or surviving a car accident or terror attack. Symptoms of PTSD include reliving the trauma through flashbacks, bad dreams, or scary thoughts, as well as avoiding places or thoughts that trigger reminders. Some people who have PTSD are constantly tense, easily startled, and have trouble sleeping. Anger and irritability are other symptoms.

Depressive Disorders: **Major depressive disorder** (often called *clinical depression* or **depression**) is characterized by a loss of interest in everything a person once cared about, and may interfere with the person's ability to work, sleep, and eat. It may cause intense mental, emotional, and physical pain and disability. Depression also makes other illnesses worse. If left untreated, it may result in suicide.

Clinical depression is not a normal reaction to stress. It may be caused by abnormal levels of chemicals in the brain. Depression can occur along with other illnesses. Cancer, AIDS, Alzheimer's disease, diabetes, and heart attack may be associated with increased rates of depression. Depression can also happen after a woman gives birth (called *postpartum depression*) or after the death of a loved one. Sadness is only one sign of this illness. Not all people who have depression complain of sadness or appear sad.

Bipolar and Related Disorders: **Bipolar disorder** causes a person to have mood swings and changes in energy levels and the ability to function. A person may swing from periods of extreme activity or excitement (a manic episode) to periods of deep depression or sadness (a depressive episode). Characteristics of manic episodes include high energy, little sleep, big speeches, rapidly changing thoughts and moods, inflated self-esteem, overspending, and poor judgment.

Schizophrenia and Other Psychotic Disorders: **Schizophrenia** is a mental health disorder that affects a person's ability to think and communicate clearly. It also affects the ability to manage emotions, make decisions, and understand reality. It affects a person's ability to interact with other people.

Hallucinations and delusions are symptoms of schizophrenia. **Hallucinations** are false or distorted sensory perceptions. A person may see someone or something that is not really there, or hear a conversation that is not real. **Delusions** are persistent false beliefs. For example, a person may believe that other people are controlling his thoughts.

Other symptoms of schizophrenia include disorganized thinking and speech. This makes a person unable to express logical thoughts. Disorganized behavior means a person moves slowly, repeating gestures or movements. People with schizophrenia may also show less emotion. They may seem to have less interest in the things around them and have a lack of energy.

It is extremely important to remember that mental health disorders can be treated. Medication and psychotherapy are common treatment methods. Medication is widely used for several disorders. It may allow people to function more completely.

Psychotherapy is a method of treating mental health disorders that involves working with trained, licensed professionals, such as clinical psychologists, therapists, and social workers. They use different techniques to help clients learn more about themselves and to teach them new ways to handle problems and be more in control of their lives.

Cognitive behavioral therapy (**CBT**) is a type of psychotherapy that is often used to treat anxiety disorders and depression. This type of therapy is usually short-term and focuses on skills and solutions that a person can use to modify negative thinking and behavior patterns.

Guidelines: Mental Health Disorders

- **G** Do not talk to adults as if they were children.
- **G** Use simple, clear statements and a normal tone of voice.
- **G** Be sure that what you say and how you say it show respect and concern.
- **G** Sit or stand at a normal distance from the patient. Be aware of your body language.
- **G** Be honest and direct, as you would with any patient.
- **G** Avoid arguments.
- **G** Maintain eye contact and listen.

5. List the signs of substance use disorder (SUD)

Substance use disorder (**SUD**) is the repeated or uncontrolled use of legal or illegal substances in a way that is harmful to oneself or others. SUD is a complex condition with various causes. People may use substances as a way to cope with stress, reduce pain, mask symptoms, or to feel "high." They may be trying to improve performance or to escape difficult thoughts.

Many types of substances are abused, including alcohol, tobacco, legal and illegal drugs, glue, and paint. It is not necessary for a substance to be illegal for it to be abused (Fig. 4-9). Alcohol and cigarettes are legal for adults but are often abused. Medications can be addictive and harmful if used incorrectly.

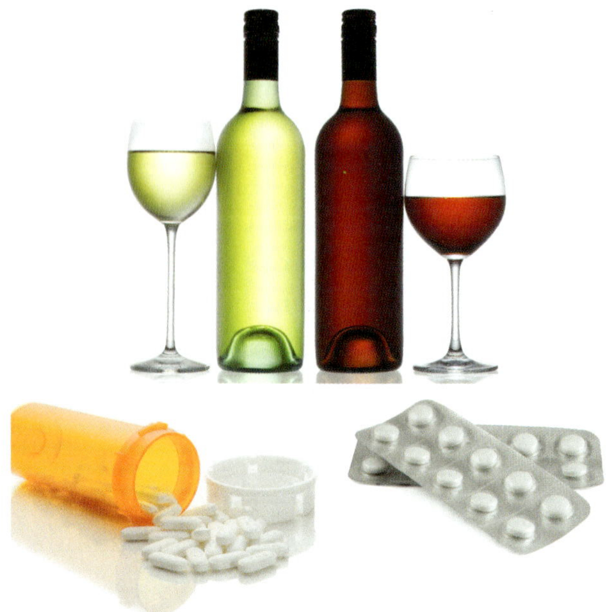

Fig. 4-9. *Prescription drugs and alcohol are examples of legal substances that may be abused.*

The harm caused by SUD may come in many forms: damage to the person's health, legal problems, and damage to the person's relationships with family and friends. **Chemical dependency** can result from substance use. It involves needing greater amounts of the drug to get the same effect and having symptoms when the drug is stopped (withdrawal). It often goes along with addiction. It affects a person physically, mentally, and emotionally. Chemical dependency and addiction are treatable but may require diagnosis and care by specialists. Treatment is not as simple as just stopping the drug.

Some medications are available legally by prescription but may also be abused. *Opioids* are drugs used to relieve severe pain, such as from surgery, cancer, or serious injuries. They are also sometimes prescribed to treat chronic pain. They work to block pain signals to the brain and boost feelings of relaxation, happiness, and pleasure. Opioid abuse has become increasingly widespread in the United States over the last few decades. Some opioids, such as oxycodone, morphine, codeine, hydrocodone, and fentanyl, are legally prescribed. Heroin and illegally made fentanyl are types of illegal opioids.

Taking prescribed opioid medication can put a person at risk for dependence on the drug and addiction. Because of the positive feeling opioids create, some people continue to want to take them and even seek illegal drugs once they can no longer obtain prescriptions from doctors. In addition, when taking prescribed opioids, a person's tolerance for the drug increases, requiring higher doses of the medication to achieve the same effects. High doses of opioids can cause breathing to slow and even stop, which can cause death. When a person overdoses on opioids, an antidote called naloxone may be given during a certain time frame to reverse the potentially fatal effects.

A PCT may be in a position to observe signs of SUD in patients. These signs should be reported to the nurse. Observations can be made without accusing anyone. The PCT should simply report what she sees, not what she thinks the cause may be.

Observing and Reporting: Substance Use Disorder

- O/R Red eyes, dilated pupils, or lack of coordination
- O/R Moodiness, strange behavior, or lying
- O/R Irritability
- O/R Smell of alcohol, cigarettes, or other substances on breath or on clothing
- O/R Unexplained changes in vital signs
- O/R Patient reports any of the following:
  - Diminished sense of smell
  - Loss of appetite
  - Inability to function normally
  - Confusion or forgetfulness
  - Blackouts or memory loss
  - Frequent accidents
  - Problems with family or friends

Some of the same signs listed above may also indicate other problems. Depression, dementia, medication issues, and medical conditions can also produce many of these same symptoms.

Chapter Review

1. Name 2 physiological and 2 psychosocial needs.
2. During what developmental stage do children develop a conscience, morals, and self-esteem?
3. At what stage of development may a person have difficulty maintaining his weight or experience a decrease in strength or metabolism?
4. What do the abilities to adapt to change, get along with others, and take responsibility for one's decisions, feelings, and actions show?
5. What types of legal substances may be abused?
6. Bipolar disorder can cause a person to cycle between what 2 extremes?
7. What are 2 types of treatment for mental health disorders?
8. How might a person who has been legally prescribed an opioid painkiller become addicted to illegal drugs?
9. What should a PCT do if he observes signs of substance use disorder in a patient?

5 Infection Prevention and Control

1. Define *infection prevention* and discuss types of infections

Infection prevention is the set of methods practiced in healthcare facilities to prevent and control the spread of disease. Facilities employ health professionals called *infection preventionists* to help with infection prevention. These team members help to manage their facilities' infection prevention measures. Preventing the spread of infection is very important and is the responsibility of all care team members. PCTs are part of the care team and are also responsible for preventing the spread of infection. They must know and follow their facility's policies relating to infection prevention. These policies help protect staff members, patients, visitors, and others from disease.

A **microorganism** (**MO**), also called a *microbe*, is a living thing that is so small that it is only visible under a microscope. Microorganisms are always present in the environment (Fig. 5-1). **Infections** occur when harmful microorganisms, called **pathogens**, invade and multiply within the body.

There are 2 main types of infections: localized and systemic. A **localized infection** is an infection that is limited to a specific location in the body. It has local symptoms, which means the symptoms are near the site of infection. For example, if a wound becomes infected, the area around it may become red, swollen, warm, and painful. A **systemic infection** affects the entire body. This type of infection travels through the bloodstream and is spread throughout the body. It causes general symptoms, such as fever, chills, or mental confusion.

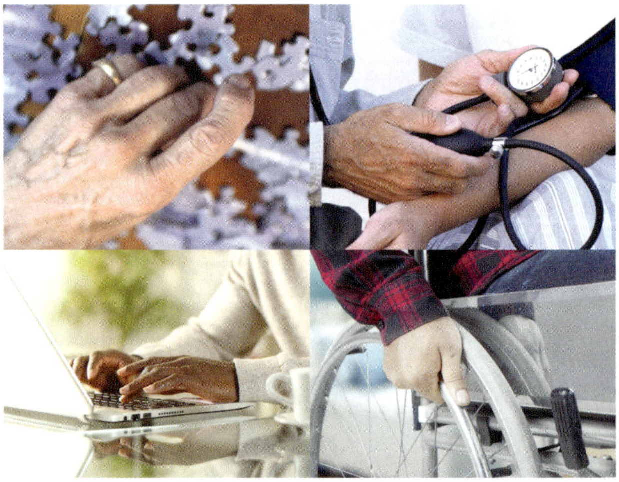

Fig. 5-1. Microorganisms are always present in the environment. They are on almost everything a person touches.

A type of infection that can be localized or systemic is a **healthcare-associated infection** (**HAI**). A healthcare-associated infection is an infection acquired in a healthcare setting during the delivery of medical care. Healthcare settings include hospitals, long-term care facilities, and outpatient surgery centers, among others.

PCTs need to be able to recognize signs and symptoms of infections so that they can report them to the nurse promptly.

Observing and Reporting: Infections

Signs and symptoms of a localized infection include the following:

- O/R Pain
- O/R Redness
- O/R Swelling
- O/R Pus
- O/R Drainage (fluid from a wound or cavity)
- O/R Heat

Signs and symptoms of a systemic infection include the following:

- O/R Fever
- O/R Body aches
- O/R Chills
- O/R Nausea
- O/R Vomiting
- O/R Weakness
- O/R Headache
- O/R Confusion or agitation
- O/R Drop in a person's normal blood pressure
- O/R Elevated heart rate
- O/R Rapid breathing

2. Describe the chain of infection

To understand how to prevent disease, it is helpful to first understand how it is spread. The **chain of infection** is a way of describing how disease is transmitted from one human being to another (Fig. 5-2). Definitions and examples of each of the 6 links in the chain of infection follow.

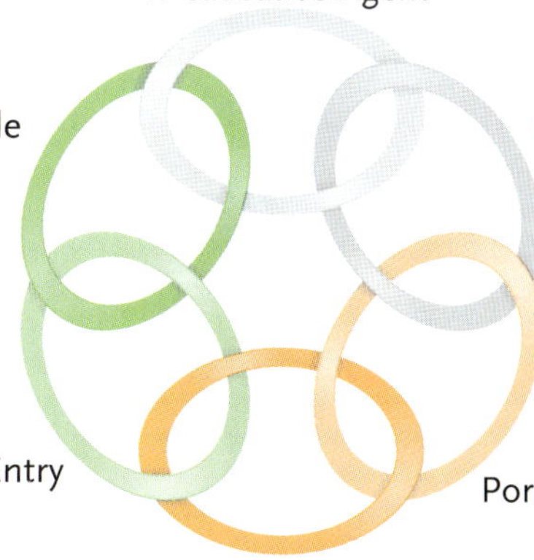
1. Causative Agent
2. Reservoir
3. Portal of Exit
4. Mode of Transmission
5. Portal of Entry
6. Susceptible Host

Fig. 5-2. *The chain of infection.*

Chain Link 1: The **causative agent** is a pathogenic microorganism that causes disease. Microorganisms are small living bodies that cannot be seen without a microscope. They are everywhere—on skin, in food, in the air, and in water. Causative agents include bacteria, viruses, fungi, and parasites.

Normal flora are the microorganisms that live in and on the body and normally do not cause harm to a healthy person, as long as the flora remain in that particular area. When they enter a different part of the body, they may cause an infection.

Chain Link 2: A **reservoir** is where the pathogen lives and multiplies. A reservoir can be a human, animal, plant, soil, or substance. Warm, dark, and moist places are the ideal environments for microorganisms to live, grow, and multiply. Some microorganisms need oxygen to survive while others do not. Examples of reservoirs include the lungs, blood, and the large intestine.

Chain Link 3: The **portal of exit** is any body opening on an infected person that allows pathogens to leave (Fig. 5-3). These include the nose, mouth, eyes, or a cut in the skin.

Chain Link 4: The **mode of transmission** describes how the pathogen travels. The main routes of transmission are contact, droplet, and airborne transmission. **Direct contact** happens by touching the infected person or their secretions. **Indirect contact** results from touching an object contaminated by the infected person, such as a needle, dressing, tissue, or bed linen. Learning Objective 6 contains more information about the routes of transmission. In the healthcare setting, the primary route of disease transmission is via the hands of healthcare workers.

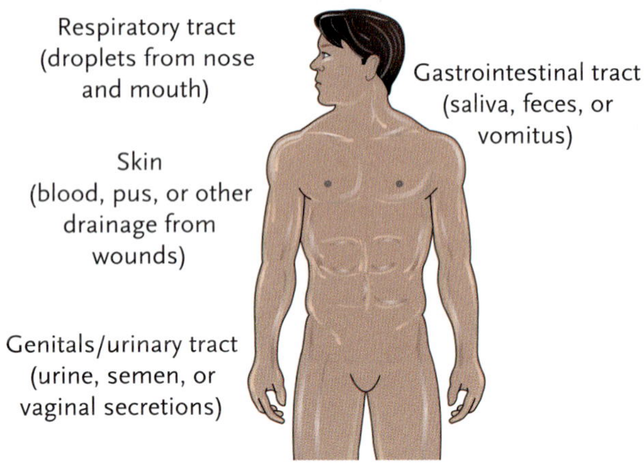

Fig. 5-3. *Portals of exit.*

Chain Link 5: The **portal of entry** is any body opening on an uninfected person that allows pathogens to enter (Fig. 5-4). These include the nose, mouth, eyes, and other mucous membranes, cuts in the skin, and cracked skin. **Mucous membranes** are the membranes that line body cavities that open to the outside of the body. These include the linings of the mouth, nose, eyes, rectum, and genitals.

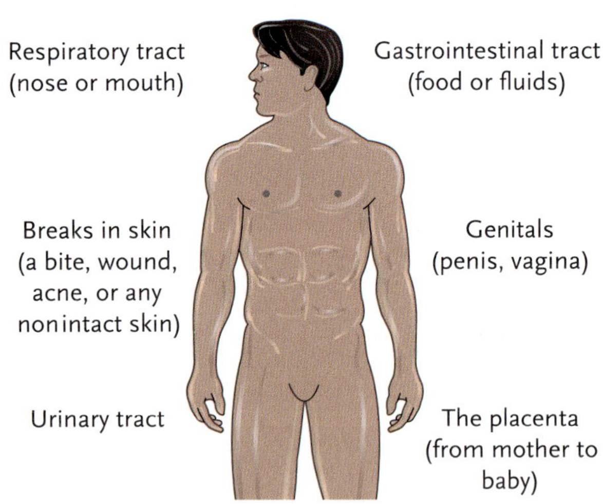

Fig. 5-4. *Portals of entry.*

Chain Link 6: A **susceptible host** is an uninfected person who could become ill. Examples include all healthcare workers and anyone in their care who is not already infected with that particular disease.

If one of the links in the chain of infection is broken, then the spread of infection is stopped. Infection prevention practices help stop pathogens from traveling (Link 4) and from getting on a person's hands, nose, eyes, mouth, skin, etc. (Link 5). Immunizations (Link 6) reduce a person's chances of getting sick from diseases such as hepatitis B and influenza (flu).

Transmission (passage or transfer) of most **infectious** diseases can be blocked by using proper infection prevention practices, such as handwashing. Handwashing is the most important way to stop the spread of infection. All healthcare workers should wash their hands often.

Handwashing is a part of medical asepsis. **Medical asepsis** refers to measures used to reduce and prevent the spread of pathogens. Medical asepsis is used in all healthcare settings. **Surgical asepsis**, also known as *sterile technique,* makes an object or area completely free of all microorganisms (not just pathogens). Surgical asepsis is used for many types of procedures, such as changing catheters.

3. Explain Standard Precautions

State and federal government agencies have guidelines and laws concerning infection prevention and control. The **Occupational Safety and Health Administration** (**OSHA**, osha.gov) is a federal government agency that makes rules to protect workers from hazards on the job. The **Centers for Disease Control and Prevention** (**CDC**, cdc.gov) is a federal government agency that issues guidelines to protect and improve the health of individuals and communities. Through education, the CDC aims to prevent and control disease, injury, and disability, as well as to promote public health.

The CDC created an infection prevention system to reduce the risk of contracting infectious diseases in healthcare settings. There are 2 levels of precautions within the infection prevention system: Standard Precautions and Transmission-Based Precautions.

Following **Standard Precautions** means treating blood and other body fluids, nonintact skin (like abrasions, pimples, or open sores), and mucous membranes as if they were infected. Body fluids include blood, tears, saliva, sputum (mucus coughed up), urine, feces, semen, vaginal secretions, pus or other wound drainage, and vomit. They do not include sweat.

Standard Precautions must be used with every patient; this promotes safety. A PCT cannot tell by looking at patients or even by reading their medical charts whether they have a contagious disease such as tuberculosis, hepatitis, or influenza. Many diseases can be spread even before the infected person shows signs or has been diagnosed.

Standard Precautions and Transmission-Based Precautions (Learning Objective 6) are ways to stop the spread of infection by interrupting the mode of transmission. In other words, these guidelines do not stop an infected person from giving off pathogens. However, PCTs help prevent those pathogens from infecting them or those in their care by following these guidelines:

- Standard Precautions must be practiced with every person in a PCT's care.
- Transmission-Based Precautions vary based on how an infection is transmitted. When indicated, these precautions are used **in addition** to Standard Precautions. More information about these precautions is located later in the chapter.

Guidelines: Standard Precautions

G **Wash your hands** before putting on gloves. Wash your hands immediately after removing your gloves. Be careful not to touch clean objects with your used gloves.

G **Wear gloves** if you may come into contact with any of the following: blood or other body fluids; secretions or excretions; broken or open skin, such as abrasions, acne, cuts, stitches, or staples; or mucous membranes. Such contact occurs during mouth care; toilet assistance; perineal care (care of the genital and anal area); helping with a bedpan or urinal; ostomy care; cleaning up spills; cleaning basins, urinals, bedpans, and other containers that have held body fluids; changing linens; and disposing of wastes.

G **Remove gloves** immediately when finished with a procedure and wash your hands.

G **Immediately wash all skin surfaces that have been contaminated** with blood or other body fluids.

G **Wear a disposable gown** that is resistant to body fluids if you may come into contact with blood or other body fluids, secretions or excretions, or when splashing or spraying of blood or other body fluids is likely. If a patient has a contagious illness, wear a gown even if it is not likely you will come into contact with blood or other body fluids.

G **Wear a mask and protective goggles and/or a face shield** if you may come into contact with blood or other body fluids, secretions or excretions, or when splashing or spraying of blood or other body fluids is likely (for example, when emptying a bedpan).

G **Wear gloves and use caution when handling razor blades, needles, and other sharps.** **Sharps** are needles or other sharp objects. Avoid nicks and cuts when shaving patients. Place sharps carefully in a biohazard container for sharps. Biohazard containers used for sharps are puncture-resistant, leakproof containers. They are clearly labeled and warn of the danger of the contents inside (Figs. 5-5 and 5-6). They must close and must be kept in an upright position to keep items inside from spilling out. They should not be filled past the line indicating that the container is full. Biohazard bags are used for biomedical waste that is not sharp, such as soiled dressings, contaminated tubing, and other items. OSHA recommends that biomedical/biohazard waste be disposed of at the *point of origin*, or where the waste occurs.

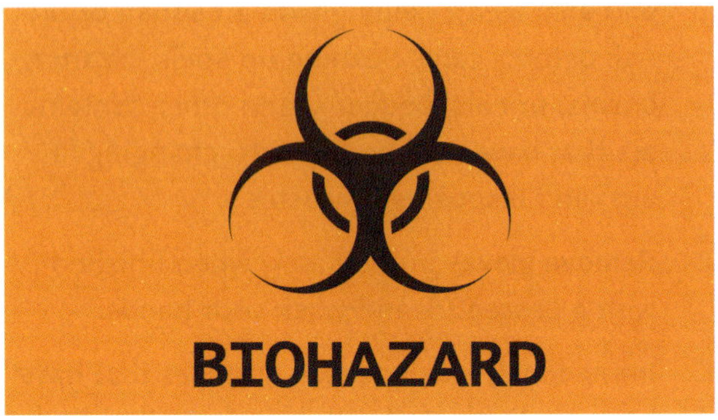

Fig. 5-5. *This label indicates that the material is potentially infectious.*

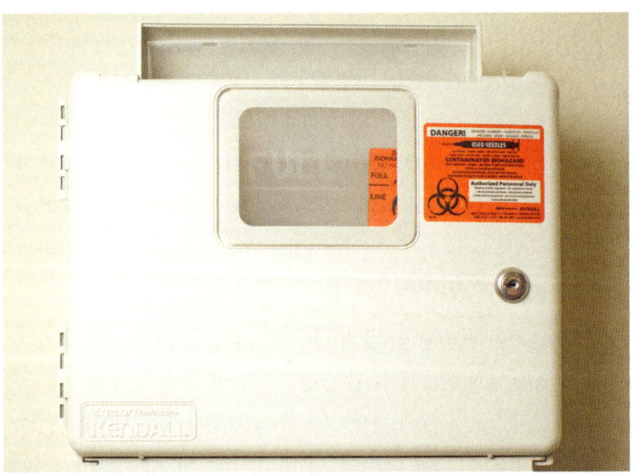

Fig. 5-6. *One type of container for sharps.*

- **G** **Never attempt to recap needles or sharps after use**. You might stick yourself. Dispose of them in a biohazard container for sharps.
- **G** **Carefully bag all contaminated supplies**. Dispose of them according to facility policy.
- **G** **Clearly label body fluids that are being saved for a specimen** with the patient's name, date of birth, date, and a biohazard label. Keep them in a container with a lid. Put them in a biohazard specimen bag for transportation if required.
- **G** **Dispose of contaminated wastes according to your facility's policy**. Waste containing blood or other body fluids is considered biohazardous waste. Liquid body wastes other than blood can usually be disposed of through the regular sewer system as long as there is no splashing, spraying, or aerosolizing of the waste as it is being disposed. Appropriate personal protective equipment needs to be worn, followed by proper removal and handwashing. Follow instructions.

Standard Precautions should always be practiced on all patients, regardless of their infection status. This greatly reduces the risk of transmitting infection. There is more information about Standard Precautions in the next several learning objectives.

4. Explain hand hygiene and identify when to wash hands

PCTs use their hands constantly while they work. Microorganisms are on everything they touch. The single most common way for healthcare-associated infections (HAIs) to be spread is via the hands of healthcare workers. Handwashing is the most important thing PCTs can do to prevent the spread of disease (Fig. 5-7).

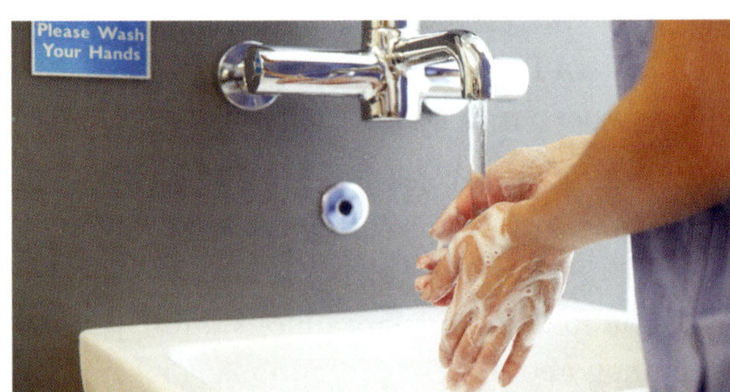

Fig. 5-7. *All people working in health care must wash their hands often. Handwashing is the most effective way to prevent the spread of disease.*

The CDC has defined **hand hygiene** as washing hands with soap and water or using an alcohol-based hand sanitizer (ABHS). Alcohol-based hand sanitizers (often called *hand sanitizer* or *hand rub*) include gels, rinses, and foams that do not require the use of water.

Alcohol-based hand sanitizers have proven effective in reducing bacteria on the skin. However, they are not a substitute for frequent, proper handwashing. When hands are visibly soiled, they should be washed with soap and water. Hand sanitizers can be used in addition to handwashing any time hands are not visibly soiled. When using a hand sanitizer, the hands must be rubbed together until the product has completely dried. Hand lotion can help prevent dry, cracked skin.

PCTs should avoid wearing rings and bracelets while working because they may increase the risk of contamination. (Smooth, plain bands may be acceptable.) Fingernails should be short, smooth, and clean. Artificial nails (acrylic, gel, sculptured, or wraps) should not be worn because they harbor bacteria and increase the risk of contamination even if hands are washed often. PCTs should wash their hands at these times:

- When first arriving at work
- Whenever hands are visibly soiled
- Before, between, and after all contact with patients
- Before putting on gloves and after removing gloves
- After contact with any body fluid, mucous membrane, nonintact skin, or wound dressing
- After handling contaminated items
- After contact with any object in the patient's room (care environment)
- Before and after touching meal trays and/or handling food
- Before and after assisting patients with meals
- Before getting clean linen
- Before and after using the toilet
- After touching garbage or trash
- After picking up anything from the floor
- After blowing or wiping the nose or coughing or sneezing into the hands
- Before and after eating
- After smoking
- After touching areas on the body, such as the mouth, face, eyes, hair, ears, or nose
- Before and after applying makeup
- Before leaving the facility

Washing hands (hand hygiene)

Equipment: soap, paper towels

1. Turn on the water at the sink. Keep your clothes dry because moisture breeds bacteria. Do not let your clothing touch the outside portion of the sink or counter.
2. Wet your hands and wrists thoroughly (Fig. 5-8).

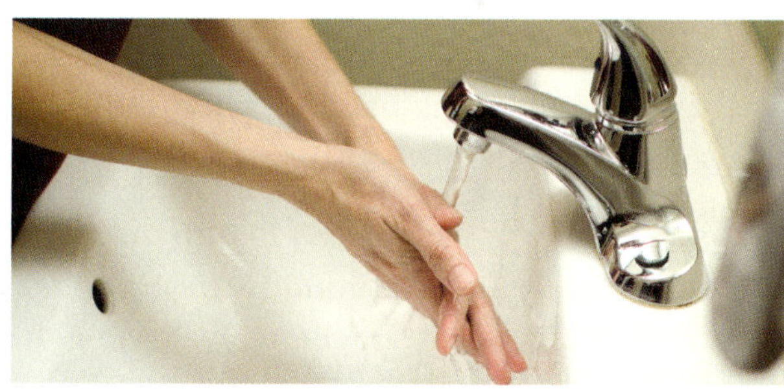

Fig. 5-8. *Keeping arms angled downward, wet your hands and wrists thoroughly.*

3. Apply soap to your hands.
4. Keep your hands lower than your elbows and your fingertips down. Rub your hands together and fingers between each other to create a lather. Lather all surfaces of your wrists, hands, and fingers, using friction for at least 20 seconds. Friction helps clean (Fig. 5-9).
5. Clean your fingernails by rubbing them in the palm of your other hand.

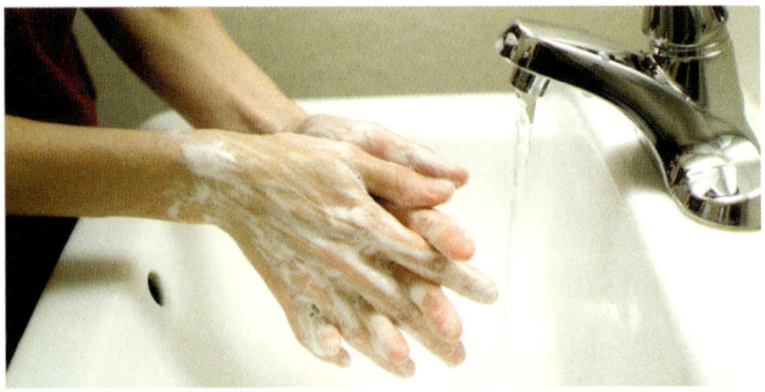

Fig. 5-9. *Using friction for at least 20 seconds, lather all surfaces of your wrists, hands, and fingers.*

6. Keep your hands lower than your elbows and your fingertips down. Being careful not to touch the sink, rinse thoroughly under running water. Rinse all surfaces of your wrists, hands, and fingers. Run water down from your wrists to your fingertips. Do not run water over unwashed arms down to clean hands.
7. Use a clean, dry paper towel to dry all surfaces of your fingers, hands, and wrists, starting at the fingertips. Do not wipe the towel on your unwashed forearms and then wipe your clean hands. Discard the paper towel into the waste container without touching the container. If your hands touch the sink or wastebasket, start over.
8. Use a clean, dry paper towel to turn off the faucet (Fig. 5-10). Discard the towel into the waste container. Do not contaminate your hands by touching the surface of the sink or faucet.

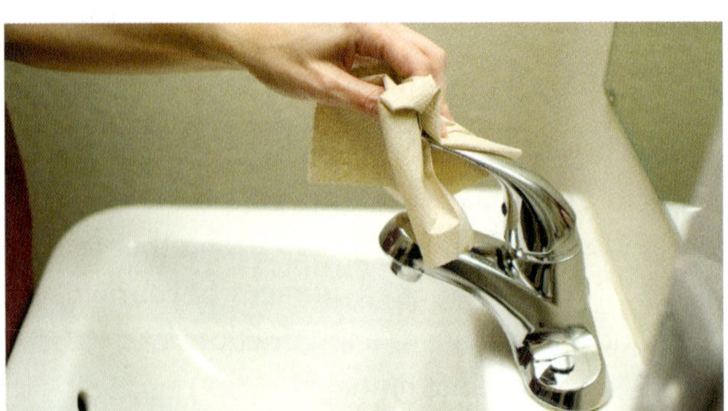

Fig. 5-10. *Use a clean, dry paper towel to turn off the faucet so that you do not contaminate your hands.*

5. Discuss the use of personal protective equipment (PPE)

Personal protective equipment (**PPE**) is equipment that helps protect employees from serious injuries or illnesses resulting from contact with workplace hazards. In hospitals and other healthcare facilities, PPE helps protect PCTs from contact with potentially infectious material. Employers are responsible for providing PCTs with the appropriate PPE to wear.

Personal protective equipment includes gowns, masks, goggles, face shields, and gloves. (Some healthcare facilities may also use shoe covers and/or hair covers in some situations.) Gowns protect the skin and/or clothing. Masks protect the mouth and nose. Goggles protect the eyes. Face shields protect the entire face—the eyes, nose, and mouth. Gloves protect the hands. Gloves are used most often by all healthcare workers.

PCTs must wear PPE if there is a chance of coming into contact with blood or other body fluids, secretions or excretions, mucous membranes, or open wounds. They should put on, or **don**, gowns, masks, goggles, and face shields when splashing or spraying of blood or other body fluids could occur. Hand hygiene should be performed before donning PPE and after removing and discarding PPE.

Gowns

Clean, nonsterile gowns protect exposed skin. They also prevent the soiling of clothing. Gowns should fully cover the torso. They should fit comfortably over the body, and have long sleeves that fit snugly at the wrists. OSHA requires fluid-resistant gowns if fluid penetration is likely. If a gown becomes wet or soiled during care, it should be discarded and a new gown should be donned. When finished with a procedure, the PCT should remove, or **doff**, the gown as soon as possible and wash her hands.

Gowns may have ties at the neck and waist and are donned by placing the arms through the sleeves before fastening the ties. Over-the-head gowns are another style. They are donned over the head and may be tied at the waist. This skill shows donning a gown with ties at the neck and waist.

Putting on (donning) and removing (doffing) a gown

1. Wash your hands.
2. Open the gown. Hold it out in front of you and allow it to open/unfold (Fig. 5-11). Do not shake the gown or touch it to the floor. Facing the back opening of the gown, place your arms through each sleeve.

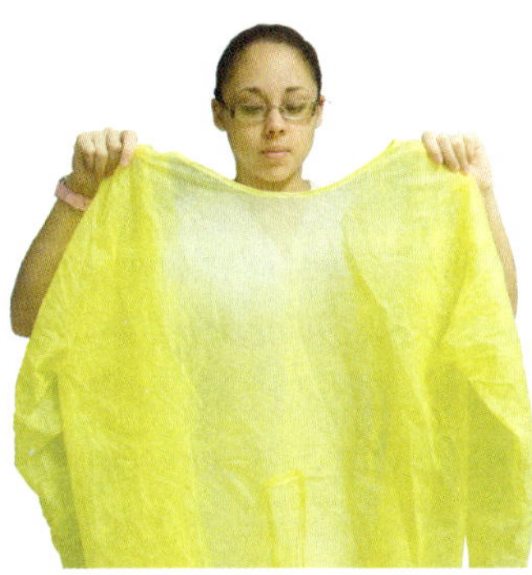

Fig. 5-11. *Let the gown unfold without shaking it.*

3. Fasten the neck opening.
4. Reaching behind you, pull the gown until it completely covers your clothing. Secure the gown at your waist (Fig. 5-12).

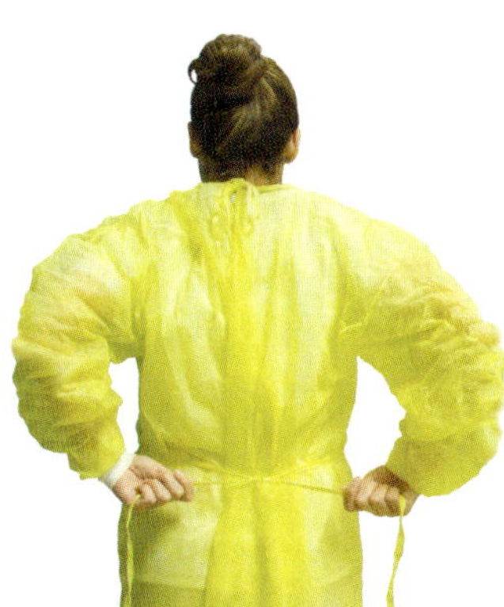

Fig. 5-12. *Reaching behind you, secure the gown at the waist.*

5. Put on your gloves after putting on the gown. The cuffs of the gloves should overlap the cuffs of the gown (Fig. 5-13).

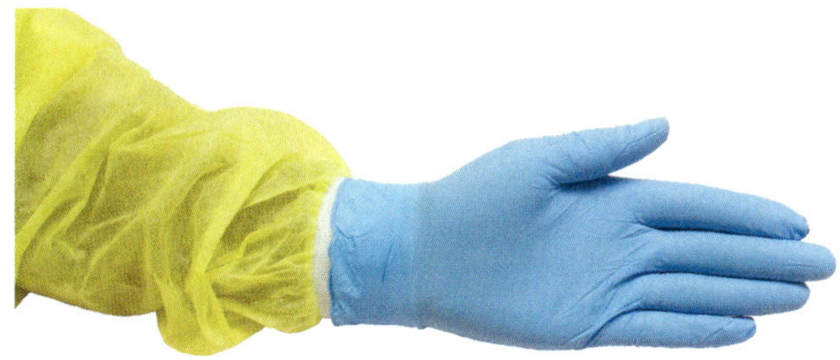

Fig. 5-13. *The cuffs of the gloves should overlap the cuffs of the gown.*

6. When removing a gown, first remove and discard your gloves properly, then unfasten the gown at the neck and waist. Remove the gown without touching the outside of the gown. Roll the dirty side in, while holding the gown away from your body. Discard the gown properly and wash your hands.

Masks and Goggles

Masks can prevent inhalation of microorganisms through the nose or mouth. Masks should be worn when caring for patients with respiratory illnesses. They should also be worn when it is likely that contact with blood or other body fluids may occur. Sometimes special masks called respirators are used. The fit of these masks must be tested for each employee before use. The next learning objective has more information about respirators. All masks should fully cover the nose and mouth and prevent fluid penetration. Masks should fit snugly over the nose and mouth.

When worn during care of a patient with a respiratory illness, masks can only be worn once before they need to be discarded. Masks that become wet or soiled must be changed immediately without touching the outside of the soiled mask. PCTs must always change their masks when moving between patients; the same mask should not be worn from one patient to another.

Although wearing a mask or respirator for source control (to prevent the possible spread) of COVID-19 is no longer required, some health-care workers may choose to do so. In this case, the same mask or respirator may be used for a full shift. It should be changed, however, if it becomes wet, soiled, or difficult to breathe through.

Goggles are worn with a mask and are used whenever it is likely that blood or other body fluids may be splashed or sprayed into the eye area or into the eyes. Eyeglasses alone do not provide proper eye protection. Goggles should fit snugly over and around the eyes or eyeglasses.

Putting on (donning) a mask and goggles

1. Wash your hands.
2. For a respirator, hold the mask in your cupped hand with the top end at your fingertips.

   For other masks, pick up the mask by the top strap, top strings, or ear loops. Do not touch the mask where it touches your face.
3. If using a respirator, place the mask over your nose and mouth. Pull the top elastic strap over your head and place it on the crown of your head. Pull the bottom strap over your head and place it on the base of your neck. Do not crisscross the straps.

   If the mask has strings, tie the top strings first on the crown of your head, then the bottom strings on the base of your neck. If the mask has loops, hook them securely around your ears. Do not wear a mask hanging from only the bottom strap or ties.
4. Pinch the metal strip at the top of the mask (if part of the mask) tightly around your nose so that it feels snug (Fig. 5-14). Fit the mask snugly around your face and below the chin. If using a respirator, always perform a user seal check according to facility training.

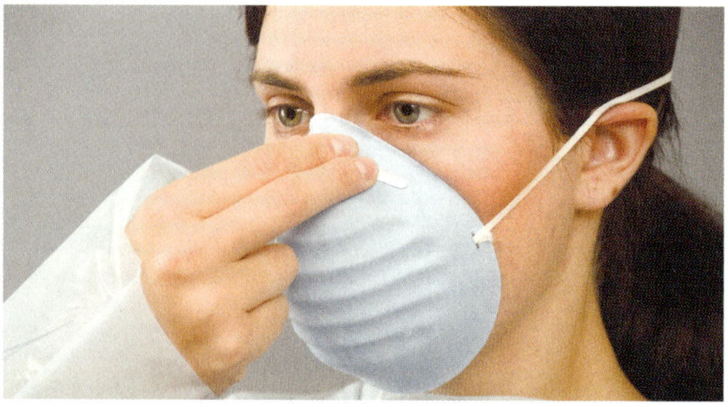

Fig. 5-14. *Adjust the metal strip until the mask fits snugly around your nose.*

5. Put the goggles on over your eyes or eyeglasses. Use the headband or earpieces to secure them to your head. Make sure they fit snugly.
6. Put on your gloves after putting on the mask and goggles.

Face Shields

Face shields may be worn when blood or body fluids may be splashed or sprayed into the eyes or eye area. A face shield can be substituted for a mask or goggles, or it can be worn with a mask. The face shield should cover the forehead, go below the chin, and wrap around the sides of the face. The headband secures it to the head.

Gloves

Nonsterile gloves are used for basic care. They are available in different sizes and may be made of nitrile, vinyl, or latex. However, due to allergy issues, some facilities have banned the use of latex gloves. In addition, in 2017 the US Food & Drug Administration (FDA, fda.gov) banned the use of all powdered patient examination gloves. This is due to the powder posing numerous risks to patients and workers.

Gloves should fit the hands comfortably and should not be too loose or too tight. Facilities have specific policies for when to wear gloves. PCTs must learn and follow these rules. Gloves must always be worn for the following tasks:

- Any time the healthcare worker might come into contact with blood or any body fluid, secretions or excretions, open wounds, or mucous membranes
- When performing or helping with mouth care or care of any mucous membrane
- When performing or helping with **perineal care** (care of the genital and anal area)
- When performing care on **nonintact skin**—skin that is broken by abrasions, cuts, rashes, acne, pimples, lesions, surgical incisions, or boils
- When the healthcare worker has open sores or cuts on her hands
- When shaving a patient
- When disposing of soiled bed linens, gowns, dressings, and pads
- When touching surfaces or equipment that is either visibly contaminated or may be contaminated

Disposable gloves can be worn only once; they cannot be washed or reused. Gloves should be changed immediately if they become wet, worn, soiled, or torn. Gloves should also be changed before contact with mucous membranes or broken skin. After removing gloves, the PCT should wash his hands before donning new gloves. Nonintact areas on the hands should be covered with bandages or gauze before putting on gloves.

Putting on (donning) gloves

1. Wash your hands.
2. If you are right-handed, slide one glove on your left hand (reverse if left-handed).
3. Using your gloved hand, slide the other hand into the second glove.
4. Interlace your fingers to smooth out folds and create a comfortable fit.
5. Carefully look for tears, holes, cracks, or discolored spots. Replace the glove if needed.
6. Adjust the gloves until they are pulled up over your wrist and fit correctly. If wearing a gown, pull the cuffs of the gloves over the sleeves of the gown (Fig. 5-15).

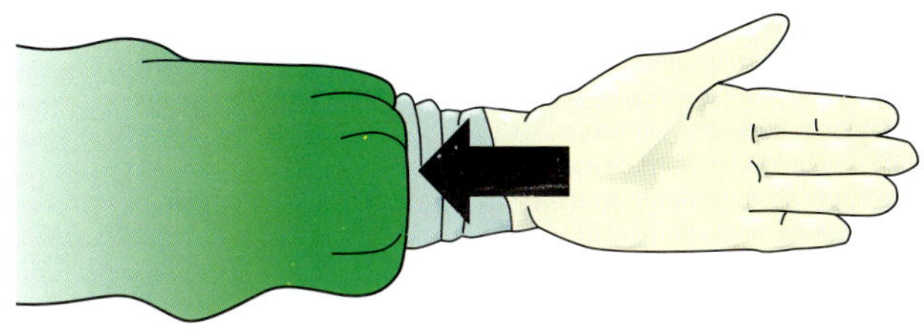

Fig. 5-15. *Adjust gloves until they are pulled up over the sleeves of the gown.*

The procedure for donning sterile gloves is located in Chapter 10.

Gloves should be removed, or doffed, promptly after use, and the PCT should wash his hands directly after removing gloves. He should be careful not to contaminate his skin or clothing when removing gloves. Gloves are worn to protect the skin from becoming contaminated. After giving care, gloves are contaminated. If a PCT opens a door with the gloved hand, the doorknob becomes contaminated. Later, anyone who opens the door with an ungloved hand will be touching a contaminated surface. Before touching surfaces or leaving patients' rooms, the PCT must remove gloves and wash his hands. Afterward, new gloves can be donned if necessary.

Removing (doffing) gloves

1. Touch only the outside of one glove. With one gloved hand, grasp the other glove at the palm and pull the glove off (Fig. 5-16).
2. With the fingertips of your gloved hand, hold the glove you just removed. With your ungloved hand, slip 2 fingers underneath the cuff of the remaining glove at the wrist. Do not touch any part of the outside of the glove (Fig. 5-17).

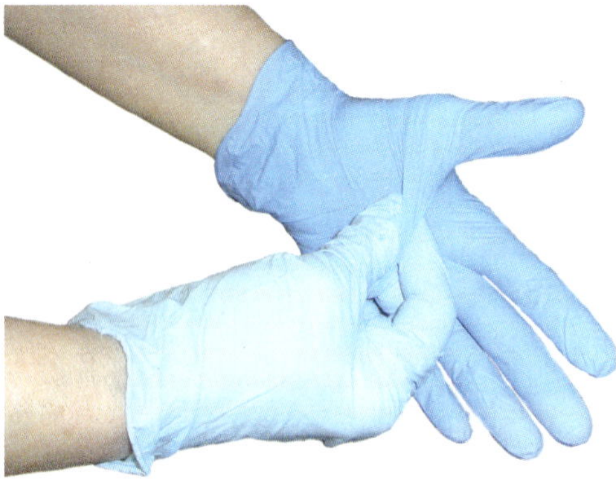

Fig. 5-16. *Grasp the glove at the palm and pull it off.*

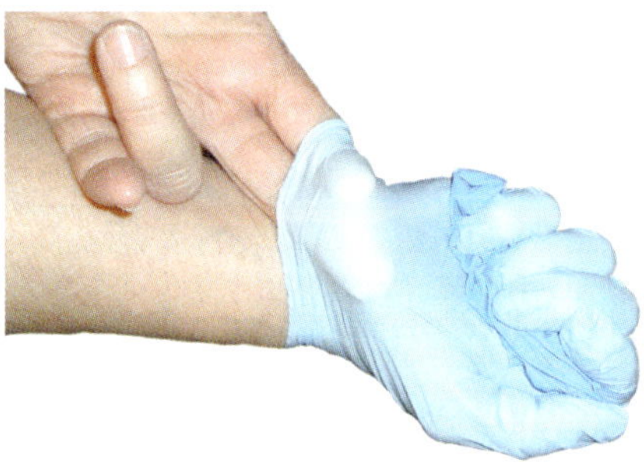

Fig. 5-17. *Reach inside the glove at the wrist, without touching any part of the outside of the glove.*

3. Pull down, turning this glove inside out and over the first glove as you remove it.
4. You should now be holding one glove from its clean inner side and the other glove should be inside it.
5. Drop both gloves into the proper container without contaminating yourself.
6. Wash your hands.

The PCT's employer will provide personal protective equipment as needed. PPE will be readily available and accessible in a variety of sizes. It is the PCT's responsibility to know where it is kept and how to use it. A specific order must be followed when donning and doffing PPE.

Donning a full set of PPE

1. Wash your hands.
2. Put on the gown.
3. Put on the mask or respirator.
4. Put on the goggles or face shield.
5. Put on gloves.

Doffing a full set of PPE

All personal protective equipment, except a respirator (if worn), must be removed before exiting the patient's room. A respirator is removed after leaving the room and closing the door.

1. Remove and discard your gloves.
2. Remove and discard the goggles or face shield.
3. Remove and discard the gown.
4. Remove and discard the mask.
5. Wash your hands. Washing hands is always the final step after removing and discarding PPE.

OSHA and PPE

OSHA states that it is the employer's responsibility to instruct the staff on how to properly don PPE, how to wear PPE effectively, and how to safely doff PPE. This instruction needs to be given before the employee is in a situation where PPE is indicated, and as an annual review.

6. Explain Transmission-Based Precautions

The CDC outlines a second level of precautions beyond Standard Precautions. These guidelines are used for persons who are infected or may be infected with certain infectious diseases. These precautions are called **Transmission-Based Precautions**. When ordered, these precautions are used in addition to Standard Precautions. These precautions will always be listed in the patient's care plan and on the PCT's assignment sheet. Following these precautions promotes the PCT's safety, as well as the safety of others.

There are 3 categories of Transmission-Based Precautions: Airborne Precautions, Droplet

Precautions, and Contact Precautions. The category used depends on what type of pathogen or disease the person has or may have and how it spreads. They may also be used in combination for diseases that have multiple routes of transmission. Conditions that require Transmission-Based Precautions in addition to Standard Precautions include the following:

- *Clostridioides difficile (C. diff or C. difficile)*
- Rotavirus (a virus that causes diarrhea and vomiting)
- Scabies (a skin disease that causes itching)
- Lice
- Influenza (during an outbreak)
- COVID-19
- **Multidrug-resistant organisms** (**MDROs**) are microorganisms, mostly bacteria, that are resistant to one or more antimicrobial agents that are commonly used for treatment. An **antimicrobial** agent destroys, resists, or prevents the development of pathogens. Two common types of MDROs are methicillin-resistant *Staphylococcus aureus* (MRSA) and vancomycin-resistant *Enterococcus* (VRE).

Airborne Precautions

Airborne Precautions prevent the spread of pathogens that can be transmitted through the air after being expelled (Fig. 5-18). The pathogens are so small they are able to remain floating in the air for some time. They are carried by moisture, air currents, and dust. An example of an airborne disease is tuberculosis. Precautions include wearing a special mask, such as an N95 respirator, to avoid being infected. More information on tuberculosis may be found in Chapter 16.

Droplet Precautions

Droplet Precautions are used for diseases that are spread by droplets in the air. Droplets normally do not travel more than 6 feet. Talking, coughing, sneezing, laughing, singing, or suctioning can spread droplets (Fig. 5-19). An example of a droplet disease is influenza (flu).

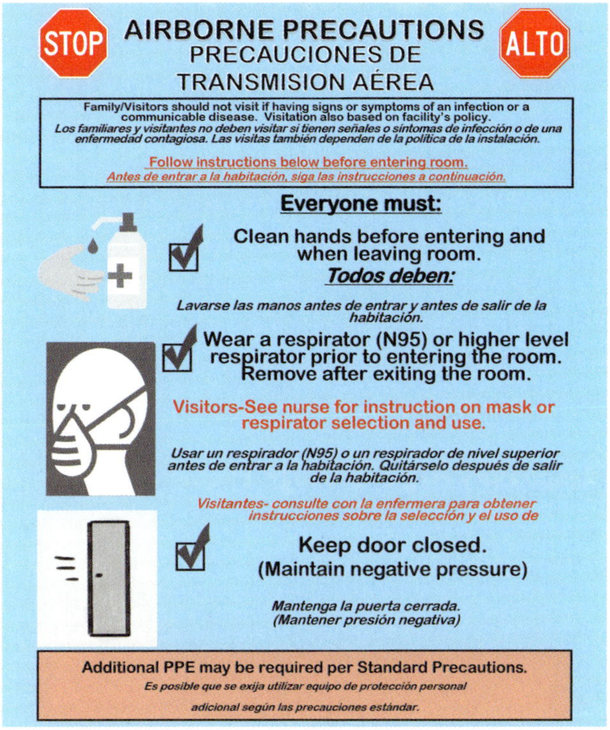

Fig. 5-18. *Airborne Precautions are used for diseases that can be transmitted through the air.* (IMAGE COURTESY OF THE NORTH CAROLINA STATEWIDE PROGRAM FOR INFECTION CONTROL AND EPIDEMIOLOGY [SPICE], UNC, CHAPEL HILL, SPICE.UNC.EDU)

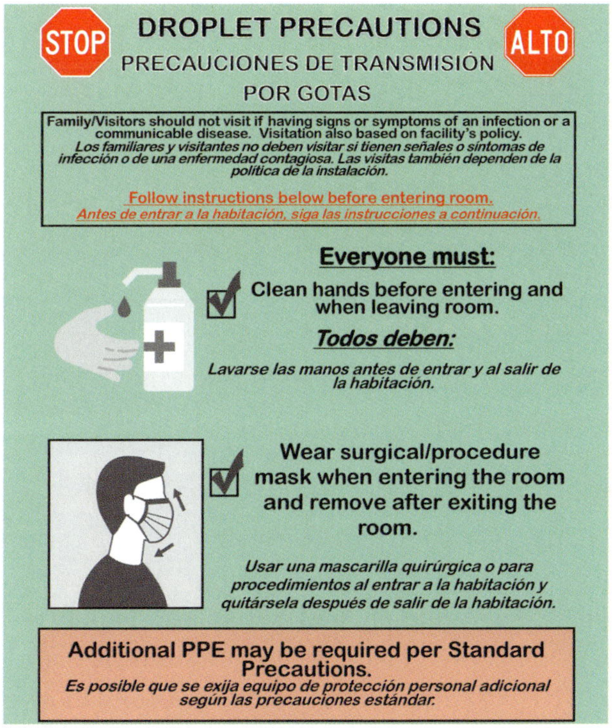

Fig. 5-19. *Droplet Precautions are followed when the disease-causing microorganism does not remain in the air.* (IMAGE COURTESY OF THE NORTH CAROLINA STATEWIDE PROGRAM FOR INFECTION CONTROL AND EPIDEMIOLOGY [SPICE], UNC, CHAPEL HILL, SPICE.UNC.EDU)

Droplet Precautions include wearing a face mask when providing care and restricting visits from uninfected people. In addition, PCTs should cover their noses and mouths with a tissue when they sneeze or cough and ask others to do the same. Used tissues should be disposed of in the nearest waste container. Used tissues should not be placed in a pocket for later use. If a tissue is not available, PCTs should cough or sneeze into their upper sleeve or elbow, not their hands. They should wash their hands immediately afterward. Patients should wear masks when being moved from room to room.

Respiratory Hygiene/Cough Etiquette

The CDC has set forth special infection prevention measures to prevent the transmission of all respiratory infections in healthcare settings. They are a part of Standard Precautions and include the following:

- Covering the nose and mouth with a tissue when coughing or sneezing
- Disposing of used tissues in the nearest waste container after use
- Performing hand hygiene (washing hands with soap and water, using an alcohol-based hand rub or an antiseptic handwash) after contact with respiratory secretions and contaminated objects
- Offering masks to people who are coughing
- Encouraging people who are coughing to sit at least 3 feet away from others in common waiting areas

Contact Precautions

Contact Precautions are used when the patient may spread an infection by direct contact with a person or object. The infection can be spread by touching a contaminated area on the patient's body or her blood or body fluids (Fig. 5-20). It may also be spread by touching contaminated items, linen, equipment, or supplies. Conjunctivitis (pink eye), rotavirus, and *Clostridioides difficile* (*C. diff*) infection are examples of situations that require Contact Precautions. *Clostridioides difficile* is discussed later in the chapter.

Contact Precautions include wearing gloves and a gown and patient isolation. To **isolate** means to keep something separate, or by itself. Contact Precautions require washing hands with soap and not touching infected surfaces with ungloved hands or uninfected surfaces with contaminated gloves.

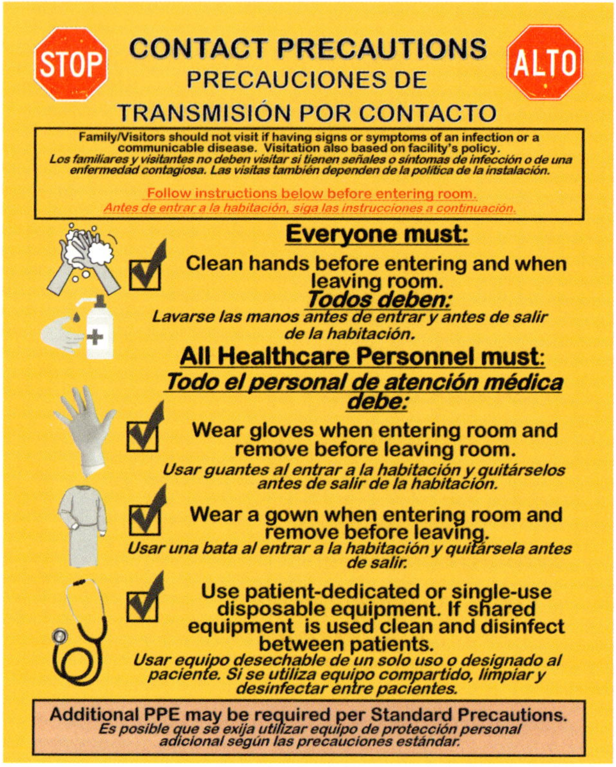
STOP
CONTACT PRECAUTIONS
PRECAUCIONES DE TRANSMISIÓN POR CONTACTO
ALTO
Family/Visitors should not visit if having signs or symptoms of an infection or a communicable disease. Visitation also based on facility's policy.
Los familiares y visitantes no deben visitar si tienen señales o síntomas de infección o de una enfermedad contagiosa. Las visitas también dependen de la política de la instalación.
Follow instructions below before entering room.
Antes de entrar a la habitación, siga las instrucciones a continuación.
Everyone must:
Clean hands before entering and when leaving room.
Todos deben:
Lavarse las manos antes de entrar y antes de salir de la habitación.
All Healthcare Personnel must:
Todo el personal de atención médica debe:
Wear gloves when entering room and remove before leaving room.
Usar guantes al entrar a la habitación y quitárselos antes de salir de la habitación.
Wear a gown when entering room and remove before leaving.
Usar una bata al entrar a la habitación y quitársela antes de salir.
Use patient-dedicated or single-use disposable equipment. If shared equipment is used clean and disinfect between patients.
Usar equipo desechable de un solo uso o designado al paciente. Si se utiliza equipo compartido, limpiar y desinfectar entre pacientes.
Additional PPE may be required per Standard Precautions.
Es posible que se exija utilizar equipo de protección personal adicional según las precauciones estándar.

Fig. 5-20. *Contact Precautions are followed when a person is at risk of transmitting a microorganism by touching an object or person.* (IMAGE COURTESY OF THE NORTH CAROLINA STATEWIDE PROGRAM FOR INFECTION CONTROL AND EPIDEMIOLOGY [SPICE], UNC, CHAPEL HILL, SPICE.UNC.EDU)

Epidemic, Pandemic, and Endemic

An *epidemic* is a disease outbreak that affects a large number of people within a specific geographical area. A *pandemic* is a global outbreak of a disease; it affects a large number of people in many countries. For example, COVID-19 was declared a pandemic in March 2020 by the World Health Organization. A disease outbreak becomes *endemic* when it is always present, but is generally limited to a specific area. An endemic disease has become more manageable and spreads at an expected level. There may be specific, additional infection prevention measures related to an epidemic or pandemic that must be followed. PCTs will be informed of these measures and trained as needed.

Staff often refer to patients who need Transmission-Based Precautions as being "in isolation." A sign should be on the door indicating the type of precaution in place and alerting people to the safety measures required. Other guidelines for PCTs to follow include the following:

Guidelines: Isolation

- **G** When they are indicated, Transmission-Based Precautions are always used **in addition** to Standard Precautions.
- **G** PCTs may be assigned to set up an isolation room. Some facilities have a special room where isolation supplies are kept. They may have carts set up with all of the necessary supplies. The PCT takes the cart to the assigned room and places it in the ordered location. Isolation supplies consist of gloves, masks, gowns or aprons, and, if indicated, goggles, face shields, respirators, or other forms of specialized personal protective equipment (PPE).
- **G** You will be told the proper PPE to wear for care of each patient in isolation. Make sure to put on PPE properly and remove it safely. Remove PPE and place it in the appropriate container before exiting a patient's room. PPE cannot be worn outside the patient's room, except for a respirator, which is removed after leaving the room and closing the door. Perform hand hygiene following the removal of PPE and again after exiting the patient's room. In addition to handwashing areas within the patient's room, there may be an alcohol-based hand sanitizer dispenser on the wall inside the room as you exit the door.
- **G** Do not share equipment between patients. Use disposable supplies that can be discarded after use whenever possible. Use dedicated equipment (only for use by one patient) when disposable is not an option. For example, a patient in isolation has her own (dedicated) blood pressure cuff and stethoscope. When using disposable supplies, discard them in the patient's room before leaving. Be careful not to contaminate reusable equipment by setting it on furniture or counters in the patient's room. When the patient is discharged or no longer needs the additional precautions, properly discard dedicated equipment if required. If the dedicated equipment is to be used for other patients, it should be cleaned and disinfected.
- **G** Wear the proper PPE, if indicated, if you are assigned to serve food and drink to patients in isolation. Do not leave uneaten food uncovered in the patient's room. When the meal is completed, remove the meal tray and take it to the designated area, or put it back on the food cart. When the food carts are returned to the kitchen, all soiled trays will be handled with gloves by the dietary staff, and the tray and dinnerware will be cleaned and sanitized.
- **G** Follow Standard Precautions when dealing with body waste removal. Wear gloves when touching or handling waste. Wear gowns and goggles when indicated. The waste must be disposed of in such a manner as to minimize splashing and spraying.
- **G** If required to take a specimen from a patient in isolation, wear the proper PPE. Collect the specimen and place it in the appropriate container without the outside of the container coming into contact with the specimen. Properly remove your PPE and dispose of it in the room. Perform hand hygiene before leaving the room and follow facility procedures for delivering the specimen for testing.
- **G** Patients need to feel that their circumstances and feelings are appreciated and understood by members of the care team without criticism or judgment. Listen to what patients are telling you and allow time to talk with patients about concerns. Reassure patients. Explain why these steps are being taken. Relay any requests outside your scope of practice to the nurse.

Connected Care

Isolation

Patients' basic needs remain the same while in isolation. Basic human needs do not change, even though physical conditions may change. Do not avoid a patient in isolation. Do not rush through care tasks or make the patient feel that they should be avoided. Being professional, caring, and competent may help lessen a patient's worries or concerns and feelings about being isolated. If a PCT has questions about the care he is providing, he should talk to the charge nurse.

7. Define *bloodborne pathogens* and describe 2 major bloodborne diseases

Bloodborne pathogens are microorganisms found in human blood that can cause infection and disease in humans. They may also be found in certain other body fluids, draining wounds, and mucous membranes. These pathogens are transmitted by infected blood entering the bloodstream, or if infected semen or vaginal secretions contact mucous membranes. Having sexual contact with someone carrying a bloodborne disease can also transmit the disease. Sexual contact includes sexual intercourse (vaginal and anal), contact of the mouth with the genitals or anus, and contact of the hands with the genital area. Sharing infected drug needles is another way to spread bloodborne diseases. Infected pregnant women may transmit bloodborne diseases to their babies in the womb or at birth.

In the healthcare setting, contact with infected blood or other body fluids is the most common way to be infected with a bloodborne disease. Infections can be spread through contact with contaminated blood or other body fluids, needles or other sharp objects, or contaminated supplies or equipment. Standard Precautions, handwashing, isolation, and using PPE are all methods of preventing transmission of bloodborne diseases. Employers are required by law to help prevent exposure to bloodborne pathogens. Following Standard Precautions and other procedures help protect healthcare workers from bloodborne diseases.

Bloodborne diseases cannot be spread by casual contact. PCTs can safely touch and spend time with patients who have a bloodborne disease (Fig. 5-21). These patients need the same thoughtful, personal attention given to all patients. PCTs need to follow Standard Precautions, but should never isolate patients emotionally because they have a bloodborne disease.

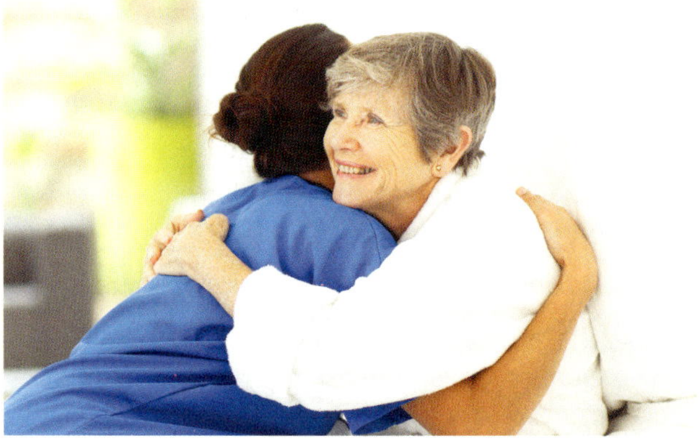

Fig. 5-21. *Hugs and touches cannot spread a bloodborne disease.*

Two major bloodborne diseases in the United States are acquired immunodeficiency syndrome (AIDS) and the viral hepatitis family. **HIV** stands for **human immunodeficiency virus**, and it is the virus that can cause AIDS. Over time, HIV weakens the immune system so that the body cannot effectively fight infections. The final stage of HIV infection is AIDS. People with AIDS lose all ability to fight infection and can die from illnesses that a healthy immune system could handle. Chapter 21 contains more information about HIV and AIDS.

Hepatitis is inflammation of the liver caused by certain viruses and other factors, such as alcohol abuse, some medications, and trauma. Liver function can be permanently damaged by hepatitis. Several different viruses can cause hepatitis. The most common types of hepatitis are

A, B, and C. Hepatitis B and C are bloodborne diseases that can cause death. Many more people have hepatitis B than HIV. In the United States today, the risk of getting hepatitis is greater than the risk of acquiring HIV.

The virus causing hepatitis A (HAV) is spread through fecal-oral contamination, which means through food or water contaminated by stool from an infected person.

Hepatitis B (HBV) is a bloodborne disease. It is spread through sexual contact, by sharing infected needles, and from a mother to her baby during delivery. It can be spread through improperly sterilized needles used for tattoos and piercings and through grooming supplies, such as razors, nail clippers, and toothbrushes. It is also spread by exposure at work from accidental contact with infected needles or other sharps or from splashing blood.

The hepatitis B virus can survive outside the body for at least 7 days and can still cause infection in others during that time. HBV may cause few symptoms or may become a severe infection. At its most severe, HBV can cause liver damage, liver cancer, and death.

HBV is a serious threat to healthcare workers. Employers must offer PCTs a free vaccine to protect them from hepatitis B. The hepatitis B vaccine is usually given as a series of 3 shots. Prevention is the best option for dealing with this disease, and employees should take the vaccine when it is offered.

Hepatitis C (HCV) is also transmitted through blood or other body fluids. Hepatitis C can lead to cirrhosis and liver cancer; it can even cause death. There is no vaccine for hepatitis C. The virus can survive, and remain potentially infectious, for as long as 6 weeks on surfaces.

Less common types of hepatitis in the United States are hepatitis D (HDV) and hepatitis E (HEV). Hepatitis D is transmitted by blood. It is only found in people who carry the hepatitis B virus. Hepatitis E (HEV) is transmitted by the fecal-oral route, usually through contaminated water. Although HEV is rare in the United States, it is more common in many other parts of the world. There is no vaccine for hepatitis D or hepatitis E.

8. Explain OSHA's Bloodborne Pathogens Standard and the Needlestick Safety and Prevention Act

OSHA sets standards that must be followed in healthcare facilities. One of these is the **Bloodborne Pathogens Standard**. This law requires that healthcare facilities protect employees from bloodborne health hazards. By law, employers must follow these rules to reduce or eliminate the risk of exposure to infectious diseases. The standard also guides employers and employees through the steps to follow if exposed to infectious material. Significant exposures include the following:

- Exposure by injection; a needle stick
- Mucous membrane contact
- A cut from an object containing a potentially infectious body fluid (includes human bites)
- Having nonintact skin (OSHA includes acne in this category)

Due to the growing number of sharps-related injuries in care facilities, the Needlestick Safety and Prevention Act was passed in 2000. It is an amendment to the Bloodborne Pathogens Standard. Research has shown that many of these injuries could be prevented by using safer devices. **Engineering controls** are features of medical devices that make their use less hazardous. Needles that can be pulled back into a cover or that have a cover that swings into place are examples (Fig. 5-22). The Needlestick Safety and Prevention Act requires the use of safer devices like these.

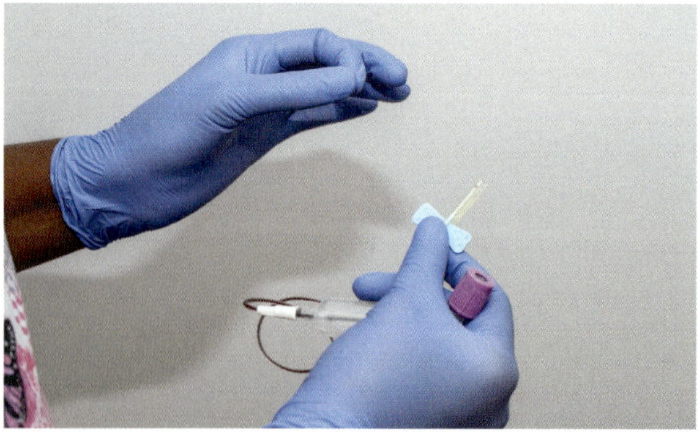

Fig. 5-22. *Engineering controls like needle sheaths/covers can prevent accidental exposure to bloodborne pathogens.*

Guidelines employers must follow according to the Bloodborne Pathogens Standard and Needlestick Safety and Prevention Act include the following:

- Employers must have a written **exposure control plan** designed to eliminate or reduce employee exposure to infectious material. This plan identifies, step by step, what to do if an employee is exposed to infectious material (for example, if a PCT is stuck by a needle). This includes medical treatment and plans to prevent any similar exposures. It also includes specific work practices that must be followed. This plan must be accessible to all employees, and they must receive training on the plan.
- Employers must give all employees, patients, and visitors to the facility proper PPE to wear when needed, at no cost. Employers must make sure PPE is available in the appropriate sizes and is readily accessible.
- Employers must make biohazard containers available for disposal of sharps and other infectious waste. Sharps containers must be puncture resistant, labeled, or color coded, and leakproof. Infectious waste containers must be emptied often to prevent overfilling.
- Employers must provide a free hepatitis B vaccine to all employees after hire.
- Warning labels must be affixed to waste containers, refrigerators, and freezers that contain blood or any other potentially infectious material.
- Employers must keep a log of injuries from contaminated sharps. The information recorded must protect the confidentiality of the injured employee. Employers are also required to select safer needle devices and to involve employees in choosing these devices.
- Employers must provide in-service training on bloodborne pathogens and updates on any new safety standards at the time of hire and annually to all employees.
- When an employee is exposed to blood or other potentially infectious material, an incident report or a special exposure report form must be completed. OSHA provides incident report forms and logs for tracking injuries or exposures in the workplace. Tests and follow-up care may be needed. The employer will take steps to prevent the employee from becoming sick. Steps will also be taken to help keep similar incidents from occurring again. PCTs must report any potential exposures immediately. Doing this helps protect their health and that of others. OSHA's website, osha.gov, has more information.

9. List guidelines for handling linens and equipment

In health care, an object is called **clean** if it has not been contaminated with pathogens. An object that is **dirty** has been contaminated with pathogens. Measures like disinfection and sterilization decrease the spread of pathogens that could cause disease.

Disinfection is a process that destroys most, but not all, pathogens. It reduces the pathogen count to a level that is considered not infectious. Disinfection is carried out with pasteurization or chemical germicides. In order for disinfectants to work properly, surfaces must remain wet for the entire time recommended (called *contact time*). Most hospital disinfectants have a contact time of 10 minutes, although it may be shorter. Examples of items that are usually disinfected are reusable oxygen tanks, wall-mounted blood pressure devices, and any reusable patient care equipment.

Sterilization is a cleaning measure that destroys all microorganisms, including those that form spores. Spore-forming microorganisms are a special group of organisms that produce a protective covering that is difficult to penetrate. Sterilization is part of surgical asepsis and is accomplished through the use of special machines and devices. An autoclave is a machine that sterilizes objects by using hot steam under pressure. Liquid or gas chemicals and dry heat may also be used to sterilize objects. Items that need to be sterilized are ones, such as surgical instruments, that go directly into the bloodstream or into other normally sterile areas of the body. Chapter 10 has more information about disinfection and sterilization.

Facilities have special rooms or areas for clean and dirty items, such as equipment, linen, and supplies. There are separate rooms for supplies that are considered clean and for supplies that are considered dirty or contaminated (Fig. 5-23). PCTs will be told where these rooms are located and what types of equipment and supplies are found in each room. PCTs should wash their hands before entering clean rooms and before leaving dirty rooms. This helps prevent the spread of pathogens.

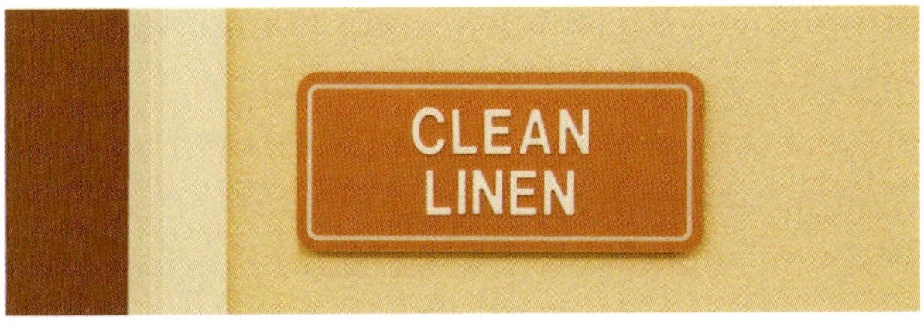

Fig. 5-23. *There are separate rooms in facilities for clean and dirty equipment, linen, and supplies.*

Guidelines: Handling Equipment, Linen, and Clothing

G Handle all equipment in a way that prevents
- Skin/mucous membrane contact
- Contamination of your clothing
- Transfer of disease to other patients or areas

G Do not use reusable equipment again until it has been properly cleaned and reprocessed.

G Dispose of all single-use, or disposable, equipment properly. **Disposable** equipment is designed to be discarded after a single use. Disposable razors are examples of disposable equipment.

G Follow facility policy to clean and disinfect
- All environmental surfaces
- Beds, bed rails, and all bedside equipment
- All frequently touched surfaces (such as doorknobs, call lights, and handles on dressers and tables)

G Handle, transport, and process soiled linens and clothing in a way that prevents
- Skin and mucous membrane exposure
- Contamination of clothing (Hold linen and clothing away from your uniform.)
- Transfer of disease to other patients and areas (Do not shake linen or clothes. Fold or roll linen so that the dirtiest area is inside; do not put soiled linen on floor.)

G Bag soiled linen at the point of origin.

G Sort soiled linen away from patient care areas.

G Use the linen bag required for your facility, which may be color coded. Place wet linen in leakproof bags.

More information about cleaning equipment and supplies is located in Chapter 7.

10. Discuss MRSA, VRE, CRE, and *C. difficile*

Multidrug-resistant organisms (MDROs) are microorganisms, mostly bacteria, that are resistant to one or more antimicrobial agents that are commonly used for treatment. There has been an increase in MDROs, and this is a serious problem. Hospital patients who have invasive medical devices (devices that are inserted into the body) are at high risk for infections with this type of pathogen. Two common types of MDROs are methicillin-resistant *Staphylococcus aureus,* commonly referred to as MRSA, and vancomycin-resistant *Enterococcus,* called VRE. A third type of MDRO, carbapenem-resistant Enterobacterales (CRE), is a growing problem in hospitals and other inpatient facilities.

Staphylococcus aureus is a common type of bacteria that can cause infection. Methicillin is a powerful antibiotic often used in healthcare facilities. **Methicillin-resistant *Staphylococcus aureus***, or **MRSA**, is a strain of this bacterium that has developed resistance to methicillin. This type of MRSA is also known as HA-MRSA, which stands for hospital-associated MRSA.

Community-associated methicillin-resistant *Staphylococcus aureus* (CA-MRSA) is a type of MRSA infection that occurs in people who have not recently been admitted to healthcare facilities and who have no past diagnosis of MRSA. Often CA-MRSA manifests as skin infections, such as boils or pimples. This type of infection is becoming more common.

MRSA is almost always spread by direct physical contact with infected people. This means if a person has MRSA on his skin, especially on his hands, and touches another person, he may spread MRSA. Spread also occurs through indirect contact by touching equipment or supplies (for example, towels, sheets, wound dressings, or clothes) contaminated by a person with MRSA. Symptoms of MRSA infection include drainage, fever, chills, and skin discoloration. PCTs can help prevent the spread of MRSA by practicing proper hygiene. Handwashing, using soap and warm water, is the single most important measure to control the spread of MRSA. PCTs must always follow Standard Precautions, along with Transmission-Based Precautions as ordered. Cuts and abrasions should be kept clean and covered with a proper dressing (e.g., bandage) until healed. Contact with other people's wounds or material that is contaminated from wounds should be avoided. Hospitals may have additional measures to prevent the spread of MRSA and other MDROs. Bathing patients, especially those in intensive care units, with an antiseptic agent called chlorhexidine is one way to try to reduce the spread of MDROs. PCTs may be assigned to assist with this or other measures, depending on facility policy.

Enterococci are bacteria that live in the digestive and genital tracts. Although they normally do not cause problems in healthy people, they can sometimes cause infection. Vancomycin is a powerful antibiotic used to treat infections caused by enterococci. If the enterococci become resistant to vancomycin, then it is called **vancomycin-resistant *Enterococcus***, or **VRE**.

VRE is spread through direct and indirect contact. Symptoms of VRE infection include fever, fatigue, chills, and drainage. VRE infections are often difficult to treat and may require the use of several medications. VRE infections can cause life-threatening infections in those with compromised immune systems—the very young, the very old, and the very ill.

Preventing VRE is much easier than trying to treat it. Proper hand hygiene can help prevent the spread of VRE. PCTs should wash their hands often and wear PPE as directed. PCTs must always follow Standard Precautions, along with Transmission-Based Precautions as ordered. Other measures, such as disinfection of the patient's room or items in the patient's room, may be part of facility policy or may be ordered for specific patients. PCTs must follow all assigned infection prevention and control measures carefully.

A growing number of healthcare-associated infections is caused by carbapenem-resistant Enterobacterales (CRE). Enterobacterales are bacteria that include *Escherichia coli* (*E. coli*), a type of bacteria that is part of the normal flora of the intestines, but which can also multiply and cause infection. Carbapenems are a type of very strong antibiotic. Because CREs are resistant to these powerful medications, CRE infection is very difficult to treat. If CRE infections enter a patient's blood, they can be deadly about 50% of the time. Although there are some antibiotics that can be used to treat CRE infection, prevention is very important. PCTs must wash hands often and follow Standard Precautions, along with Transmission-Based Precautions as ordered. This affects the safety of specific patients, as well as the entire facility. It is very dangerous for MDROs to spread in an inpatient setting.

Clostridioides difficile (formerly known as *Clostridium difficile*) infection (CDI) is commonly known as *C. diff* or *C. difficile*. It is not an MDRO, but using antibiotics too often or using them when they are not needed greatly increases the risk of infection. *C. difficile* is a spore-forming bacterium which can be part of the normal intestinal flora. When the normal intestinal flora is altered, *C. difficile* can flourish in the intestinal tract and can cause infection. It produces a toxin that causes watery diarrhea. Enemas, nasogastric tube insertion, and GI tract surgery increase a person's risk of developing the infection. The elderly are at a higher risk of getting *C. difficile* infection. The overuse of antibiotics may alter the normal intestinal flora and increase the risk of developing *C. difficile*. It can also cause colitis, a more serious intestinal condition.

When released in the environment, *C. difficile* can form a spore that makes it difficult to kill. This makes it especially dangerous in healthcare facilities. *C. difficile* spores can be carried on the hands of people who have direct contact with infected patients or with environmental surfaces (floors, bedpans, toilets, etc.) contaminated with *C. difficile*. Touching an object contaminated with *C. difficile* can transmit *C. difficile*. Alcohol-based hand sanitizer is not considered effective on *C. difficile*. Soap and water must be used each time hand hygiene is performed.

Symptoms of *C. difficile* include frequent, foul-smelling, watery stools. Other symptoms are fever, diarrhea that contains blood and mucus, nausea, lack of appetite, and abdominal cramps. Proper handwashing with soap and water is vital in preventing the spread of the infection. Handling contaminated wastes properly can help prevent the spread of the infection. Cleaning surfaces with an appropriate disinfectant, such as a bleach solution, can also reduce transmission. Limiting the use of antibiotics helps lower the risk of developing *C. difficile* infection.

11. List employer and employee responsibilities for infection prevention

Several state and federal government agencies have guidelines and laws concerning infection prevention. OSHA requires employers to provide for the safety of their employees through rules and suggested guidelines. The CDC issues guidelines for healthcare workers to follow on the job. Some states have additional requirements. Facilities consider these rules very carefully when writing their policies and procedures. It is important that PCTs learn these policies and procedures and follow them. They exist to protect all staff members and patients. Employers and employees both have key roles in infection prevention.

The **employer's** responsibilities for infection prevention include the following:

- Establish infection prevention procedures and an exposure control plan to protect workers
- Provide continuing in-service education on infection prevention and control, including education on bloodborne and airborne pathogens and updates on any new safety standards
- Have written procedures to follow should an exposure occur, including medical treatment and plans to prevent similar exposures
- Provide personal protective equipment (PPE) for employees to use, and teach them when and how to properly use it
- Provide free hepatitis B vaccinations for all employees

The **employee's** responsibilities for infection prevention include the following:

- Follow Standard Precautions
- Follow all facility policies and procedures
- Follow patient care plans and assignments
- Use provided personal protective equipment as indicated or as appropriate
- Take advantage of the free hepatitis B vaccination
- Immediately report any exposure to infection or blood or other body fluids
- Participate in annual education programs covering the prevention of infection

Chapter Review

1. What does infection prevention mean?
2. Which link in the chain of infection is broken by wearing gloves, and why?
3. Under Standard Precautions, what substances are considered body fluids?
4. On whom should Standard Precautions be practiced?
5. What is the single most important thing a PCT can do to prevent the spread of disease?
6. What is hand hygiene?
7. For how long should a PCT use friction when washing her hands?
8. How many times can disposable gloves be worn?
9. In what order should personal protective equipment (PPE) be put on and removed?
10. Define *sterilization*. Define *disinfection*.
11. How should soiled linen be carried?
12. When blood or other body fluids are spilled, what should the PCT do first, before starting to clean the spill?
13. What are Transmission-Based Precautions?
14. How should the mouth and nose be covered when a person coughs or sneezes?
15. How are bloodborne diseases transmitted? What is the most common way to be infected with a bloodborne disease in a healthcare setting?
16. How is hepatitis B (HBV) contracted?
17. Describe an exposure control plan.
18. What are multidrug-resistant organisms (MDROs)?
19. What is one of the best ways to prevent the spread of MDROs and other hospital-associated infections?
20. What is an employer required to do with regard to the hepatitis B vaccination?

6 Emergency Care, Safety, and Disaster Response

1. Demonstrate how to recognize and respond to medical emergencies

Medical emergencies may be the result of accidents or sudden illnesses. This chapter discusses how to respond appropriately to medical emergencies. Heart attacks, strokes, diabetic emergencies, choking, automobile accidents, and gunshot wounds are all medical emergencies. Falls, burns, and cuts can also be emergencies. In an emergency situation, it is important for responders to remain calm, act quickly, and communicate clearly. The following steps illustrate the correct response to emergencies:

Assess the situation. The responder should try to determine what has happened. She must make sure she is not in danger and notice the time.

Assess the victim. The responder should ask the injured or ill person what has happened. If the person is unable to respond, he may be unconscious. Being **conscious** means being mentally alert and having awareness of surroundings, sensations, and thoughts. Tapping the person and asking if he is all right helps to determine if a person is conscious. The responder should speak loudly and use the person's name if she knows it. If there is no response, she should assume the person is unconscious and that an emergency situation exists. She should call for help right away or send someone else to call.

If a person is conscious and able to speak, then he is breathing and has a pulse. The responder should talk with the person about what happened. She should get the person's permission to touch him. Anyone who is unable to give consent for treatment, such as a child with no parent nearby or an unconscious or seriously injured person, may be treated with *implied consent*. The person should be checked for the following:

- Severe bleeding
- Changes in consciousness
- Irregular breathing
- Unusual color or feel to the skin
- Swollen places on the body
- Medical alert tags
- Pain

If any of these conditions exists, professional medical help may be needed. When a PCT is responding to an emergency, she should always get help before doing anything else. If the injured or ill person is conscious, he may be frightened. The responder should listen to the person and tell him what is being done to help him. A calm and confident response will help reassure him.

Hospitals and other healthcare facilities have policies and procedures to guide responses to emergencies that happen in the facility. Patients, visitors, or employees may experience medical emergencies. PCTs must know and follow the procedures for medical emergencies.

After an emergency is over, the PCT may be involved in documenting the emergency and completing an incident report. It is important to include as many details as possible and report only facts. For example, if the PCT thinks a patient had a heart attack, she should only document the signs she observed and the actions she took. Knowing the kind of information to document will help the PCT remember the important facts during the emergency. For instance, it is especially important to remember the time at which a patient became unconscious.

Emergency Response

Each facility's emergency response procedures may be different, but in most cases a **code team** is called to provide care. This team includes one or more doctors, nurses, and respiratory therapists. When a PCT encounters a medical emergency, they should follow facility policy for calling the code team. When the team is called, the type of emergency is usually indicated by a color. *Code blue* is used for cardiac arrest or other serious medical emergencies. Other codes are called for other emergencies (e.g., *code red* for a fire in the facility). PCTs should know the codes used at their facility.

2. Demonstrate knowledge of first aid procedures

Emergency situations can happen to anyone at any time. **First aid** is emergency care given immediately to an injured person by the first people to respond to an emergency. **Cardiopulmonary resuscitation** (**CPR**) refers to medical procedures used when a person's heart or lungs have stopped working. CPR is used until medical help arrives. Quick action is necessary. CPR must be started immediately to help prevent or lessen brain damage. Brain damage can occur within 4 to 6 minutes after the heart stops beating and breathing stops. The person can die within 10 minutes.

PCTs must be trained in CPR. Most hospitals only hire PCTs who have completed Basic Life Support (BLS) training from the American Heart Association (heart.org). BLS is a course specifically for people who work in healthcare facilities. In addition to CPR, it includes instruction about using an AED, working as part of a resuscitation team, and responding to airway obstruction (choking).

PCTs need to know their facility's policies on initiating CPR. Some facilities do not allow PCTs to begin CPR without the direction of a licensed healthcare professional. This is due, in part, to patients' advance directives. Some people have made the decision that they do not want CPR. The facility's emergency alert procedures should be followed immediately if an emergency occurs.

Guidelines: Performing CPR

- **G** Assess the situation and assess the victim for unconsciousness.
- **G** Call for help.
- **G** Check for signs of circulation (breathing and a pulse). Use the **carotid pulse** in the neck for adults and children (Fig. 6-1). Use the **brachial pulse** in infants (Fig. 6-2).

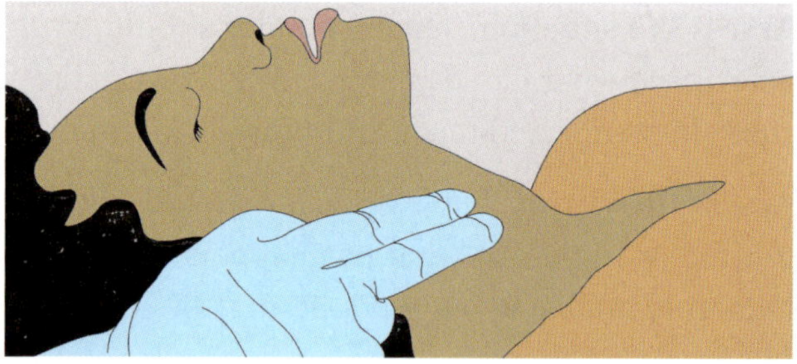

Fig. 6-1. *The carotid pulse is located in the neck.*

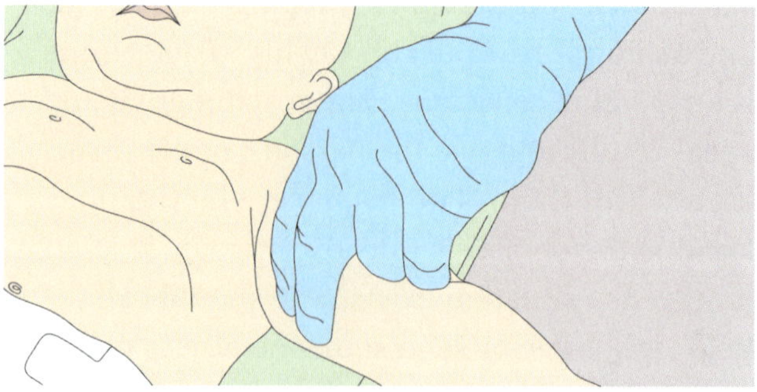

Fig. 6-2. *The brachial pulse is located in the upper arm.*

- If there is no breathing and no pulse, start CPR if you are trained to do so. Begin with 30 compressions. Check the airway and give 2 rescue breaths. Remember *CAB:* **c**ompressions, **a**irway, **b**reaths. Facility policy may require compression-only CPR until a barrier device (a form of PPE to protect healthcare workers from exposure to infection) can be used.
- Use an **automated external defibrillator (AED)** if available and if you are trained and allowed to use it. This is a device that can shock the heart and restore its normal rhythm if certain dangerous rhythms are present.
- Continue CPR until someone else takes over or the patient becomes conscious.
- Report and document the procedure properly.

The following information and procedures can help PCTs recognize and respond to medical emergencies. It is always very important, however, to first call for help. The PCT should not provide any care that she is not trained or allowed to provide.

Choking

When something is blocking the tube through which air enters the lungs, the person has an **obstructed airway**. When people are choking, they usually put their hands to their throats (Fig. 6-3). PCTs may encounter patients who are choking or seem to be choking. As long as the patient can speak, breathe, or cough, the PCT should only encourage her to cough as forcefully as possible to get the object out. The PCT should stay with the patient until she stops choking or can no longer speak, breathe, or cough. If a patient can no longer speak, breathe, or cough, the PCT should call for help immediately. The choking victim should not be left alone.

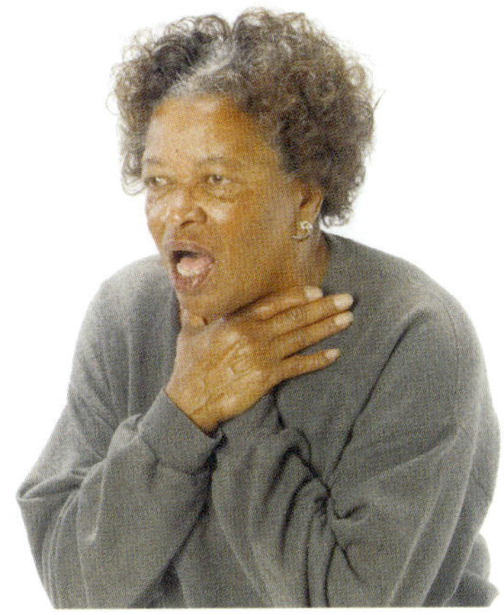

Fig. 6-3. *People who are choking usually put their hands to their throats.*

Abdominal thrusts are a method of attempting to remove an object from the airway of someone who is choking. These thrusts work to remove the blockage upward, out of the throat. The PCT should make sure the patient needs help before starting to give abdominal thrusts. The patient must show signs of a severely obstructed airway. These signs include poor air exchange; an increase in trouble breathing; silent coughing; pale, gray, bluish (cyanotic), or discolored skin; or an inability to speak, breathe, or cough. The PCT should ask, "Are you choking? I know what to do. Can I help you?" If the patient nods her head yes, she has a severe airway obstruction and needs immediate help. The PCT should begin giving abdominal thrusts. This procedure should never be performed on a person who is not choking. Abdominal thrusts risk injury to the ribs or internal organs.

Performing abdominal thrusts for the conscious person

1. Stand behind the person and bring your arms under her arms. Wrap your arms around the person's waist.
2. Make a fist with one hand. Place the thumb side of the fist against the person's abdomen, above the navel but below the breastbone (Fig. 6-4).

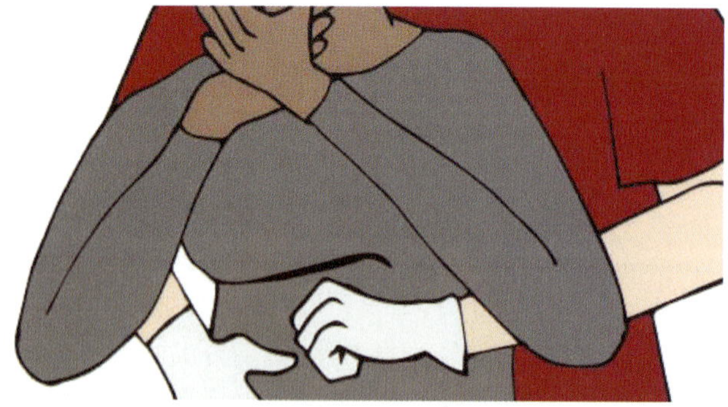

Fig. 6-4. *The flat, thumb side of the fist against the person's abdomen is the correct placement for abdominal thrusts.*

3. Grasp the fist with your other hand. Pull both hands toward you and up, quickly and forcefully.
4. Repeat until the object is pushed out or the person loses consciousness.
5. Report and document the incident properly.

If the patient becomes unconscious while choking, she should be helped to the floor gently so she is lying on her back on a hard surface with her face up.

The PCT should begin CPR for an unconscious person if trained and allowed to do so. The patient may have a completely blocked airway and needs professional medical help immediately. The PCT should make sure help is on the way and should stay with the patient until help arrives.

Shock

Shock occurs when organs and tissues in the body do not receive an adequate blood supply. Bleeding, heart attack, severe infection, and falling blood pressure can lead to shock. Shock can become worse when the person is frightened or in severe pain.

Shock is a dangerous, life-threatening situation. Signs of shock include pale, gray, bluish, or discolored skin; staring; increased pulse and respiration rates; low blood pressure; and extreme thirst. A PCT should always call for help if she suspects a patient is experiencing shock.

Responding to shock

1. Follow facility policy to call for help. Victims of shock should always receive medical care as soon as possible.
2. If you need to control bleeding, put on gloves first. The procedure for controlling bleeding is described later in the chapter.
3. Have the person lie down on her back. If the person is bleeding from the mouth or vomiting, place her on her left side. Elevate the legs about 8 to 12 inches unless the person has a head, neck, back, spinal, or abdominal injury; breathing difficulties; or fractures (Fig. 6-5). Elevating the legs allows blood to flow back to the brain (and other vital areas). Never elevate a body part if the person has a broken bone or if it causes pain.

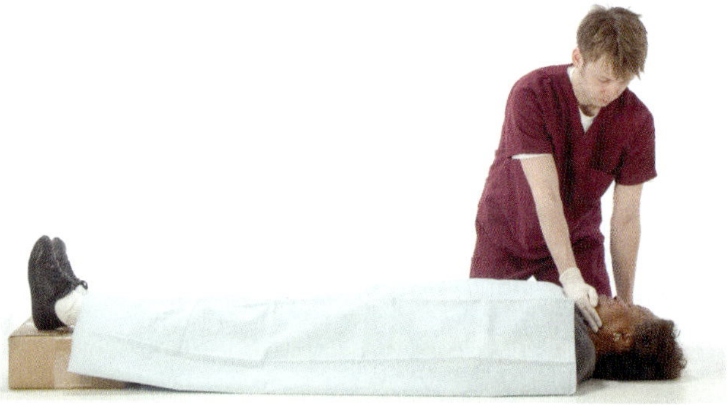

Fig. 6-5. *If a person is in shock, elevate the legs unless the person has head, neck, back, spinal, or abdominal injuries; breathing difficulties; or fractures.*

4. Check pulse and respirations if possible (Chapter 10). Begin CPR if breathing and pulse are absent and if you are trained and allowed to do so.
5. Keep the person as calm and comfortable as possible.
6. Maintain normal body temperature. If the weather is cold, place a blanket around the person. If the weather is hot, provide shade.

7. Do not give the person food or liquids.
8. Report and document the incident properly.

Myocardial Infarction or Heart Attack

Myocardial infarction (MI), or heart attack, occurs when the heart muscle itself does not receive enough oxygen because blood vessels are blocked. (Chapter 15 contains more information.) A myocardial infarction is an emergency that can result in serious heart damage or death. The following are signs and symptoms of MI:

- Sudden, severe pain, pressure, or squeezing in the chest, usually on the left side or in the center, behind the breastbone
- Pain or discomfort in other areas of the body, such as one or both arms, the back, neck, jaw, or stomach
- Indigestion or heartburn
- Nausea and vomiting
- Shortness of breath
- Dizziness
- Pale, gray, blue, or discolored skin or mucous membranes, indicating lack of oxygen
- Perspiration
- Cold and clammy skin
- Weak and irregular pulse rate
- Low blood pressure
- Anxiety and a sense of doom
- Denial of a heart problem

The pain of a heart attack is commonly described as a crushing, pressing, squeezing, stabbing, piercing pain, or "like someone is sitting on my chest." The pain may go down the inside of the left arm. A person may also feel it in the neck and/or in the jaw. The pain usually does not go away.

As with men, women may experience chest pain or discomfort. Women, though, can have heart attacks without chest pressure. Women are more likely to have shortness of breath, nausea, vomiting, light-headedness, fainting, dizziness, stomach pain, sweating, fatigue, and back, neck, or jaw pain. Some women's symptoms seem more flu-like, and women are more likely to deny that they are having a heart attack. A PCT must take immediate action if a patient experiences any of these symptoms.

Responding to a myocardial infarction

1. Follow facility policy to call for help.
2. Place the person in a comfortable position. Encourage him to rest, and reassure him that you will not leave him alone.
3. Loosen clothing around the person's neck as needed (Fig. 6-6).

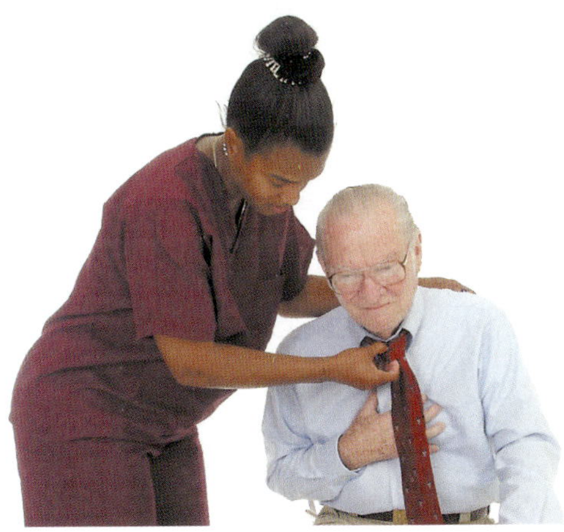

Fig. 6-6. *Loosen clothing around the person's neck if you suspect he is having an MI.*

4. Do not give the person food or liquids.
5. Monitor the person's breathing and pulse. If the person stops breathing and has no pulse, begin CPR if trained and allowed to do so.
6. Stay with the person until help arrives.
7. Report and document the incident properly.

Bleeding

Severe bleeding can cause death quickly and must be controlled.

Controlling bleeding

1. Follow facility policy to call for help.
2. Put on gloves. Take the time to do this. If the person is able, he can hold his bare hand over the wound until you can put on gloves.
3. Hold a thick sterile pad, clean cloth, or clean towel against the wound.
4. Press down hard directly on the bleeding wound until help arrives. Do not decrease pressure (Fig. 6-7). Put additional pads or cloths over the first pad if blood seeps through. Do not remove the first pads.

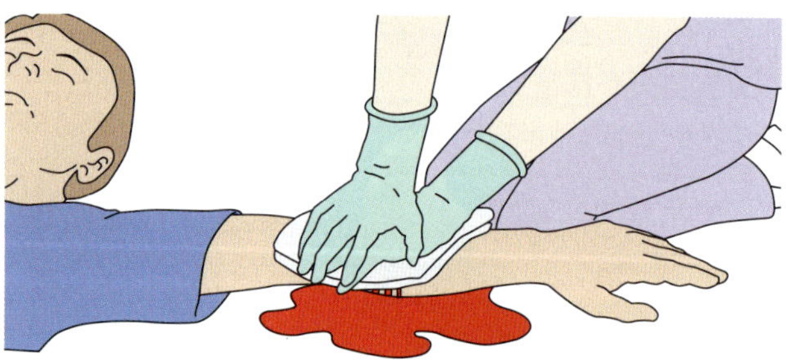

Fig. 6-7. *Press down hard directly on the bleeding wound; do not decrease pressure.*

5. If you can, raise the wound above the level of the heart to slow the bleeding. Prop up the limb if the wound is on an arm, leg, hand, or foot, and if there are no head, neck, back, spinal, or abdominal injuries; breathing difficulties; or fractures. Use towels or other absorbent material.
6. When bleeding is under control, secure the dressing to keep it in place. Check for symptoms of shock (pale skin, staring, increased pulse and respiration rates, low blood pressure, and extreme thirst). Stay with the person until help arrives.
7. Remove and discard your gloves and wash your hands thoroughly when finished.
8. Report and document the incident properly.

Poisoning

Signs and symptoms of poisoning vary widely. They depend on the substance that the person ate or drank. Poisoning may be suspected when a person vomits; has heavy, difficult breathing; is very drowsy; is confused; or has burns or red areas around the mouth. If a PCT suspects poisoning, he should follow facility policy to call for help.

Burns

Care of a burn depends on its depth, size, and location. There are 3 types of burns: first degree (superficial), second degree (partial thickness), and third degree (full thickness) (Fig. 6-8). First-degree burns involve just the outer layer of skin. The skin becomes discolored, painful, and swollen, but no blisters appear. Second-degree burns extend from the outer layer of skin to the next deeper layer of skin. The skin is discolored, painful, and swollen, and blisters appear. Third-degree burns involve all 3 layers of the skin and may extend to the bone. The skin is shiny and appears hard. It may look white, deep red, or charred black.

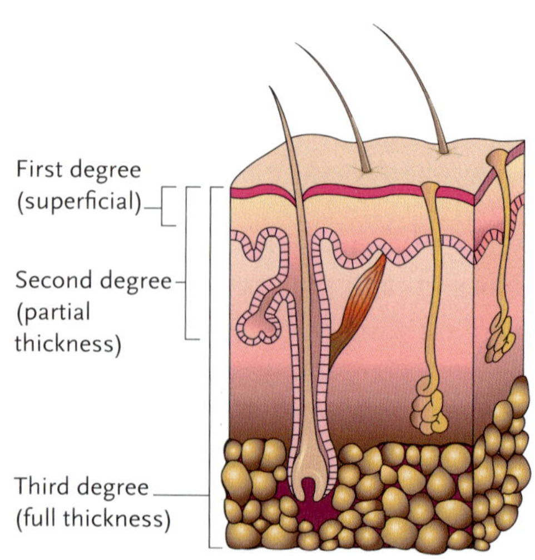

Fig. 6-8. *Different degrees of burns.*

Treating burns

To treat a minor burn:

1. Follow facility policy to call for help.
2. Put on gloves.
3. Use cool, clean water to decrease the skin temperature and prevent further injury (Fig. 6-9). Do not use ice or ice water, as ice may cause further skin damage. Dampen a clean cloth with cool water and place it over the burn.

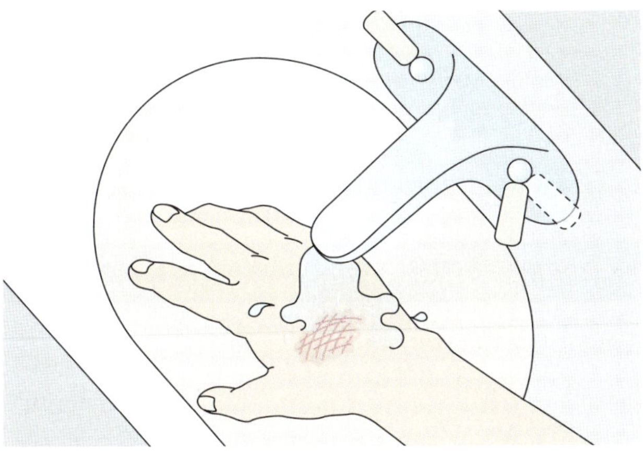

Fig. 6-9. *Use cool, clean water, not ice, on burned skin.*

4. Once the pain has eased, you may cover the area with a dry, clean dressing or nonadhesive sterile bandage.
5. Remove and discard your gloves. Wash your hands.
6. Never use any kind of ointment, salve, or grease on a burn.
7. Report and document the incident properly.

For more serious burns:

1. Remove the person from the source of the burn. If clothing has caught fire, have the person stop, drop, and roll, or smother the fire with a blanket or towel to put out flames. Protect yourself from the source of the burn.
2. Follow facility policy to call for help. Put on gloves.
3. Check for breathing, pulse, and severe bleeding. If the person is not breathing and has no pulse, begin CPR if trained and allowed to do so.
4. Do not use any type of ointment, water, salve, or grease on the burn.
5. Do not try to pull away any clothing from burned areas. Cover the burn with sterile gauze or a clean sheet. Apply the gauze or sheet lightly. Do not rub the burned area.
6. Do not give the person food or liquids.
7. Monitor vital signs and wait for further instructions.
8. Remove and discard your gloves. Wash your hands.
9. Report and document the incident properly.

Chemical burns require special care. The PCT should call for help immediately. The chemical must be washed away thoroughly. A shower or a hose may be needed when the burns cover a large area.

Fainting

Fainting, called **syncope**, occurs as a result of decreased blood flow to the brain, causing a temporary loss of consciousness. Fainting may be the result of an abnormal heart rhythm, hunger, hypoglycemia, dehydration, fear, pain, fatigue, standing for a long time, poor ventilation, certain medications, pregnancy, or overheating. Fainting may sometimes be caused by orthostatic hypotension (also called *postural hypotension*). **Orthostatic hypotension** is a sudden drop in blood pressure that occurs when a person stands or sits up. Signs and symptoms of fainting include dizziness, light-headedness, nausea, perspiration, pale skin, weak pulse, shallow respirations, and blackness in the visual field.

Responding to fainting

1. Follow facility policy to call for help.
2. Have the person lie down or sit down before fainting occurs.
3. If the person is in a sitting position, have him bend forward (Fig. 6-10). He can place his head between his knees if he is able. If the person is lying flat on his back, and there are no head, neck, back, spinal, or abdominal injuries; breathing difficulties; or fractures, elevate his legs about 12 inches.

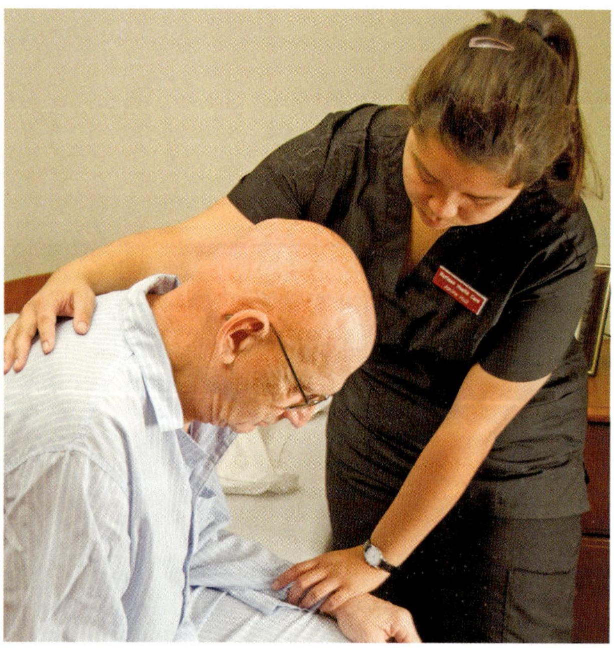

Fig. 6-10. *Have the person bend forward if he is sitting.*

4. Loosen any tight clothing.
5. Have the person stay in position for at least 5 minutes after symptoms disappear.
6. Help the person get up slowly. Continue to observe him for symptoms of fainting. Stay with him until he feels better. If you need help but cannot leave him, use the call light.
7. If a person does faint, lower him to the floor or other flat surface. Position him on his back. If he has no head, neck, back, spinal, or abdominal injuries; breathing difficulties; or fractures, elevate his legs about 12 inches. If unsure about injuries, leave him flat on his back. Loosen any tight clothing. Check to make sure he is breathing. (If he is not breathing and has no pulse, begin CPR if you are trained and allowed to do so.) He should recover quickly, but keep him lying down for several minutes. Report the incident to the nurse immediately. Fainting may be a sign of a more serious medical condition.
8. Report and document the incident properly.

Nosebleed

A nosebleed can occur suddenly when the air is dry, when injury has occurred, or when a person has taken certain medications. The medical term for a nosebleed is **epistaxis**.

Responding to a nosebleed

1. Notify the nurse immediately.
2. Elevate the head of the bed, or tell the person to remain in a sitting position, leaning forward slightly. Offer tissues or a clean cloth to catch the blood. Do not touch blood or bloody clothes, tissues, or cloths without gloves.
3. Put on gloves. Apply firm pressure on both sides of the nose, on the soft part up near the bridge. Squeeze the sides with your thumb and forefinger (Fig. 6-11). (Have the patient do this until you are able to put on gloves.)

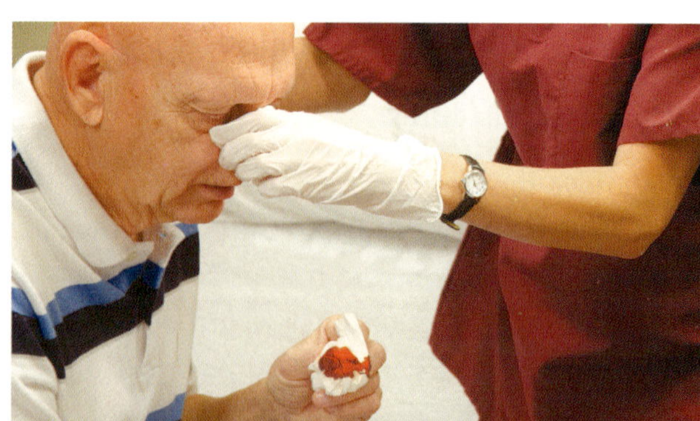

Fig. 6-11. *With gloves on, squeeze near the bridge of the nose on both sides, using your thumb and forefinger.*

4. Apply pressure until the bleeding stops. This may take several minutes.
5. Use a cool cloth or ice wrapped in a cloth on the bridge of the nose to slow the flow of blood. Never apply ice directly to skin.
6. Remove and discard your gloves. Wash your hands.
7. Report and document the incident properly.

Hypoglycemia and Diabetic Ketoacidosis

Hypoglycemia and diabetic ketoacidosis are complications of diabetes that can be life-threatening. **Hypoglycemia** (also called *insulin reaction*) can result from either too much insulin or too little food. It occurs when insulin is given and the person skips a meal or does not eat all the food required. Even when a regular amount of food is eaten, physical activity may rapidly metabolize the food so that too much insulin is in the body. Vomiting and diarrhea may also lead to hypoglycemia in people who have diabetes.

The first signs of hypoglycemia include feeling weak or different, nervousness, dizziness, and perspiration. The PCT should immediately report these signs to the nurse. These signs signal that the patient needs food in a form that can be rapidly absorbed. A glass of milk, fruit juice, or water with sugar dissolved in it should be consumed right away. A glucose tablet is another quick source of sugar. A fingerstick blood glucose test may need to be done right away. (Chapter 22 has more information on testing.) The PCT should follow her facility's policies. Signs and symptoms of hypoglycemia include the following:

- Hunger
- Headache
- Rapid pulse
- Low blood pressure
- Cold, clammy skin
- Confusion
- Trembling
- Blurred vision
- Numbness of the lips and tongue
- Unconsciousness

Diabetic ketoacidosis (**DKA**) is caused by having too little insulin in the body. Blood glucose levels become very high. It can result from undiagnosed diabetes, infection, going without insulin or not taking enough insulin, eating too much, not getting enough exercise, or physical or emotional stress. The signs of the onset of diabetic ketoacidosis include increased hunger, thirst, or urination; abdominal pain; deep or labored breathing; and breath that smells sweet or fruity. The nurse should be notified immediately if a patient shows signs of diabetic ketoacidosis. Other signs and symptoms include the following:

- Headache
- Weakness
- Rapid, weak pulse
- Low blood pressure
- Dry skin
- Flushed cheeks
- Drowsiness
- Nausea and vomiting
- Shortness of breath or air hunger (person gasping for air and being unable to catch his breath)
- Unconsciousness

Chapter 19 has more information about diabetes.

Seizures

Seizures are involuntary, often violent, contractions of muscles. They can involve a small area or the entire body. Seizures are caused by abnormalities in the brain. They can occur in young children who have a high fever. Older children and adults who have a serious illness, fever, head injury, or a seizure disorder such as **epilepsy** may also have seizures.

The main goal during a seizure is to make sure the patient is safe. During a seizure, a person may shake severely and thrust his arms and legs uncontrollably. He may clench his jaw, drool, and be unable to swallow. Most seizures last only a short time.

Responding to a seizure

1. Note the time. Put on gloves. Remove eyeglasses if the person is wearing them.
2. If the person is walking or standing, lower him to the floor. Cradle and protect his head. If a pillow is nearby, place it under his head. Loosen clothing to help with breathing. Try to turn him to one side to help lower the risk of choking. This may not be possible during a violent seizure.
3. Have someone call the nurse immediately or use the call light. Do not leave a person during a seizure unless you must do so to get medical help.
4. Move furniture away to prevent injury.
5. Do not try to stop the seizure or restrain the person.
6. Do not force anything between the person's teeth. Do not place your hands in his mouth for any reason. You could be bitten.
7. Do not give the person food or liquids.
8. When the seizure is over, note the time. Gently turn the person to his left side unless he has a head, neck, back, spinal, or abdominal injury; breathing difficulties; or fractures. Turning the person reduces the risk of choking on vomit or saliva. If the person begins to choke, get help immediately. Check for adequate breathing and pulse. If the person is not breathing and has no pulse, begin CPR if you are trained and allowed to do so. Do not begin CPR during a seizure.
9. Remove and discard your gloves. Wash your hands.
10. Report and document the incident properly, including how long the seizure lasted.

If the person is in a wheelchair when a seizure starts, move him to a clear, safe area, while keeping him in the sitting position. If the person is sitting on a couch or chair, keep him in the sitting position and remove nearby furniture that could cause injury. If the person is in bed, make sure the side rails (if present) are covered and remove any other items that could cause injury.

CVA or Stroke

The medical term for a stroke is a **cerebrovascular accident** (**CVA**). CVA (sometimes called *brain attack*) occurs when blood supply to a part of the brain is blocked or a blood vessel leaks or ruptures within the brain. A quick response to a CVA is critical. Tests and treatment need to be given within a short time of the stroke's onset (ideally within an hour). Early treatment may be able to reduce the severity.

A **transient ischemic attack** (**TIA**) is a warning sign of a CVA. It is the result of a temporary lack of blood supply to the brain. Symptoms may last up to 24 hours. They include difficulty speaking, weakness on one side of the body, temporary loss of vision, and numbness or tingling. These symptoms should not be ignored; the PCT should immediately follow facility policy to call for help. These are also signs that a TIA or stroke is occurring:

- Facial numbness, weakness, or drooping, especially on one side
- Paralysis on one side of the body (hemiplegia)

- Arm numbness or weakness, especially on one side (hemiparesis)
- Slurred speech or inability to speak (expressive aphasia)
- Inability to understand spoken or written words (receptive aphasia)
- Use of inappropriate words
- Loss of balance or new trouble walking
- Severe headache
- Vision changes, including blurred vision, double vision, or loss of vision
- Ringing in the ears
- Redness in the face
- Noisy breathing
- Elevated blood pressure
- Slow pulse rate
- Nausea or vomiting
- Loss of bowel and bladder control
- Seizures
- Dizziness
- Loss of consciousness

These symptoms may also be related to TIA, especially in women:

- Pain in the face, arms, and legs
- Hiccups
- Weakness
- Chest pain
- Shortness of breath
- Palpitations

B.E.F.A.S.T.

The acronym **B.E.F.A.S.T.** can be used as a way to remember the sudden signs that a stroke is occurring.

(B)alance: Is the person having balance issues? Is the person dizzy or walking differently?

(E)yes: Is the person having blurred vision, double vision, or a loss of vision?

(F)ace: Is one side of the face drooping? Is it numb? Ask the person to smile. Is the smile uneven?

(A)rms: Is one arm numb or weak? Ask the person to raise both arms. Check to see if one arm drifts downward.

(S)peech: Is the person's speech slurred? Is the person unable to speak? Can the person be understood? Ask the person to repeat a simple sentence and see if the sentence is repeated correctly.

(T)ime: Time is of the utmost importance when responding to a stroke. If the person shows any of the symptoms listed above, report to the nurse immediately.

The website for the American Stroke Association (stroke.org) has more information. Chapter 14 contains more information about strokes.

Vomiting

Vomiting, or **emesis**, is the act of ejecting stomach contents through the mouth and/or nose. It may be a sign of illness, injury, or a reaction to medication. Some patients, such as those with cancer who are undergoing chemotherapy, may vomit frequently as a result of treatment. Because a PCT may not know when a patient is going to vomit, she may not have time to explain what she will do and assemble supplies ahead of time. Vomiting is unpleasant. The PCT should talk to the patient soothingly as she helps him clean up. She should tell the patient what she is doing to help him.

Responding to vomiting

1. Notify the nurse immediately.
2. Put on gloves.
3. Make sure the head is up or turned to one side. Place an emesis basin under the chin. Remove it when vomiting has stopped.
4. Remove soiled linens or clothes and set aside. Replace with fresh linens or clothes.
5. If the patient's intake and output (I&O) is being monitored (Chapter 11), measure and note the amount of vomitus.

6. Flush vomit down the toilet unless vomit is red, has blood in it, looks like wet coffee grounds, or has medication in it. If these signs are observed, show the vomit to the nurse before discarding it. After disposing of the vomit, wash, dry, and store the basin.
7. Remove and discard your gloves. Wash your hands.
8. Put on clean gloves.
9. Provide comfort to the patient: wipe the face and mouth, position comfortably, and offer a drink of water (if patient does not have an NPO order) or mouth care (Chapter 9) (Fig. 6-12). Mouth care helps get rid of the taste of vomit in the mouth.

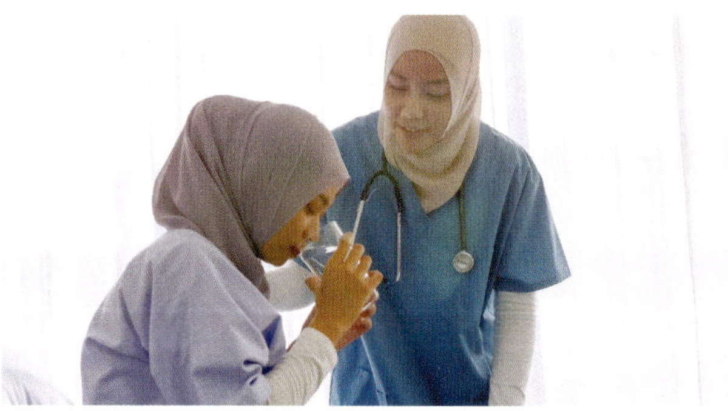

Fig. 6-12. *Be calm and comforting when helping a patient who has vomited.*

10. Put soiled linen in proper containers.
11. Remove and discard your gloves. Wash your hands again.
12. Document time, amount, color, odor, and consistency of vomitus.

Falls

Falls can be minor or severe. All falls should be reported to the nurse immediately, even if the patient says he feels fine. In the case of a severe fall, the PCT may need to call for emergency help, following facility policy. If a patient starts to fall, the PCT should not try to reverse or stop the fall. Doing this may cause more injury. The PCT should notify the nurse immediately after the fall and not attempt to get the patient up. Whenever a patient falls, an incident report must be completed. Learning Objective 7 contains more information about falls and fall prevention.

3. Discuss workplace safety and identify OSHA's categories of common hazards

Workplace hazards vary, but all healthcare settings can pose dangers to workers and patients alike. All staff members, including PCTs, are responsible for safety in a facility. Recognizing and working to reduce risks results in fewer accidents and a safer environment for everyone. OSHA identifies the following 4 categories of hazards in a healthcare environment:

Chemical. Chemicals used in healthcare settings may create dangerous fumes. They may also be caustic (damaging to the skin or other tissues) or flammable (able to catch fire easily).

Biological. Bloodborne pathogens are one significant biological hazard PCTs may encounter. Disease-causing bacteria, viruses, and fungi, spread through the air by droplets or through direct contact, are also biological hazards.

Physical. **Ergonomics** is the science of designing equipment, areas, and work tasks to make them safer and to suit workers' abilities. Physical hazards include poor ergonomic practices. They also include exposure to radiation or to excessive noise.

Safety. General safety hazards include electrical hazards, fire, hot equipment, and uneven or slippery floors. Disaster situations can also create safety hazards.

PCTs encounter all of these types of hazards. They work with patients with a range of health conditions. PCTs care for patients with infectious diseases. They may draw blood or collect other specimens, which means they are exposed to biological hazards. PCTs may also work with equipment that could pose a risk of burns or electrical shock. They may work with harmful chemicals, including products used to disinfect surfaces or clean up spills (Fig. 6-13).

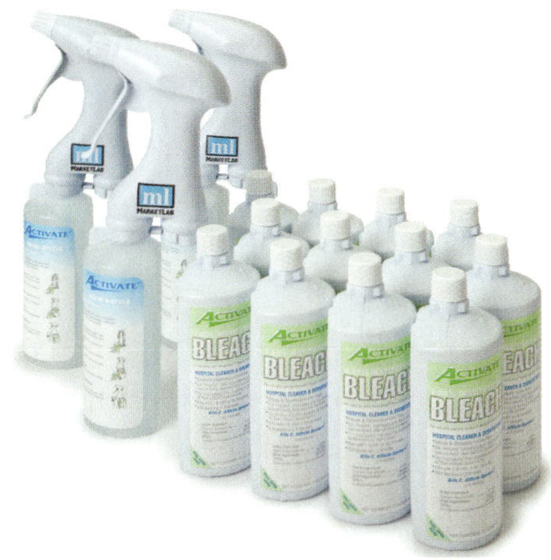

Fig. 6-13. *Cleaning products often contain potentially hazardous chemicals and should be used exactly as directed.* (PHOTO COURTESY OF MARKETLAB, INC., WWW.MARKETLAB.COM)

Every workplace has its own ergonomic challenges. The height of patient beds, the location of linens and supplies, and the amount of space in patient rooms can all affect safety. Fires are a concern in any healthcare setting, but laboratories and other areas where flammable chemicals are stored are at higher risk.

OSHA emphasizes being prepared to deal with safety hazards. All healthcare facilities have policies and procedures for responding to hazards. Training on this topic must be given at least once a year. Drills for fire evacuation and disaster response should be done regularly. Healthcare workers should review and practice safety responses often so that they become automatic.

Safety of Healthcare Workers

In recent years there has been an increased focus on the dangers healthcare workers face from angry or hostile patients and visitors. Coworkers may also sometimes pose a threat. OSHA statistics show that healthcare workers experience workplace violence at a rate about 4 times as high as workers in private industry in general.

If a patient, visitor, or coworker says or does anything that makes a PCT uncomfortable, it is important to report this to a supervisor. PCTs should not confront or argue with hostile or abusive patients, visitors, or coworkers. They should try to remove themselves from the situation and immediately report the incident. Threats of violence and physical or sexual assault should always be reported according to the facility's chain of command. They must also be reported to law enforcement. If action is not taken, the PCT should keep reporting up the chain of command until action is taken. If no appropriate action is taken at the facility, the PCT has the right and responsibility to report to law enforcement.

4. Explain the Safety Data Sheet (SDS)

The Occupational Safety and Health Administration (OSHA, osha.gov) requires that all hazardous chemicals have a **Safety Data Sheet** (**SDS**) (formerly called *Material Safety Data Sheet*, or *MSDS*). The SDS details the chemical ingredients, chemical dangers, and safe handling, storage, and disposal procedures for a product. Information about emergency response actions to be taken is also included. Some facilities use a toll-free number to access SDS information. These sheets must be accessible in work areas for all employees. Important information about the SDS includes the following:

- Employers must have an SDS for every chemical used.
- Employers must provide easy access to the SDS.
- Staff members must know where these sheets are kept and how to read them. They should ask for help if they do not know how to do this.

The list of hazardous chemicals that must have an SDS will be updated as new chemicals are purchased. The chemicals themselves must also be clearly labeled to identify hazards. OSHA's Hazard Communication Standard (often called *HazCom*) uses simple pictograms to illustrate the dangers posed by chemicals (Fig. 6-14).

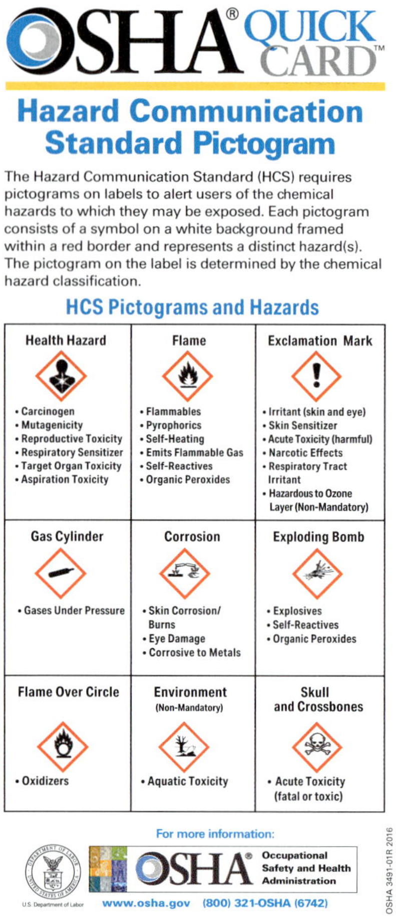
OSHA® QUICK CARD™

Hazard Communication Standard Pictogram

The Hazard Communication Standard (HCS) requires pictograms on labels to alert users of the chemical hazards to which they may be exposed. Each pictogram consists of a symbol on a white background framed within a red border and represents a distinct hazard(s). The pictogram on the label is determined by the chemical hazard classification.

HCS Pictograms and Hazards

Health Hazard	Flame	Exclamation Mark
• Carcinogen • Mutagenicity • Reproductive Toxicity • Respiratory Sensitizer • Target Organ Toxicity • Aspiration Toxicity	• Flammables • Pyrophorics • Self-Heating • Emits Flammable Gas • Self-Reactives • Organic Peroxides	• Irritant (skin and eye) • Skin Sensitizer • Acute Toxicity (harmful) • Narcotic Effects • Respiratory Tract Irritant • Hazardous to Ozone Layer (Non-Mandatory)
Gas Cylinder	**Corrosion**	**Exploding Bomb**
• Gases Under Pressure	• Skin Corrosion/ Burns • Eye Damage • Corrosive to Metals	• Explosives • Self-Reactives • Organic Peroxides
Flame Over Circle	**Environment (Non-Mandatory)**	**Skull and Crossbones**
• Oxidizers	• Aquatic Toxicity	• Acute Toxicity (fatal or toxic)

For more information:

OSHA® Occupational Safety and Health Administration

U.S. Department of Labor www.osha.gov (800) 321-OSHA (6742)

OSHA 3491-01R 2016

Fig. 6-14. *These pictograms alert healthcare workers, patients, and visitors to potential hazards in a facility.* (REPRINTED FROM WWW.OSHA.GOV/SITES/DEFAULT/FILES/PUBLICATIONS/OSHA3491QUICK-CARDPICTOGRAM.PDF)

OSHA requires that emergency eyewash stations be placed in all hazardous areas in case an eye injury occurs (Fig. 6-15). Employees must know where the closest eyewash station is and how to get there with restricted vision.

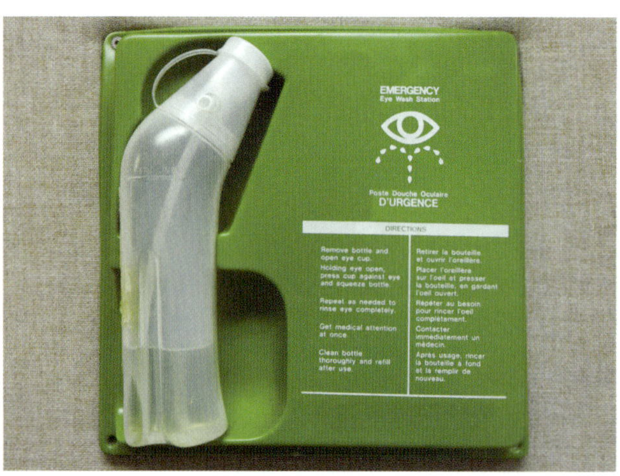

Fig. 6-15. *This is one type of eyewash station.*

5. Describe guidelines for responding to common hazards

The best way to avoid danger in the workplace is to develop what the CDC calls a *culture of safety.* This means the healthcare facility's policies emphasize safety and identify and address potential hazards. Healthcare workers are encouraged to speak up about possible hazards and share their ideas for avoiding them. When hazardous situations do occur, PCTs need to know how to respond.

Chemical exposure may result in harm to the skin, eyes, or mucous membranes (linings of body cavities that open to the outside of the body, such as the linings of the mouth, nose, and eyes). It can also cause breathing difficulties and many other symptoms, depending upon the specific chemical. PCTs work with antiseptics, which are used to reduce the number of pathogens on the body, and with disinfectants, which are used to reduce the number of pathogens on environmental surfaces. Some disinfectants can cause damage if spilled or used improperly. This is why PCTs should understand how and where to access Safety Data Sheets.

Guidelines: Chemical Hazards

- **G** Do not use any chemical agents you are not trained or allowed to use.
- **G** Wear appropriate gloves when using disinfectants, per facility policy. Change gloves if you are in contact with disinfectants for longer than 30 minutes. These chemicals can damage gloves over time.
- **G** Do not store food or drink in an area where hazardous chemicals are used or stored.
- **G** Do not drink or eat anything in the workplace if you do not know where it came from. (Food and drink should be limited to break areas and never consumed in patient care or other work areas.)

- Do not place pens or pencils in your mouth, apply makeup, or touch your face or eyes while working.
- Keep all liquids in their original containers. Do not remove or cover labels, instructions, or warnings.
- Always know how to access SDS information.
- Know where eyewash stations, sinks, and showers are located and the quickest way to reach them.
- In the case of exposure, flush with running water or wash the exposed area immediately. The length of time required for washing depends on the chemical. It ranges from 5 minutes for mildly irritating chemicals to an hour for highly corrosive chemicals. The SDS provides guidance on this topic.
- Report any known or suspected exposure to hazardous chemicals to your supervisor.
- Seek medical attention if needed, as directed by your supervisor.

Chapter 5 includes information about biological hazards and infection prevention. In addition to accidental needle sticks or contact with an infected patient, PCTs may also be exposed to biological hazards through spills, leaking specimen containers, or through the air during cleaning. This can happen when small particles of liquid or dried blood or other body fluids are **aerosolized**, or spread through the air in such a way that they might be inhaled.

Guidelines: Biological Hazards

- Seal specimen containers properly to prevent leaks or spills. No part of the specimen should be on the outside of the container.
- Place specimens to be carried to another area in a hard, latching container that can contain spills (Fig. 6-16).

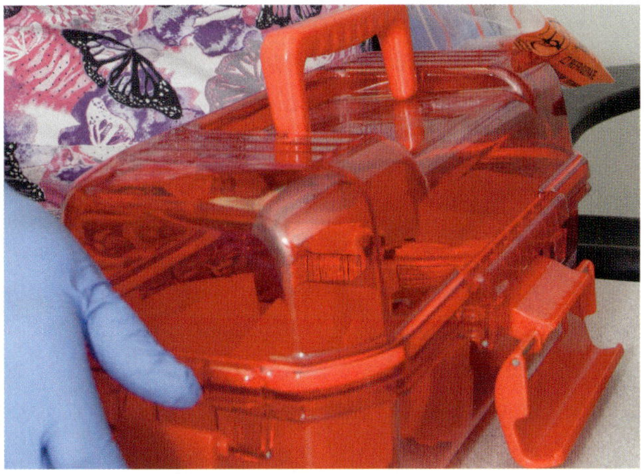

Fig. 6-16. *Specimen containers should be rigid and have latches. Latch the container before transporting specimens.*

- Follow facility policy for cleaning broken specimen containers and/or spills. Notify your supervisor or the appropriate person or department. Don gloves before cleaning. Special heavy-duty gloves may be required. Do not pick up any pieces of broken glass, no matter how large, with your hands. Use a dustpan and broom or other tools. Absorb the spill with whatever product is used by the facility. Apply the proper disinfectant and follow instructions regarding the amount of time it must stand before cleaning. Nonsharp waste (tissues, gauze, cloths, etc.) containing blood or other body fluids should be properly bagged in a special biohazard waste bag. Anything that could pierce a biohazard bag (such as broken glass) must be placed in a puncture-proof sharps container. Follow facility policy.
- Never scrape dried blood or other body fluids off of any surface or floor. The dried material can become aerosolized and then inhaled. Follow facility policy for cleaning dried blood and other body fluids. This usually involves soaking the dried materials in an antimicrobial cleaner before cleaning.
- In the case of exposure to blood or other body fluids (e.g., accidental needle stick), wash

or flush the area immediately with soap and water for 15 minutes, report the exposure, and get immediate medical attention.

PCTs may also encounter physical hazards at work. Poor ergonomic practices can cause injury. (Learning Objective 6 includes more information about this.) Exposure to X-rays or radioactive chemicals is a potential hazard. Specimens from patients who have received certain treatments may have low levels of radioactivity. Loud noise from machinery can also be a danger.

Guidelines: Physical Hazards

- **G** Pay attention to ergonomics. You should be able to provide care without stooping or bending. Supplies should be easy to reach. If not, talk to a supervisor about possible changes.
- **G** Standard Precautions protect against exposure to low-level radiation that might be present in patient specimens. Wear gloves when handling any specimen containers.
- **G** Pay attention to signs, lights, or other warnings about X-ray and other radiation exposure. Do not enter an area in which X-rays or radioactive substances are used without following the required precautions (Fig. 6-17).

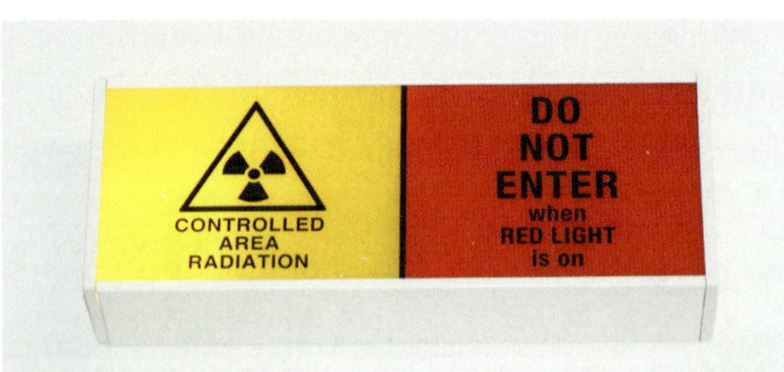

Fig. 6-17. *Lights and/or warning signs are used to indicate areas where radiation is used.*

- **G** Follow facility policies about tracking radiation exposure. If you often work in areas where radiation is common, you will need to wear a dosimeter. This is a small clip-on badge that measures radiation exposure. It is turned in after a certain amount of time to check exposure levels.
- **G** Use ear protection when working with noisy machines or entering rooms in which loud machines are operating.

Many PCTs work near electrical equipment that can produce dangerous levels of heat. Damaged or improperly used electrical equipment can cause injuries or fires. PCTs should never use equipment they have not been trained and assigned to use.

Guidelines: Electrical and Burn Hazards

- **G** Immediately report frayed electrical cords or electrical equipment that looks unsafe. Do not use this equipment. Report it to a supervisor.
- **G** Do not put combustible (able to burn) material near any appliance or machine that generates heat.
- **G** Do not touch the surface of any appliance or machine if it might be hot (e.g., an autoclave) (Fig. 6-18).

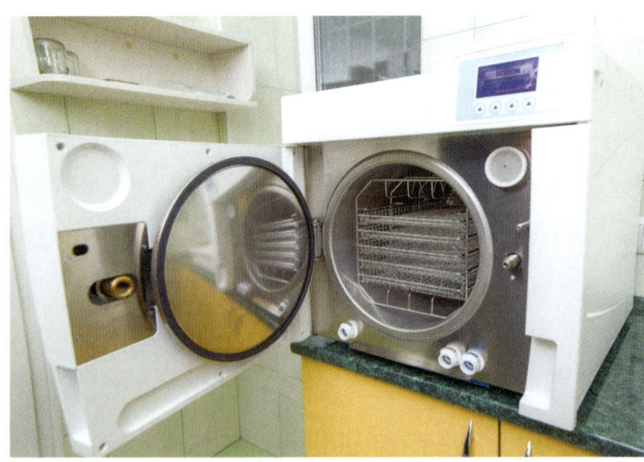

Fig. 6-18. *Autoclaves are used to sterilize equipment. The outer surfaces of some models may become hot during operation.*

- **G** Do not overload electrical sockets. Report overloaded sockets if you see them.

- Do not use extension cords or 2-prong electrical plugs. Only 3-prong plugs protect against electrical surges.
- Report damaged equipment or equipment that is not working properly to the appropriate person right away.

Learning Organizations

The Joint Commission encourages healthcare facilities to adopt the qualities of a *learning organization* to promote workplace safety. It recommends creating an atmosphere where employees "report to learn." This means encouraging employees to speak up about risks and dangers so that processes can be improved. Reports of problems or potential problems should be welcomed. Blame and punishment for errors should be avoided. Facilities are less safe if employees think they will be punished for reporting mistakes. Knowing about mistakes helps supervisors see where procedures can be improved. PCTs should watch for ways to promote safety at work.

6. Explain the principles of body mechanics

Back strain or injury can be a serious problem for all healthcare workers. **Body mechanics** is the way the parts of the body work together when a person moves. Using proper body mechanics helps save energy and prevent injury. PCTs can keep themselves and their patients safer if they understand the basic principles of body mechanics.

Alignment: Alignment is based on the word *line*. When a person stands up straight, a vertical line could be drawn through the center of his body and his center of gravity (Fig. 6-19). When the line is straight, the body is in alignment. Whether standing, sitting, or lying down, the body should be in alignment and should have good posture. This means that the 2 sides of the body are mirror images of each other, with body parts lined up naturally. **Posture** is the way a person holds and positions his body. A person can maintain correct body alignment when lifting or carrying an object by keeping the object close to his body. His feet and body should be pointed in the direction he is moving. He should avoid twisting at the waist.

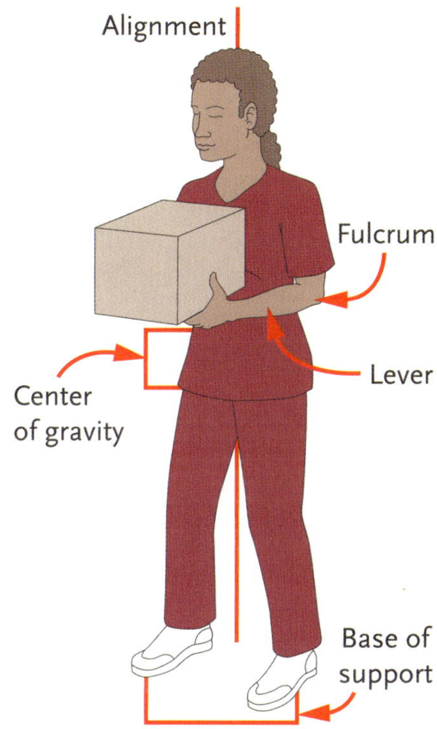

Fig. 6-19. *Proper body alignment is important when standing and sitting.*

Base of support: The base of support is the foundation that supports an object. The feet are the body's base of support. The wider the support, the more stable a person is. Standing with legs shoulder-width apart allows for a greater base of support. This is more stable than standing with the feet together.

Center of gravity: The center of gravity in the body is the point where the most weight is concentrated (Fig. 6-20). This point will depend on the position of the body. When a person stands, weight is centered in the pelvis. A low center of gravity gives a more stable base of support. Bending the knees when lifting an object lowers the pelvis and, therefore, lowers a person's center of gravity. This gives more stability and makes the person less likely to fall or strain the working muscles.

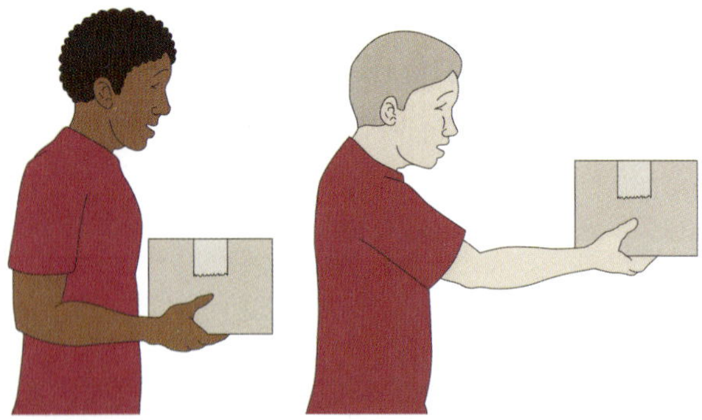

Fig. 6-20. Holding things close to the body moves weight toward the center of gravity. In this illustration, who is more likely to strain his back muscles?

By applying the principles of body mechanics to daily activities, injury can be avoided and less energy used. The following guidelines are helpful:

Guidelines: Using Proper Body Mechanics

- Assess the situation first. Clear the path and remove any obstacles.
- Use both arms and hands to lift, push, or carry objects.
- When lifting a heavy object from the floor, spread your feet shoulder-width apart. Bend your knees. Use the strong, large muscles in your thighs, upper arms, and shoulders to lift the object. Raise your body and the object together (Fig. 6-21).

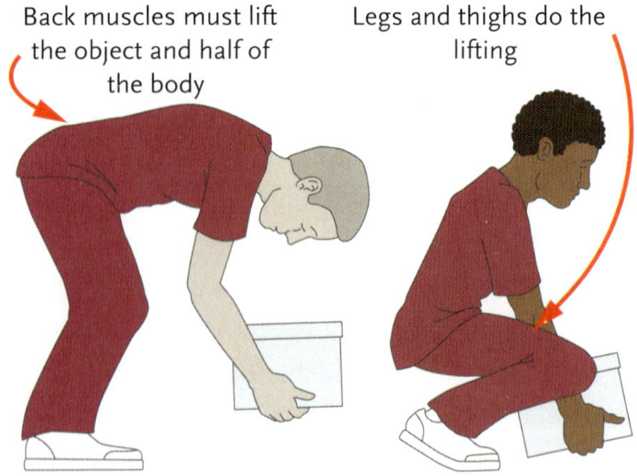

Fig. 6-21. In this illustration, which person is lifting correctly?

- Hold objects close to you when you are lifting or carrying them. This keeps the object closer to your center of gravity and base of support.
- Push or slide objects rather than lifting them.
- Avoid bending and reaching as much as possible.
- When a task requires bending, use a good stance. Bend your knees to lower yourself (squat), rather than bending from the waist. This uses the big muscles in your legs and hips rather than the smaller muscles in your back.
- Do not twist when you are lifting or moving an object. Instead, turn your whole body. Pivot your feet instead of twisting at the waist. Your feet should point toward what you are lifting or moving.
- Get help from coworkers when possible for lifting heavy objects or helping patients who have limited mobility. Many facilities have guidelines about the number of staff members needed to move patients and when to use lift equipment.
- Never try to catch a falling patient. If you try to reverse a fall in progress, you could injure yourself and/or the patient.
- Report to the provider any task you feel that you cannot safely do. Never try to lift an object or a patient that you feel you cannot handle.

7. Provide for patient safety in an inpatient setting

Hospitals and other healthcare facilities can pose dangers to patients as well as to employees. Every member of the care team is responsible for protecting patients from harm. Each year the Joint Commission outlines National Patient Safety Goals for different healthcare settings (jointcommission.org/standards/national-patient-safety-goals). These goals help facilities try to improve patient safety. Policies and procedures should reflect these goals, and all employees should be trained to follow them.

The National Patient Safety Goals for 2023 are as follows:

Identify patients correctly. Two identifiers (e.g., full name and date of birth) should always be used to identify patients. Facilities should have special procedures for identifying newborns. These may include identification bands on 2 different body sites and naming systems that include the baby's full name and gender. Babies with similar names should have extra measures in place (e.g., a sign on the bassinets alerting staff to the situation). PCTs should always carefully follow all patient identification procedures.

Improve staff communication. This goal relates to communicating critical, potentially life-threatening test results. PCTs may be trained to perform some point-of-care tests such as fingerstick blood glucose testing. They should know critical ranges (results that may mean the patient is in danger) for any tests they are trained to perform. They should also know their facility's procedures for communicating critical results. Critical results must be reported immediately.

Use medicines safely. PCTs do not give medications to patients. However, they still have an important role in observing and reporting. If PCTs see that a patient has not taken an ordered medication (for example, that the patient has placed or lost a tablet in her bedding or has pocketed it in her mouth), it should be reported immediately. If a patient has his own medication or if a visitor brings medication of any kind to a patient (this includes vitamins, supplements, and herbal medications), the PCT should also report this immediately.

Use alarms safely. Hospitals are noisy. Alarms are often sounding. Cardiac monitors, pulse oximeters (which measure blood oxygen), and IV infusion pumps are used for most hospital patients. In an intensive care unit, ventilators may breathe for patients. A capnography monitor may be used to measure carbon dioxide in exhaled air. Care team members may become less alert to alarm sounds because they happen so often.

Prevent infection. MDROs and other HAIs are a serious threat to safety. PCTs must follow all facility guidelines related to hand hygiene, PPE use, and other infection prevention and control methods. All facilities require frequent hand hygiene, but healthcare workers do not always follow hand hygiene policies. PCTs must wash their hands properly and/or use alcohol-based hand sanitizer every time it is required. Not doing so puts patients at risk for deadly infections.

Identify patient safety risks. This goal relates to recognizing suicide risk and protecting patients from self-harm while they are in the hospital. A patient who is considered to be at risk for suicide may have *one-to-one monitoring* ordered. This means that a healthcare worker must stay with the patient at all times. If a PCT is assigned this task, they will be trained in their facility's policies and procedures. These may include limiting access to certain items that could be used for self-harm and never allowing the patient to be alone. PCTs should follow guidelines for one-to-one monitoring carefully and should understand how and when to notify a nurse.

Improve health care equity. This goal relates to making sure all patients receive the highest level of care, regardless of age, gender, preferred language, race, ethnicity, or any other factor. All healthcare workers must treat patients without bias. PCTs have frequent contact with patients. If a PCT becomes aware of a patient need that is not being met, she should report it to a nurse.

Prevent mistakes in surgery. This goal relates to care that is beyond the PCT's scope of practice. Even so, PCTs who assist with preoperative care can promote patient safety. PCTs protect patients having surgery by following patient identification policies carefully and doing all assigned preoperative tasks correctly.

Although the National Patient Safety Goals may change with time, all of these concerns remain important. Another important issue is the patient's physical safety while in the facility. Patient falls are a serious problem in all healthcare facilities, including hospitals. AHRQ estimates that 700,000 to 1,000,000 people fall each year in hospitals. A *fall* is any sudden, uncontrollable descent from a higher to a lower level, with or without injury resulting. Falls can be caused by an unsafe environment, loss of abilities, diseases, and medications. In a hospital, equipment such as IV tubing and poles can increase fall risk. Problems resulting from falls range from minor bruises to fractures (broken bones) and life-threatening injuries.

When a patient is admitted to a hospital, nursing staff complete a fall risk assessment. The assessment considers factors such as the following:

- The patient's ability to walk and balance independently and the need for aids such as a walker or cane
- Any medications or conditions that may cause dizziness or weakness, or may limit the patient's judgment
- Confusion, disorientation, or cognitive impairment
- Age (elderly patients are at a higher risk for falls)
- Changes in elimination caused by medications or conditions (e.g., taking a drug that increases the need to urinate)

If the assessment tool shows that a patient has an elevated fall risk, precautions are put in place. These may be different in each facility, but they always involve clear visual communication of the fall risk. Yellow wristbands, signs on patient doors and/or at the foot of the bed, and alerts within a patient's records are all ways to communicate fall risk (Fig. 6-22). Some facilities may use alarms that sound when a patient leaves her bed. Falls may be prevented if healthcare workers respond quickly to help the patient.

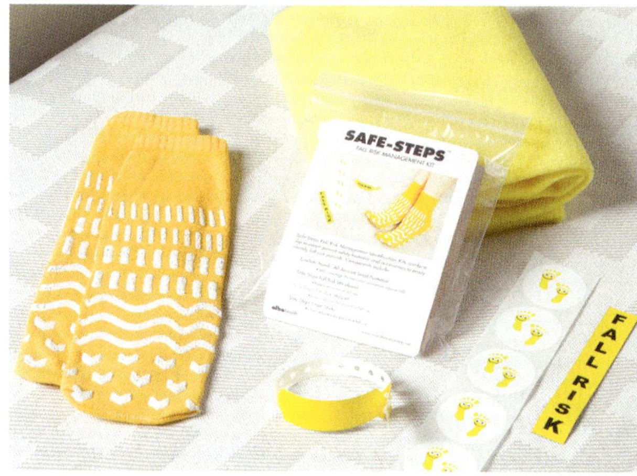

***Fig. 6-22.** Yellow is often used to alert healthcare workers to a patient's elevated fall risk.* (IMAGE COURTESY OF ENCOMPASS GROUP, LLC)

All team members must work together to prevent falls. The guidelines listed below apply to all patients, regardless of fall risk.

Guidelines: Preventing Falls

G Keep a patient's room free of clutter and trash. Make sure cords, tubes, and wires are kept as tidy as possible. Remind patients to be aware of these items.

G Make sure patients are wearing nonskid footwear if they leave their beds. Hospitals generally provide nonskid socks to patients on admission.

G Report to a nurse if a patient's gown seems too long. This could trip the patient.

G Keep personal items that are used often close to patients, including call lights. Call lights are very important to all patients, but especially to patients who have an elevated fall risk.

- G Answer call lights right away. If nobody is responding to a call light, the patient may try to get up. This can result in falls.
- G Immediately clean up spills on the floor.
- G Report loose handrails immediately.
- G Lock wheels and move footrests out of the way before helping patients into or out of wheelchairs.
- G Lock the bed wheels before helping the patient into and out of bed and when giving care.
- G Raise the bed to a safe level, usually waist high, before you provide care. This allows for proper body mechanics while you work. After completing care, return the bed to its lowest position.
- G Get help when moving a patient; do not assume you can do it alone. When in doubt, ask for help. Keep any walking aids, such as canes or walkers, within the patient's reach.
- G Offer help with elimination regularly. Respond to requests for help immediately.
- G Know which patients are at risk for falls and pay attention so that you can give help often. Follow any facility fall prevention measures and report any changes in patients to the nurse. Changes may require extra fall precautions.
- G If a patient starts to fall, do not try to catch her or reverse the fall in progress. If you try to reverse a fall, you may hurt yourself and/or the patient. If you are able to do this without hurting yourself, use your body to slide her to the floor. Always try to protect the patient's head. Move objects out of the way if possible.
- G Whenever a patient falls, it must be reported to the nurse. Follow facility policy for completing an incident report.

Connected Care

Restraints

A **restraint** is a physical or chemical way to restrict voluntary movement or behavior. In the past, restraints were commonly used to prevent confused patients from wandering, to prevent falls, to keep patients from injuring themselves or others, or to prevent patients from pulling out tubing. Restraints were overused, especially in long-term care and psychiatric care settings. This led to new laws restricting the use of restraints.

Today, restraints may only be used when they are considered medically necessary. They are only used as a last resort and only after less restrictive measures have been tried. If a restraint is needed, a doctor must order it. It is against the law for healthcare workers to apply a restraint for convenience or to discipline a patient. Very specific guidelines apply to carrying out a restraint order, including frequent monitoring of the patient. This is important because patients have been severely injured and have died due to improper restraint use and lack of monitoring. PCTs must carefully follow all facility guidelines if assigned to care for a patient on whom restraints are used. If any problems occur with the restraint, especially injury, the PCT must notify the nurse and complete an incident report as soon as possible.

8. Describe response to emergency and disaster situations

Emergencies such as natural disasters or active shooter situations also pose a danger to patients, visitors, and healthcare workers. Workers must know how best to protect patients and themselves from these risks.

Disasters can include fire, flood, earthquake, hurricane, tornado, or other severe weather. Human-created dangers, such as acts of terrorism, bomb threats, and active shooter/assailant situations, can also threaten safety in a facility. PCTs must participate in any training or drills regarding disaster response. Emergency medical personnel, fire departments, and police may attend these drills. Taking an active role in drills can help PCTs understand what to do if disasters occur.

Fires are a risk at any healthcare facility. Laboratories can be especially dangerous in a fire because of chemicals and heat-generating equipment. All facilities have a fire safety plan, and all workers need to know this plan. Guidelines regarding fires and evacuations are explained to all employees. Evacuation routes are posted in facilities. PCTs should read and review them often and should attend fire and disaster response trainings when they are offered.

Guidelines: Responding to Fires

- **G** Fire alarms and exit doors should not be blocked. If they are, report this to a supervisor.
- **G** Know the facility's fire evacuation plan.
- **G** Stay calm. Do not panic.
- **G** Every facility will have multiple fire extinguishers (Fig. 6-23). Learn where they are located. The PASS acronym will help you understand how to use an extinguisher:
    - **P**ull the pin.
    - **A**im at the base of the fire when spraying.
    - **S**queeze the handle.
    - **S**weep back and forth at the base of the fire.
- **G** In case of fire, the RACE acronym is a good rule to follow:
    - **R**emove anyone in danger if you are not in danger.
    - **A**lert by activating the fire alarm system or calling 911.
    - **C**ontain the fire if possible by closing all doors and windows.
    - **E**xtinguish the fire, or the fire department will extinguish it. Evacuate the area if instructed to do so.

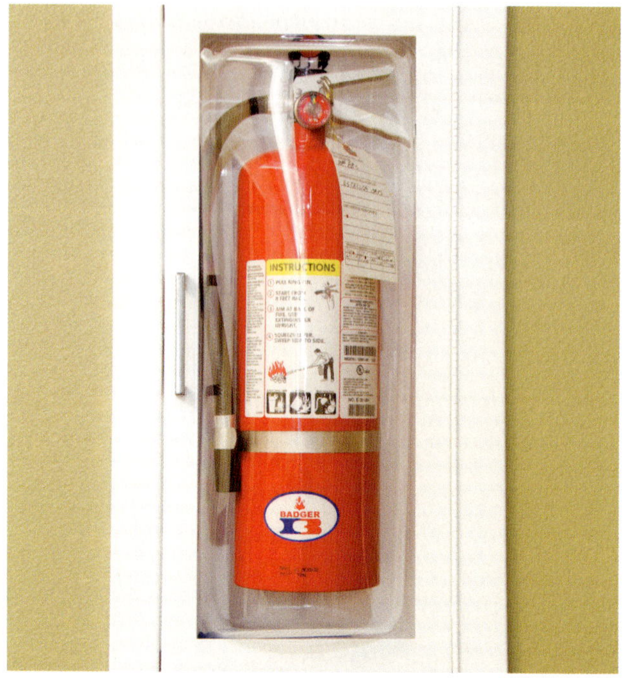

Fig. 6-23. *Know the locations of your facility's fire extinguishers and know how to use them.*

- **G** Follow the directions of the fire department.
- **G** Do not get into an elevator during a fire. In certain situations, firefighters may direct people into an elevator. This is the only exception to the guideline. If firefighters do not direct you to enter an elevator, always use the stairs.
- **G** Stay low in a room to escape a fire.
- **G** If the door of the room you are in is closed, check for heat coming from it before opening it. If the door or doorknob feels hot, stay in the room if there is no safe exit. Plug the doorway (use wet towels or clothing) to prevent smoke from entering. Stay in the room until help arrives.
- **G** Use the stop, drop, and roll fire safety technique to extinguish a fire on clothing or hair. Stop running or stay still. Drop to the ground, lying down if possible. Roll on the ground to try to extinguish the flames.
- **G** Use a damp covering over the mouth and nose to reduce smoke inhalation.
- **G** After leaving the building, move away from it.

Preparing and practicing for emergencies is the best way to respond appropriately if one occurs. In the case of a disaster, PCTs should follow their facility's response plan and the instructions of first responders. The following guidelines apply to many disaster situations:

Guidelines: Disasters

- Remain calm.
- Know the locations of all exits and stairways.
- Know where the fire alarms and extinguishers are located.
- Know the appropriate action to take in various situations based on facility training. If you are supposed to direct patients or visitors to safety, stay calm and follow the training you have received.
- Use the internet to stay informed, or keep the radio or television tuned to a local station to get the latest information.

PCTs should also be aware of specific emergency guidelines for the geographic area in which they work. For example, a PCT working where hurricanes may occur needs to know the guidelines for hurricane preparedness. The following guidelines are listed by the type of disaster:

Tornadoes

- Seek shelter inside, ideally in a steel-framed or concrete building.
- Stay away from windows.
- Stay in a hallway or basement, or take cover under heavy furniture.
- Crouch on the ground, head down. Cover your head and neck with your arms.

Power Outages

- Keep calm and take prompt action to provide light.
- Use a backup pack for electrical medical equipment as needed.
- Backup packs do not last more than 24 hours, so contact emergency services when instructed.

Hurricanes

- Know the hurricane's category and track its expected path.
- Evacuate if advised to do so.

Earthquakes

- Drop to the ground.
- Get under a sturdy piece of furniture, such as a heavy table, if possible. Hold on until the shaking stops.
- If no table or desk is available, stay crouched down in the inside corner of a building. Cover your face and head with your arms.
- Stay away from windows, outside walls, and anything that might fall over or fall down.
- Do not exit a building during the shaking.
- Do not use elevators.
- If trapped under debris after an earthquake, do not light a match or ignite a lighter. Avoid kicking up dust. Breathe through a handkerchief or clothing. Make tapping noises or use a whistle, if available, to get rescuers' attention. Do not shout. Shouting could cause you to inhale dangerous amounts of dust.

Active Shooter/Assailant

- Follow the facility's emergency notification procedures.
- If there is an escape path, try to evacuate.
- If you cannot get out safely, stay where you are.
  - Turn off the lights and stay hidden from outside view.

- Lock the door if possible. Move heavy furniture to barricade the door and cover any openings or windows in the door.
- If you cannot find a safe room or area with a door, hide behind a large object.
- Turn off all cell phone ringers. Remain quiet.
- If safe to do so, call 911 and notify the operator of your exact location in the building.
- Provide information on the number and description of assailant(s), the number and type(s) of weapons in use, the number of victims and nature of their injuries, and their locations if known.

G If there is no way to escape or hide, fight. Confront the assailant with the goal of taking him down. Be aggressive and decisive. Improvise weapons if possible.

G When police arrive on the scene, do not move toward any police vehicle until directed to do so by the officers. Move with hands on top of your head and follow all directions given by police.

G Remain in the area until released by police.

Chapter Review

1. List 2 steps to follow when encountering an emergency situation.
2. What is one reason PCTs may not be allowed to start CPR without the direction of a licensed healthcare professional?
3. How are abdominal thrusts used to help someone who is choking?
4. If the person becomes unconscious while choking, what should the PCT do?
5. In what position should a person be placed if he is in shock?
6. What symptoms are women more likely to experience than men if they are having a myocardial infarction (heart attack)?
7. What can be done to a wounded limb to slow bleeding?
8. Why should ice not be applied to burns?
9. If a person feels like they are going to faint, in what position should they be placed?
10. What must a PCT do before helping a patient with a nosebleed?
11. What are the first signs that a person is experiencing diabetic ketoacidosis?
12. Why should a PCT not force anything into the mouth of a person who is having a seizure?
13. What is a transient ischemic attack (TIA)?
14. What should a PCT do if a patient starts to fall?
15. When would a PCT need to show the nurse a patient's vomit before discarding it?
16. Give an example for each of the following OSHA common hazard categories: chemical, biological, physical, and safety.
17. Explain what a *culture of safety* is.
18. What is body mechanics?
19. What is the name for the point in the body where the most weight is concentrated?
20. When lifting a heavy object from the floor, how should the feet be placed?
21. What is one-to-one monitoring in health care and when might it be ordered?
22. What factors are considered in a fall risk assessment?
23. Explain what the PASS and RACE acronyms stand for.
24. What are 4 general guidelines that apply to many disaster situations?

7 The Patient's Environment

1. Describe inpatient care settings

A typical hospital has several departments and units where patients receive care. The equipment in patient rooms and the type of care a PCT may provide differs, depending on the area. Patients may be admitted to a hospital in many ways. One way is through the facility's **emergency department** (**ED**), sometimes called the *emergency room* (*ER*) (Fig. 7-1). Patients may also be admitted for planned operations, testing, or treatment, or they may be transferred to the hospital from another facility, such as an urgent care center or a long-term care facility. Patients who are giving birth are generally admitted directly to a facility's labor and delivery department.

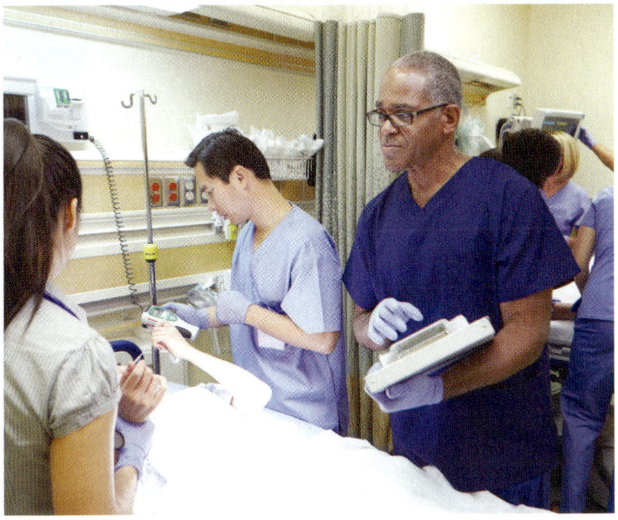

Fig. 7-1. *Often patients are admitted through a hospital's emergency department.*

An emergency department provides immediate medical care 24 hours a day, 7 days a week. Patients may arrive at an ED on their own, with help from others, or in an ambulance. Strokes, seizures, heart attacks, sudden illnesses, and **trauma**, or injuries due to accidents or acts of violence, are some conditions that may be treated in an emergency department. Since patients may need a wide range of care, the first step is **triage**, or deciding how urgently the patient needs care. Triage is usually performed by a nurse.

EDs have areas and equipment for resuscitation of patients experiencing cardiac arrest. They can also manage major trauma such as from a serious car accident or a shooting. There are rooms for performing major and minor surgical procedures. There are also consultation and observation rooms for patients with less immediate needs.

PCTs who work in emergency rooms may draw blood, set up EKG monitoring, and insert or remove IVs and urinary catheters. A **catheter** is a thin tube inserted into the body that is used to drain or inject fluids. A **urinary catheter** is used to drain urine from the bladder. (Not all states allow PCTs to insert IVs or catheters.) They may perform point-of-care tests, including tests on blood drawn by finger stick and tests on urine. They may assist providers with care and procedures. They also perform routine tasks such as measuring vital signs and assisting patients with elimination and other activities of daily living.

Other units in a hospital include the following:

- The **medical/surgical unit** (often called *med/surg*) is for patients who are admitted to the hospital for surgery, testing, observation, or treatment of an illness that does not require constant, intensive care. This unit cares for the general patient population. In hospitals that serve all ages, there may be a separate **pediatric unit**. (Many cities also have pediatric hospitals.)
- The **intensive care unit** (**ICU**) provides care to patients who are critically ill. These patients require constant skilled care. They may be receiving care such as artificial ventilation. In addition to general ICUs, hospitals may have ICUs for neonatal patients (NICU), pediatric patients (PICU), and patients who need intensive cardiac care (CICU). Some hospitals may provide ICU care for patients who have experienced physical trauma or burns. They have special beds and other equipment to aid in healing.
- Patients who no longer need intensive care but need more care than is given in the medical/surgical unit may be moved to a **step-down unit**. The care given in these units is an intermediate level, between ICU and general care. The specific type of care provided depends on the patient's diagnosis and/or condition. Cardiac **telemetry**, or monitoring that allows a trained healthcare worker to observe the heart activity of several patients at once in a special monitoring room, is often part of this care. Some may still be on a ventilator, but are stable enough to require less frequent monitoring and adjustment.
- A **labor and delivery unit** is where patients give birth and where they and their infants stay until they are discharged from the hospital.
- Some hospitals have dedicated **psychiatric units**. These units provide care for acute needs related to mental health.
- Some hospitals have **subacute care units**. Patients who do not need the level of care provided in the med/surg unit, but who are not ready to go home, may be treated in a subacute care unit.
- Although it is not always a separate unit, **hospice care** may be provided to patients who are dying. Hospice care is a compassionate way to care for people who are dying and their families. It emphasizes a holistic, person-centered approach. PCTs who work with patients receiving hospice care must understand that recovery is not the goal. Instead, goals relate to the comfort and dignity of the patient. Chapter 24 has more information.

Hospitals have many other departments that relate to patient care. X-rays and other types of imaging are done in the radiology department. These give providers more information on patients' conditions. A hospital laboratory performs diagnostic tests on patient specimens. The pharmacy department provides ordered medications. Patient meals are made by the dietary department, and dietitians/nutritionists work with providers to ensure that the meals meet patients' needs. The environmental services department of a hospital (sometimes called *housekeeping* or *custodial/janitorial services*) has the very important job of keeping the facility clean. Proper cleaning of patient rooms, equipment, and the common areas of a facility promotes health and prevents infection.

2. Explain why a comfortable environment is important for the patient's well-being

Illness and disability cause great stress. It helps patients feel better physically and psychologically if their environments are clean and comfortable. A comfortable and clean environment aids in relaxation and helps to reduce stress. A soothing environment may also help relieve pain and promote healing. Many things affect patients' comfort within their hospital rooms. The more PCTs try to improve patients' environments, the more positive impact it may have on health and well-being.

Hospitals are noisy and busy. Many things can affect patients' comfort level, such as noise, odors, temperature, lighting, diet, medications, illness, fear, and anxiety. PCTs can use the following guidelines to promote comfort:

Guidelines: Promoting Comfort

G Common noises in facilities can upset and/or irritate patients. Some noise is unavoidable, but PCTs can reduce excess noise by doing the following:

- Do not bang equipment or meal trays.
- Keep your voice low.
- Promptly answer ringing telephones and call lights.
- Close doors when patients ask you to if you are allowed to do so. In some cases, patients' doors must be kept open for observation.
- Turn off televisions when they are not in use.

G Odors may be caused by urine, feces, vomit, certain diseases, and wound drainage. Body and breath odors may be offensive too. Help control odors by doing the following:

- Empty and clean bedpans, urinals, commodes, and emesis basins immediately.
- Change soiled bed linens and clothing as soon as possible.
- Give regular oral care and personal care to help avoid body and breath odors.
- Promptly clean up after episodes of incontinence.
- If a patient uses incontinence briefs, assist with changing them as soon as they are soiled and discard them properly. Incontinence briefs may be used by patients who are unable to control their bladder or bowels. These briefs help keep wastes away from the skin to keep the skin clean and dry.

G Temperature can affect comfort. Certain illnesses can cause a person to feel cold, as can being anxious or scared. Help patients stay comfortable by doing the following:

- Layer bed covers for warmth.
- Check that patients in drafty areas, such as areas near doors and windows, have enough blankets to feel comfortable.
- Offer blankets to patients in wheelchairs.
- Keep patients covered while giving personal care.
- If patients control the heat and air conditioning in their rooms, do not change the temperature for your comfort.

G Adequate lighting promotes safety and prevents falls. It also helps make a room pleasant. Patients may prefer darker rooms when they are ill, have a headache, or are sleeping. Keep lighting controls within the patient's reach.

G Foods ordered in special diets may cause discomfort. Heavy meals can also cause discomfort. Report patient complaints about food to the nurse.

G Foods and drinks that contain caffeine can prevent sleep or interfere with sleeping well. Caffeine may need to be decreased to promote better rest (Fig. 7-2).

G Help the patient to keep as normal a daily routine as possible. Open window coverings during the day if the patient agrees. Encourage as normal a wake/sleep schedule as possible.

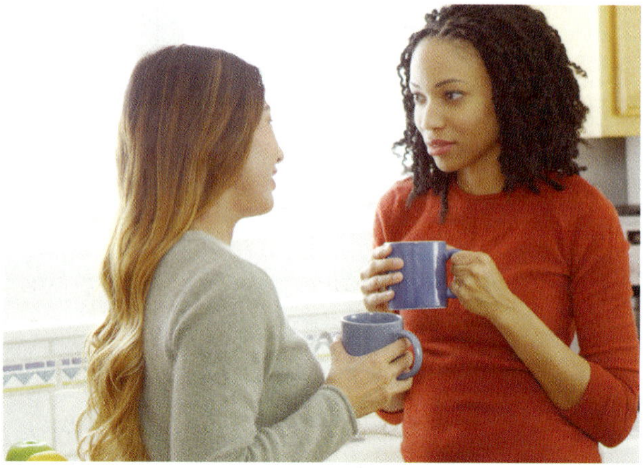

Fig. 7-2. Caffeinated drinks, such as coffee and some teas, can prevent sleep and cause fatigue and irritability.

G If patients seem sad, anxious, or fearful, help them by talking with them and listening to their concerns. Provide emotional support. If you think patients require more help than you can give, discuss this with the nurse. Hospital social workers or religious leaders may be called to help if the patient wishes.

Connected Care

Supporting Children and Their Families

Hospitals can be scary and confusing places for all patients. This is especially true for children. Medical environments can cause emotional trauma for children. Small adjustments to how PCTs and other healthcare workers care for children can make a big difference. It is very important to tell children and their parents/guardians what to expect. The language used should be right for the child's age. PCTs must be honest, even if that means telling the child that something might hurt or that they do not know an answer. Giving children choices, even in small things that do not seem important, can help them feel more in control. Whenever possible, healthcare workers should focus on the child's strengths. Recognizing that a child asked a good question, or was helpful with a task (such as holding a bandage or telling the PCT when something beeps), can increase the child's comfort. It is normal and expected for children to have a strong emotional response to being in the hospital. It may seem like talking about these emotions will make the situation worse, but that is not true. It is much better to let children talk about how they feel. They should know that what they feel is normal.

3. Describe a standard patient room and how to care for equipment

A patient's room must be kept neat and clean. After providing care, the PCT will clean the area and put equipment away. Providing a clean, safe, and orderly environment is an essential part of the PCT's job.

PCTs should always knock and wait to receive permission before entering. However, this may not always be possible. Certain patients, such as those who are confused, intubated or unconscious, or have problems speaking, may not be able to give this permission.

Equipment that is generally found in each patient's room includes the following:

Bed: An electric bed, also called a *hospital bed,* is adjustable and can be raised and lowered (Fig. 7-3). Electric beds are operated by controls that hang on or near the side of the bed (Fig. 7-4). Buttons are used to raise and lower the head of the bed, the foot of the bed, sections of the bed, and the bed height. Most electric beds have a way to insert a crank so that they can be adjusted if there is a power failure. Manual beds have cranks to adjust height and to raise and lower the head of the bed.

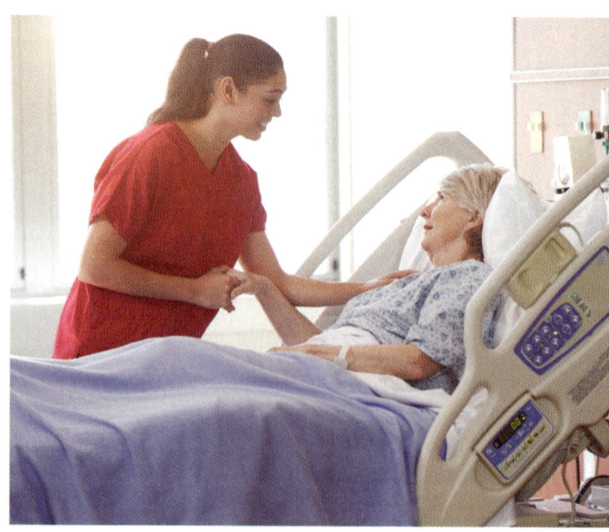

Fig. 7-3. One type of electric bed.

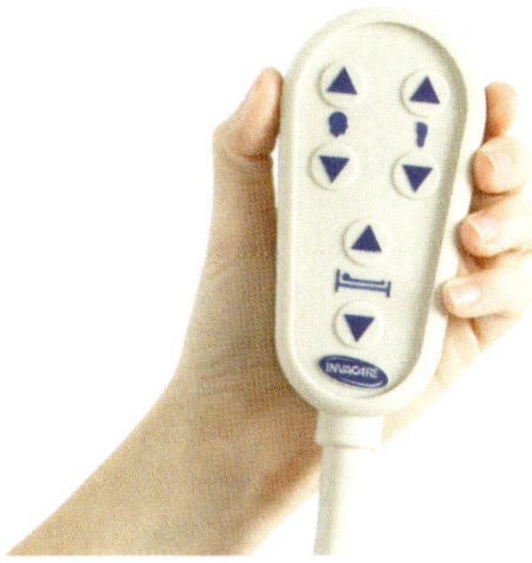

Fig. 7-4. Controls for an electric bed may look like this.

Normally beds are kept in their lowest horizontal position. They may be raised while care is provided, but should be lowered again immediately after. Lowering the bed provides for patients' safety and helps reduce the risk of falls. Cranks should be placed back under the bed after a manual bed has been moved to reduce the risk of injury.

A bariatric bed is used for patients who are obese and has weight ranges set by the manufacturer. They usually accommodate patients who weigh from 250 to 1,000 pounds.

An alternating pressure bed is used to prevent or treat pressure injuries (Chapter 12). The mattress has tubes that alternate deflating and inflating to relieve pressure under the body and to promote circulation. It helps ensure that one area of the body does not rest on one spot for too long and has increased air circulation under the body. It may also have temperature control/cooling features.

A pulmonary therapy bed is also used to prevent or treat pressure injuries, as well as pulmonary complications. It provides pressure redistribution along with percussion (tapping) and vibration therapies in the area under the patient's chest. It may also have a feature that continuously turns the patient from side to side to prevent breathing complications.

A bassinet is for an infant. It is on a wheeled cart with drawers for care items. Beds for infants in a NICU may be enclosed and include warmers or special lights to treat jaundice, a common condition for newborns. Babies who do not need special care are usually placed in bassinets that can be wheeled between the parent's room and other care areas.

Bedside stand: Small items are usually stored in a bedside stand. The water pitcher and cup are often placed on top of the bedside stand. A telephone and other items may also be placed there.

These items may be stored inside the bedside stand or may be stored in the bathroom:

- Wash basin
- Emesis basin (Fig. 7-5)

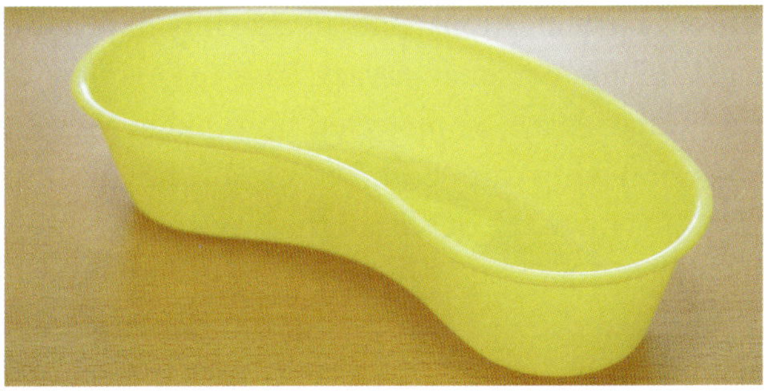

Fig. 7-5. An emesis basin is a kidney-shaped basin often used when giving mouth care.

- Soap dish and soap
- Bath blanket
- Toilet paper
- Personal hygiene items

Overbed table: The overbed table may be used for meals or personal care. It is considered a clean area and must be kept clean and free of clutter (Fig. 7-6). Bedpans, urinals, soiled linen, waste bags, and other contaminated items should not be placed on overbed tables.

Call light: The intercom system is the most common call system used. When the patient presses the button, a light will be seen and/or a bell will be heard at the nurses' station. The call light allows the patient to communicate with staff whenever necessary. It is important for PCTs to always place the call light within the patient's reach and to answer all call lights immediately.

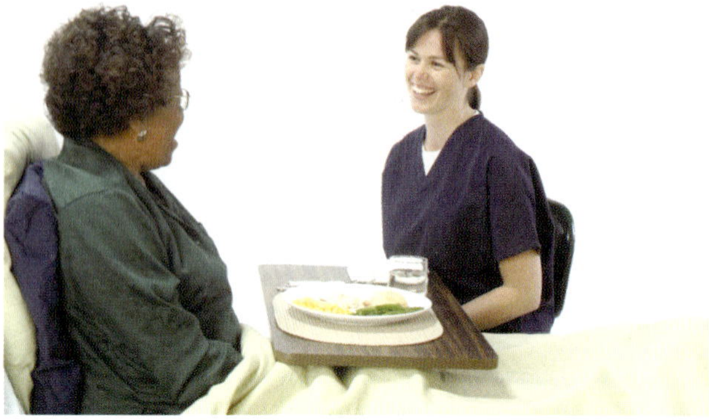

Fig. 7-6. *Overbed tables are often used for patients' meals; they must be kept clean. PCTs should never place bedpans, urinals, or soiled linens on overbed tables.*

Privacy curtain: All patients in a facility have a legal right to personal privacy. This means that they must always be protected from public view when receiving care. Each bed usually has a privacy curtain that extends all the way around the bed (Fig. 7-7). Curtains keep others from seeing a patient undressed or while having care procedures done. To protect each patient's privacy, PCTs must keep this curtain closed when giving care. Although curtains and screens block vision, they do not block sound. PCTs should keep their voices low and not discuss a patient's care near others. Closing the door when possible provides more complete privacy.

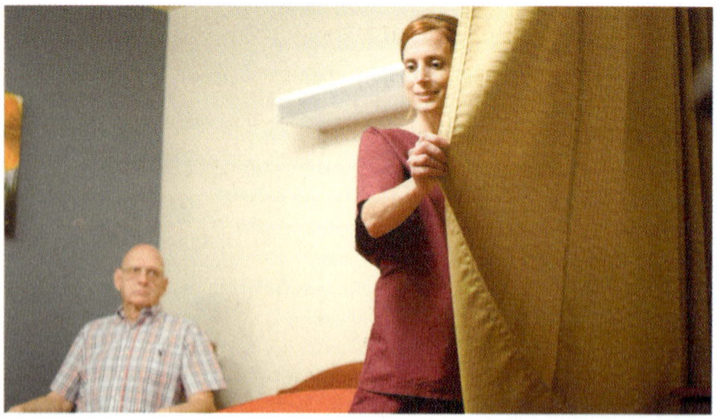

Fig. 7-7. *PCTs should pull the privacy curtain around the bed before giving care.*

There are many types of equipment in a care facility, and PCTs must know how to use and care for all equipment properly. This helps prevent infection and injury. If a PCT does not know how to use a particular piece of equipment, she should ask for assistance. A PCT should not try to use equipment that she does not know how to use.

Equipment that is discarded after one use is called *disposable*, or *single-use*, equipment. Disposable razors and nitrile gloves are examples of this type of equipment. Disposable equipment is used to prevent the spread of microorganisms. PCTs should discard disposable equipment in the proper containers.

Some equipment, such as bedpans, urinals, and basins, needs to be cleaned after each use. When handling this equipment, PCTs must wear gloves so that they do not come into contact with infectious wastes. PCTs may need to clean and disinfect this equipment themselves or place it in the proper area for cleaning.

Guidelines: Patient's Room

- **G** Keep patients' rooms neat and clean. Clean the overbed table after use. Place the table within the patient's reach before leaving.
- **G** Keep the call light within the patient's reach. Check to see that it is within the patient's reach before you leave the room.
- **G** Keep equipment clean and in good condition. If any equipment appears damaged, report it to the nurse and/or file the proper paperwork to get it repaired. Do not use broken or damaged equipment.
- **G** Remove meal trays right after meals. Check to make sure that there are no crumbs in the bed. Straighten bed linens as needed. Change linens if they become wet, soiled, or wrinkled.
- **G** Restock supplies. Make sure the patient has fresh drinking water and a clean cup within reach and is able to lift the pitcher and the cup. Make sure that tissues, paper towels, toilet paper, soap, and other supplies that are used daily are stocked before you leave.

- If trash needs to be emptied or the bathroom needs to be cleaned, notify the housekeeping department. Trash should be emptied at least daily. Remove the trash when you leave the room if cleaning staff is not available.
- Report signs of insects or pests immediately.
- Do not move a patient's belongings or discard any personal items. Respect the patient's things. Ask patients where they want items stored.
- Clean equipment and return it to proper storage. Tidy the area. Providing a clean, safe, and orderly environment is part of your job.

4. Describe how patients may feel when entering a hospital or other inpatient facility

Entering a hospital can be overwhelming. Patients may be experiencing fear, anxiety, loss, and uncertainty, along with the illness or injury being treated. Reactions to serious health problems can also include denial, withdrawal, anger, hostility, and depression. Each person responds to illness and change in their own way. It is important for PCTs to be supportive and encouraging. PCTs should be patient, understanding, and empathetic.

Entering a hospital involves a tremendous loss of independence for a patient, and this can be very difficult. Hospital schedules focus on meeting patients' medical needs. Although measures are taken to promote comfort, it is hard for patients to rest. There is equipment noise in the room and the noise of healthcare workers' activities in and outside the room. In rooms with more than one bed, there are noises from the roommate's care, visitors, and television. Patients who are not able to get out of bed without assistance must use the call light every time they need to use the bathroom or get up for any reason.

PCTs should try to imagine what it would be like to be in a hospital. They should think about the fear patients might feel for their health and well-being. They should also consider the lack of control a patient has over his environment and situation. Allowing patients to make choices is an important way to promote independence and person-centered care. For example, patients are often given menus from which to choose their meals. They may also be able to choose to have visits from religious leaders. Patient choice should be encouraged whenever possible.

Connected Care

Dignity and Independence

Patients have the right to refuse care and to make their own choices. They should not be rushed. Promoting dignity and independence is part of protecting their legal rights. It is also the proper and ethical way for PCTs to work. If an adult patient refuses care, the PCT can gently ask if there are questions or concerns that the PCT, nurse, or provider could address. If the patient still refuses, the PCT should document the refusal and report it to the nurse right away. A child's parent or guardian has a legal right to refuse care. If a child is refusing or resisting care, PCTs must behave with patience and compassion. It is never appropriate to shame, scold, or threaten a patient of any age. Parents/guardians may be able to help a child understand why care is needed.

The loss of a familiar environment or the loss of control can be upsetting. A new patient may cry or may yell at healthcare workers. He may want to talk and ask questions. However a patient responds, PCTs should remain calm and professional. They should answer patients' questions honestly, within their scope of practice, or get answers from a nurse or provider. They should respond to call lights and requests.

PCTs play an important role in helping patients feel as comfortable as they can in a facility. By giving emotional support such as listening, as well as being compassionate and helpful, PCTs can help patients adjust to being in the hospital. This can help promote healing and recovery.

Connected Care

LGBTQ Patients

Entering a hospital can be especially difficult for patients who are lesbian, gay, bisexual, transgender, or queer (LGBTQ). In addition to the challenges all patients face when dealing with illness, these patients may fear that they will not be treated with dignity and acceptance.

In addition, paperwork, such as the admission form, is often written with the assumption that a patient is straight and cisgender (that their gender identity is the same as their birth sex). There may be no way to indicate on the form if the patient is nonbinary or if a spouse or partner is nonbinary or is of the same gender as the patient. All healthcare workers should make every effort to make all patients feel comfortable and welcome. They should use the name and pronouns a patient wants them to use. If the patient's preferred name is not the same as the name that is in the patient's medical record, the name in the medical record must be used for identification purposes, but the preferred name should be used at all other times. PCTs should greet and welcome patients' loved ones and spouses without bias.

5. Explain the patient care technician's role in admission, transfer, and discharge

During a planned hospital admission, the patient is first directed to the admitting office. Paperwork is signed. The admission staff member makes copies of insurance information, Medicare cards, and identifying information. Both parties sign an agreement or contract agreeing to the services provided. This may include acknowledging an estimated cost (as in the case of a planned surgery). Consent forms may also be signed at this time, both general consent for routine care a patient may receive and informed consent for any planned procedures. Emergency contact information and names of doctors are obtained. The Patient Self-Determination Act (PSDA) requires staff to explain information about advance directives and to find out whether the patient has advance directives in place or wants to create them. A copy of the patient's legal rights is given to the new patient and his family. The rights are explained in language the patient can understand. The patient also receives and acknowledges the hospital's notification of privacy practices. This form describes how patients' protected health information is handled to maintain confidentiality.

Before being taken to her room, a wristband is placed on the patient. It is usually printed with the patient's full name and date of birth. It may also show the name of a provider who will be overseeing the patient's care. Some wristbands have barcodes that can be scanned to open the patient's medical record.

If a patient is admitted to the hospital from the emergency room, all of these administrative processes still must happen. They may happen in the admitting office if the patient is well enough to be taken there. They may also happen in the emergency department or in a patient's room. In some cases, a family member or other designated legal representative may complete the paperwork for the patient.

PCTs often help with patient admission after paperwork has been completed. The PCT should try to make sure the patient has a positive impression of her and her facility. PCTs can explain what to expect during the process and answer any questions that are within their scope of practice. If a new patient has questions that a PCT cannot answer, she should find the nurse.

Each facility will have a procedure for admitting patients. These general guidelines will help make the experience successful:

Guidelines: Admission

G Prepare the room before the patient arrives. Make sure the bed is made and the room is tidy. If you know that the patient needs any special equipment, be sure it is in the room and ready for use. Restock supplies that are low. Make sure there is an admission kit available if used. Admission kits often contain personal care items, such as a bath basin, an emesis basin, a water pitcher and cup, toothpaste, soap, a comb, lotion, and tissues (Fig. 7-8). Admission kits may also contain a urine specimen cup, label, and transport bag.

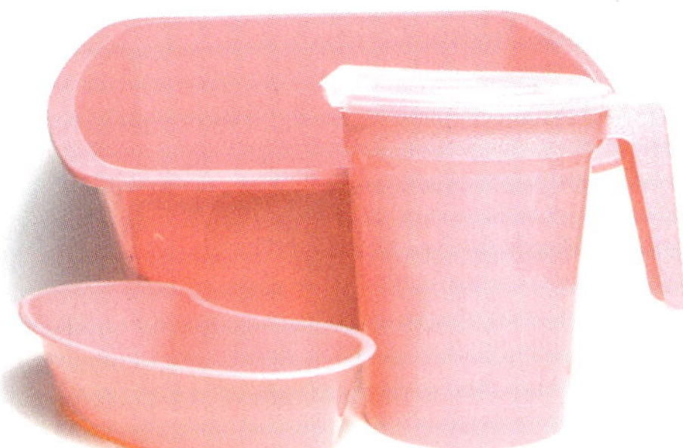

***Fig. 7-8.** An admission kit is usually placed in a patient's room before she is admitted. It may contain personal care items that the patient will need.*

- **G** Be alert to a new patient's condition. Is she using a wheelchair, is she on a stretcher, or is she walking? If you know that the patient will be arriving on a stretcher, the bed should be in its highest position. If the patient will be walking or in a wheelchair, the bed should be in its lowest position. Is anyone with the patient? Observe the patient for level of consciousness and signs of confusion. A patient who is admitted from the ED may already be receiving medications or other care. Note any tubes she has, such as IVs or catheters.
- **G** Introduce yourself and state your position. Smile and be friendly. Always call an adult patient by their formal name until they tell you what they want to be called.
- **G** Never rush the process or the new patient. The patient should not feel like she is an inconvenience.
- **G** If a patient has brought any personal items with her, handle them with care and respect. Facilities may have inventory forms to complete showing what the patient brought with her. Some items may be stored in bags marked specifically for personal belongings.

  Facilities discourage patients from keeping valuables or money with them. If the patient has valuables or money, however, offer to have them safely stored according to your facility's policy. If she refuses, follow the procedure to write an inventory and get the necessary signatures.
- **G** Give the patient a hospital gown and nonslip socks (or other clothing used at your facility). Show the patient how to put on the gown, including how to tie or snap it. Help the patient as needed, while providing privacy. Show the patient where to store her clothing.
- **G** Orient the patient and any family members/visitors to the room and the facility. Review processes for ordering meals and tell visitors where the cafeteria is and when it is open. Describe the location of waiting rooms/lounges, vending machines, gift shops, and rooms for prayer, meditation, or reflection.
- **G** Tell the patient who is taking care of them and for how long (i.e., when the shift ends). Many facilities have whiteboards in patients' rooms to help with orientation (Fig. 7-9). They show the date, the names of healthcare workers caring for the patient, and may also show any scheduled testing or appointments for the day. The information is changed with each shift and at other times as needed. Some of these boards are "smart" boards that are linked to patient records and can be updated automatically.

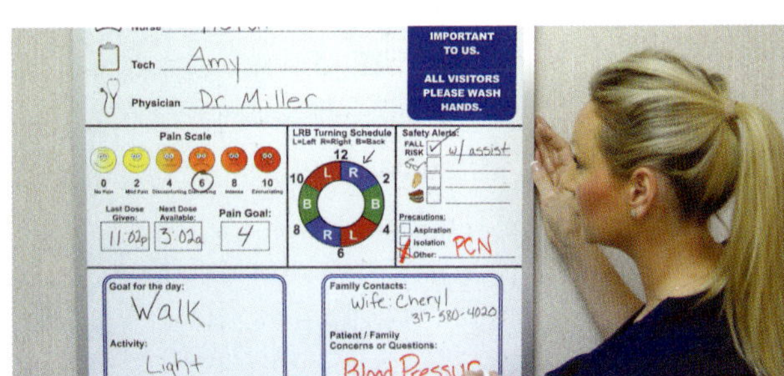

***Fig. 7-9.** A whiteboard in a patient's room shows the date, the names of healthcare workers caring for the patient, and may also show tests to be done or other information.* (IMAGE COURTESY OF MAGNETIC CONCEPTS © 2023, WWW.MAGNETICCONCEPTS.COM)

G If the patient is a child, encourage exploration as much as possible. Tell the child and any adults what equipment can or cannot be touched. Using language that is right for the age of the child, answer any questions that are within your scope of practice. Describe what any machines do (e.g., "These wires hook the stickers on your chest to this machine. It shows us how your heart is beating.") Explain noises they may hear, such as beeps or alarms.

G Admission is a stressful time. Observe the patient, as she could have a problem or issue that is missed during the process of arriving, completing paperwork, and settling in to the room. It is important to observe the new patient's condition in order to recognize any changes that may take place later. Report to the nurse if you notice any of the following:

- Disconnected tubing
- Patient seems confused, combative, and/or unaware of surroundings
- Patient is having difficulty breathing, pain, or shows any other signs of distress
- Patient has bruises or wounds
- Patient has missed a meal during the admission process
- Patient has medications, hearing aids, eyeglasses, or dentures

G Follow facility policy about any other required tasks during the admission process.

Connected Care

Admission

Most states have laws requiring that patients be told of their legal rights at admission. They must be provided with a written copy of these rights. This includes rights about privacy, consent, and receiving information in a language the patient can understand. Patients must also be provided with information about their rights related to advance directives.

Admitting a patient

Equipment: gloves, vital signs equipment, gown and socks or other facility-issued clothing

1. Identify yourself by name. Identify the patient according to facility policy.
2. Wash your hands.
3. Explain the procedure to the patient. Speak clearly, slowly, and directly. Maintain face-to-face contact whenever possible.
4. Provide for the patient's privacy with a curtain, screen, or door (Fig. 7-10). If the family is present, ask them to step outside until the admission process is over if an adult patient prefers. Some patients may find it reassuring to have family members stay. If family members leave the room, show them where they can wait, and let them know approximately how long the process will take.

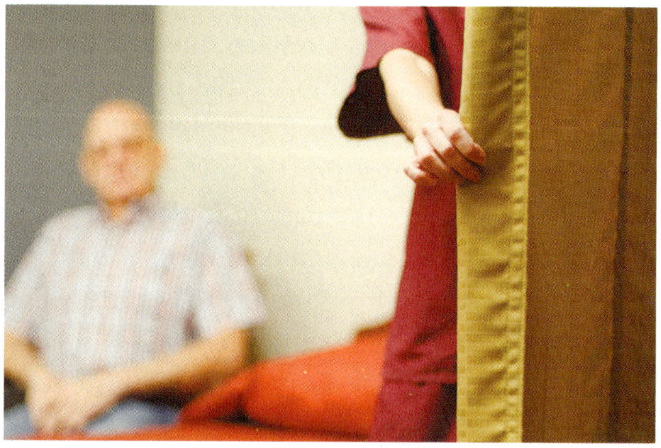

Fig. 7-10. *All patients have a legal right to privacy, and providing privacy is part of doing your job professionally. Your professional, respectful behavior can help put a new patient at ease.*

5. Give the patient his gown and socks. Explain how to put the gown on and provide privacy while he changes. Assist as needed.
6. If part of facility policy, do these things:

- Measure the patient's height and weight (see procedures that follow).

- Measure the patient's baseline vital signs (see Chapter 10). **Baseline** signs are initial values that can then be compared to future measurements.
- Obtain a urine specimen if required (see Chapter 17).
- Help the patient put personal items away. Make an inventory of personal items if part of facility policy.
- Provide fresh water (and ice if requested). Providing fresh water is something you should do every time you leave a patient's room, unless he is on a fluid restriction. Doing this helps prevent dehydration. Make sure the pitcher and cup are light enough for the patient to lift.

7. Show the patient the room and bathroom. Explain how to work the bed controls and the call light. Show the patient the telephone, lights, and television controls. Help as needed to plug in phone, computer, and other equipment chargers.
8. Use the whiteboard or other communication system in the patient's room to show the patient who will be caring for him. Tell him when shifts will change. Show him how and where to find important information on the board.
9. Make sure the patient is comfortable. Remove privacy measures. Bring the family back in if they were outside the room.
10. Place the call light within the patient's reach.
11. Wash your hands.
12. Document the procedure using facility guidelines.

Patients who need more or less care than they are receiving are often transferred to a unit or facility that can better meet their needs. Staff should make the transfer as smooth as possible for the patient. A patient should be informed of the transfer as soon as possible. A nurse or provider will inform the patient about the transfer, and should explain how, where, when, and why the transfer will occur. Any questions the patient has should be answered. The unit or facility that will be receiving the patient must also be informed. This allows them to be ready to welcome and care for the patient.

PCTs help patients gather their personal items before transferring. Patients may worry about losing their belongings. PCTs can reassure them by involving them in the process. For example, the PCT can let the patient see the empty closet, drawers, etc. If facility policy allows, the patient can carry the bag containing their belongings as they are transferred.

The patient may be transferred in a bed, stretcher, or wheelchair. Infants are usually transferred in wheeled bassinets or enclosed incubators. If the transfer is to a new facility or building, an adult patient may be transferred by stretcher and transported in an ambulance. If the patient is transferred to a new room in the same facility, the PCT should introduce her to any healthcare workers who will be caring for her. This can help make the patient feel welcome, settled, and comfortable.

Transferring a patient

Equipment: may include a wheelchair, bag for belongings, any of the patient's personal care items and packed personal items that will be transferred with the patient

1. Identify yourself by name. Identify the patient according to facility policy.
2. Wash your hands.
3. Explain the procedure to the patient. Speak clearly, slowly, and directly. Maintain face-to-face contact whenever possible.
4. Collect the patient's clothing and any personal belongings in a bag.

5. Help the patient into the wheelchair (or stretcher if one is used). Take him to the proper area. If the patient is transferring to a different building or facility, stay with the patient until staff involved in the transfer have taken control. Steps 6 through 11 apply to transfers within the same facility.
6. Follow facility policy for handing off care of the patient to staff in the new unit. Introduce healthcare workers who will be caring for the patient if possible.
7. Help the patient to put personal items away.
8. Make sure that the patient is comfortable.
9. Place the call light within the patient's reach.
10. Wash your hands.
11. Report any changes in the patient to the nurse in the new unit.
12. Document the procedure using facility guidelines.

To discharge a patient from a facility, a doctor must give the discharge order. The nurse then completes instructions for the patient to follow after discharge. The nurse will review these instructions and important information with the patient and any family members or other visitors who are helping the patient. Some of the following areas may be discussed:

- Future doctor or physical, speech, and occupational therapy appointments
- Home care, skilled nursing care
- Medications
- Ambulation instructions
- Medical equipment needed
- Medical transportation
- Any restrictions on activities
- Special exercises to keep the patient functioning at the highest level (Fig. 7-11)

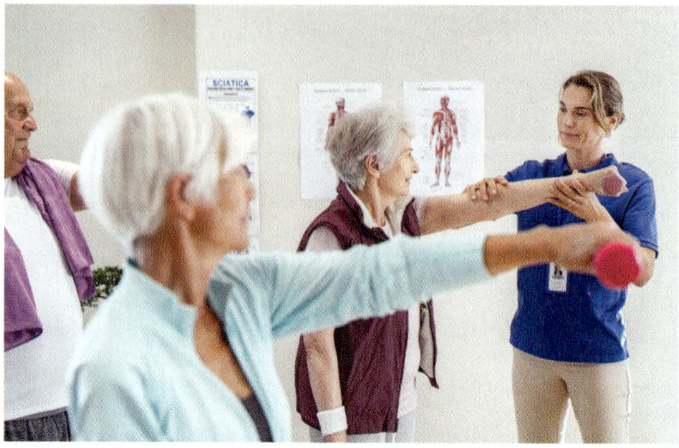

Fig. 7-11. *When a patient is discharged, she may receive instructions to exercise.*

- Special nutrition or dietary requirements
- Community resources

PCTs help by collecting the patient's belongings and personal care items and packing them carefully. Final vital sign measurements may be taken. The PCT may also be assigned to remove IVs or other tubes from the patient's body. (More information about removing IVs is in Chapter 22.) The patient may need help with bathing, personal hygiene, or changing from gown to clothes. The PCT should know what the patient's condition is at the time of discharge and find out whether the patient will be using a wheelchair or stretcher. If the patient is discharged close to a meal time, it may be possible to arrange for an early meal.

Discharge is often a happy time for patients who are going home. However, some patients may experience uncertainty or fear about leaving the facility. They may worry that they are not ready to be away from the regular medical care they have received. PCTs can help by being positive and reassuring. They can remind patients that their doctors believe they are ready to leave. However, if a patient has specific questions about care, the PCT should inform the nurse.

Discharging a patient

Equipment: may include a wheelchair, bag for belongings, discharge paperwork, the patient's care items, vital signs equipment

1. Identify yourself by name. Identify the patient according to facility policy.
2. Wash your hands.
3. Explain the procedure to the patient. Speak clearly, slowly, and directly. Maintain face-to-face contact whenever possible.
4. Provide for the patient's privacy with a curtain, screen, or door.
5. Measure the patient's vital signs.
6. Remove and properly discard EKG electrodes, IV needle and tubing, and any other equipment as assigned.
7. Put the personal items to be taken into the bag.
8. Help the patient dress and then into the wheelchair or onto the stretcher if used.
9. Help the patient if he wants to say goodbye to staff or other patients.
10. If assigned to do so, take the patient to the pick-up area. Help him into the vehicle. You are responsible for the patient until he is safely in the vehicle and the door is closed. If the patient is an infant or small child, there may be facility policy and/or state laws about child seats that the PCT must follow. Infants and small children should only be transported in a vehicle with an appropriate seat that is properly installed.
11. Wash your hands.
12. Document the procedure using facility guidelines. Information may include the following:

- The patient's vital signs at discharge
- Time of discharge
- Method of transport
- Who was with the patient
- What items the patient took with him (using your facility's inventory checklist if this is part of facility policy)

Connected Care

Privacy during Discharges

It is important for PCTs to always provide privacy for patients. The PCT should close the door before talking about medical matters or other private things. He should pull the privacy curtain before the patient changes clothes or is bathed prior to the transfer or discharge.

6. Explain the importance of sleep and factors affecting sleep

Sleep is a natural period of rest for the mind and body. As a person sleeps, the mind and body's energy is restored. During sleep, vital functions are performed. These include repairing and renewing cells, processing information, and organizing memory. Sleep is essential to a person's health and well-being.

The circadian rhythm is an important factor in determining sleep patterns of humans. The **circadian rhythm** is the 24-hour day-night cycle. It also affects body temperature and hormone production, among other things.

When a person is sleep-deprived or suffers from **insomnia** (inability to fall asleep or remain asleep) or other sleep disorders, problems result. These include decreased mental function, reduced reaction time, and irritability. Sleep deprivation also decreases immune system function.

It can be very hard for patients in a hospital to fall asleep and stay asleep. Many factors can affect patients' sleep, such as fear, anxiety, stress, noise, diet, medications, and illness. Sharing a room with another person can also disturb sleep, as can hearing staff care for other patients or talk in the hallways or at a nurses' station. Hospital patients may be awakened to take medications or check vital signs. All of these factors can contribute to serious sleep deprivation. It may even cause temporary cognitive difficulties. It is important for PCTs to do what they can to promote rest and sleep.

Observing and Reporting: Sleep Issues

When a patient mentions that he is not sleeping well, observe and report the following:

- O/R Eating or drinking items that contain too much caffeine late in the day
- O/R Patient reports of side effects from new medications
- O/R Having the TV, radio, computer, phone, or light on late at night (or roommate doing the same)
- O/R Experiencing pain
- O/R Alarms sounding often in the patient's room or nearby
- O/R Patient reports excessive noise from hallways, nurses' station, etc.

7. Describe bedmaking guidelines and perform proper bedmaking

Some patients spend much or all of their time in bed at an inpatient facility. Careful bedmaking is essential for comfort, cleanliness, and health. It is one way a PCT can improve the quality of patients' rest. Linens should always be changed after personal care, such as after a bed bath. They should also be changed any time bedding or sheets are damp, soiled, or in need of straightening. Bed linens should be changed often for these reasons:

- Sheets that are damp, wrinkled, or bunched up are uncomfortable. They may keep the patient from sleeping well. They can also cause skin breakdown.
- Microorganisms thrive in moist, warm places. Bedding that is damp or unclean may cause infection and disease.
- Patients who spend long hours in bed are at risk for pressure injuries. Sheets that do not lie flat increase this risk by cutting off circulation.

Guidelines: Bedmaking

- G Keep linens wrinkle-free and tidy. Change linen whenever it is wet, damp, wrinkled, or dirty.
- G Wash your hands before handling clean linen (Fig. 7-12).

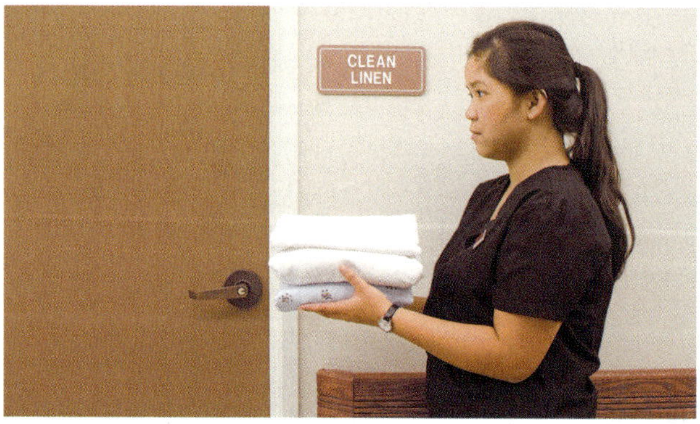

Fig. 7-12. *Make sure you have washed your hands before gathering clean linen.*

- G Place clean linen on a clean surface within reach, such as a bedside stand, overbed table, or chair. Do not place clean linen on the floor or on a contaminated area.
- G Don (put on) gloves before removing bed linen from the bed.
- G Look for personal items, such as phones, tablets, dentures, hearing aids, jewelry, and eyeglasses, before removing linen.
- G When removing linen, fold or roll linen so that the dirtiest area is inside. Rolling puts the dirtiest surface of the linen inward. This lessens contamination.

G Do not shake linen or clothes. It may spread airborne contaminants.

G Bag soiled linen at the point of origin. Do not take it to other patients' rooms.

G Sort soiled linen away from patient care areas.

G Place wet linen in leakproof bags.

G Wear gloves when handling soiled linen. Hold soiled linen away from your body. Place it in the proper container or area immediately. If dirty linen touches your uniform, your uniform becomes contaminated.

G Change disposable bed protectors whenever they become soiled or wet. Discard them in the proper container. Put a clean bed protector on the bed when you change linen.

If a patient cannot get out of bed, a PCT must change the linens with the patient in bed. An **occupied bed** is a bed made while the patient is still in the bed. When making the bed, the PCT should use a wide stance and bend her knees. Bending from the waist should be avoided, especially when tucking sheets under the mattress. The height of the bed should be raised to make the job easier and safer.

Making an occupied bed

Equipment: clean linen—mattress pad, fitted or flat bottom sheet, disposable bed protector (if needed), cotton draw sheet, flat top sheet, blanket(s), bath blanket, pillowcase(s); gloves

1. Identify yourself by name. Identify the patient according to facility policy.
2. Wash your hands.
3. Explain the procedure to the patient. Speak clearly, slowly, and directly. Maintain face-to-face contact whenever possible.
4. Provide for the patient's privacy with a curtain, screen, or door.
5. Place clean linen on a clean surface within reach (e.g., bedside stand, overbed table, or chair).
6. Adjust the bed to a safe level, usually waist high. Lower the head of the bed. Lock the bed wheels.
7. Put on gloves.
8. Loosen top linen from the end of the bed on the working side.
9. Unfold the bath blanket over the top sheet to cover the patient. Remove the top sheet. Keep the patient covered at all times with the bath blanket. Be aware of any tubing, such as from an IV line or catheter, and take care not to dislodge it.
10. You will make the bed one side at a time. Raise the far side rail. Then go to the other side of the bed. Help the patient to turn onto her side, toward the raised side rail.
11. Loosen the bottom soiled linen, mattress pad, and protector, if present, on the working side.
12. Roll the bottom soiled linen toward the patient, soiled side inside. Tuck it snugly against the patient's back.
13. Place the mattress pad (if used) on the bed, attaching elastic at corners on the working side.
14. Place and tuck in the clean bottom linen. If a flat sheet is used, leave enough overlap on each end to tuck under the mattress. Make hospital corners to keep the bottom sheet wrinkle-free (Fig. 7-13). If a fitted sheet is used, tightly pull the 2 fitted corners on the working side. Finish with the bottom sheet free of wrinkles.
15. Smooth the bottom sheet out toward the patient. Be sure there are no wrinkles in the mattress pad. Roll the extra material toward the patient. Tuck it under the patient's body (Fig. 7-14).

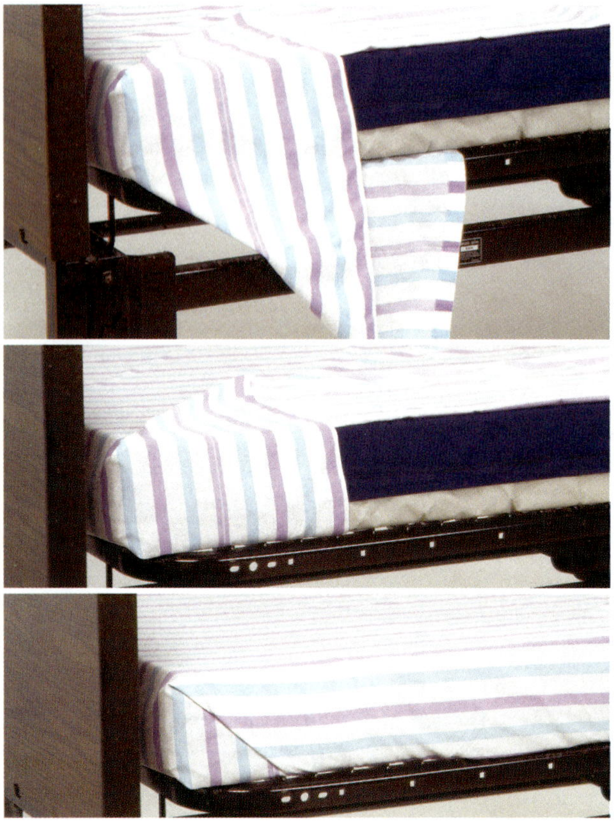

Fig. 7-13. *Hospital corners help keep the flat sheet smooth under the patient.*

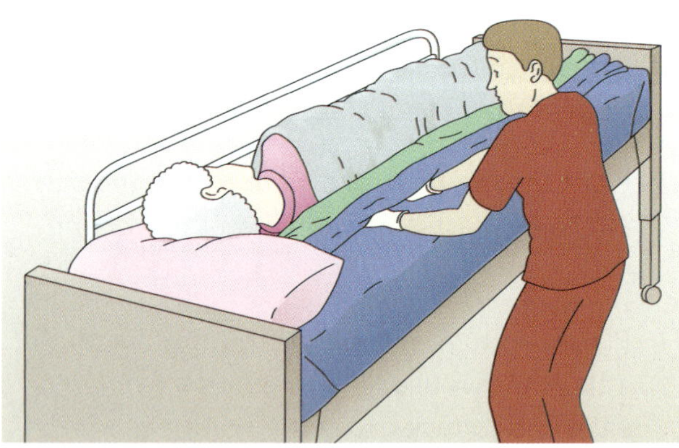

Fig. 7-14. *Tuck extra material under the patient's body.*

16. If using a disposable bed protector, unfold it and center it on the bed. Tuck the side near you under the mattress. Smooth it out toward the patient. Tuck as you did with the sheet.

17. If using a draw sheet, place it on the bed. Tuck in on your side, smooth, and tuck as you did with the other bedding.

18. Raise the side rail nearest you. Go to the other side of the bed and lower that side rail. Help the patient roll or turn onto the clean bottom sheet, toward the raised side rail. Protect the patient from any soiled matter on the old linens.

19. Loosen the soiled linen. Check for any personal items. Roll the linen from the head to the foot of the bed. Avoid contact with your skin or clothes. Place it in a hamper or bag. Do not put it on the floor or furniture. Do not shake it. Soiled linens are full of microorganisms that should not be spread to other parts of the room.

20. Pull the clean linen through as quickly as possible. Start with the mattress pad and wrap it around corners. Pull and tuck in the clean bottom linen just like the other side. Pull and tuck in the bed protector and draw sheet (if used). Make hospital corners with the bottom sheet. Finish with bottom sheet free of wrinkles.

21. Ask the patient to turn onto her back. Help as needed. Keep the patient covered and comfortable, with a pillow under her head. Raise the side rail nearest you.

22. Unfold the top sheet. Place it over the patient and center it. Ask the patient to hold the top sheet. Slip the bath blanket out from underneath (Fig. 7-15). Put it in the hamper or bag.

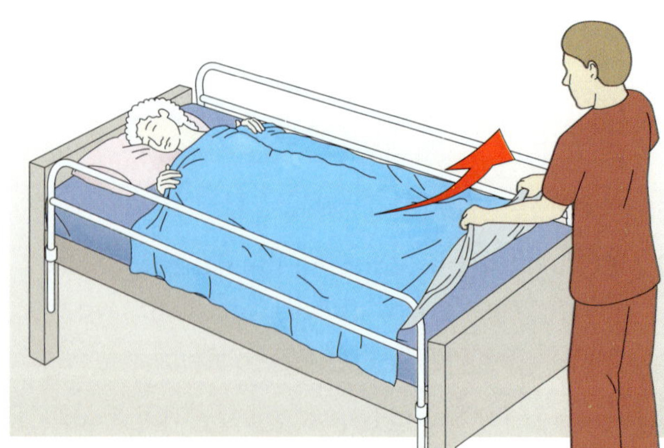

Fig. 7-15. *With the patient holding on to the top sheet, pull the bath blanket out.*

23. Place a blanket over the top sheet. Match the top edges. Tuck the bottom edges of the top sheet and blanket under the foot of the bed. Make hospital corners on each side. Loosen the top linens over the patient's feet. At the head of the bed, fold the top sheet over the blanket about 6 inches.
24. Remove the pillow. Do not hold it near your face. Remove the soiled pillowcase by turning it inside out. Place it in the hamper or bag.
25. Remove and discard your gloves. Wash your hands.
26. With one hand, grasp the clean pillowcase at the closed end. Turn it inside out over your arm. Next, using the same hand that has the pillowcase over it, grasp the center of the end of the pillow. Pull the pillowcase over it with your free hand (Fig. 7-16). Do the same for any other pillows. Place them under the patient's head with the open end away from the door.

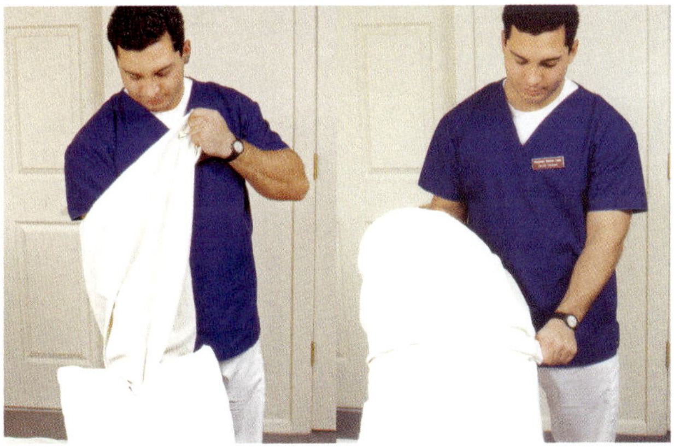

Fig. 7-16. *After the pillowcase is turned inside out over your arm, grasp the center of the end of the pillow. Pull the pillowcase over the pillow.*

27. Make the patient comfortable.
28. Return the bed to its lowest position. Leave the side rails in the ordered position.
29. Place the call light within the patient's reach.
30. Take the laundry bag or hamper to the proper area.
31. Wash your hands.
32. Report any changes in patient to the nurse.
33. Document the procedure using facility guidelines.

Mattresses can be heavy. It is easier to make an empty bed than one with a patient in it. An **unoccupied bed** is a bed made while no patient is in the bed. If the patient can be moved, the PCT's job will be easier.

Making an unoccupied bed

Equipment: clean linen—mattress pad, fitted or flat bottom sheet, disposable bed protector (if needed), blanket(s), cotton draw sheet, flat top sheet, pillowcase(s); gloves

1. Wash your hands.
2. Place clean linen on a clean surface within reach (e.g., bedside stand, overbed table, or chair).
3. Adjust the bed to a safe level, usually waist high. Put the bed in its flattest position. Lock the bed wheels.
4. Put on gloves.
5. Loosen the soiled linen. Roll it (soiled side inside) from the head to the foot of the bed. Avoid contact with your skin or clothes. Place it in a hamper or bag. Do not put it on the floor or furniture. Do not shake it. Remove pillows and pillowcases and place pillowcases in the hamper or bag.
6. Remove and discard your gloves. Wash your hands.
7. Remake the bed. Place the mattress pad (if used) on the bed, attaching elastic at corners on the working side. If a flat sheet is used, leave enough overlap on each end to tuck under the mattress. Make hospital corners to keep the bottom sheet wrinkle-free. If a fitted sheet is used, tightly pull the 2 fitted corners on the working side. Finish with the bottom

sheet free of wrinkles. Put on the disposable bed protector and draw sheet (if used), smooth, and tuck under the sides of the bed.

8. Place the top sheet and blanket over the bed. Center these, tuck under the foot of the bed, and make hospital corners on each side. Fold down the top sheet over the blanket about 6 inches. Fold both the top sheet and blanket down (open bed) so the patient can easily get into bed. If the patient will not be returning to bed immediately, leave the bedding up (closed bed).
9. Put on clean pillowcases. Replace the pillows.
10. Return the bed to its lowest position.
11. Take the laundry bag or hamper to the proper area.
12. Wash your hands.
13. Document the procedure using facility guidelines.

A **surgical bed** is made to accept patients who are returning to bed on stretchers, or gurneys. These patients may be returning from surgery or testing. A surgical bed is opened to receive patients by loosening the linens on one side and folding them to the other side. This leaves one side open.

Making a surgical bed

Equipment: clean linen, gloves

1. Wash your hands.
2. Place clean linen on a clean surface within reach (e.g., bedside stand, overbed table, or chair).
3. Adjust the bed to a safe level, usually waist high. Lock the bed wheels.
4. Put on gloves.
5. Remove all soiled linen, rolling it (soiled side inside) from the head to the foot of the bed. Avoid contact with your skin or clothes. Do not shake soiled linen. Place it in a hamper or bag.
6. Remove and discard your gloves. Wash your hands.
7. Make an unoccupied bed, but do not fold the sheet and blanket down. See previous procedure: *Making an unoccupied bed.*
8. Loosen linens on the side of the bed that is closer to the door (where the stretcher will be).
9. Fanfold linens lengthwise to the side away from the door (Fig. 7-17). Fanfolded means folded several times into pleats.

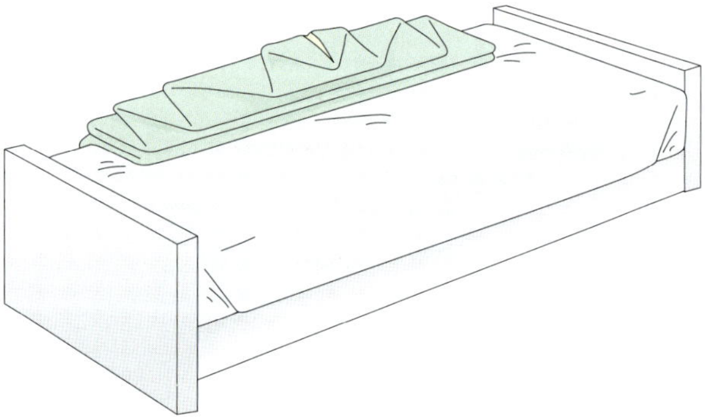

Fig. 7-17. *Fanfold the linen so that it is in pleated layers and position linen opposite the stretcher side of the bed.*

10. Put on clean pillowcases. Replace the pillows.
11. Leave the bed in its locked position with both side rails down.
12. Make sure the pathway to the bed is clear.
13. Take the laundry bag or hamper to the proper area.
14. Wash your hands.
15. Document the procedure using facility guidelines.

Chapter Review

1. List 6 units in a typical hospital. For each unit, give an example of a patient who might be treated in that unit.
2. What are 3 ways that PCTs can keep the noise level low in facilities?
3. What are 3 ways that PCTs can help control odors in facilities?
4. Where should call lights always be placed?
5. How do privacy curtains help protect patients' privacy?
6. What is disposable equipment? Why is it used?
7. List 8 guidelines for PCTs to follow to help patients during the admission process.
8. Name a type of equipment the PCT may use during an in-house transfer of a patient.
9. List 5 types of information that the nurse may cover with the patient and her family and friends during the discharge process.
10. List 2 functions that sleep performs for the body.
11. What problems can result from a lack of sleep?
12. When should bed linens be changed?
13. List 3 reasons why it is important to change bed linens frequently.
14. Which way should pillows face while under patients' heads?

8 Positioning, Transfers, and Ambulation

1. Explain positioning and describe how to safely position patients

Patients in a hospital spend a lot of time in bed. They may need help getting into comfortable positions. They also need to change positions periodically to avoid muscle stiffness and skin breakdown. Too much pressure on one area for too long can cause a decrease in circulation, which can lead to pressure injuries and other problems like muscle contractures. (Chapter 12 contains information about pressure injuries.)

Positioning means helping patients into positions that promote comfort and health. Bedbound patients should be repositioned at least every 2 hours. Patients in wheelchairs or chairs should be repositioned at least every hour. Each time there is a change of position, the PCT should document the position and the time.

The position used depends on the diagnosis, the condition, and the patient's preference. The care plan will give specific instructions. It is important that even immobile patients not remain in the same position for long. They should be checked regularly. When positioning patients, PCTs must use proper body mechanics to help prevent injury. They must be aware of surgical/wound drains and any other tubing the patient has. PCTs should also check the skin for any discoloration or warm spots, especially around bony areas, each time they reposition patients.

The following are guidelines for positioning patients in the 5 basic body positions:

Supine: In this position, the patient lies flat on her back. To maintain correct body position, the head and shoulders should be supported with a pillow (Fig. 8-1). Pillows, rolled towels, or washcloths can also be used to support her arms (especially a weak or immobilized arm) or hands. A pillow should be placed under the calves so the heels are elevated ("floating") and do not touch the bed. Pillows or a footboard (padded board placed against the patient's feet) can keep the feet positioned properly.

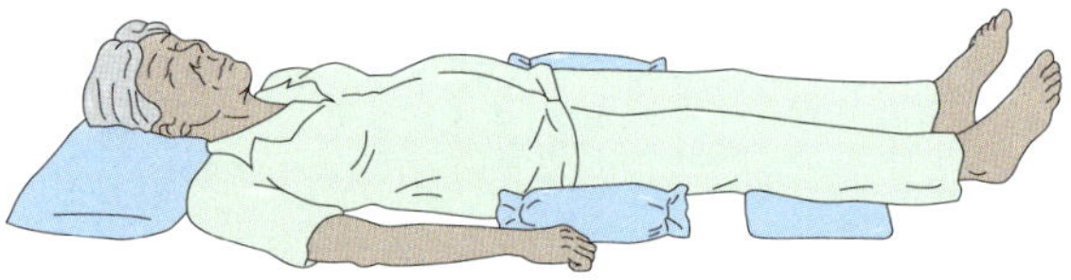

Fig. 8-1. A person in the supine position is lying flat on her back.

Lateral/side: A patient in the lateral position is lying on either side (Fig. 8-2). There are many variations of this position. Pillows can support the arm and leg on the upper side, the back, and the head. Ideally, the knee on the upper side of the body should be flexed. The leg is brought in front of the body and supported on a pillow. There should be a pillow under the bottom foot so that the toes and ankles are not touching the bed. If the top leg cannot be brought forward, it should be placed slightly behind the bottom leg, not resting directly on it. Pillows should be used between the 2 legs and ankles to relieve pressure and avoid skin breakdown.

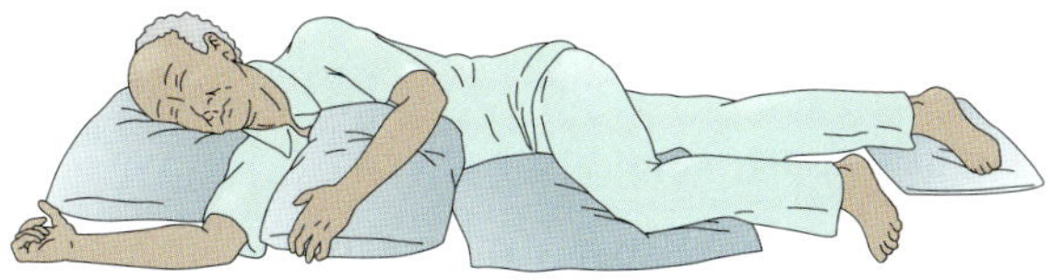

Fig. 8-2. A person in the lateral position is lying on his side.

Prone: A patient in the prone position is lying on the stomach, or front side of the body (Fig. 8-3). This is not comfortable for many people, especially elderly people. A PCT should not leave a patient in the prone position for very long and should check the care plan before using this position. In the prone position, the arms are either placed at the sides or raised above the head, or one is raised and one is by the side. The head is turned to one side and a small pillow may be used under the head and legs. A pillow under the legs helps keep the feet from touching the bed.

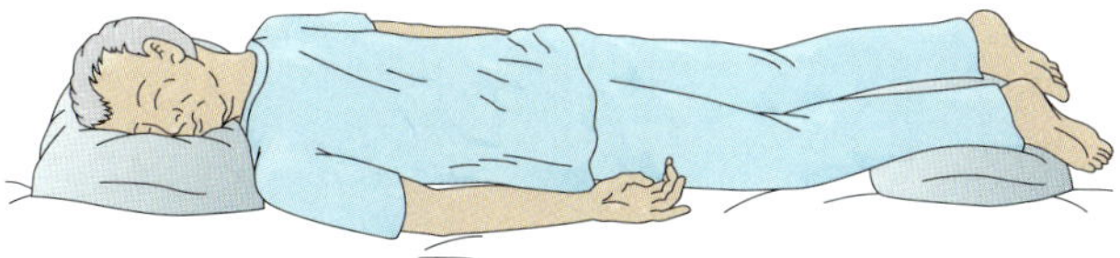

Fig. 8-3. A person in the prone position is lying on his stomach.

Fowler's: A patient in the Fowler's position is in a semisitting position (45 to 60 degrees) (Fig. 8-4). The head and shoulders are elevated. The patient's knees may be flexed and elevated, using a pillow or rolled blanket as a support. The feet may be supported using a footboard or other support. The spine should be straight. In a high-Fowler's position, the upper body is sitting nearly straight up (60 to 90 degrees). In a semi-Fowler's position, the upper body is not raised as high (30 to 45 degrees). In a low-Fowler's position, the body is raised 15 to 30 degrees.

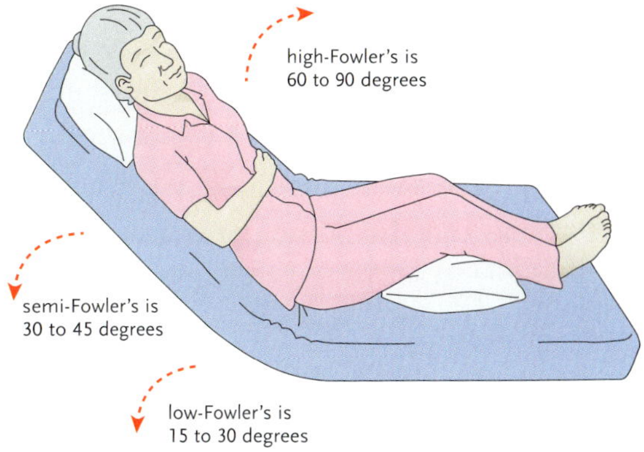

Fig. 8-4. A person in the Fowler's position is partially reclined.

Sims': The Sims' position is a left side-lying position (Fig. 8-5). The lower arm is behind the back, and the upper knee is flexed and raised toward the chest, using a pillow as support. There should be a pillow under the bottom foot so that the toes and ankle do not touch the bed.

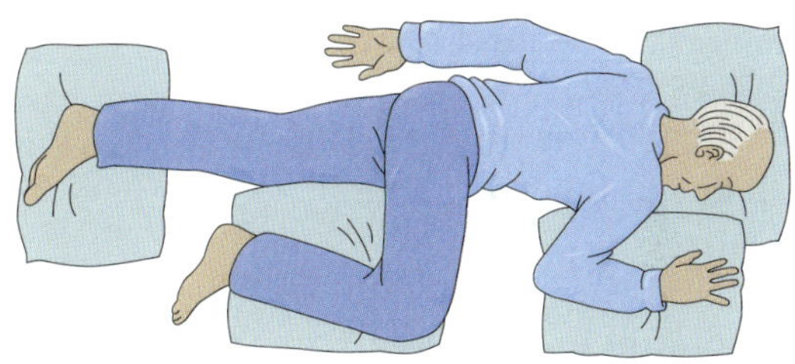

Fig. 8-5. A person in the Sims' position is lying on his left side with one leg drawn up.

Bed Positions

PCTs may be asked to position electric beds in specific positions. To position the bed in the Fowler's position, the head of the bed should be raised 45 to 60 degrees. For semi-Fowler's the head of the bed should be raised 30 to 45 degrees. For low-Fowler's, it should be raised 15 to 30 degrees.

Helping a patient move up in bed helps prevent skin irritation that can lead to pressure injuries. A PCT should get help if she thinks it is not safe to move the patient by herself. A draw sheet, turning sheet, transfer sheet, or glide sheet should be used (Fig. 8-6). A **draw sheet** is an extra sheet placed on top of the bottom sheet when the bed is made. Draw sheets help prevent skin damage caused by shearing. **Shearing** is rubbing or friction that results from the skin moving one way and the bone underneath it remaining fixed or moving in the opposite direction. The draw sheet should lie flat under the patient's body and should not be wrinkled.

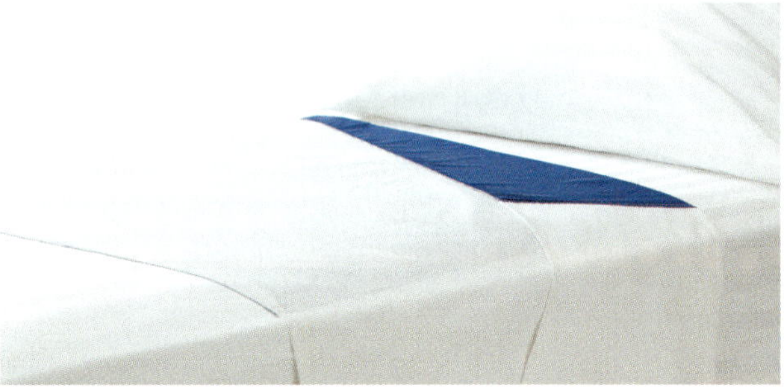

Fig. 8-6. *There are different types of devices used for positioning and transferring. This photo shows a glide sheet that needs to be removed after repositioning.* (IMAGE COURTESY OF MEDLINE INDUSTRIES, LP. USED WITH PERMISSION.)

Moving a patient up in bed

Equipment: draw sheet or other device

When the patient can help you move her up in bed, take the following steps:

1. Identify yourself by name. Identify the patient according to facility policy.
2. Wash your hands.
3. Explain the procedure to the patient. Speak clearly, slowly, and directly. Maintain face-to-face contact whenever possible.
4. Provide for the patient's privacy with a curtain, screen, or door.
5. Adjust the bed to a safe level, usually waist high. Lock the bed wheels (Fig. 8-7).

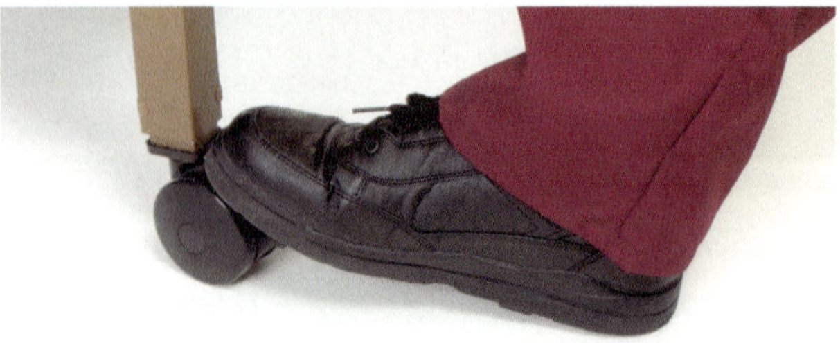

Fig. 8-7. *Always lock bed wheels before positioning or transferring a patient.*

6. Lower the head of the bed to make it flat. Move the pillow to the head of the bed.
7. If the bed has side rails, raise the rail on the far side of the bed.
8. Stand by the bed with your feet shoulder-width apart. Face the patient.
9. Place one arm under the patient's shoulder blades. Place the other arm under the patient's thighs. Use proper body mechanics.
10. Ask the patient to bend her knees, place her feet firmly on the mattress, and push with her feet and hands on the count of 3.
11. On 3, shift your body weight to help move the patient while she pushes with her feet (Fig. 8-8).

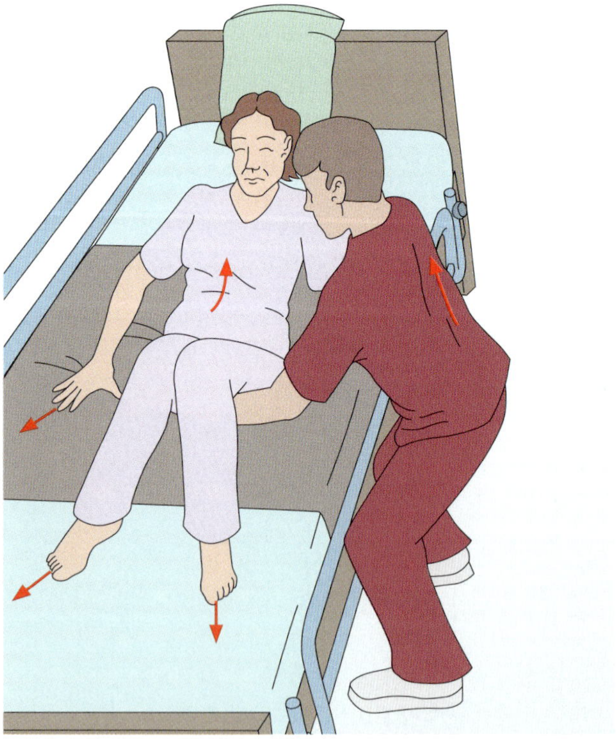

Fig. 8-8. *Keep your back straight and your knees bent.*

12. Make the patient comfortable. Put the pillow back under the patient's head and arrange the blankets for her.
13. Return the bed to its lowest position. Return the side rails to the ordered position. Remove privacy measures.

14. Place the call light within the patient's reach.
15. Wash your hands.
16. Report any changes in the patient to the nurse. Document the procedure using facility guidelines.

When you have help from another person, you can modify the procedure as follows:

1. Follow steps 1 through 6 above.
2. Stand on one side of the bed with your feet shoulder-width apart. Face the head of the bed. The foot that is closer to the head of the bed should be pointed toward the head of the bed. Bend your knees. Keep your back straight. Your helper should be standing on the other side of the bed.
3. Both of you should roll the draw sheet up to the patient's side and grasp the sheet. One hand should be at the patient's shoulders, the other about level with the patient's hips. Use proper body mechanics.
4. Let the patient know you will be moving her on the count of 3. Shift your weight to your back foot (the foot closer to the foot of the bed). Have your helper do the same. On the count of 3, you and your helper both shift your weight to the forward foot. Slide the draw sheet and patient toward the head of the bed (Fig. 8-9).

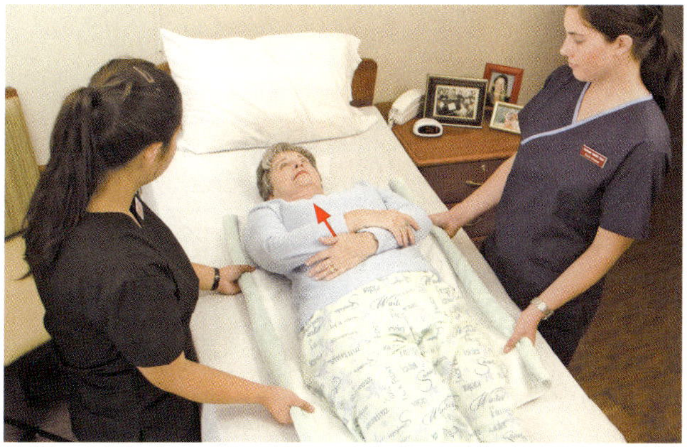

Fig. 8-9. *The patient and draw sheet are moved up toward the head of the bed.*

5. Make the patient comfortable. Put the pillow back under the patient's head and arrange the blankets. Unroll the draw sheet and leave it in place for the next repositioning (Fig. 8-10). If using another type of device (other than a draw sheet), you will need to remove it.

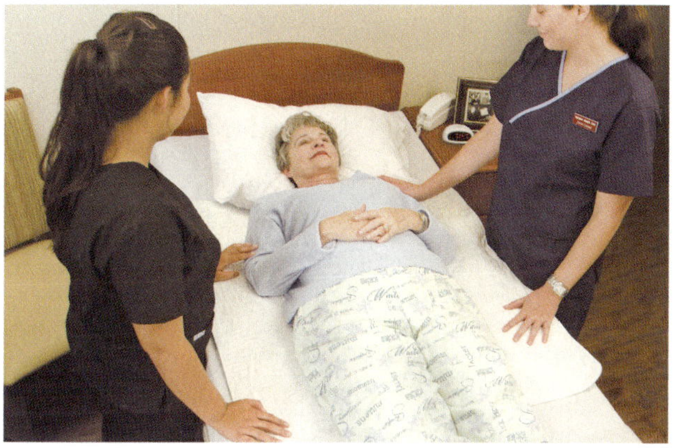

Fig. 8-10. *Unroll the draw sheet and leave it in place.*

6. Return the bed to its lowest position. Remove privacy measures.
7. Place the call light within the patient's reach.
8. Wash your hands.
9. Report any changes in the patient to the nurse.
10. Document the procedure using facility guidelines.

Moving a patient to the side of the bed

Equipment: draw sheet or other device

1. Identify yourself by name. Identify the patient according to facility policy.
2. Wash your hands.
3. Explain the procedure to the patient. Speak clearly, slowly, and directly. Maintain face-to-face contact whenever possible.
4. Provide for the patient's privacy with a curtain, screen, or door.
5. Adjust the bed to a safe level, usually waist high. Lock bed wheels.

6. Lower the head of the bed.
7. Stand on the side of the bed to which you are moving the patient. Stand with feet shoulder-width apart. Bend your knees and keep your back straight.
8. **With a draw sheet**: Roll the draw sheet up to the patient's side and grasp the sheet. One hand should be at the patient's shoulders, the other about level with the patient's hips. Place one knee against the side of the bed, and lean back with your body. Let the patient know you will be moving her on the count of 3. On 3, pull the draw sheet and patient toward you. Unroll the draw sheet and leave it in place for the next repositioning. If using another type of device (other than a draw sheet), you will need to remove it.

   Without a draw sheet: Gently slide your hands under the patient's head and shoulders and move them toward you (Fig. 8-11). Gently slide your hands under her midsection and move it toward you. Gently slide your hands under the hips and legs and move them toward you.

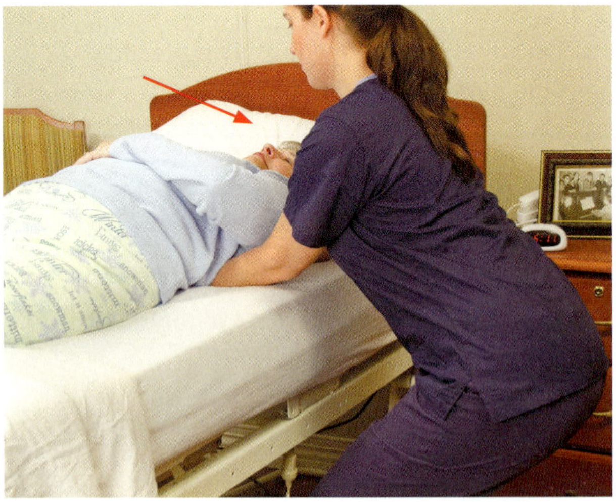

Fig. 8-11. *First, gently move the patient's head and shoulders toward you.*

9. Make the patient comfortable.
10. Return the bed to its lowest position. Remove privacy measures.
11. Place the call light within the patient's reach.
12. Wash your hands.
13. Report any changes in the patient to the nurse.
14. Document the procedure using facility guidelines.

Patients may be turned on their sides in preparation for sitting up or to change position and to take pressure off their backs. This helps prevent skin irritation and pressure injuries.

Positioning a patient on his side

1. Identify yourself by name. Identify the patient according to facility policy.
2. Wash your hands.
3. Explain the procedure to the patient. Speak clearly, slowly, and directly. Maintain face-to-face contact whenever possible.
4. Provide for the patient's privacy with a curtain, screen, or door.
5. Adjust the bed to a safe level, usually waist high. Lock the bed wheels.
6. Lower the head of the bed to make it flat.
7. Move the patient toward the side of the bed near you, using the previous procedure.
8. If the bed has side rails, raise the far side rail.

Turning a patient away from you:

a. Cross the patient's arms over his chest. Cross the near leg over the far leg.
b. Stand with feet shoulder-width apart. Bend your knees.
c. Place one hand on the patient's near shoulder. Place the other hand on the near hip.

d. While supporting the body, gently roll the patient onto his side as one unit, toward the raised side rail.

Turning a patient toward you:

a. Cross the patient's far arm over his chest. Move the arm on the side the patient is being turned to out of the way. Cross the far leg over the near leg.

b. Stand with feet shoulder-width apart. Bend your knees.

c. Place one hand on the patient's far shoulder. Place the other hand on the far hip.

d. While supporting the body, gently roll the patient onto his side as one unit, toward you. Use your body to block him to prevent him from rolling out of bed.

9. Position the patient properly and comfortably. Proper positioning includes the following:

- Head supported by a pillow (the patient's face should not be obstructed by the pillow)
- Shoulder adjusted so the patient is not lying on his arm or hand
- Top arm supported by a pillow
- Back supported by a supportive device
- Hips properly aligned
- Supportive device between legs with top knee flexed; knee and ankle supported
- Pillow under the bottom foot so that toes and ankle are not touching the bed

10. Return the bed to its lowest position. Return side rails to their ordered position. Remove privacy measures.

11. Place the call light within the patient's reach.

12. Wash your hands.

13. Report any changes in the patient to the nurse.

14. Document the procedure using facility guidelines.

Some patients' spinal columns must be kept in alignment. These patients must be turned in bed by logrolling. **Logrolling** means moving a patient as a unit, without disturbing the alignment of the body. The head, back, and legs must be kept in a straight line. This is necessary in cases of neck or back problems, spinal cord injuries, or after back or hip surgeries. It is safer for 2 or more people to perform this procedure together. A draw sheet helps with moving.

Logrolling a patient

Equipment: draw sheet or other device

1. Identify yourself by name. Identify the patient according to facility policy.

2. Wash your hands.

3. Explain the procedure to the patient. Speak clearly, slowly, and directly. Maintain face-to-face contact whenever possible.

4. Provide for the patient's privacy with a curtain, screen, or door.

5. Adjust the bed to a safe level, usually waist high. Lock the bed wheels.

6. Lower the head of the bed.

7. Both of you stand on the same side of the bed. One person stands at the patient's head and shoulders. The other stands near the patient's midsection.

8. Place a pillow under the patient's head to support the neck during the move.

9. Place the patient's arms across his chest. Place a pillow between the knees.

10. Stand with your feet shoulder-width apart. Bend your knees.

11. Grasp the draw sheet on the far side (Fig. 8-12).

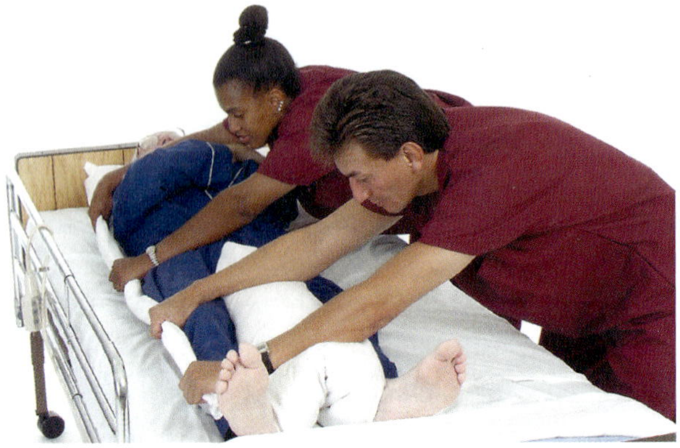

Fig. 8-12. *Both of you grasp the draw sheet on the far side.*

12. Let the patient know you will be moving him on the count of 3. On 3, gently roll the patient toward you. Turn him as a unit (Fig. 8-13). Use your bodies to block him to prevent him from rolling out of bed.

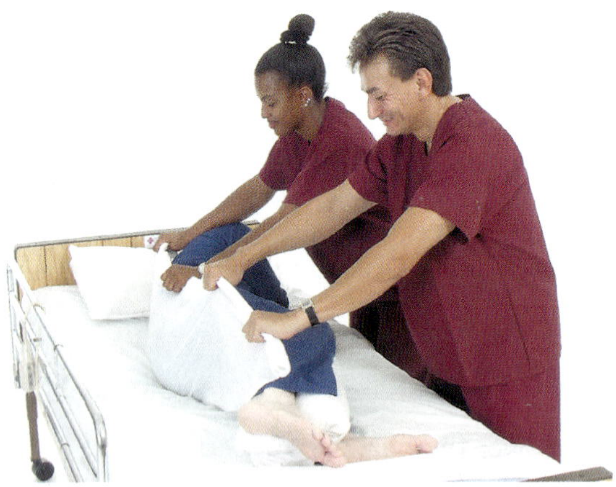

Fig. 8-13. *On the count of 3, both workers should roll the patient toward them, turning him as a unit.*

13. Make the patient comfortable. Arrange pillows and covers for comfort. If you used a draw sheet, unroll it and leave it in place for the next repositioning. If using another type of device (other than a draw sheet), remove it.

14. Return the bed to its lowest position. Remove privacy measures.

15. Place the call light within the patient's reach.

16. Wash your hands.

17. Report any changes in the patient to the nurse.

18. Document the procedure using facility guidelines.

Before a patient who has been lying down stands up, he should dangle. To **dangle** means to sit up on the side of the bed with the legs hanging over the side. This helps patients regain balance before standing up and allows blood pressure to stabilize. It helps prevent dizziness and lightheadedness that can cause fainting. For some patients who are unable to walk, sitting up and dangling the legs for a few minutes may be ordered in the care plan.

Assisting a patient to sit up on side of bed: dangling

1. Identify yourself by name. Identify the patient according to facility policy.

2. Wash your hands.

3. Explain the procedure to the patient. Speak clearly, slowly, and directly. Maintain face-to-face contact whenever possible.

4. Provide for the patient's privacy with a curtain, screen, or door.

5. Adjust the bed to its lowest position. Lock the bed wheels.

6. Raise the head of the bed to a sitting position. Fanfold (fold into pleats) the top covers to the foot of the bed.

7. Tell the patient to reach across his chest with his top arm and place his hand on the edge of the bed near his opposite shoulder. Ask him to push down on that hand to raise his shoulders up while swinging his legs over the side of the bed (Fig. 8-14).

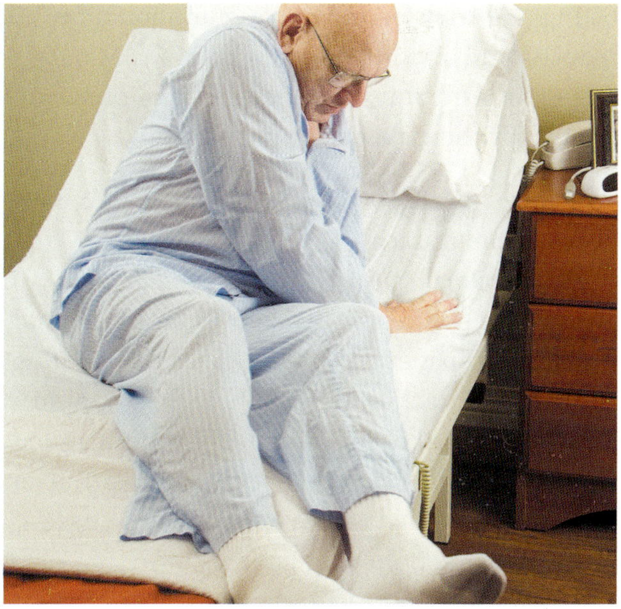

Fig. 8-14. Have the patient push himself up while swinging his legs over the side of the bed.

8. Always allow the patient to do all he can for himself. However, if the patient needs assistance, follow these steps:

a. Stand with your legs shoulder-width apart. Bend your knees. Keep your back straight.

b. Place one arm under the patient's shoulder blades. Place the other arm under the patient's thighs (Fig. 8-15).

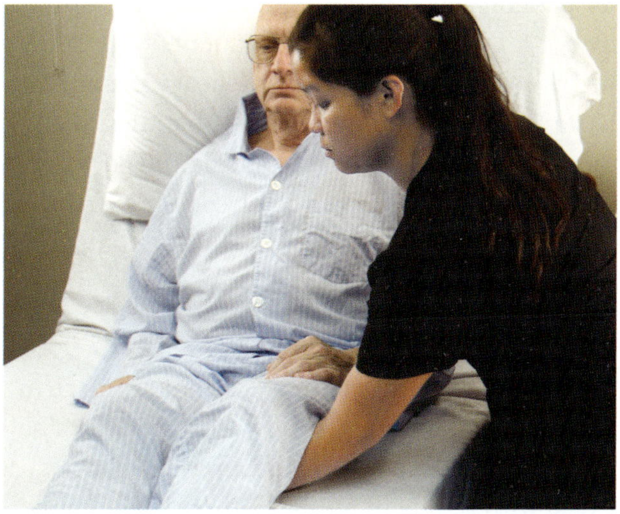

Fig. 8-15. One arm should be under the patient's shoulder blades and the other arm should be under the thighs.

c. Let the patient know you will be moving him on the count of 3. On 3, slowly move the patient into a sitting position with his legs dangling over the side of the bed. The weight of his legs hanging down from the bed helps the patient sit up (Fig. 8-16).

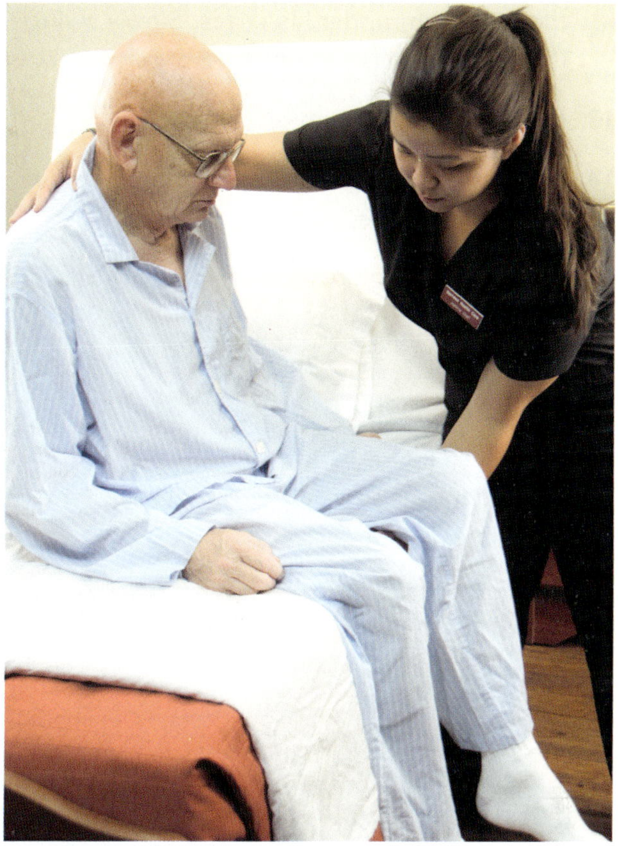

Fig. 8-16. The weight of the patient's legs hanging down from the bed helps the patient sit up.

9. Ask the patient to sit up as straight as possible and to hold on to the edge of the mattress with both hands. Help him to put on nonskid footwear if he is not wearing it and is going to get out of bed.

10. Have the patient dangle as long as ordered. The care plan may direct you to allow the patient to dangle for several minutes and then assist him to lie down again, or it may direct you to allow him to dangle in preparation for walking or a transfer. Follow the care plan. Do not leave the patient alone. If he is dizzy for more than a minute, have him lie down again. Count his pulse and respiration rates and report to the nurse. (You will learn how to measure vital signs in Chapter 10.)

11. Remove the patient's footwear if he wishes to have it removed.
12. Gently assist the patient back into bed. Place one arm around the patient's shoulders and the other arm under his knees. Slowly swing the patient's legs onto the bed.
13. Make the patient comfortable.
14. Leave the bed in its lowest position. Remove privacy measures.
15. Place the call light within the patient's reach.
16. Wash your hands.
17. Report any changes in the patient to the nurse.
18. Document the procedure using facility guidelines.

Connected Care

Positioning and Moving

When positioning and moving patients, PCTs should make sure patients are not unnecessarily exposed. They should be kept properly covered, dressed, or draped to protect their privacy and to promote dignity. PCTs should pull the privacy curtain around the bed when moving patients in bed.

2. Describe how to safely transfer patients

Transferring a patient means that a PCT is moving him from one place to another. Transfers can move patients from beds to chairs or wheelchairs, from wheelchairs to showers or toilets, and so on.

Safety is one of the most important factors to consider during transfers. The Occupational Safety and Health Administration (OSHA, osha.gov) set specific ergonomic guidelines to help avoid injuries during transfers. A person's back is especially prone to injury. OSHA's ergonomic guidelines address ways to help avoid work-related injuries. OSHA states that manual lifting and transferring of patients should be reduced and eliminated when possible. Manual lifting, transferring, and repositioning of patients may increase risk of injury.

To reduce the risk of injury, some hospitals have adopted *no-lift*, *zero-lift*, or *lift-free* policies. Many more hospitals have *safe patient handling* policies. These policies set guidelines for lifting and transferring patients. Lift-free and safe handling policies vary; facilities decide how they want to address the goal of reducing lifting and transferring of patients. Some do not allow any lifting at all and require that equipment always be used when lifting and moving patients.

The more restrictions placed on lifting, the less chance there is of injury. The amount and type of equipment available also factor into reducing workplace injuries. The following procedures are for manual lifting and transferring of patients. It is important for PCTs to carefully follow facility policies on lifting and to use equipment properly. If PCTs are unsure how to use equipment, they should ask for help and always get help when they need it.

A **transfer belt** is a safety device used to transfer patients who are weak, unsteady, or uncoordinated. It is also used to help patients walk. The belt is made of canvas or other heavy material. It has a buckle and sometimes has handles. It fits around the patient's waist, outside the gown or clothing. It should never be placed on bare skin. It is important for the PCT to check female patients to make sure their breasts are not caught under the belt.

The transfer belt gives the PCT something firm to hold on to when assisting with transfers. The PCT should grasp the belt securely on both sides, with hands in an upward position. Transfer belts cannot be used if a patient has fragile bones, fractures, or has had certain kinds of surgery recently.

Connected Care

Transfers

Any time a PCT helps a patient transfer, she should talk to the patient about what she would like to do. The PCT can promote independence by letting the patient do what he can. The PCT and patient must work together, especially during transfers.

Applying a transfer belt

Equipment: transfer belt, nonskid footwear

1. Identify yourself by name. Identify the patient according to facility policy.
2. Wash your hands.
3. Explain the procedure to the patient. Speak clearly, slowly, and directly. Maintain face-to-face contact whenever possible.
4. Provide for the patient's privacy with a curtain, screen, or door.
5. Adjust the bed to its lowest position. Lock the bed wheels.
6. Assist the patient to a sitting position with feet flat on the floor.
7. Put nonskid footwear on the patient as needed.
8. Place the transfer belt over the patient's gown or clothing and around the waist. Do not put it over bare skin.
9. Tighten the buckle until it is snug. Leave enough room to insert flat fingers/hand comfortably under the belt.
10. Check to make sure that skin or skin folds (for example, breasts) are not caught under the belt.
11. Position the buckle slightly off-center in the front or back for comfort.

A **slide board**, or transfer board, may be used to transfer patients who are unable to bear weight on their legs. Slide boards can be used for almost any transfer that involves moving from one sitting position to another (for example, from a bed to a chair). Slide boards should not be used against bare skin. Before beginning the transfer, the PCT should make sure that the patient's fingers are not under the board.

Wheelchairs are used to move or transport patients who are unable to walk or who find walking difficult due to injury, illness, or disability. In a hospital, wheelchairs may be used to move patients from their units to other areas of the facility for testing or treatment.

Guidelines: Wheelchairs

G Know how to apply and release the brake and how to operate the armrests and footrests. Always lock a wheelchair before helping a patient into or out of it (Fig. 8-17). After a transfer, unlock the wheelchair.

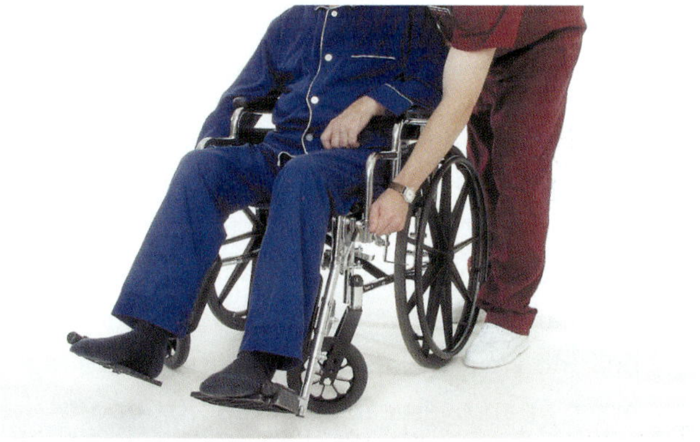

Fig. 8-17. *Always lock the wheelchair before a patient gets into or out of it.*

G To unfold a standard wheelchair, tilt the chair slightly to raise the wheels on the opposite side. Press down on one or both seat rails until the chair opens and the seat is flat. To fold a standard wheelchair, lift up under the center edge of the seat.

G To remove an armrest, release the arm lock by the armrest, and lift the arm from the center. To replace the armrest, simply reverse the procedure.

G To move a footrest out of the way, press or pull the release lever. Swing the footrest out toward the side of the wheelchair. To remove the footrest, lift it off when it is toward the side of the wheelchair (Fig. 8-18). To replace a footrest, simply put it back in the side position, then swing it back to the front position. It should lock into place.

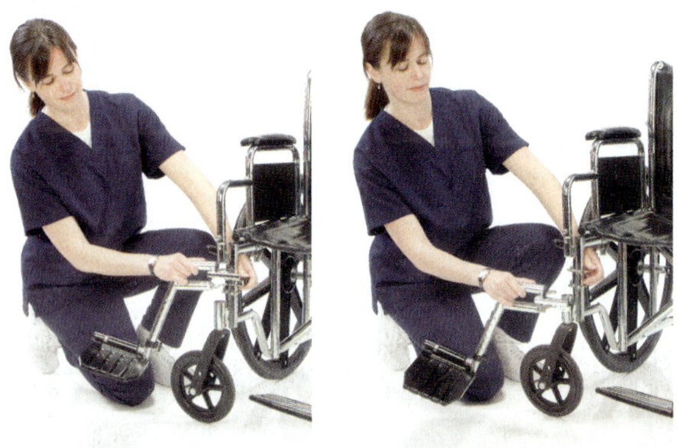

Fig. 8-18. *To remove a footrest, swing the footrest toward the side of the wheelchair and lift it off.*

G To lift or lower a footrest, support the leg or foot. Squeeze the lever and pull up or push down.

G To transfer to or from a wheelchair, the patient must use the side of the body that can bear weight to support and lift the side that cannot bear weight. A patient who can bear no weight with their legs may use a leg brace or an overhead trapeze for support.

G Before any transfer, make sure the patient is wearing nonskid footwear. This promotes patient safety and reduces the risk of falls.

G During wheelchair transfers, make sure the patient is safe and comfortable. Ask the patient how you can help. Some may only want you to bring the chair to the bedside. Others may want you to be more involved. (Always assist patients who are considered a fall risk with transfers.) Always be sure the chair is as close as possible to the patient and is locked in place. Use a transfer belt if you are going to assist with the transfer. Be sure the transfer is done slowly, allowing time for the patient to rest. Upon standing, check to see if the patient is dizzy. If he is, help him sit back down. Measure vital signs as ordered and report to the nurse.

G Check that the patient is in proper alignment in the chair once the transfer is complete. Make sure that the patient is not sitting on any tubing. Special cushions and pillows can be used for support. The hips should be well-positioned back in the chair. If the patient needs to be moved back in the wheelchair, lock wheelchair wheels. Stand in front of the wheelchair and ask the patient to grasp the armrests while his feet are flat on the floor. Brace one or both knees against the patient's knee(s). On the count of 3, ask the patient to push with his feet into the floor and move himself toward the back of the chair. Gently assist as needed.

Falls

If a patient starts to fall during a transfer or while walking, the PCT should not try to reverse or stop a fall because she or the patient can suffer worse injuries if she tries to stop a fall. The PCT should try to protect the patient's head and move objects out of the way if possible. If a patient has fallen, the PCT should call for help. She should not try to get the patient up after the fall.

Some patients have one-sided weakness due to paralysis or stroke. When transferring a patient with one-sided weakness, the PCT should move the stronger side first. The weaker (also called **affected**, or **involved**) side follows.

Transferring a patient from bed to wheelchair

Equipment: wheelchair, transfer belt, nonskid footwear

1. Identify yourself by name. Identify the patient according to facility policy.

2. Wash your hands.

3. Explain the procedure to the patient. Speak clearly, slowly, and directly. Maintain face-to-face contact whenever possible.

4. Provide for the patient's privacy with a curtain, screen, or door. Check the area to be certain it is uncluttered and safe.

5. Place the wheelchair at the head of the bed, facing the foot of the bed, or at the foot of the bed, facing the head of the bed. The arm of the wheelchair should be almost touching the bed. The wheelchair should be placed on the patient's **stronger**, or unaffected, side.

6. Remove both wheelchair footrests close to the bed.

7. Lock the wheelchair wheels.

8. Raise the head of the bed. Adjust the bed to its lowest position. Lock the bed wheels.

9. Assist the patient into a sitting position. Make sure his feet are flat on the floor. Adjust the bed height if needed. Let the patient sit for a few minutes to adjust to the change in position.

10. Put nonskid footwear on the patient if he is not already wearing it.

11. Stand in front of the patient with your feet about shoulder-width apart. Bend your knees. Keep your back straight.

12. Place the transfer belt around the patient's waist over his gown or clothing (not on bare skin). Tighten the buckle until it is snug. Grasp the belt securely on both sides, with hands in an upward position.

13. Provide instructions to allow the patient to help with the transfer. Instructions may include: "When you start to stand, push with your hands against the bed." "Once standing, if you're able, you can take small steps in the direction of the chair." "Once standing, reach for the chair with your stronger hand."

14. With your legs, brace (support) the patient's lower legs to prevent slipping (Fig. 8-19). This can be done by placing one or both of your knees against the patient's knees. You can also stand toe to toe with the patient. Bend your knees and keep your back straight.

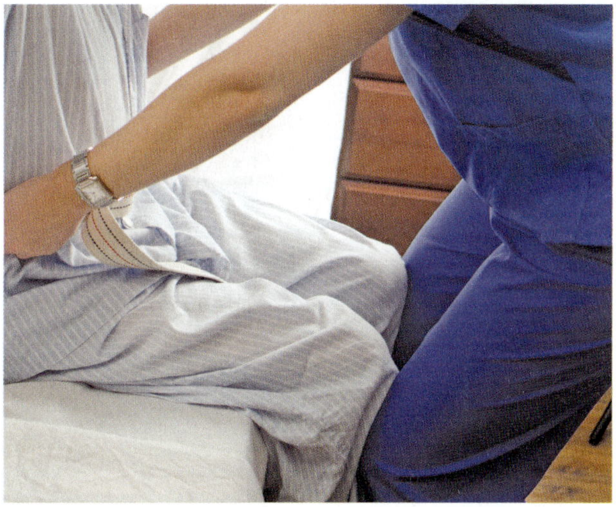

Fig. 8-19. *Brace the patient's lower legs to prevent slipping by placing either one or both knees (shown) against the patient's knees.*

15. Let the patient know you will be moving him on the count of 3. If possible, have the patient rock while counting to 3. On 3, with hands still grasping the transfer belt on both sides and moving upward, slowly help the patient to stand.

16. Tell the patient to take small steps in the direction of the wheelchair while turning his back toward the chair. If more help is needed, help the patient pivot (turn) to stand in front of the wheelchair with the back of the patient's legs against the wheelchair (Fig. 8-20). Always allow the patient to do all he can for himself.

17. Ask the patient to put his hands on the wheelchair armrests if he is able. When the chair is touching the back of the patient's legs, help him lower himself into the chair.

18. Reposition the patient so that his hips touch the back of the wheelchair seat.

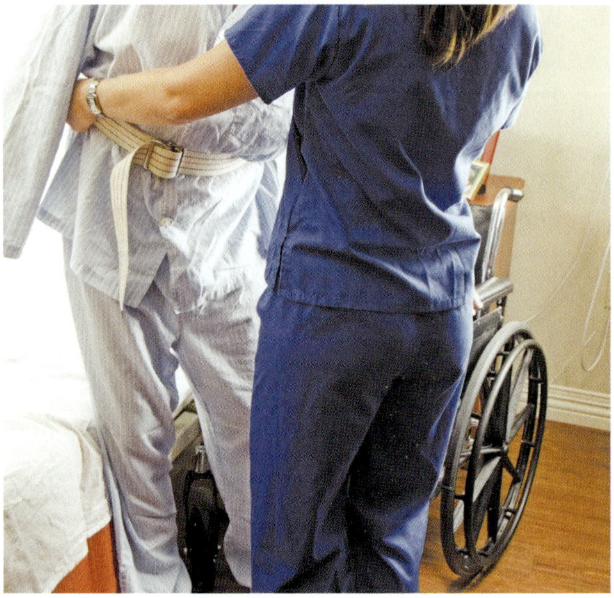

Fig. 8-20. *Help the patient pivot to the front of the wheelchair. Pivoting is safer than twisting.*

19. Attach the footrests and place the patient's feet on the footrests. Check that the patient's body is in proper alignment. Gently remove the transfer belt. Make the patient comfortable.
20. Remove privacy measures.
21. Place the call light within the patient's reach.
22. Wash your hands.
23. Report any changes in the patient to the nurse.
24. Document the procedure using facility guidelines.

When transferring back to bed from a wheelchair, the height of the bed should be equal to or slightly lower than the chair. Help the patient pivot to the bed. When the patient feels the bed with the back of his legs, help him sit down slowly.

Stretchers

A stretcher, also called a *gurney*, is a medical device used to move injured or ill persons from one place to another. Stretchers may be used for serious injuries and illnesses and/or when a person cannot or should not walk but needs to be transported somewhere. Stretchers transfer patients within facilities or to other facilities.

Guidelines: Safe Use of Stretchers

G Lock the stretcher's wheels before transferring a patient onto or off a stretcher.

G Secure the patient with safety belts (if available) while in the stretcher.

G Raise the safety rails.

G Cover the patient with a sheet. Hands, feet, fingers, etc., should remain inside the sheet during transport.

G Keep the wheels locked at all times except when moving the stretcher.

G Get help if you cannot move the stretcher alone.

G Move slowly and carefully.

G Push the stretcher from the head end.

G Go through doorways by opening the door, entering first, and pulling the stretcher through.

G Avoid hitting walls or doorways.

G Be cautious going down sloping areas.

G Stay with the patient at all times.

A draw sheet is used to transfer a patient to a stretcher. The procedure below shows how to transfer a patient to a stretcher from a bed using 4 staff members. At least 3 people are necessary to safely transfer a patient to a stretcher.

Transferring a patient from bed to stretcher

Equipment: stretcher, blanket, draw sheet

1. Identify yourself by name. Identify the patient according to facility policy.
2. Wash your hands.

3. Explain the procedure to the patient. Speak clearly, slowly, and directly. Maintain face-to-face contact whenever possible.
4. Provide for the patient's privacy with a curtain, screen, or door.
5. Lower the head of the bed so that it is flat. Lock the bed wheels.
6. Fold linens to the foot of the bed. Cover the patient with a blanket.
7. Move the patient to the side of the bed. Have your coworkers help you do this. Refer to the procedure *Moving a patient to the side of the bed* earlier in this chapter.
8. Place the stretcher solidly against the bed, and lock the stretcher wheels. Bed height should be equal to or slightly above the height of the stretcher. Move any safety belts out of the way.
9. At least 2 workers should be on one side of the bed opposite the stretcher. At least 2 more workers should be on the other side of the stretcher.
10. Each worker should roll up the sides of the draw sheet and prepare to move the patient (Fig. 8-21). Protect the patient's arms and legs during the transfer.

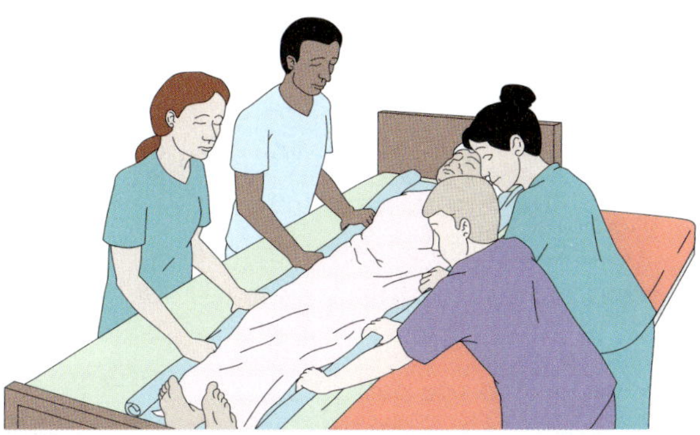

Fig. 8-21. *With 2 workers on each side, roll up the sides of the draw sheet and prepare to move the patient.*

11. Let the patient know you will be moving him on the count of 3. On 3, the workers lift and move the patient to the stretcher (Fig. 8-22). All should move at once. Make sure the patient is centered on the stretcher.

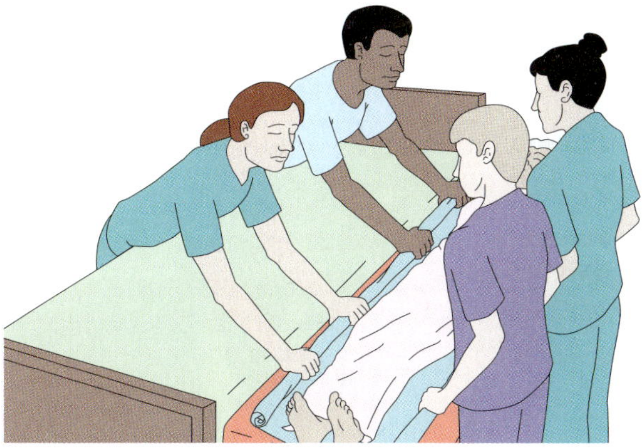

Fig. 8-22. *On the count of 3, all workers should lift and move at once.*

12. Place a pillow under the patient's head. Make sure the patient is still covered with the blanket.
13. Secure the safety straps across the patient. Raise side rails on the stretcher.
14. Unlock the stretcher's wheels. Move the patient to the proper place, staying with him until another staff member takes over.
15. Wash your hands.
16. Report any changes in the patient to the nurse.
17. Document the procedure using facility guidelines.

To return the patient to bed, the bed height should be equal to or slightly below the stretcher.

Mechanical Lifts

Facilities often have mechanical (also called *hydraulic, power,* or *standing*) lifts available to transfer patients. This equipment helps prevent injury to patients and healthcare workers. PCTs may assist patients with many types of transfers using a mechanical or hydraulic lift. Using these lifts requires special training. PCTs should not use equipment they have not been trained to use, as doing this could cause injury.

There are many different types of mechanical lifts (Fig. 8-23). Using these devices helps prevent common workplace injuries and may be mandatory at facilities that have no-lift policies. PCTs should always ask for help if there is anything that they do not understand about the provided lift equipment.

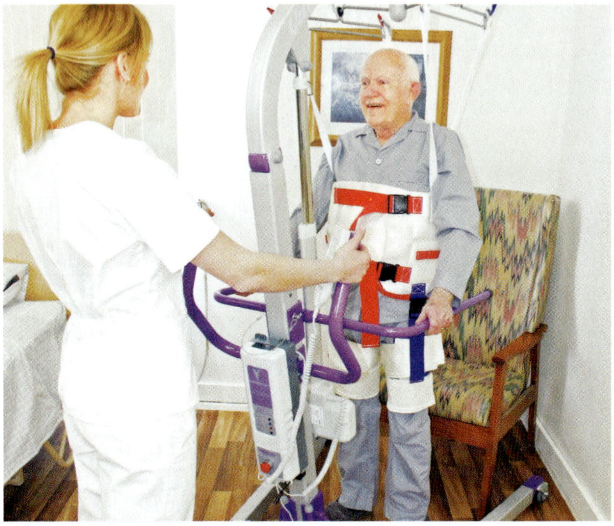

Fig. 8-23. *There are different types of lifts for transferring both completely dependent patients and patients who can bear some weight. This patient can bear some weight on his legs.* (PHOTO COURTESY OF VANCARE INC., WWW.VANCARE.COM)

Guidelines: Mechanical or Hydraulic Lifts

G Be careful when moving a patient using a mechanical lift. Have another person assist you when transferring with these lifts. It is safer for at least 2 people to do these types of transfers.

G Keep the chair to which the patient is to be moved close to the bed so that the patient is only moved a short distance in the lift. Lock the wheels on the chair if it has wheels.

G Check that the valves on the lift are working before using it.

G Use the correct sling for the lift that is being used. Using an incorrect sling may result in serious injury or death. If you have questions about the sling, talk to the nurse.

G Check the sling and straps for any fraying or tears. Do not use the lift if there are tears or holes.

G Open the legs of the stand to the widest position before helping the patient into the lift.

G Once the patient is in the sling and the straps are connected, pump up the lift only to the point where the patient's body clears the bed or chair.

G Electric/battery-powered lifts have emergency releases. Be aware of where the release is located and how to operate this function. Talk to the nurse if you do not know how to do this.

Transferring a patient using a mechanical lift

Equipment: wheelchair or chair, coworker, mechanical or hydraulic lift

The following is a basic procedure for transferring using a mechanical lift. Ask a coworker to help you before starting.

1. Identify yourself by name. Identify the patient according to facility policy.
2. Wash your hands.
3. Explain the procedure to the patient. Speak clearly, slowly, and directly. Maintain face-to-face contact whenever possible.
4. Provide for the patient's privacy with a curtain, screen, or door.
5. Lock the bed wheels.
6. Position the wheelchair next to the bed. Lock the brakes.
7. Help the patient turn to one side of the bed. Position the sling under the patient, with the edge next to the patient's back. Fanfold if necessary. Adjust the bottom of the sling so that it is even with the patient's knees. Help the patient roll back to the middle of the bed, and then spread out the fanfolded edge of the sling.
8. Roll the mechanical lift to the bedside. Make sure the base is opened to its widest point. Push the base of the lift under the bed.

9. Position the overhead bar directly over the patient (Fig. 8-24).

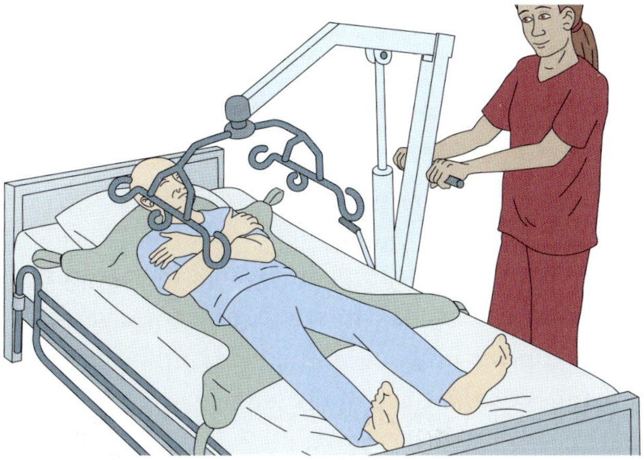

Fig. 8-24. *Position the overhead bar directly over the patient.*

10. With the patient lying on his back, attach one set of straps to each side of the sling. Attach one set of straps to the overhead bar. If available, have a coworker support the patient's head, shoulders, and knees while being lifted. The patient's arms should be folded across his chest (Fig. 8-25). If the device has S hooks, they should face away from the patient. Make sure all straps are connected properly and are smooth and straight.

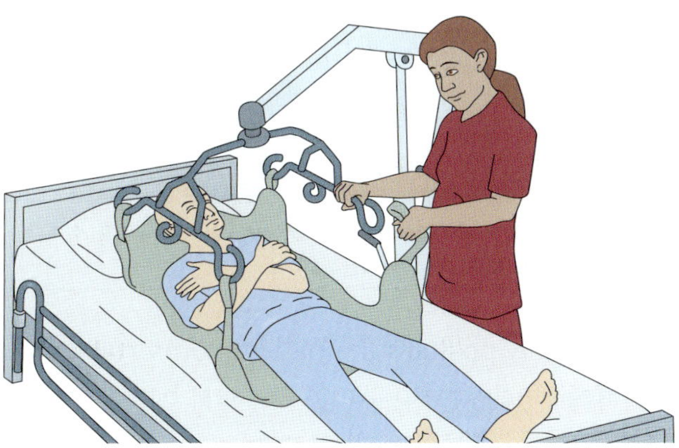

Fig. 8-25. *With the patient's arms folded across his chest, attach the straps to the sling.*

11. Following manufacturer instructions, raise the patient 2 inches above the bed. Pause a moment for the patient to gain balance.

12. Have your coworker support and guide the patient's body while you roll the lift so that the patient is positioned over the chair or wheelchair (Fig. 8-26).

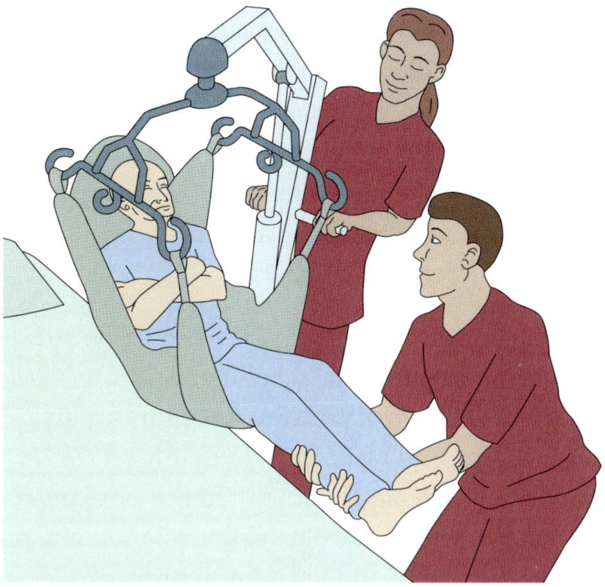

Fig. 8-26. *Having another person help to support and guide the patient promotes safety during the transfer and reduces the chance of injury.*

13. Slowly lower the patient into the chair or wheelchair. Push down gently on the patient's knees to help the patient into a sitting, rather than reclining, position.

14. Undo the straps from the overhead bar on the sling. Remove the sling or leave it in place for the transfer back to bed.

15. Be sure the patient is seated comfortably and correctly in the chair or wheelchair. Remove privacy measures.

16. Place the call light within the patient's reach.

17. Wash your hands.

18. Report any changes in the patient to the nurse.

19. Document the procedure using facility guidelines.

A stand-up, or standing, lift is used when a person can bear some weight on his legs, but has poor leg strength and/or balance. The patient must be able to stand and have some arm strength in order to use this lift. There are different types of stand-up lifts, including manual and battery-powered. The stand-up lift consists of both user and operator support bars (the user support bars may consist of 2 vertical bars or 1 crossbar), padded swivel swing-out seats (and/or straps, vest, or belt for some models), knee pads, a platform base with foot plate, and 4 small wheels with locking brakes.

If using a stand-up lift, the PCT should be sure that the brakes are locked before beginning the transfer. The patient should begin in a sitting position and place his feet firmly on the foot plate of the platform, with knees pressing against the knee pads. The patient should grasp the support bar(s) and gently pull himself to a standing position, using his own strength. Then the PCT can lower both sides of the padded swing-out seat into position. The PCT should adjust straps, vest, or belt if these are used. The patient should slowly lower himself onto the seat while holding the support bars and pressing his knees against the knee pads. The PCT should unlock the wheel brakes and use the operator bars to transfer the patient to the location desired and then perform these steps in reverse order to release the patient from the lift.

Vehicle Transfers

When a patient is leaving a facility, he may need help getting into a vehicle. The front seat is wider and is usually easier to get into. PCTs should understand that patients leaving the hospital may be weaker than they realize. They may need more help than they expect.

Transferring a patient into a vehicle

Equipment: wheelchair

1. Identify yourself by name. Identify the patient according to facility policy.
2. Wash your hands.
3. Explain the procedure to the patient. Speak clearly, slowly, and directly. Maintain face-to-face contact whenever possible.
4. Place the wheelchair close to the vehicle at a 45-degree angle. Open the door on the patient's stronger side if possible.
5. Lock the wheelchair wheels.
6. Ask the patient to push against the armrests of the wheelchair to stand, grasp the vehicle, and pivot his foot so the side of the seat touches the back of his legs.
7. The patient should then sit in the seat and lift one leg, and then the other, into the vehicle (Fig. 8-27). Assist as needed.

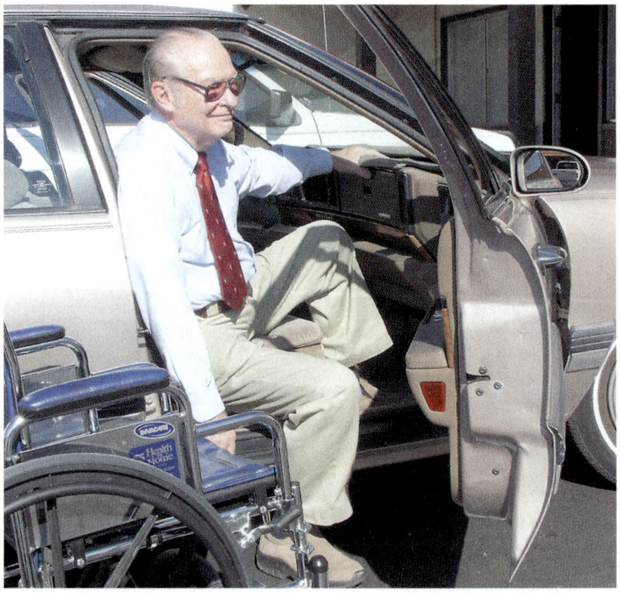

Fig. 8-27. *After the patient sits in the vehicle seat, he should put his legs in one at a time.*

8. Carefully position the patient comfortably in the vehicle. Help fasten the seat belt.
9. Safely shut the door.
10. Return the wheelchair to the appropriate place for cleaning.
11. Wash your hands.
12. Document the procedure using facility guidelines.

3. Discuss how to safely assist patients with ambulation

Ambulation means moving or walking, with or without an assistive device. A patient who is **ambulatory** is one who can get out of bed and move or walk. Many patients are ambulatory, but need help to walk safely. Several tools, including transfer belts, canes, walkers, and crutches, help with ambulation. The PCT should check the care plan before helping a patient ambulate. It is important to know the patient's abilities, limitations, and disabilities. The PCT should communicate what she would like to do and allow the patient to do what he can.

Assisting a patient to ambulate

Equipment: transfer belt, nonskid footwear

1. Identify yourself by name. Identify the patient according to facility policy.
2. Wash your hands.
3. Explain the procedure to the patient. Speak clearly, slowly, and directly. Maintain face-to-face contact whenever possible.
4. Provide for the patient's privacy with a curtain, screen, or door.
5. Adjust the bed to its lowest position. Lock the bed wheels. Assist the patient into a sitting position. Make sure his feet are flat on the floor. Adjust the bed height if needed.
6. Before ambulating, put nonskid footwear on the patient if he is not already wearing it.
7. Stand in front of and face the patient. Place your feet about shoulder-width apart.
8. Place the transfer belt around the patient's waist over his clothing (not on bare skin). Grasp the belt securely on both sides, with hands in an upward position.
9. If the patient is unable to stand without help, brace (support) the patient's lower extremities. This can be done by placing one or both of your knees against the patient's knees (Fig. 8-28). Or you can stand toe to toe with the patient. Bend your knees. Keep your back straight.

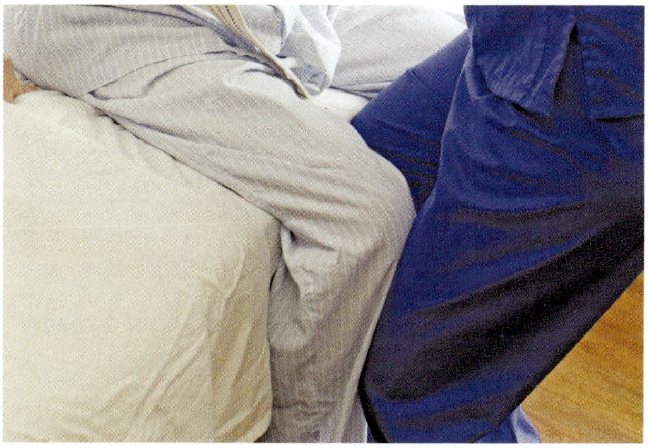

Fig. 8-28. *Use one or both of your knees to brace the patient's knee.*

10. Hold the patient close to your center of gravity. Provide instructions to allow the patient to help with standing. Tell the patient to lean forward, push down on the bed with his hands, and stand on the count of 3. When you start to count, begin to rock. On 3, with hands still grasping the transfer belt on both sides and moving upward, rock your weight onto your back foot. Slowly help the patient to stand.
11. Walk slightly behind and to one side of the patient for the full distance, while holding on to the transfer belt (Fig. 8-29). If the patient has a weaker side, stand on the weaker side. Use the hand that is not holding the belt to offer support on the weak side. Ask the patient to look forward, not down at the floor, during ambulation.
12. After ambulation, return the patient to the bed or chair and remove the transfer belt. Check that the patient's body is in proper alignment. Make the patient comfortable.

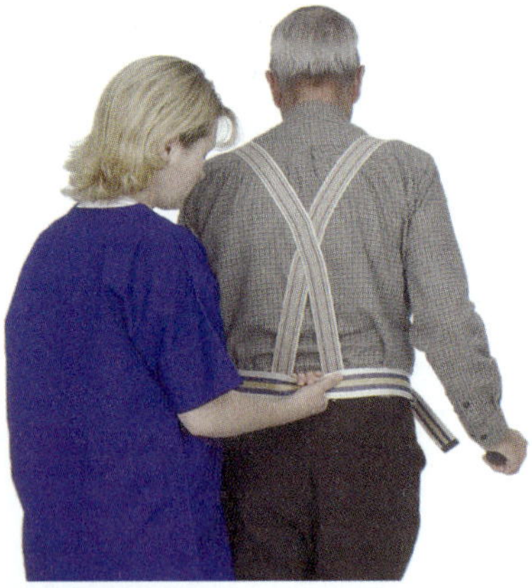

Fig. 8-29. *Standing on the weaker side, walk behind the patient while holding on to the transfer belt.*

13. Leave the bed in its lowest position.
14. Place the call light within the patient's reach.
15. Wash your hands.
16. Report any changes in the patient to the nurse.
17. Document the procedure using facility guidelines.

When helping a patient who has a visual impairment walk, the PCT should be beside and slightly ahead of the patient. The patient should be able to place his hand on the PCT's elbow. The PCT should walk at a normal pace. She should let the patient know when they are about to turn a corner or when a step is approaching. The PCT should state whether they will be stepping up or down.

Patients who have trouble walking may use canes, walkers, or crutches to help themselves. Canes help with balance. Patients using canes should be able to bear weight on both legs. If one leg is weaker, the cane should be held in the hand on the stronger side.

Types of canes are the C cane, the functional grip cane, and the quad cane. The C cane is a straight cane with a curved handle at the top. It has a rubber-tipped bottom to prevent slipping. A C cane is used to improve balance. A functional grip cane is similar to the C cane, except that it has a straight grip handle rather than a curved handle. The grip handle helps improve grip control. It provides more support than the C cane. A quad cane has 4 rubber-tipped feet and a rectangular base (Fig. 8-30). It is designed to bear more weight than the other canes.

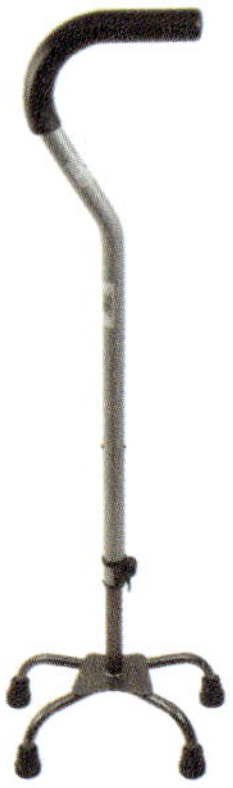

Fig. 8-30. *A quad cane has 4 rubber-tipped feet and can bear more weight than other canes.*

A walker is used when the patient can bear some weight on both legs. The walker gives stability for patients who are unsteady or lack balance. The metal frame may have rubber-tipped feet and/or wheels (Fig. 8-31). Crutches are used for patients who can bear no weight or limited weight on one leg. Crutches have rubber-tipped feet to prevent sliding. Some people use 1 crutch, and some use 2.

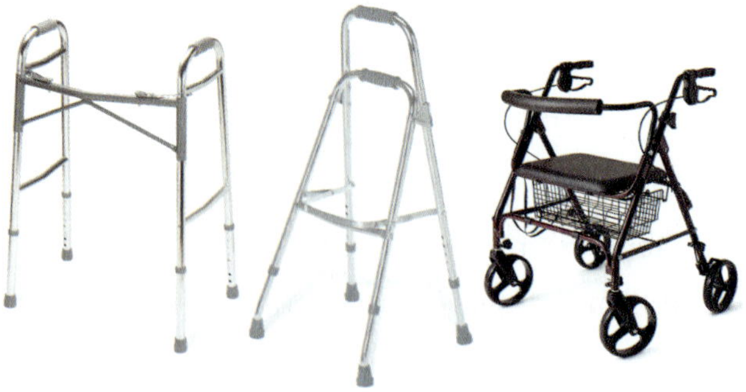

Fig. 8-31. *The photo on the left shows a standard walker. The photo in the middle shows a "hemi walker," which is a walker that is designed for people who have difficulty using an arm or a hand. The photo on the right shows a walker with a seat and basket.* (IMAGES COURTESY OF MEDLINE INDUSTRIES, LP. USED WITH PERMISSION.)

Guidelines: Cane or Walker Use

G Be sure the walker or cane is in good condition. It must have rubber tips on the bottom. The tips should not be cracked. Walkers may have wheels. If so, roll the walker to make sure the wheels are moving properly.

G Be sure the patient is wearing securely fastened, nonskid shoes before ambulating.

G When using a cane, the patient should place it on his stronger side.

G When using a walker, have the patient place both hands on the walker. The walker should not be overextended. It should be placed no more than 6 inches in front of the patient.

G Stay near the patient on the weaker side.

G Do not hang purses or clothing on the walker.

G If the height of the cane or walker does not appear to be correct (too short, too tall, etc.), tell the nurse.

Assisting with ambulation for a patient using a cane, walker, or crutches

Equipment: transfer belt; nonskid footwear; cane, walker, or crutches

1. Identify yourself by name. Identify the patient according to facility policy.
2. Wash your hands.
3. Explain the procedure to the patient. Speak clearly, slowly, and directly. Maintain face-to-face contact whenever possible.
4. Provide for the patient's privacy with a curtain, screen, or door.
5. Adjust the bed to its lowest position. Lock the bed wheels. Assist the patient into a sitting position. Make sure his feet are flat on the floor. Adjust the bed height if needed.
6. Before ambulating, put nonskid footwear on the patient if he is not already wearing it.
7. Stand in front of and face the patient. Place your feet about shoulder-width apart.
8. Place the transfer belt around the patient's waist over his clothing (not on bare skin). Grasp the belt securely on both sides, with hands in an upward position.
9. If the patient is unable to stand without help, brace (support) the patient's lower extremities. Bend your knees. Keep your back straight. Help the patient to stand as described in the previous procedure.
10. Help as needed with ambulation.

a. **Cane**: Patient places the cane about 6 inches, or a comfortable distance, in front of his stronger leg. He brings his weaker leg even with the cane. He then brings his stronger leg forward slightly ahead of the cane. Repeat.

b. **Walker**: Patient picks up or rolls the walker. He places it about 6 inches, or a comfortable distance, in front of him. All 4 feet or wheels of the walker should be on the ground before the patient steps forward to the walker. The walker should not be moved again until the patient has moved both feet forward and is steady. The patient should never put his feet ahead of the walker.

c. **Crutches**: The patient should be fitted for crutches and taught to use them correctly by a physical therapist or a nurse. The patient may use the crutches in different ways. It depends on his weakness. No matter how they are used, the patient's weight should be on his hands and arms. Weight should not be on the underarm area.

11. Walk slightly behind and to one side of the patient for the full distance, while holding on to the transfer belt. If the patient has a weaker side, stand on the weaker side.

12. Watch for obstacles in the patient's path. Ask the patient to look forward, not down at the floor, during ambulation.
13. Encourage the patient to rest if he is tired. Being tired increases the risk of a fall. Let the patient set the pace. Discuss how far he plans to go based on the care plan.
14. After ambulation, return the patient to the bed or chair and remove the transfer belt. Check that the patient's body is in proper alignment. Make the patient comfortable.
15. Leave the bed in its lowest position.
16. Place the call light within the patient's reach.
17. Wash your hands.
18. Report any changes in the patient to the nurse.
19. Document the procedure using facility guidelines.

Chapter Review

1. What is positioning?
2. How often should patients who are bed-bound be repositioned?
3. In which position is a patient lying on his side?
4. In which position is a patient lying on his stomach?
5. In which position is a patient lying flat on his back?
6. In which position is a patient lying on his left side with the lower arm behind the back and the upper knee flexed and raised toward the chest?
7. In which position is a patient in a semisitting position (45 to 60 degrees) with the head and shoulders elevated?
8. What is a draw sheet?
9. What is shearing?
10. When is logrolling necessary?
11. Why is it a good idea for a patient to dangle before standing up and getting out of bed?
12. Describe how a transfer belt is applied.
13. Before helping a patient into or out of a wheelchair, what should a PCT do?
14. If a patient has a weaker side, which side should move first in a transfer—the weaker or stronger side?
15. When may stretchers be used for patients?
16. List 5 guidelines for using a mechanical lift.
17. Define *ambulation*.
18. What is the purpose of canes?
19. How many feet does a quad cane have?
20. Which type of assistive device for walking can be used when a patient can bear no weight on one leg—cane, walker, or crutches?
21. Which side should a PCT stand near when a patient is using assistive equipment—the weaker or stronger side?

9 Personal Care Skills

1. Explain personal care of patients

Personal care is different from other tasks that PCTs may perform for patients, such as measuring vital signs or tidying a room. The term *personal* refers to tasks that are concerned with the person's body, appearance, and hygiene. It suggests privacy may be important. **Hygiene** is the term used to describe ways to keep bodies clean and healthy. Bathing and brushing teeth are examples. **Grooming** refers to practices like caring for fingernails and hair. Hygiene and grooming activities, as well as dressing, eating, drinking, transferring, and eliminating, are called *activities of daily living* (*ADLs*).

The way PCTs help patients with personal care plays a large part in promoting patients' dignity. The help PCTs give will be different for each patient. It will depend on each patient's abilities. For example, a patient who has recently had a stroke may need more help than one who is in the hospital for testing or observation.

Many people have been doing personal care tasks for themselves their entire lives. They may feel uncomfortable about having anyone help them with these tasks. Some patients may not like to be touched by someone else. PCTs must be sensitive to these issues. They should be professional when helping with these tasks.

Before beginning any task, the PCT should explain to the patient exactly what she will be doing. Explaining care is a patient's legal right. It may also help lessen anxiety. The PCT should ask if the patient would like to use the bathroom or bedpan first. She should provide privacy by pulling the privacy curtain around the bed and closing the door. Although facility schedules may require that care be given at a certain time, patients should be allowed to make as many decisions as possible about when and how a procedure is done (Fig. 9-1). This is part of providing person-centered care. Other ways for PCTs to promote respect, dignity, and privacy include the following:

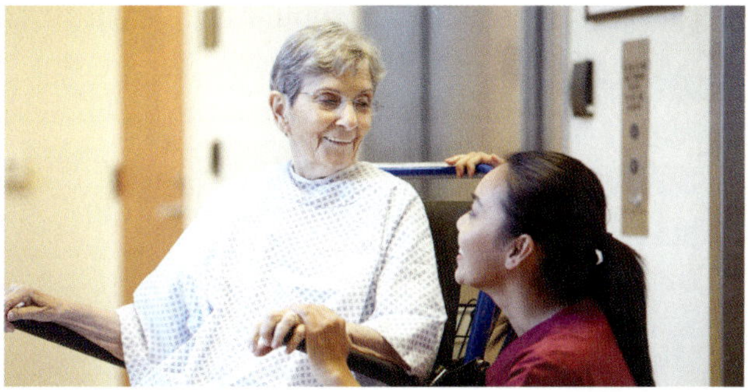

Fig. 9-1. *Allowing patients to make as many choices as possible promotes person-centered care.*

- Encourage patients to do as much as they are able to do and be patient.
- Knock and wait for permission to enter the patient's room if the patient is able to give permission.
- Do not interrupt patients while they are in the bathroom.
- Leave the room when patients receive or make phone calls.

- Keep patients covered whenever possible when helping with bathing or other personal care.
- If scheduling allows, give patients private time with visitors and come back later to give care.

Communication is very important during personal care. Some patients will share symptoms, feelings, and concerns with the PCT. The PCT should have a way to note exactly how the patient describes these symptoms (for example, a small notepad). These comments should be reported to the nurse and documented. The patient's environment should be checked for anything unsafe. These issues should also be reported.

During the procedure, if the patient appears tired, the PCT should stop and take a short break. The patient should not be rushed. After care, the PCT should always ask if the patient would like anything else. She should leave the patient's area clean and tidy. Before leaving, the PCT must make sure all ordered safety measures are in place. The call light should be left within reach of the patient's stronger hand. The room should be at a comfortable temperature. The walkways must be clear. The bed should be left in its lowest position unless the care plan instructs otherwise.

Observing and Reporting: Personal Care

O/R Skin color, temperature, and texture/feel

O/R Mobility

O/R Flexibility

O/R Comfort level, or pain or discomfort

O/R Strength and the ability to perform ADLs

O/R Mental and emotional state

O/R Patient's complaints

2. Explain guidelines for assisting with bathing

Bathing promotes health and well-being. It removes perspiration, dirt, oil, and dead skin cells from the skin. It helps to prevent skin irritation and body odor. Bathing can also be relaxing. The bed bath is an excellent time for moving arms and legs. It increases circulation. Bathing gives PCTs an opportunity to observe patients' skin carefully.

Some patients are able to shower on their own or with assistance. Others need to be bathed in bed. They may have a **partial bath**, which is a bath given on days when a complete bed bath or shower is not done. It includes washing the face, hands, axillae (underarms), and perineum. The **perineum** is the genital and anal area.

Guidelines: Bathing

G The face, hands, underarms, and perineum should be washed every day. A complete bath can be taken every other day or less often.

G Older skin produces less perspiration and oil. Elderly people may have dry and fragile skin. Be gentle when bathing elderly patients.

G Use only products approved by the facility.

G Before bathing a patient, make sure the room is warm enough.

G Be familiar with available safety and assistive devices.

G Gather supplies before giving a bath so the patient is not left waiting.

G Before bathing, make sure the water temperature is safe and comfortable. Test the water temperature against the inside of your wrist to make sure it is not too hot. Then have the patient test the water temperature. The patient is best able to choose a comfortable temperature.

G Wear gloves while bathing a patient and change your gloves before performing perineal care.

G Some facilities use bath wipes rather than soap and water. There may be different wipes used for the perineum and for the rest of the body. When using bath wipes, the process of bathing described below is the same, but the wipes are used in place of a washcloth. The skin does not need to be rinsed after cleaning with wipes. If soap and water are used, make sure all soap is removed from the skin before completing the bath.

G Follow the care plan and bathe a patient when it is assigned. Tell the nurse if a patient requests bathing or help with bathing.

Giving a complete bed bath

Equipment: bath blanket; bath basin, soap, and 2–4 washcloths or bath wipes for body and perineal care; 2–4 bath towels; disposable absorbent pads; clean gown or clothes; 2 pairs of gloves; barrier cream (if ordered); orangewood stick; lotion; deodorant; brush or comb

When bathing, move the patient's body gently and naturally. Avoid force and overextension of limbs and joints. Be careful not to dislodge any tubing.

1. Identify yourself by name. Identify the patient according to facility policy.
2. Wash your hands.
3. Explain the procedure to the patient. Speak clearly, slowly, and directly. Maintain face-to-face contact whenever possible.
4. Provide for the patient's privacy with a curtain, screen, or door. Be sure the room is at a comfortable temperature and there are no drafts.
5. Adjust the bed to a safe level, usually waist high. Lock the bed wheels.
6. Place a bath blanket or towel over the patient (Fig. 9-2). Ask him to hold on to it as you fold back the top bedding to the foot of the bed. Remove top clothing or gown, while keeping the patient covered with the bath blanket. Place gown or clothing in the proper container.

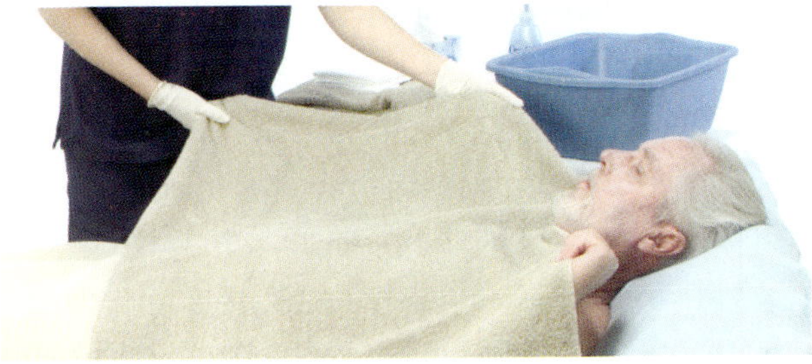

Fig. 9-2. *Cover the patient with a bath blanket or towel before removing the top bedding.*

7. Fill the basin with warm water (if used). Test the water temperature against the inside of your wrist. Ask the patient to check the water temperature to see if it is comfortable. Adjust if necessary. The water will cool quickly. Change the water when it becomes too cool, soapy, or dirty.
8. Put on gloves.
9. Ask the patient to participate in washing. Help him do this when needed.
10. Uncover only one part of the body at a time. Place a towel or absorbent pad under the part being washed.
11. Wash, rinse, and dry one part of the body at a time. Start at the head. Work down, and complete the front first. When washing, use a clean area of the washcloth for each stroke.

    Eyes, Face, Ears, and Neck: With a wet washcloth (no soap), begin with the eye farther away from you. Wash inner to outer area (Fig. 9-3). Use a different area of the washcloth for each stroke. Repeat for the other eye. Wash the face from the middle outward. Use firm but gentle strokes. Wash the ears and behind the ears. Wash the neck. Rinse and pat dry.

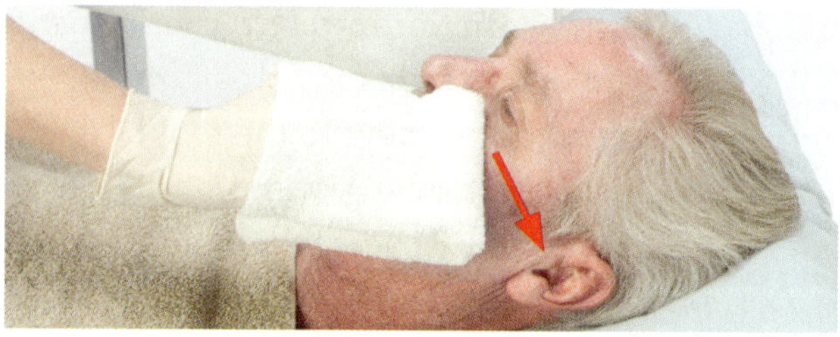

Fig. 9-3. *First wash the far eye from the inner to outer area, using a different area of the washcloth for each stroke.*

Arms and Axillae: Begin with the arm farther away from you. Remove the arm from under the towel. With a soapy washcloth, wash the upper arm and underarm. Use long strokes from the shoulder down to the wrist. Rinse and pat dry. Repeat for the other arm (Fig. 9-4).

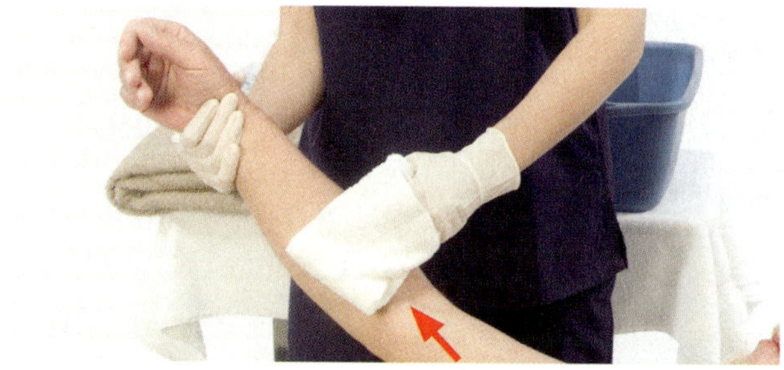

Fig. 9-4. *Support the wrist while washing the shoulder, arm, underarm, and elbow.*

Hands: Wash the far hand, including the fingers and fingernails. Clean under the nails with an orangewood stick. Rinse and pat dry. Make sure to dry between the fingers. Give nail care. (See procedure later in this chapter.) Repeat for the other hand. Put lotion on the patient's elbows and hands.

Chest: Place the towel across the patient's chest. Pull the blanket down to the waist. Lift the towel only enough to wash the chest. Rinse it and pat dry. For a female patient, wash, rinse, and dry breasts and under breasts. Check the skin in this area for signs of irritation.

Abdomen: Keep the towel across the patient's chest. Fold the blanket down so that it still covers the genital area. Wash the abdomen, rinse, and pat dry. If the patient has an ostomy, give skin care around the opening.

Cover with the towel. Pull the bath blanket up to the patient's chin. Remove the towel.

Legs and Feet: Expose the far leg. Place a towel under it. Wash the thigh. Use long, downward strokes. Rinse and pat dry. Do the same from the knee to the ankle (Fig. 9-5).

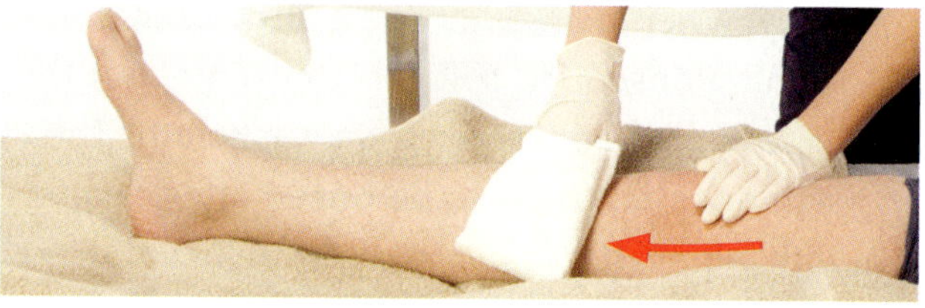

Fig. 9-5. *Use long, downward strokes when washing the legs.*

Place another towel under the far foot. Move the basin to the towel. Place the foot into the basin. Wash the foot and between the toes (Fig. 9-6). Rinse the foot and pat dry. Make sure the area between the toes is dry. Apply lotion to the foot if ordered, especially at the heels. Do not apply lotion between the toes. Repeat the steps for the other leg and foot.

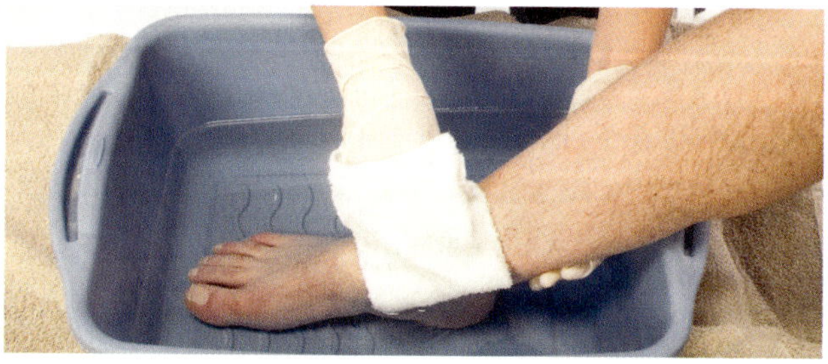

Fig. 9-6. *Washing the feet includes cleaning between the toes.*

Back: Help the patient move to the center of the bed. Raise the far side rail for safety. Help the patient to turn onto his side, toward the raised side rail. Return to the working side of the bed. His back should be facing you. Fold the blanket away from the back. Place a towel lengthwise next to the back. Wash the back and neck with long, downward strokes (Fig. 9-7). Rinse and pat dry. Apply lotion if ordered.

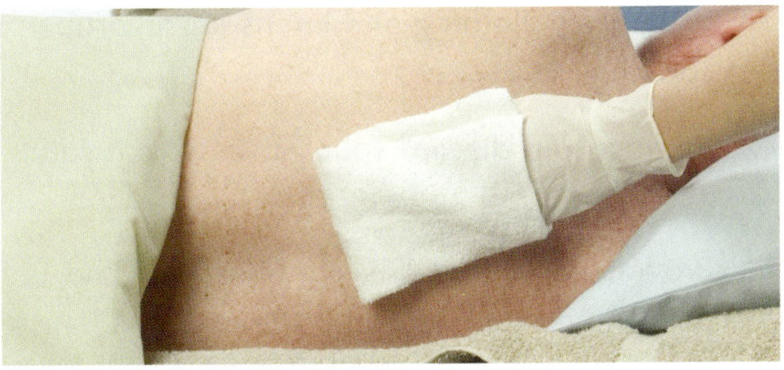

Fig. 9-7. *Wash the back with long, downward strokes.*

12. Place the towel under the buttocks and upper thighs. Help the patient turn onto his back. If the patient is able to wash his perineal area, place a basin of clean, warm water, a washcloth, and a towel within reach. Hand items to the patient as needed. If the patient wants you to leave the room, remove and discard your gloves. Wash your hands. Leave side rails up. Return the bed to its lowest position. Leave supplies and the call light within reach.

13. If the patient cannot provide perineal care, you will do so. Remove and discard your gloves. Wash your hands and put on clean gloves. Provide privacy at all times.

14. **Perineal area and buttocks**: Change the bath water. Place a towel or pad under the perineal area, including the buttocks. Wash, rinse, and dry the perineal area. Work from front to back (clean to dirty). Expose the perineal area only.

    For a female patient: Using water and a small amount of soap, wash from front to back. Use single strokes (Fig. 9-8). Use a clean area of washcloth or a clean washcloth for each stroke.

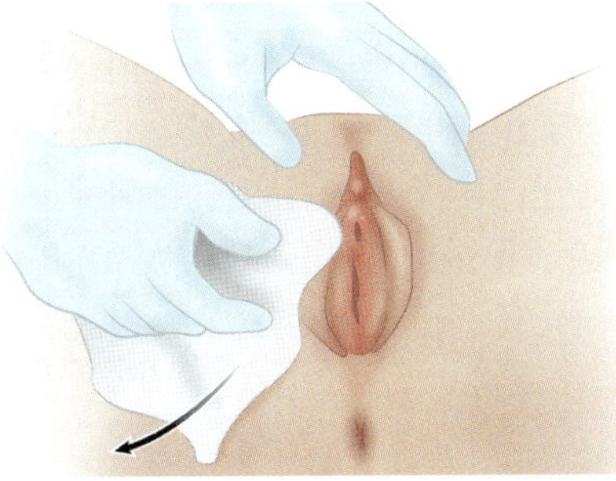

Fig. 9-8. *Always work from front to back when performing perineal care. This helps prevent infection.*

Working from front to back, wipe one side of the labia majora, the outside folds of perineal skin that protect the urinary meatus and the vaginal opening. Then wipe the other side, using a clean part of the washcloth. With your thumb and forefinger, gently separate the labia majora. Wipe from front to back on one side with a clean washcloth, using a single stroke. Using a clean area of the washcloth, wipe from front to back on the other side. Using another clean area of the washcloth, wipe from front to back down the center. Clean the perineum (area between the vagina and anus) last with a front-to-back motion. Rinse the area thoroughly in the same way. Make sure all soap is removed. With a clean, dry towel or washcloth, dry the entire perineal area. Move from front to back, using a blotting motion.

Ask the patient to turn on her side. Using a clean washcloth, wash and rinse the buttocks and anal area. Work from front to back. Clean the anal area without contaminating the perineal area. With a clean, dry towel or washcloth, dry the buttocks and anal area. If ordered, apply a barrier cream (a nonmedicated cream) to help prevent skin breakdown from incontinence.

For a male patient: If the patient is uncircumcised, pull back the foreskin first. Gently push the skin toward the base of the penis. Hold the penis by the shaft. Wash in a circular motion from the tip down to the base (Fig. 9-9). Use a clean area of washcloth or clean washcloth for each stroke.

Thoroughly rinse the penis and pat dry with a clean, dry towel or washcloth. If the patient is uncircumcised, gently return the foreskin to its normal position. Then wash the scrotum and groin. The groin is the area from the pubis (area around the penis and scrotum) to the upper thighs. Rinse and pat dry. Ask the patient to turn on his side.

Using a clean washcloth, wash and rinse the buttocks and anal area. Work from front to back. Clean the anal area without contaminating the perineal area. With a clean, dry towel or washcloth, dry the buttocks and anal area. If ordered, apply a barrier cream (a nonmedicated cream) to help prevent skin breakdown from incontinence.

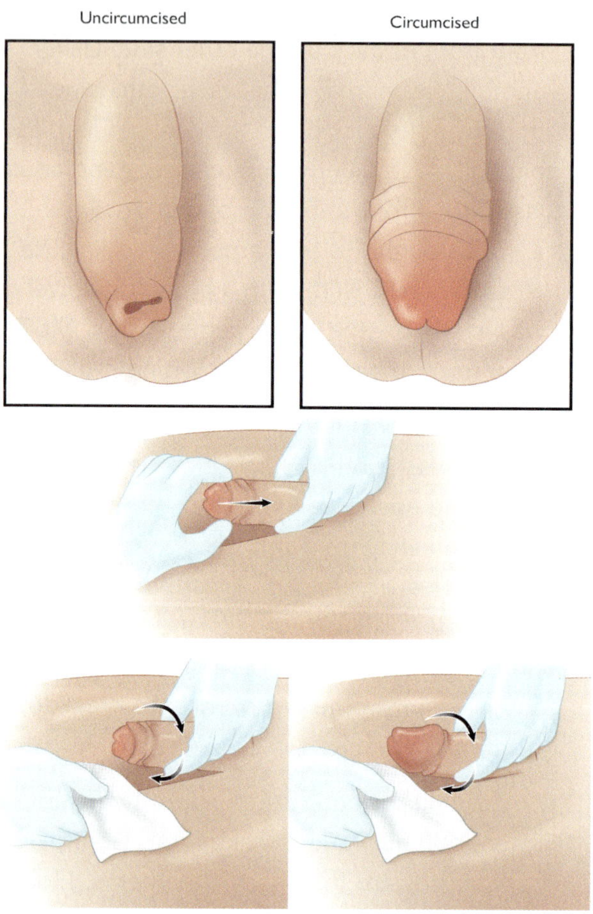

***Fig. 9-9.** The top illustration shows an uncircumcised penis on the left and a circumcised penis on the right. If the penis is uncircumcised, gently push back the foreskin toward the base of the penis (middle illustration). Then wash the penis in a circular motion from the tip down to the base. (Bottom illustration shows an uncircumcised penis on the left and a circumcised penis on the right.)*

15. Cover the patient with the bath blanket.
16. Empty, rinse, and dry the bath basin. Place the basin in the dirty supply area or return to storage, depending on facility policy.
17. Place used clothing and linens in the proper containers.
18. Remove and discard your gloves. Wash your hands.
19. Provide deodorant. Place a towel over the pillow and brush or comb the patient's hair. (See procedure later in this chapter.) Help the patient put on a clean gown or clothing. Help the patient into a comfortable position with proper body alignment.
20. Return the bed to its lowest position. Leave side rails in the ordered position. Remove privacy measures.
21. Place the call light within the patient's reach.
22. Wash your hands.
23. Report any changes in the patient to the nurse.
24. Document the procedure using facility guidelines.

Hair care is an important part of cleanliness. Shampooing the hair removes dirt, bacteria, oils, and other materials from the hair. Depending on the patient's hair type, shampooing may be needed between once and 3–4 times per week. Patients who can get out of bed may shampoo their hair in the shower, with or without help from a PCT. For patients who cannot get out of bed, there are several options. A basin or trough may be used to shampoo the patient's hair in bed. There are also special types of shampoo that do not require the use of water. This type of shampoo is available in a cap that can be placed on the patient's head. The PCT then massages the hair through the cap to activate the shampoo and clean the hair and scalp (Fig. 9-10). Gloves should be worn if a patient has open sores on his scalp.

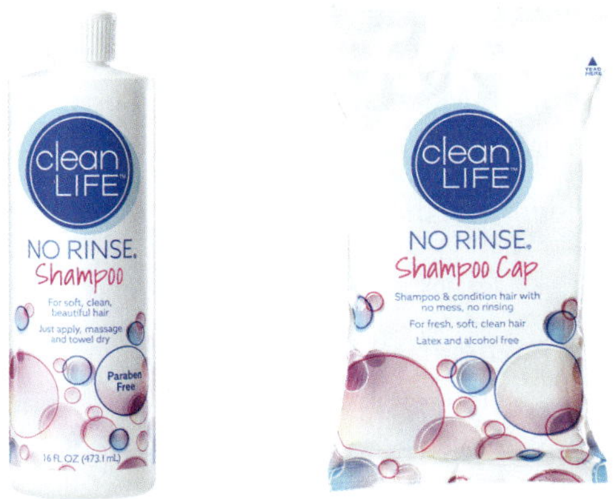

Fig. 9-10. *These are examples of shampoos that do not require the use of water.* (PHOTOS COURTESY OF CLEANLIFE PRODUCTS, WWW.CLEANLIFEPRODUCTS.COM)

Connected Care

Hair Types

Every person's hair is different, and most people have more than one type of hair. Hair can be coily (very tightly curled), curly, wavy, or straight. It can be thick or thin, and the hair itself can be more or less able to absorb oils and moisture.

Different types of hair require different care. Hair that is curly or coily is sometimes called *textured hair*. Black patients are more likely to have textured hair. Patients with textured hair do not need their hair washed as often as patients with straight hair, which becomes oily more quickly. Textured hair dries out easily and may break more easily than other types of hair. If conditioners or hair oils are available, they may be used during combing to help prevent drying. A silk or satin bonnet or kerchief can protect hair while the patient is in bed. Combs with thicker, wider teeth are better for textured hair.

Hospitals may not have products and equipment to care for all hair types. Patients' families may be able to bring these products for the patient. Some hospital volunteers collect hair care items for patients whose hair requires care that hospital products cannot provide. PCTs who care for patients' hair should honor their preferences about hair care whenever they can. If the patient has a need that is not being met, it should be reported to the nurse.

Shampooing hair in bed

Equipment: shampoo, hair conditioner (if requested and available), 2 bath towels, washcloth, pitcher or handheld shower or sink attachment, waterproof pad, bath blanket, shampoo basin, comb and brush

1. Identify yourself by name. Identify the patient according to facility policy.
2. Wash your hands.
3. Explain the procedure to the patient. Speak clearly, slowly, and directly. Maintain face-to-face contact whenever possible.
4. Provide for the patient's privacy with a curtain, screen, or door. Be sure the room is at a comfortable temperature and there are no drafts.
5. Arrange the supplies within reach.
6. Test the water temperature against the inside of your wrist. Have the patient check the water temperature. Adjust if necessary.
7. Remove all pillows and place the patient in a flat position. Adjust the bed to a safe level, usually waist high. Lock the bed wheels.
8. Place the waterproof pad under the patient's head and shoulders. Cover the patient with the bath blanket. Fold back the top sheet and regular blankets.
9. Place the basin under the patient's head. Place a towel across the patient's shoulders. Protect the patient's eyes with a dry washcloth.
10. Using the pitcher, wet the hair thoroughly. Apply a small amount of shampoo to your hands and rub them together.
11. Using both hands, massage the shampoo into a lather in the patient's hair. With your fingertips (not fingernails), massage the scalp in a circular motion, from front to back. Do not scratch the scalp.
12. Rinse the hair until water runs clear. Use conditioner if the patient wants it. Rinse as directed on the container. Rinse the hair thoroughly to prevent the scalp from getting dry and itchy.

13. Wrap the patient's hair in a clean towel. Remove the basin. Dry his face and neck with the washcloth or a towel.
14. Raise the head of the bed.
15. Gently rub the scalp and hair with the towel.
16. Comb or brush the hair. Style the hair as the patient prefers.
17. Return the bed to its lowest position. Remove privacy measures.
18. Place the call light within the patient's reach.
19. Empty, rinse, and wipe the bath basin and pitcher. Take them to the proper area.
20. Clean and store the comb or brush.
21. Place used linen in the proper container.
22. Wash your hands.
23. Report any changes in the patient to the nurse.
24. Document the procedure using facility guidelines.

Many people prefer showers to bed baths. The PCT must check with the nurse first to make sure a shower is allowed.

Guidelines: Safety for Showers

G Make sure the floor is dry.

G Be familiar with available safety and assistive devices. Check that handrails, grab bars, and lifts are in working order.

G Have the patient use safety bars to get into the shower if the patient has limited mobility or may be unsteady.

G Place all needed items within reach.

G Do not leave the patient alone if the care plan states he needs help with showering.

G Do not use lotions or powders in showers. They make surfaces slippery.

G Test water temperature against the inside of your wrist before the patient gets into the shower. Make sure the temperature is comfortable for the patient.

G Clean the shower after use.

Connected Care

Privacy when Bathing

Privacy is very important when patients are having a shower. Doors should be kept closed. Patients should be covered when possible. Their bodies should not be unnecessarily exposed.

Giving a shower

Equipment: soap, shampoo, 2–4 washcloths, 2–4 bath towels, clean clothes or gown, nonskid footwear, gloves, lotion, deodorant

1. Identify yourself by name. Identify the patient according to facility policy.
2. Wash your hands.
3. Explain the procedure to the patient. Speak clearly, slowly, and directly. Maintain face-to-face contact whenever possible.
4. Place equipment in the shower area. Put on gloves. If the patient is using a shower chair, place a bucket under the shower chair (in case the patient has a bowel movement). Turn on the heat lamp to warm the room (if available).
5. Provide for the patient's privacy with a curtain, screen, or door.
6. Help the patient to put on nonskid footwear and go to the shower area.
7. Wash your hands. Put on clean gloves.
8. Help the patient remove clothing and shoes.
9. If using a shower chair, place it close to the patient. Lock its wheels (Fig. 9-11). Safely transfer the patient into the chair.
10. Turn on the water. Test the water temperature against the inside of your wrist. Have

the patient check the water temperature. Adjust if necessary. Check the temperature throughout the shower.

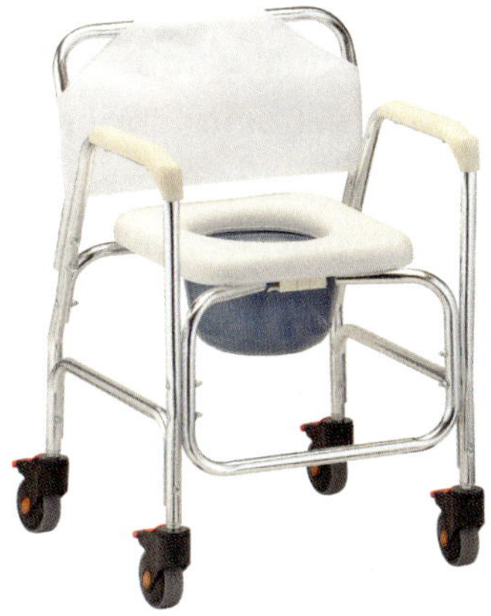

Fig. 9-11. *A shower chair is a sturdy chair designed to be placed in a shower. It is water- and slip-resistant. The chair allows a person who is too weak to stand in a shower to bathe in the shower, rather than in bed. A shower chair must be locked before transferring a patient into it.* (PHOTO COURTESY OF NOVA MEDICAL PRODUCTS, WWW.NOVAJOY.COM)

11. Unlock the shower chair and move it into the shower stall. Lock its wheels.
12. Stay with the patient during the procedure.
13. Let the patient wash as much as possible. Help to wash their face.
14. Help the patient shampoo and rinse hair.
15. Using soap, help to wash and rinse the entire body. Move from head to toe (clean to dirty).
16. Turn off the water. Unlock the chair wheels. Roll the patient out of the shower.
17. Give the patient a towel and help to pat dry. Pat dry under the breasts, between skin folds, in the perineal area, and between toes.
18. Apply lotion and deodorant as needed.
19. Place used clothing or gown in the proper containers.
20. Remove and discard your gloves. Wash your hands.
21. Help the patient put on a clean gown or clothing and comb hair before leaving the room. Put on nonskid footwear. Return the patient to bed.
22. Make sure the patient is comfortable.
23. Place the call light within the patient's reach.
24. Report any changes in the patient to the nurse.
25. Document the procedure using facility guidelines.

3. Explain guidelines for assisting with grooming

Grooming affects the way people feel about themselves and how they look to others (Fig. 9-12). When helping with grooming, PCTs should always let patients do all they can for themselves. Patients should make as many choices as possible. Patients may have particular ways of grooming themselves. They may have routines, and routines remain important even when people are in a healthcare facility. Some patients may be embarrassed, depressed, or anxious because they need help with grooming tasks. PCTs should be sensitive to this. Being respectful promotes person-centered care.

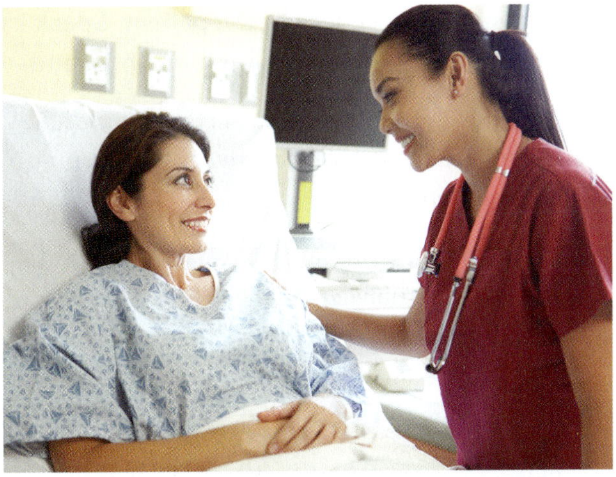

Fig. 9-12. *A well-groomed appearance helps a person feel good about herself.*

Hair Care

Pieces of hair can be accidentally pulled out of the head while combing or brushing it. PCTs must handle patients' hair very gently.

Pediculosis is an infestation of lice. Lice are tiny bugs that bite into the skin and suck blood to live and grow. Types of lice include head lice, body lice, and crab or pubic lice. Head lice are usually found on the scalp. Lice are hard to see. Symptoms include itching, bite marks on the scalp, skin sores, and matted, bad-smelling hair and scalp. Lice eggs may be visible on the hair, behind the ears, and on the neck. They are small and round and may be brown or white. Lice droppings look like a fine black powder. They may be on sheets or pillows. If PCTs notice any of these signs or symptoms, they should tell the nurse immediately. Lice can spread to others very quickly. Special creams, shampoos, lotions, sprays, or special combs may be used to treat lice.

Combing or brushing hair

Equipment: comb and/or brush suited to patient's hair, water and/or conditioner (if needed), towel

1. Identify yourself by name. Identify the patient according to facility policy.
2. Wash your hands.
3. Explain the procedure to the patient. Speak clearly, slowly, and directly. Maintain face-to-face contact whenever possible.
4. Provide for the patient's privacy with a curtain, screen, or door.
5. If the patient is in bed, adjust the bed to a safe level, usually waist high. Raise the head of the bed so that the patient is sitting up. Lock the bed wheels. If the patient is ambulatory, provide a chair.
6. Place a towel under the patient's head or around the shoulders.
7. Remove any hairpins, hair ties, or clips.
8. Remove tangles first by dividing hair into small sections. For patients with textured (curly or coily) hair, hair should be wet and a wide-toothed comb is best. Hold the lock of hair just above the tangle so you do not pull at the scalp. Gently comb or brush through the tangle. If the patient agrees, use a small amount of detangler or leave-in conditioner if it is available.
9. After tangles are removed, comb or brush 2-inch sections of hair at a time. Keep the hair wet as you work, as needed, based on hair type.
10. Return supplies to proper storage. Clean and store the comb or brush.
11. Dispose of used linen in the proper container.
12. Return the bed to its lowest position. Remove privacy measures.
13. Place the call light within the patient's reach.
14. Wash your hands.
15. Report any changes in the patient to the nurse.
16. Document the procedure using facility guidelines.

Shaving

Personal preferences for shaving must be respected. The PCT should make sure the patient wants to be shaved before beginning. In a hospital, electric razors are the first choice for shaving patients. They are the safest and easiest razors to use. They do not require soap or shaving cream. Patients who take blood thinners (anticoagulant medication that helps prevent blood clots) should always be shaved with an electric razor if one is available. If a disposable razor is used, PCTs must wear gloves due to the risk of exposure to blood. Disposable razors are discarded in a biohazard container for sharps after use. Razors should not be shared between patients.

Shaving a patient

Equipment: razor, basin filled halfway with warm water (if using a disposable razor), 2 towels, washcloth, mirror, shaving cream or soap (if using a disposable razor), gloves

1. Identify yourself by name. Identify the patient according to facility policy.
2. Wash your hands.
3. Explain the procedure to the patient. Speak clearly, slowly, and directly. Maintain face-to-face contact whenever possible.
4. Provide for the patient's privacy with a curtain, screen, or door.
5. If the patient is in bed, adjust the bed to a safe level, usually waist high. Lock the bed wheels.
6. Raise the head of the bed so that the patient is sitting up. Place a towel across the patient's chest, under his chin.
7. Put on gloves.

Shaving using an electric razor

8. Use a small brush to clean the razor. Do not use an electric razor near any water source or when oxygen is in use.
9. Turn on the razor and hold skin taut. Shave with smooth, even movements. Shave the beard with a back-and-forth motion in the direction of the beard growth.
10. Offer a mirror to the patient.

Shaving using a disposable razor

8. Soften the beard with a warm, wet washcloth on the face for a few minutes before shaving. Lather the face with shaving cream or soap and warm water.
9. Hold skin taut. Shave in the direction of hair growth. Shave in short, downward, and even strokes on the face and upward strokes on the neck (Fig. 9-13). Rinse the blade often in the basin to keep it clean and wet.

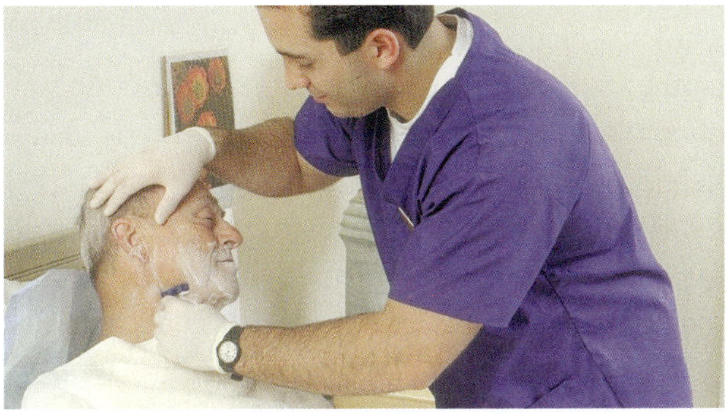

Fig. 9-13. *Holding the skin taut, shave in downward strokes on the face and upward strokes on the neck.*

10. When you have finished, wash and rinse the patient's face with a warm, wet washcloth. If he is able, let him use the cloth himself. Use the towel to dry his face. Offer a mirror.

Final steps

11. Remove the towel. Place the towel and washcloth in the proper container.
12. For an electric razor, clean the razor according to facility policy. Change the razor head according to manufacturer instructions. For a disposable razor, dispose of it in a biohazard container for sharps.
13. Remove and discard your gloves. Wash your hands.
14. Make sure that the area and the patient's skin and clothing are free of loose hairs.
15. Return the bed to its lowest position. Remove privacy measures.
16. Place the call light within the patient's reach.
17. Report any changes in the patient to the nurse.
18. Document the procedure using facility guidelines.

4. List guidelines for assisting with dressing

Although patients may wear a hospital gown most of the time they are in a facility, PCTs must know how to assist with dressing patients. They may help patients change from their clothes into a gown. They may help patients change gowns during their stay. They may also help patients dress for discharge from the facility. When helping with dressing, the PCT should know what limitations the patient has. Patients may have one side of the body that is weaker due to stroke or injury. That side is called the *weaker, affected,* or *involved* side. The PCT should not refer to the weaker side as the "bad side," or talk about the "bad" leg or arm. When dressing a patient with one-sided weakness, the PCT should begin with the weaker side of the body. This helps reduce the risk of injury. The weaker arm is placed through a sleeve first. When a leg is weak, it is easier if the patient sits down to pull the pants over both legs.

Guidelines: Dressing and Undressing

G Let the patient do as much to dress or undress himself as possible. It may take longer, but it helps maintain dignity. Ask where your help is needed. Assistive devices for dressing are available (Fig. 9-14). Use them as directed.

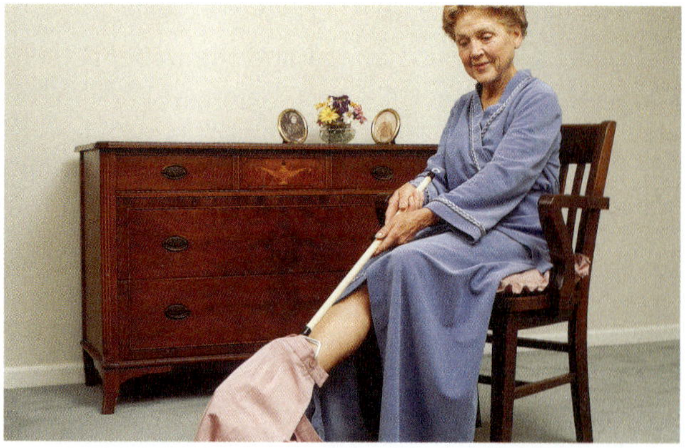

Fig. 9-14. *Special dressing aids promote independence by helping patients dress themselves.* (PHOTO COURTESY OF NORTH COAST MEDICAL, INC., WWW.NCMEDICAL.COM)

G Provide privacy and never expose more than what is necessary.

G Roll or fold socks or stockings down when putting them on. Slip over the toes and foot, then unroll them up into place.

G For a female patient, make sure bra cups fit over the breasts.

G Place the weaker arm or leg through the garment first. Then help with the stronger arm or leg. When undressing, start with the stronger, or unaffected, side (Fig. 9-15).

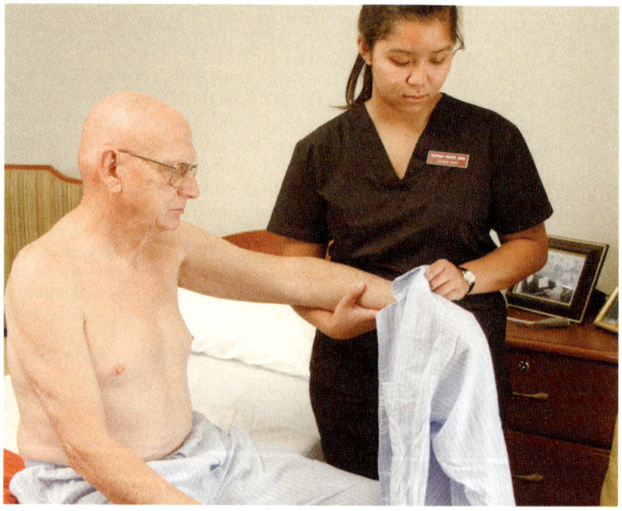

Fig. 9-15. *When dressing, the PCT should start with the affected (weaker) side first.*

Dressing a patient

Equipment: bath blanket, clean clothes or gown, nonskid footwear, gloves

When putting on items, move the patient's body gently and naturally. Avoid force and overextension of limbs and joints.

1. Identify yourself by name. Identify the patient according to facility policy.
2. Wash your hands.
3. Explain the procedure to the patient. Speak clearly, slowly, and directly. Maintain face-to-face contact whenever possible.
4. Provide for the patient's privacy with a curtain, screen, or door.

5. Adjust the bed to a safe level, usually waist high. Lock the bed wheels.
6. Raise the head of the bed so that the patient is sitting up.
7. Place a bath blanket over the patient. Ask her to hold on to it as you remove or fold back the top bedding to the foot of the bed. Remove the gown or top. Keep the patient covered with the bath blanket. Take clothes/gown off the stronger side first when undressing. Then remove from the weaker side. Place top clothing in the proper container. Move the bath blanket down to cover the lower body.
8. Help the patient put on the top or clean gown. If the top goes over the head, slide the top over the head first. Then place the weaker arm through the sleeve before placing the garment on the stronger arm. Help the patient lean forward and smooth the top down. If the top fastens in the front, slide your hand through one sleeve and grasp the patient's hand on the weaker side, pulling it through. Help the patient lean forward and arrange the top across the back. Pull the second sleeve on the stronger side as you did with the first one. Fasten the top.
9. Remove the bath blanket and place it in the proper container. Help the patient put on a skirt or pants if the patient is dressing for transfer or discharge from the facility. Put the weaker leg through the skirt or pants first. Then place the stronger leg through the skirt or pants. Have the patient raise her buttocks or turn her from side to side to pull the pants over her buttocks up to the waist. Fasten the pants or skirt if needed and make sure the clothing is comfortable.
10. Roll one sock over the weaker foot. Make sure the heel of the sock is over the heel of the foot. Make sure there are no twists or wrinkles in the sock after it is on. Repeat for the other foot.
11. If the patient is leaving the facility and will be wearing shoes, place the bed at the lowest position. Have the patient sit up on the side of the bed with her legs hanging over the side (dangle).
12. Starting with the weaker foot, help put on nonskid footwear. Fasten one shoe securely and then put on the other shoe and fasten it.
13. Finish with the patient dressed appropriately in clothing or a gown. Make sure clothing is right side out and zippers and buttons are fastened.
14. Leave the bed in its lowest position. Remove privacy measures.
15. Place the call light within the patient's reach.
16. Wash your hands.
17. Report any changes in the patient to the nurse.
18. Document the procedure using facility guidelines.

Intravenous therapy, often called *IV therapy*, is the delivery of medication, nutrition, or fluids through a vein. Medication, nutrition, or fluids either drip from a bag suspended on a pole or are pumped by a portable pump through a tube and into the vein.

Guidelines: Changing Gowns for a Patient with an IV

G Never disconnect IV lines or turn off the pump. The nurse will be responsible for unhooking IV tubing from the pump. (Some hospital gowns have snaps that allow them to be changed easily without disconnecting IV tubing.)

G Always keep the IV bag higher than the IV site on the body.

G First remove the gown from the side without the IV. Then gather the gown on the side with the IV. Lift the gown over the IV site. Move it up the tubing toward the IV bag. Lift the IV bag off its pole. Carefully slide the gown over the bag. Place the bag back on the pole.

G Lift the IV bag off its pole. Apply a clean gown to the side with the IV. Slide the gown over the bag. Place the IV bag back on the pole. Move the gown down the IV tubing, over the IV site, and onto the patient's arm. Put the other arm into the gown.

G Check that the IV is dripping properly. Make sure none of the tubing is dislodged. This should be done after every procedure when a patient has an IV. Check to see that the IV site dressing is in place. Make sure tubing is not kinked after you are finished.

5. Identify guidelines for proper oral care

Oral care, or care of the mouth, teeth, and gums, is done at least twice each day to clean the mouth. Oral care should be done after breakfast and after the last meal or snack of the day. It may also be done before a patient eats. Oral care includes brushing the teeth, tongue, and gums; flossing teeth; caring for lips; and caring for dentures (Fig. 9-16). Patients may be able to perform their own oral care. PCTs do this task if patients cannot do it on their own. When giving oral care, PCTs must wear gloves. They should follow Standard Precautions.

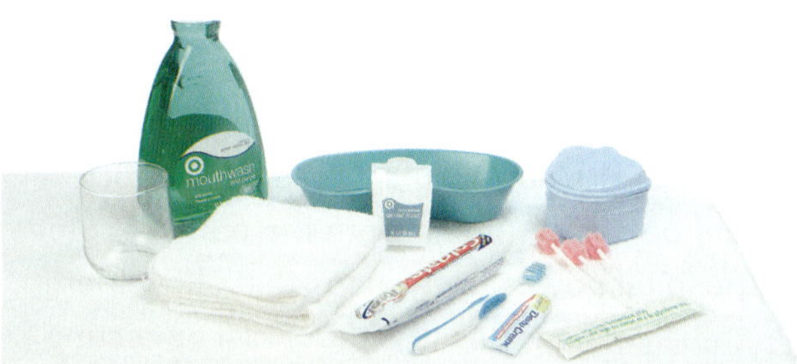

Fig. 9-16. *Some supplies needed for oral care.*

Observing and Reporting: Oral Care

When performing oral care, observe the patient's mouth carefully. Report any of these to the nurse:

O/R Irritation

O/R Raised areas

O/R Coated or swollen tongue

O/R Ulcers, such as canker sores or small, painful, white sores

O/R Flaky, white spots

O/R Dry, cracked, bleeding, or chapped lips

O/R Loose, chipped, broken, or decayed teeth

O/R Swollen, irritated, bleeding, or whitish gums

O/R Breath that smells bad or fruity

O/R Patient reports of mouth pain

Providing oral care

Equipment: toothbrush; toothpaste; emesis basin; gloves; clothing protector, towel, or washcloth; cup of water; lip moisturizer

1. Identify yourself by name. Identify the patient according to facility policy.
2. Wash your hands.
3. Explain the procedure to the patient. Speak clearly, slowly, and directly. Maintain face-to-face contact whenever possible.
4. Provide for the patient's privacy with a curtain, screen, or door.
5. If the patient is in bed, adjust the bed to a safe level, usually waist high. Raise the head of the bed to have the patient in an upright sitting position. Lock the bed wheels.
6. Put on gloves.
7. Place a clothing protector, towel, or washcloth across the patient's chest.
8. Wet the toothbrush. Put on a small amount of toothpaste.

9. Clean the entire mouth, including the tongue and all surfaces of the teeth and gumline. Use gentle strokes. First brush the inner, outer, and chewing surfaces of the upper teeth. Then do the same with the lower teeth. Use short strokes. Brush back and forth. Brush the tongue.

10. Give the patient water to rinse the mouth. Place the emesis basin under the patient's chin, with the inward curve under the chin. Have the patient spit water into the basin (Fig. 9-17). Wipe his mouth and remove the towel. Apply lip moisturizer.

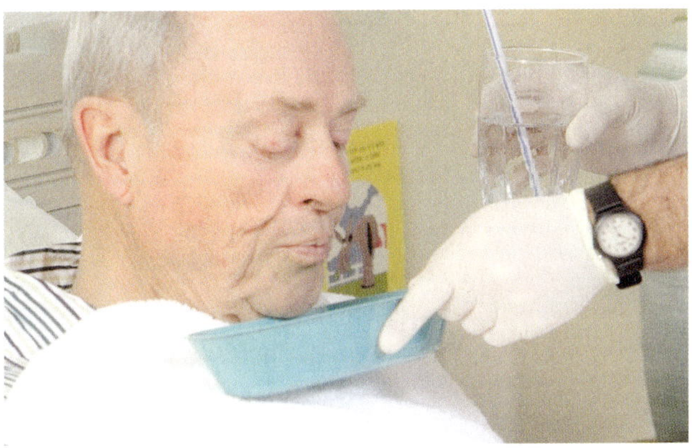

Fig. 9-17. *Rinsing and spitting removes food particles and toothpaste.*

11. Rinse the toothbrush and place it in the proper container. Empty, rinse, and dry the basin. Place the basin in the designated area or return to storage, depending on facility policy.

12. Place the used clothing protector and linens in proper containers.

13. Remove and discard your gloves. Wash your hands.

14. Return the bed to its lowest position. Remove privacy measures.

15. Place the call light within the patient's reach.

16. Report any problems with the teeth, mouth, tongue, or lips to the nurse. This includes odor, cracking, sores, bleeding, and any discoloration.

17. Document the procedure using facility guidelines.

Even though a person who is unconscious cannot eat, breathing through the mouth causes saliva to dry in the mouth. A lack of fluid intake can also cause the mouth to become dry. Regular oral care helps keep the mouth clean and moist and must be done at least every 2 hours. With unconscious patients, PCTs must use as little liquid as possible when giving mouth care. Because the person's swallowing reflex is weak, he is at risk for aspiration. **Aspiration** is the inhalation of food, fluid, or foreign material into the lungs. Aspiration can cause pneumonia or death. Turning an unconscious patient on his side before giving oral care can also help prevent aspiration. Only swabs soaked in tiny amounts of fluid should be used to clean the mouth. Oral suctioning may be used to make sure no liquid is left in the patient's mouth. Chapter 16 has more information about oral suctioning.

Providing oral care for an unconscious patient

Equipment: sponge swabs, tongue depressor, towel, emesis basin, gloves, cup of cool water, lip moisturizer, cleaning solution (check the care plan)

1. Identify yourself by name. Identify the patient according to facility policy. Even patients who are unconscious may be able to hear you. Always speak to them as you would to any patient.

2. Wash your hands.

3. Explain the procedure to the patient. Speak clearly, slowly, and directly. Maintain face-to-face contact whenever possible.

4. Provide for the patient's privacy with a curtain, screen, or door.

5. Adjust the bed to a safe level, usually waist high. Lock the bed wheels.
6. Put on gloves.
7. Turn the patient onto his side. Place a towel under his cheek and chin. Place an emesis basin next to the cheek and chin for excess fluid.
8. Hold the mouth open with the tongue depressor. (You can also use gentle pressure on the chin to open the mouth. Follow facility policy.)
9. Dip the sponge swab in the cleaning solution. Squeeze excess solution to prevent aspiration. Wipe the teeth, gums, tongue, and inside surfaces of the mouth. Remove debris with the swab. Change the swab often. Repeat this until the mouth is clean.
10. Rinse with a clean swab dipped in water. Squeeze the swab first to remove excess water.
11. Remove the towel and basin. Pat lips or face dry if needed. Apply lip moisturizer. Turn the patient onto his back.
12. Empty, rinse, and dry the basin. Place the basin in the designated area or return to storage, depending on facility policy.
13. Place used linens in the proper container.
14. Remove and discard your gloves. Wash your hands.
15. Return the bed to its lowest position. Remove privacy measures.
16. Place the call light within the patient's reach.
17. Report any problems with the teeth, mouth, tongue, or lips to the nurse. This includes odor, cracking, sores, bleeding, and any discoloration.
18. Document the procedure using facility guidelines.

Dentures are artificial teeth. They are expensive. Dentures must be handled carefully to avoid breaking or chipping them. If a patient's dentures break, the patient cannot eat. Denture care may be something a patient can do for himself. If not, the PCT will do it.

The PCT must wear gloves when handling and cleaning dentures. Dentures and denture brushes should not be placed on contaminated surfaces. Once dentures are cleaned, they should either be returned to the patient or stored in denture solution or in clean, moderate/cool water (not hot water) so that they do not dry out and warp. Dentures may crack if left uncovered. Dentures should be stored in a denture cup labeled with the patient's name when not being worn. They should not be removed from the patient's room.

Connected Care

Denture Care

Denture care is very personal. The PCT should pull the privacy curtain and close the door before beginning. Many people who have dentures do not want to be seen without their teeth in place. After teeth are removed, they should be cleaned and returned immediately.

Cleaning and storing dentures

Equipment: denture brush or toothbrush, denture cleanser, labeled denture cup, 2 towels, gloves

1. Wash your hands.
2. Put on gloves.
3. Line the sink or a basin with a towel(s) and partially fill the sink with water.
4. Handle dentures carefully. Hold them over the sink. Rinse the dentures in clean, moderate/cool running water before brushing them. Do not use hot water.
5. Apply cleanser to the brush.
6. Brush dentures on all surfaces (Fig. 9-18). This includes the inner, outer, and chew-

ing surfaces of the dentures, as well as the groove that will touch gum surfaces.

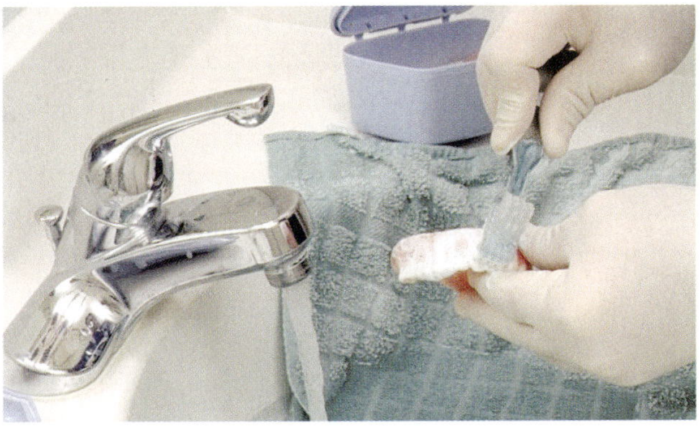

Fig. 9-18. Brush dentures on all surfaces to properly clean them.

7. Rinse all surfaces of dentures under clean, moderate/cool running water. Do not use hot water.
8. Rinse the denture cup and lid before placing clean dentures in the cup.
9. Place dentures in a clean, labeled denture cup with solution or clean, moderate/cool water. Dentures should be completely covered with solution. Place the lid on the cup. Make sure the cup is labeled with the patient's name and room number. Return the cup to where it is stored. Some patients will want to wear their dentures all of the time. They will only remove them for cleaning. If the patient wants to wear her dentures, return them to her. Do not place them in the denture cup.
10. Rinse the brush. Clean, dry, and return the equipment to storage. Drain the sink. Place used linens in the proper container.
11. Remove and discard your gloves. Wash your hands.
12. Document the procedure using facility guidelines. Report any change in the appearance of the dentures to the nurse.

Removing and Reinserting Dentures

If a patient cannot remove her dentures, the PCT must do it if trained and allowed to do so. The patient should be sitting upright before beginning. The PCT should first don gloves. The lower denture should be removed first. It is easier to remove because it floats on the gumline of the lower jaw. The PCT should grasp the lower denture with a gauze square (for a good grip) and remove it. She should place it in a denture cup filled with solution or moderate/cool water.

The upper denture is sealed by suction. The PCT should firmly grasp the upper denture with a gauze square and give a slight downward pull to break the suction. She should turn it at an angle to take it out of the mouth. It should be placed in a denture cup filled with solution or moderate/cool water.

When inserting dentures, the PCT should ask the patient to sit upright, then she should don gloves. If needed, she should apply denture cream or adhesive to the dentures. When the patient's mouth is open, the upper denture should be placed into the mouth by turning it at an angle. The PCT should straighten it and press it onto the upper gumline firmly and evenly. She should insert the lower denture onto the gumline of the lower jaw and press firmly.

Chapter Review

1. List 4 examples of activities of daily living.
2. Give 4 examples of how to promote respect, dignity, and privacy while giving personal care.
3. What are 5 observations that a PCT can make about a patient during personal care?
4. Which parts of the body should be washed every day?
5. Why is it important for the PCT to be particularly gentle when bathing an elderly patient?
6. Why should the PCT wipe from front to back when giving perineal care?

7. How might a PCT assist with washing hair for a patient who is bedbound?
8. What are 4 safety guidelines for assisting with showers?
9. What type of razor is the safest and easiest choice for shaving patients? Why?
10. Why should a PCT wear gloves while shaving patients?
11. If a patient has an affected side due to a stroke, how should the PCT refer to that side?
12. When dressing a patient with a weaker side, which arm is usually placed through the sleeve first—the weaker or stronger arm?
13. When giving oral care to a patient, what are 3 things a PCT should report about a patient's mouth?
14. How can PCTs help prevent aspiration during oral care of patients who are unconscious?
15. Why should hot water not be used on dentures?

10 Basic Nursing Skills

1. Describe patient rounding

Many people are familiar with the idea of doctors making rounds in a hospital. During these rounds, doctors, often along with medical residents (doctors in post-graduate training) or other healthcare providers, visit patients under their care. They assess the patients' progress, including response to treatment. They ask about any new concerns and adjust the care plan as needed.

PCTs may perform a type of patient rounding as well. Although procedures vary by facility, PCTs may be assigned to visit each patient every hour. The schedule may be less often at night to avoid disrupting the patient's sleep. During these visits, PCTs check for the following:

- Bathroom needs
- Pain levels, which are often measured by asking the patient to rate pain using a pain scale
- Comfort/need for repositioning
- Anything the patient needs help reaching or moving (e.g., helping the patient to plug in a cell phone to charge or moving a book within the patient's reach)
- Proper functioning of medical equipment (e.g., checking that an IV bag is not empty or that tubing is not kinked)
- Any other needs the patient may have

If the patient has needs that are beyond the PCT's scope of practice, or if the patient's condition has changed, the PCT should report to the nurse. The nurse can also be called if there are any problems with medical equipment. Vital signs (see later in the chapter) are usually measured every 4 hours, depending on the patient's condition. These procedures are added to the rounding process at the proper times. Patients who are unable to reposition themselves may also be repositioned every 2 hours.

When PCT rounding is done carefully and correctly, it provides important benefits for patients. It helps to reduce falls and pressure injuries. It reduces the need for call light use and lets patients know that they are being cared for. Rounding can reduce patient fear and anxiety. The PCT's observations can also help the care team by identifying changes that may signal a problem for the patient.

Patient rounding is not always documented in a patient's record unless vital signs are measured or a significant change is observed. There may be a rounding checklist on the patient's door or on the whiteboard/patient communication board. Some facilities also have a "turning wheel," or a display to show when a patient was last repositioned (Fig. 10-1).

If patient rounding is done at a facility, it is very important to follow facility procedures exactly. Being consistent, or doing things the same way every time, is part of what makes rounding effective. Some facilities develop a script for PCTs to use. This helps make sure that the correct information is gathered and the correct steps taken during each visit. If rounding is not consistent, the benefits to the patient are lost.

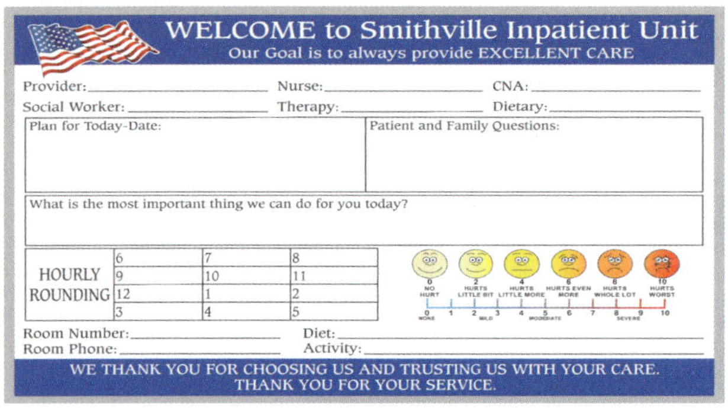
WELCOME to Smithville Inpatient Unit
Our Goal is to always provide EXCELLENT CARE
Provider: Nurse: CNA:
Social Worker: Therapy: Dietary:
Plan for Today-Date: Patient and Family Questions:
What is the most important thing we can do for you today?
HOURLY ROUNDING 6 7 8 9 10 11 12 1 2 3 4 5
Room Number: Diet:
Room Phone: Activity:
WE THANK YOU FOR CHOOSING US AND TRUSTING US WITH YOUR CARE.
THANK YOU FOR YOUR SERVICE.

Fig. 10-1. *PCTs may update some of the information on a patient's whiteboard. Positioning, pain levels, and patient rounding schedules are sometimes included on these boards.* *(IMAGE COURTESY OF MAGNETIC CONCEPTS © 2023, WWW.MAGNETICCONCEPTS.COM)*

2. Explain the importance of monitoring vital signs

PCTs monitor, document, and report patients' **vital signs**. Vital signs are important. They show how well the vital organs of the body, such as the heart and lungs, are working. They consist of the following:

- Measuring body temperature
- Counting the pulse rate
- Counting the rate of respirations
- Measuring blood pressure

Watching for changes in vital signs is very important. Changes can indicate a patient's condition is worsening. A PCT should always notify the nurse if

- The patient has a fever (temperature is above average for the patient or outside the normal range)
- The patient has a respiratory or pulse rate that is too rapid or too slow
- The patient's blood pressure changes

Many factors, such as age, medical condition, medications, mental state, room temperature, and noise levels, can affect vital signs. All of the factors should be considered, along with the patient's baseline vital signs. Baseline vital signs are the measurements that are normal for a particular person. PCTs must know the normal ranges for vital signs. Measurements that are not in normal range or that are different from a patient's baseline measurements should be reported to a nurse.

Ranges for Adult Vital Signs

Temp. Site	Fahrenheit	Celsius
Mouth (oral)	97.6°–99.6°	36.4°–37.6°
Rectum (rectal)	98.6°–100.6°	37.0°–38.1°
Armpit (axillary)	96.6°–98.6°	35.9°–37.0°
Ear (tympanic)	96.6°–99.7°	35.9°–37.6°
Temporal Artery (forehead)	97.2°–100.1°	36.2°–37.8°

Normal Pulse Rate: 60–100 beats per minute
Normal Respiratory Rate: 12–20 respirations per minute

Blood Pressure

Normal	Systolic Diastolic	90–119 mm Hg *and* 60–79 mm Hg
Low (hypotensive)	Systolic Diastolic	Below 90 mm Hg *or* Below 60 mm Hg
Elevated	Systolic Diastolic	120–129 mm Hg *and* Less than 80 mm Hg
Stage 1 hypertension	Systolic Diastolic	130–139 mm Hg *or* 80–89 mm Hg
Stage 2 hypertension	Systolic Diastolic	At or over 140 mm Hg *or* At or over 90 mm Hg
Hypertensive crisis	Systolic Diastolic	Over 180 mm Hg *and/or* Over 120 mm Hg

Connected Care

Pediatric Vital Signs

Normal body temperature stays the same throughout a person's life, but ranges for other vital signs are different for children. In general, infants and children have faster pulse and respiratory rates and lower blood pressure than adults. As children grow, pulse and respiratory rates slow and blood pressure rises. Normal ranges for children are noted in the learning objectives for each vital sign.

Most of the procedures in this chapter are written for an adult patient. The beginning steps, including identification, introductions, and explanation of the procedure, also apply to pediatric patients. The PCT should adjust communication for the age of the patient. If the patient is too young to understand or respond, the PCT should speak to the parent or guardian (if present). Children may have questions about vital signs measurements. PCTs should always answer their questions if it is within their scope of practice.

3. List guidelines for measuring body temperature

Body temperature is normally very close to 98.6°F (Fahrenheit) or 37°C (Celsius). Body temperature reflects a balance between the heat created by the body and the heat lost to the environment. Many factors affect body temperature: age, illness, stress, environment, exercise, and the circadian rhythm can all cause changes in body temperature. Average temperature readings change throughout the day. People tend to have lower temperatures in the morning. Increases in body temperature may indicate an infection or disease.

There are different sites for measuring the body's temperature: the mouth (oral), the rectum (rectal), the armpit (axillary), the ear (tympanic), and the temporal artery (the artery just under the skin of the forehead).

The different sites require different thermometers. There are several types of thermometers, including the following:

- Digital
- Electronic
- Tympanic
- Temporal artery
- Mercury-free

A digital thermometer can be used to measure an oral, rectal, or axillary temperature (Fig. 10-2). This thermometer displays the results digitally in 2 to 60 seconds. The thermometer will beep or flash when the temperature has registered. A digital thermometer is battery-operated and requires battery replacement periodically. This thermometer may require a disposable plastic sheath to cover the probe to help prevent infection. The sheath is used once and is then discarded. This type of thermometer is not commonly used in inpatient settings.

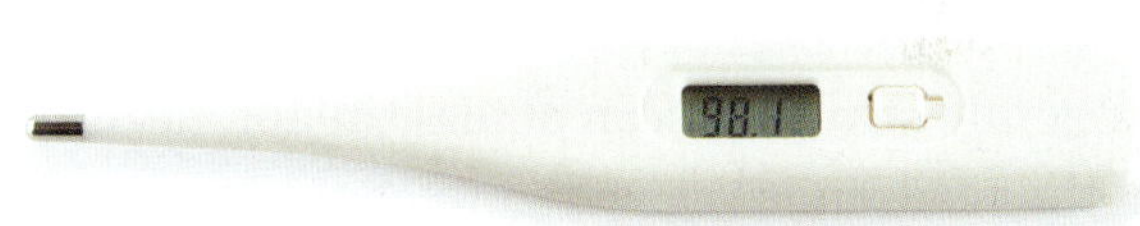

Fig. 10-2. *A digital thermometer.*

An electronic thermometer can be used to measure an oral, rectal, or axillary temperature. This thermometer registers the results digitally in 2 to 60 seconds. The thermometer flashes or makes a sound when the temperature is displayed. An electronic thermometer is battery-operated and is stored in a wall unit for recharging when it is not in use (Fig. 10-3). A probe cover is applied before use and is only used once before being discarded.

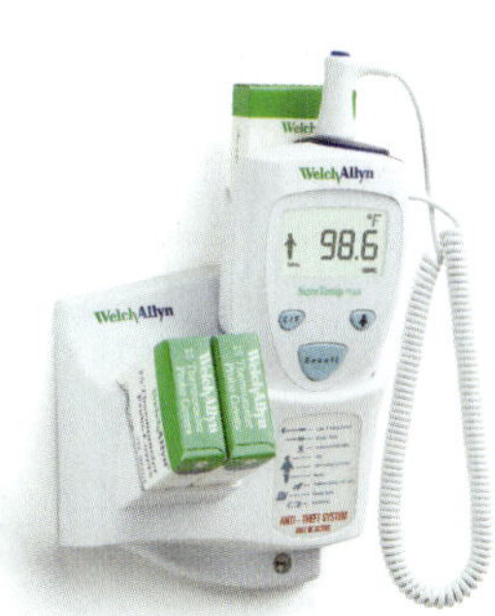

Fig. 10-3. *An electronic thermometer.* (WELCH ALLYN IS A TRADEMARK OF BAXTER INTERNATIONAL INC. OR ITS SUBSIDIARIES. © 2023 BAXTER INTERNATIONAL INC. REPRINTED WITH PERMISSION—ALL RIGHTS RESERVED.)

A tympanic thermometer is used to measure the temperature reading in the ear (Fig. 10-4). This thermometer registers the temperature in seconds. However, this thermometer may require more practice to be able to use it accurately.

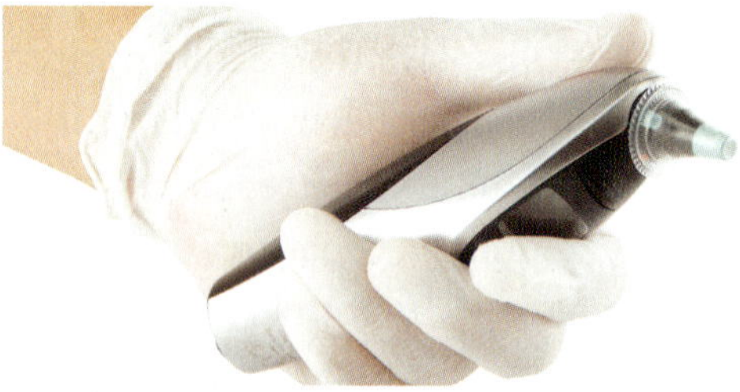

Fig. 10-4. A tympanic thermometer.

A temporal artery thermometer determines the temperature reading by measuring the heat from the skin over the temporal artery, the artery under the skin of the forehead. This is done by a gentle stroke or scan across the forehead, and the reading is registered in about 3 seconds (Fig. 10-5). A temporal artery thermometer is noninvasive, which means that it does not need to be inserted into the body.

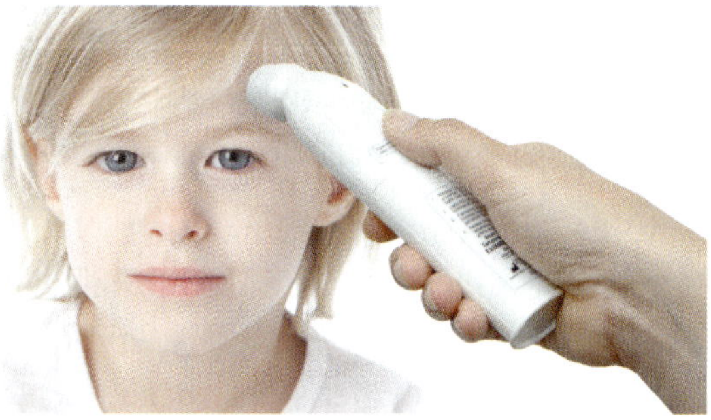

Fig. 10-5. A temporal artery thermometer. (PHOTO COURTESY OF EXERGEN CORPORATION, WWW.EXERGEN.COM)

A mercury-free thermometer can be used to measure an oral, rectal, or axillary temperature. Thermometers are usually color-coded. Oral thermometers are usually green or blue. Rectal thermometers are usually red.

Numbers on the thermometer allow the temperature to be read after it registers. Small arrows or highlighted numbers show the normal temperature: 98.6°F and 37°C. This type of thermometer is unlikely to be used in inpatient settings.

Although 98.6°F and 37°C are called normal, there is actually a range of normal temperatures. Some people's temperatures normally run low. Others in good health will run slightly higher temperatures. Normal temperature readings also vary by the method used to take the temperature. A rectal temperature is considered to be the most accurate. However, measuring a rectal temperature on an uncooperative person, such as a patient with dementia, can be dangerous. An axillary temperature is considered the least accurate.

A PCT should not measure an oral temperature on a person who

- Is unconscious
- Has recently had facial or oral surgery
- Is younger than 5 years old
- Is confused or disoriented
- Is heavily sedated
- Is likely to have a seizure
- Is coughing
- Is using an oxygen face mask
- Has facial paralysis
- Has sores, redness, swelling, or pain in the mouth
- Has an injury to the face or neck

Measuring and recording an oral temperature

Equipment: clean digital or electronic thermometer, gloves, disposable sheath/cover for thermometer, tissues

Do not take an oral temperature if the patient has smoked, eaten food or drunk fluids, chewed gum, or exercised in the last 10 to 20 minutes.

1. Identify yourself by name. Identify the patient according to facility policy.
2. Wash your hands.
3. Explain the procedure to the patient. Speak clearly, slowly, and directly. Maintain face-to-face contact whenever possible.

4. Provide for the patient's privacy with a curtain, screen, or door.
5. Put on gloves.
6. **Digital thermometer**: Put on the disposable sheath. Turn on the thermometer and wait until the *ready* sign appears.

   Electronic thermometer: Remove the probe from the base unit. Put on the probe cover.
7. Insert the end of the thermometer into the patient's mouth, under the tongue and to one side.
8. Tell the patient to hold the thermometer in her mouth with her lips closed (Fig. 10-6). Assist as necessary. The patient should breathe through her nose. Ask the patient not to bite down or talk.

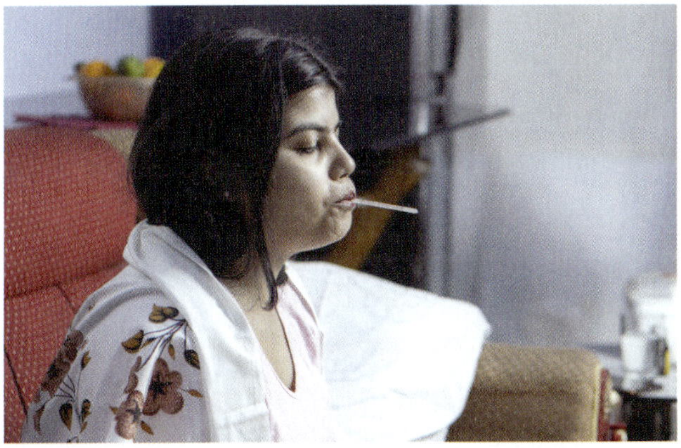

Fig. 10-6. *While the thermometer is in the patient's mouth, she should keep her lips closed.*

   Digital thermometer: Hold in place until the thermometer blinks or beeps.

   Electronic thermometer: Hold in place until you hear a tone or see a flashing or steady light.
9. **Digital thermometer**: Remove the thermometer. Read the temperature on the display screen. Remember the temperature reading.

   Electronic thermometer: Read the temperature on the display screen. Remember the temperature reading. Remove the probe.
10. **Digital thermometer**: Using a tissue, remove and discard the sheath. Replace the thermometer in the case.

    Electronic thermometer: Press the eject button to discard the cover. Return the probe to the holder.
11. Remove and discard your gloves. Wash your hands.
12. Immediately record the temperature, date, time, and method used (oral).
13. Remove privacy measures. Place the call light within the patient's reach.
14. Wash your hands.
15. Report any changes in the patient to the nurse.

Changes in Skin

As a PCT measures a patient's temperature, she can also observe the skin. Normally skin is warm and dry. The areas inside the mouth and nose are pink. Sometimes medical conditions or illness can change how the skin looks and feels.

When skin is hot and dry to the touch, but the patient is not sweating, this may be due to fever or to a heat-related emergency. *Diaphoresis* is excessive sweating. The patient's skin may also feel cool or clammy. It should be reported to a nurse right away. Diaphoresis may be caused by fever or pain, but it can also be a sign of heart attack.

Cyanosis causes a blue or gray color that can often be seen around the lips, on the nail beds, or inside the nose or mouth. It is a sign of decreased oxygen in the blood. Pallor and flushing are opposite changes in the skin. A patient with *pallor* (pale skin) has skin that is lighter than normal. In patients with dark skin, this is easier to see in nail beds and in the lining of the mouth and nose. Skin may also have an ash gray tone. Pallor may be a sign of illness or of poor circulation. *Flushing* causes skin in patients with light skin to appear red and in patients with dark skin to appear darker than normal. This may be seen as a difference between the skin on the face and on other parts of the body. Flushing may be caused by fever, pain, or an environment that is too hot.

Axillary temperatures are not as accurate as temperatures measured at other sites. However, they can be safer if a patient is confused, disoriented, uncooperative, or has dementia. They are also often used when measuring an infant's or toddler's temperature. Although rectal temperature measurements are sometimes recommended for infants and toddlers, axillary measurement is easier to perform safely. The axillary area must be clean and dry before measuring the temperature.

Measuring and recording an axillary temperature

Equipment: clean digital or electronic thermometer, gloves, tissues, disposable sheath/cover

1. Identify yourself by name. Identify the patient according to facility policy.
2. Wash your hands.
3. Explain the procedure to the patient. Speak clearly, slowly, and directly. Maintain face-to-face contact whenever possible.
4. Provide for the patient's privacy with a curtain, screen, or door.
5. Adjust the bed to a safe level, usually waist high. Lock the bed wheels.
6. Put on gloves.
7. Remove the patient's arm from the sleeve of the gown to allow skin contact with the end of the thermometer. Wipe the axillary area with tissues before placing the thermometer.
8. **Digital thermometer**: Put on the disposable sheath. Turn on the thermometer and wait until the *ready* sign appears.

   Electronic thermometer: Remove the probe from the base unit. Put on the probe cover.
9. Position the thermometer (bulb end for mercury-free) in the center of the armpit. Fold the patient's arm over his chest.
10. **Digital thermometer**: Hold in place until the thermometer blinks or beeps.

    Electronic thermometer: Hold in place until you hear a tone or see a flashing or steady light.
11. **Digital thermometer**: Remove the thermometer. Read the temperature on the display screen. Remember the temperature reading.

    Electronic thermometer: Read the temperature on the display screen. Remember the temperature reading. Remove the probe.
12. **Digital thermometer**: Using a tissue, remove and discard the sheath. Replace the thermometer in the case.

    Electronic thermometer: Press the eject button to discard the cover. Return the probe to the holder.
13. Remove and discard your gloves. Wash your hands.
14. Put the patient's arm back into the sleeve of the gown.
15. Immediately record the temperature, date, time, and method used (axillary).
16. Return the bed to its lowest position. Remove privacy measures.
17. Place the call light within the patient's reach.
18. Wash your hands.
19. Report any changes in the patient to the nurse.

Measuring and recording a temporal artery temperature

Equipment: clean temporal artery thermometer, alcohol swab

1. Identify yourself by name. Identify the patient according to facility policy.
2. Wash your hands.

3. Explain the procedure to the patient. Speak clearly, slowly, and directly. Maintain face-to-face contact whenever possible.
4. Provide for the patient's privacy with a curtain, screen, or door.
5. Adjust the bed to a safe level, usually waist high. Lock the bed wheels.
6. Turn on the thermometer. Place the thermometer flat on the forehead, usually midway between the eyebrow and the hairline.
7. Press and hold the scan button. Gently sweep the thermometer across the patient's forehead, keeping the thermometer in contact with the skin. Release the scan button.
8. Read the temperature on the display screen. Remember the temperature reading.
9. Wipe the thermometer clean using the alcohol swab. Only alcohol should be used on the lens in the center of the probe. If you do not have an alcohol wipe available, a cotton-tipped stick applicator moistened in alcohol can be used.
10. Wash your hands.
11. Immediately record the temperature, date, time, and method used (temporal artery).
12. Return the bed to its lowest position. Remove privacy measures.
13. Place the call light within the patient's reach.
14. Wash your hands.
15. Report any changes in the patient to the nurse.

A clean disposable sheath/cover can be used on a temporal artery thermometer if required for certain patients.

Information on measuring and recording a rectal temperature and a tympanic temperature is located in the instructor's guide.

4. List guidelines for measuring pulse, respirations, and oxygen saturation

The pulse is the number of heartbeats per minute. The beat that is felt at certain pulse points in the body represents the wave of blood moving through an artery as a result of the heart pumping. The most common site for monitoring the pulse in adults and children 6 and older is on the inside of the wrist, where the radial artery runs just beneath the skin. This is called the **radial pulse**. The procedure for counting this pulse rate is located later in this chapter. The brachial pulse is the pulse inside the elbow, about 1 to 1 1/2 inches above the elbow. The radial and brachial pulses are involved in measuring blood pressure, which is explained later in this chapter. Common pulse sites are shown below (Fig. 10-7).

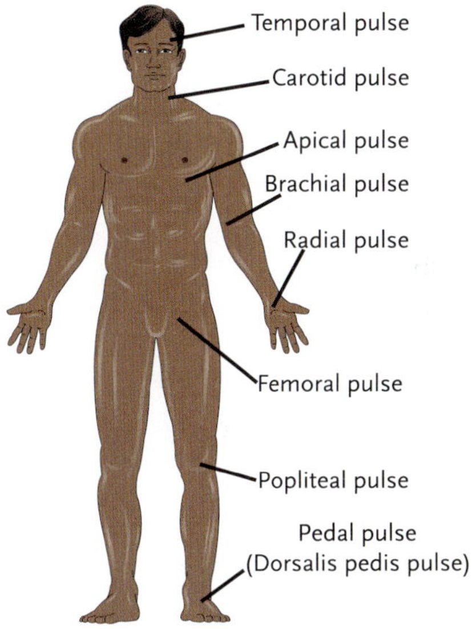

Fig. 10-7. *Common pulse sites.*

For adults, the normal pulse rate is 60 to 100 beats per minute. Small children have more rapid pulses, in the range of 100 to 120 beats per minute. A newborn baby's pulse rate may be as high as 120 to 180 beats per minute. Many things can affect pulse rate, including exercise, fear, anger, anxiety, heat, infection, illness, medications, and pain. A high (**tachycardia**) or low (**bradycardia**) rate does not necessarily indicate disease. However, sometimes the pulse rate can signal illness. For example, a rapid pulse may result from fever, dehydration, or heart failure. A slow or weak pulse may indicate infection.

The **apical pulse** is heard by listening directly over the heart with a stethoscope. A **stethoscope** is an instrument designed to listen to sounds within the body (**auscultation**), such as the heart beating or air moving through the lungs (Fig. 10-8). This is often the easiest method for counting the pulse rate in infants and young children because their pulse points are harder to find.

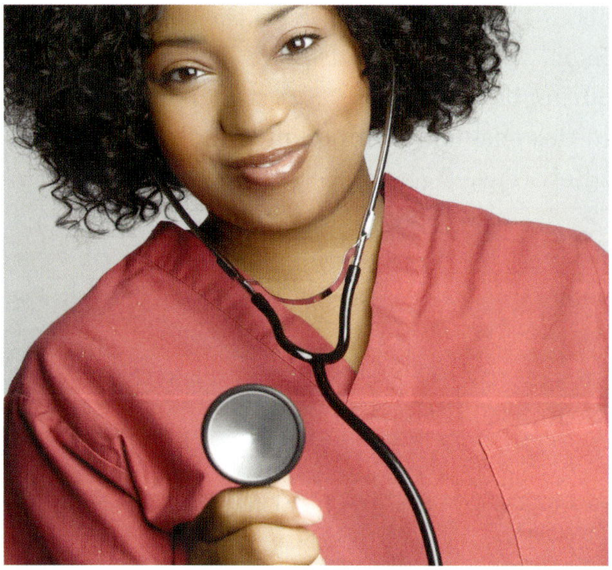

Fig. 10-8. *The diaphragm (the larger side) of the stethoscope is used to hear a pulse and to measure blood pressure.*

The apical pulse is on the left side of the chest, just below the nipple. For adult patients, the apical pulse may be checked when the person has heart disease or takes medication that affects the heart. It may also be checked if patients have a weak radial pulse or an irregular pulse.

Counting and recording apical pulse

Equipment: stethoscope, watch with second hand, alcohol swabs

1. Identify yourself by name. Identify the patient according to facility policy.
2. Wash your hands.
3. Explain the procedure to the patient. Speak clearly, slowly, and directly. Maintain face-to-face contact whenever possible.
4. Provide for the patient's privacy with a curtain, screen, or door.
5. Adjust the bed to a safe level, usually waist high. Lock the bed wheels.
6. Before using the stethoscope, wipe the diaphragm and earpieces with alcohol swabs.
7. Fit the earpieces of the stethoscope snugly in your ears. Place the flat metal diaphragm on the left side of the chest, just below the nipple. Listen for the heartbeat.
8. Use the second hand of your watch. Count the heartbeats for 1 minute (Fig. 10-9). Each *lub-dub* that you hear is counted as 1 beat. A normal heartbeat is rhythmical. Leave the stethoscope in place while counting respirations (procedure later in this chapter).

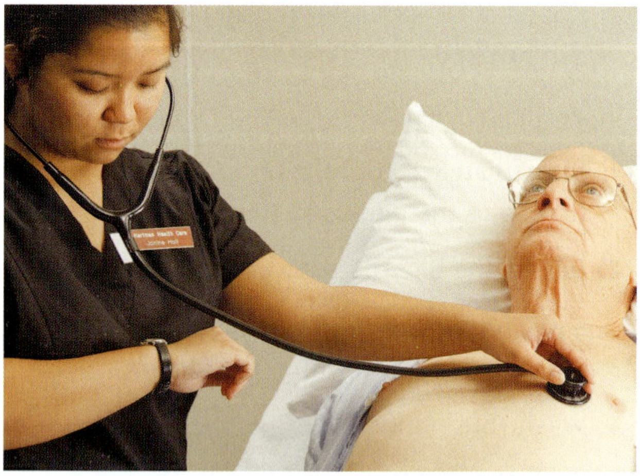

Fig. 10-9. *Count the heartbeats for 1 full minute to measure the apical pulse.*

9. Wash your hands.
10. Immediately record the pulse rate, date, time, and method used (apical). Note any irregularities in the rhythm.
11. Clean the earpieces and diaphragm of the stethoscope with alcohol swabs. Store the stethoscope.

12. Return the bed to its lowest position. Remove privacy measures.
13. Place the call light within the patient's reach.
14. Wash your hands.
15. Report to the nurse if the pulse is less than 60 beats per minute, over 100 beats per minute, or if the rhythm is irregular.

Respiration is the process of inhaling air into the lungs, or **inspiration**, and exhaling air out of the lungs, or **expiration**. Each respiration consists of an inspiration and an expiration. The chest rises during inspiration and falls during expiration.

The normal respiration rate for adults ranges from 12 to 20 breaths per minute. Infants and children have a faster respiratory rate. Infants normally breathe at a rate of 30 to 40 respirations per minute.

Different types of respirations include the following:

- **Apnea**: the absence of breathing
- **Dyspnea**: difficulty breathing
- **Eupnea**: normal respirations
- **Orthopnea**: shortness of breath when lying down that is relieved by sitting up
- **Tachypnea**: rapid respirations
- **Bradypnea**: slow respirations
- **Cheyne-Stokes**: alternating periods of slow, irregular respirations and rapid, shallow respirations, along with short periods of apnea

The respiratory rate is usually counted directly after counting the pulse rate because people tend to breathe more quickly if they know they are being observed. The PCT should keep their fingers on the patient's wrist or on the stethoscope over the heart. They should not make it obvious that they are observing the patient's breathing and should not mention that they are counting respirations.

Counting and recording radial pulse and counting and recording respirations

Equipment: watch with a second hand

1. Identify yourself by name. Identify the patient according to facility policy.
2. Wash your hands.
3. Explain the procedure to the patient. Speak clearly, slowly, and directly. Maintain face-to-face contact whenever possible.
4. Provide for the patient's privacy with a curtain, screen, or door.
5. Adjust the bed to a safe level, usually waist high. Lock the bed wheels.
6. Place the tips of your index finger and middle finger on (**palpate**) the thumb side of the patient's wrist to locate the radial pulse (Fig. 10-10). Do not use your thumb.

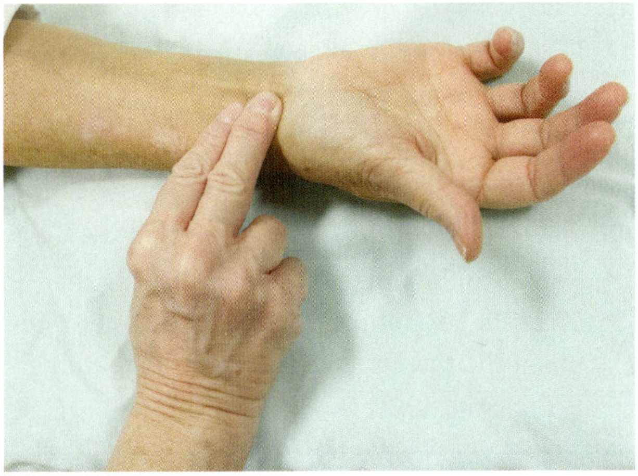

Fig. 10-10. *Count the radial pulse by placing the tips of your index finger and middle finger on the thumb side of the patient's wrist.*

7. Using your watch, count the beats for 1 full minute.
8. Keep your fingertips on the patient's wrist. Count respirations for 1 full minute (Fig. 10-11). Observe the patient's breathing. Normal breathing is smooth and quiet. If you see difficult, shallow, or noisy breathing, such as wheezing, report it to the nurse.

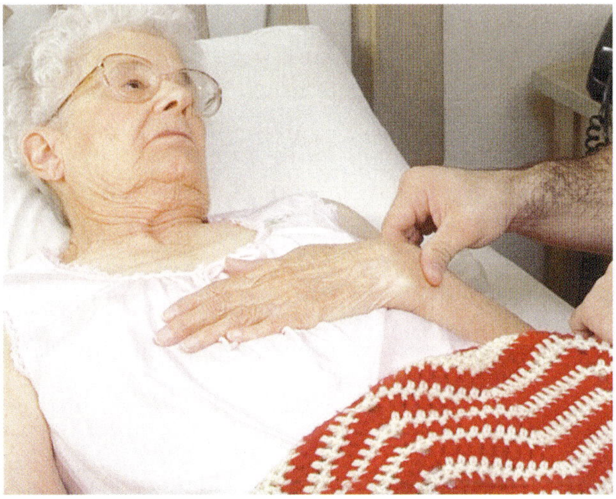

Fig. 10-11. *Count the respiratory rate directly after counting the radial pulse rate. Do not make it obvious that you are watching the patient's breathing.*

9. Wash your hands.
10. Immediately record the pulse rate, date, time, and method used (radial). Record the respiratory rate and the pattern or character of breathing.
11. Return the bed to its lowest position. Remove privacy measures.
12. Place the call light within the patient's reach.
13. Wash your hands.
14. Report to the nurse if the pulse is less than 60 beats per minute, over 100 beats per minute, if the rhythm is irregular, or if breathing is irregular.

PCTs may also be asked to obtain a pulse oximetry reading. A **pulse oximeter** is a noninvasive device that uses a light to determine the amount of oxygen in the blood (also called *oxygen saturation*). A pulse oximeter also measures a person's pulse rate. Low blood oxygen levels can affect vital sign measurements. Common symptoms of low blood oxygen are rapid breathing, shortness of breath, and a rapid pulse rate.

Most pulse oximeters have sensors that are placed on a patient's finger (most common), toe, or earlobe (Fig. 10-12). Infants and small children may have oxygen saturation measured with a sensor that wraps around the foot.

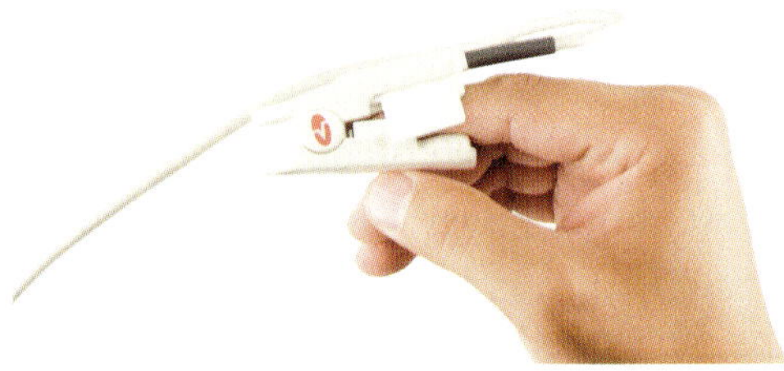

Fig. 10-12. *A pulse oximeter sensor is usually clipped on a person's finger.*

A normal pulse oximetry reading for adult and pediatric patients is 95%–100%. If the patient's blood oxygen has dramatically decreased (severe **hypoxia**) it is difficult to get an accurate reading. Readings may also be affected by poor circulation, certain diseases, skin thickness, and the use of fingernail polish and tobacco products. Pulse oximeter readings may be less accurate in people with dark skin tones. Blood oxygen is monitored constantly for some patients. In these cases, the sensor stays on the patient's finger at all times (or a wrap-style sensor may be used). An alarm sounds if oxygen saturation drops below a certain level.

Measuring and recording a pulse oximetry reading

Equipment: pulse oximeter, proper sensor type, nail polish remover if needed

1. Identify yourself by name. Identify the patient according to facility policy.
2. Wash your hands.
3. Explain the procedure to the patient. Speak clearly, slowly, and directly. Maintain face-to-face contact whenever possible.
4. Choose the proper sensor. Most machines have a reusable sensor for adult patients. Disposable probes are often used for pediatric patients.
5. Identify the site for the sensor—finger, earlobe, or toe. Remove nail polish if needed.

6. Place the sensor on the proper site.
7. Ask the patient to keep the sensor in place until a reading is displayed.
8. Wash your hands.
9. Record the pulse oximetry reading.
10. Report to the nurse if the reading is abnormal or very different from a previous reading.

5. Explain guidelines for measuring blood pressure

Blood pressure is an important indicator of a person's health. The measurement shows how well the heart is working. Blood pressure is measured in millimeters of mercury (mm Hg) and is recorded as a fraction—for example, 120/80. There are 2 parts of blood pressure: the systolic measurement and the diastolic measurement.

In the **systolic** phase, which is the top number of the blood pressure reading, the heart is at work, contracting and pushing the blood from the left ventricle of the heart. The reading shows the pressure on the walls of the arteries as blood is pumped through the body. The normal range for systolic blood pressure is below 120 mm Hg.

The second measurement reflects the **diastolic** phase, which is the bottom number of the reading. This phase is when the heart relaxes. The diastolic measurement is always lower than the systolic measurement. It shows the pressure in the arteries when the heart is at rest. The normal range for adults is below 80 mm Hg.

When blood pressure is consistently high, it may be categorized as elevated, stage 1 hypertensive, stage 2 hypertensive, or hypertensive crisis. People with high blood pressure (**hypertension** [**HTN**]) have elevated systolic and/or diastolic blood pressures. The ranges for the different categories of hypertension are listed in the orange box on page 148.

Blood pressure that is too low (below 90 mm Hg systolic or below 60 mm Hg diastolic) is called **hypotension**. A loss of blood or slowed blood flow can cause hypotension, which can be life-threatening if not corrected.

Blood pressure is affected by many factors. These include aging, exercise, stress, pain, medications, illness, obesity, alcohol intake, tobacco products, and the volume of blood in circulation.

Blood pressure is measured with either a manual or digital **sphygmomanometer**. An aneroid sphygmomanometer is a type of manual sphygmomanometer (Fig. 10-13). This sphygmomanometer consists of a cuff, a bulb, and a pressure gauge. Inside the cuff is an inflatable balloon that expands when air is pumped into the cuff. Two pieces of tubing are connected to the cuff. One leads to a rubber bulb that pumps air into the cuff. A pressure control button allows the release of air from the cuff after it is inflated. The other piece of tubing is connected to a pressure gauge with numbers that shows the blood pressure. Manual sphygmomanometers require the use of a stethoscope to determine the blood pressure reading.

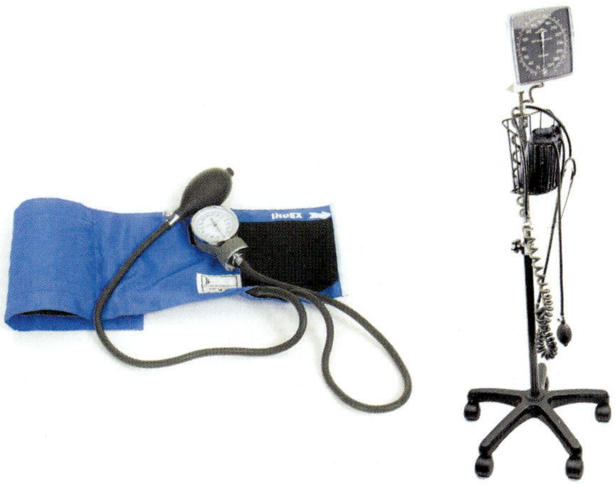

Fig. 10-13. *Two types of aneroid sphygmomanometers.*

With an electronic sphygmomanometer, the systolic and diastolic pressure readings are displayed digitally. In addition to blood pressure, an electronic sphygmomanometer may also measure other vital signs, such as pulse rate, respiratory rate, and temperature, as well as checking blood oxygen levels (Fig. 10-14). The cuff usually inflates and deflates automatically, and the use of a stethoscope is not required with electronic sphygmomanometers.

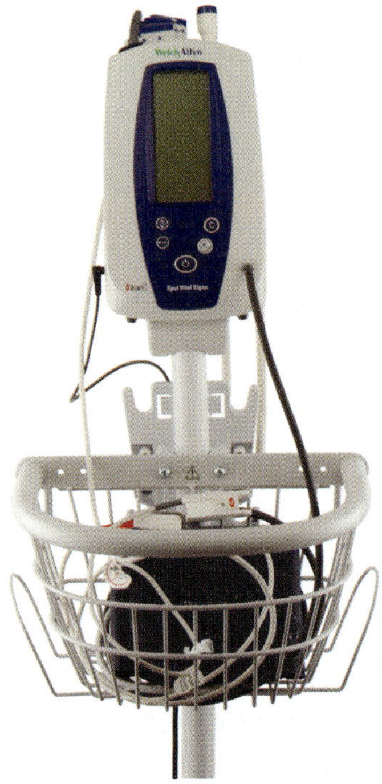

Fig. 10-14. *This type of electronic sphygmomanometer measures blood pressure, as well as other vital signs.*

When measuring blood pressure manually, the first sound heard is the systolic pressure (top number). When the sound changes to a soft muffled thump or disappears, this is the diastolic pressure (bottom number).

Blood pressure should not be measured on an arm that has an IV, a dialysis shunt, or any medical equipment. A side that has a cast, recent trauma, paralysis from a stroke, burns, or breast surgery (mastectomy) should be avoided.

It is important to use a cuff that is the correct size when measuring blood pressure. Available sizes for adults include small adult, adult, large adult, and thigh. There are also sizes available for infants and children.

Measuring and recording blood pressure manually

Equipment: manual sphygmomanometer, stethoscope, alcohol swabs

Do not check blood pressure if the patient has smoked, eaten, drunk alcohol or fluids containing caffeine, or exercised in the last 30 minutes.

1. Identify yourself by name. Identify the patient according to facility policy.
2. Wash your hands.
3. Explain the procedure to the patient. Speak clearly, slowly, and directly. Maintain face-to-face contact whenever possible.
4. Provide for the patient's privacy with a curtain, screen, or door.
5. Adjust the bed to a safe level, usually waist high. Lock the bed wheels.
6. Before using the stethoscope, wipe the diaphragm and earpieces with alcohol swabs.
7. Ask the patient to roll up his sleeve so that his upper arm is exposed. Do not measure blood pressure over clothing.
8. Position the patient's arm with his palm up. The arm should be level with the heart.
9. With the valve open, squeeze the cuff to make sure it is completely deflated.
10. Place the blood pressure cuff snugly on the patient's upper arm. The center of the cuff with the sensor/arrow is placed over the brachial artery (1–1½ inches above the elbow, toward the inside of the elbow) (Fig. 10-15).
11. Ask the patient to remain still and quiet during the measurement. Be sure the patient's legs or feet are not crossed.
12. Locate the brachial pulse with your fingertips.
13. Place the earpieces of the stethoscope in your ears.

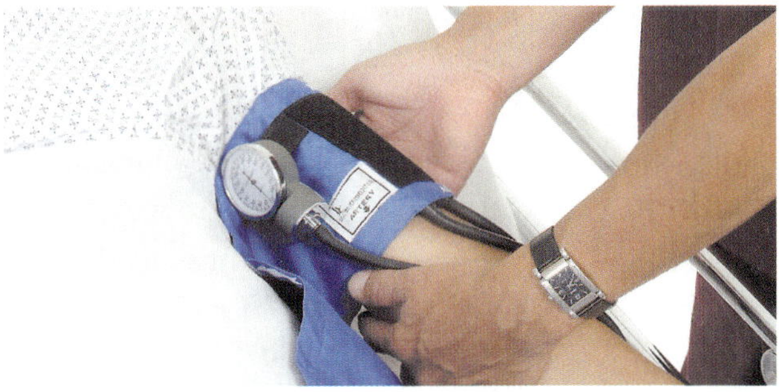

Fig. 10-15. *Place the center of the cuff over the brachial artery.*

14. Place the diaphragm of the stethoscope over the brachial artery.
15. Close the valve (clockwise) until it stops. Do not overtighten it (Fig. 10-16).

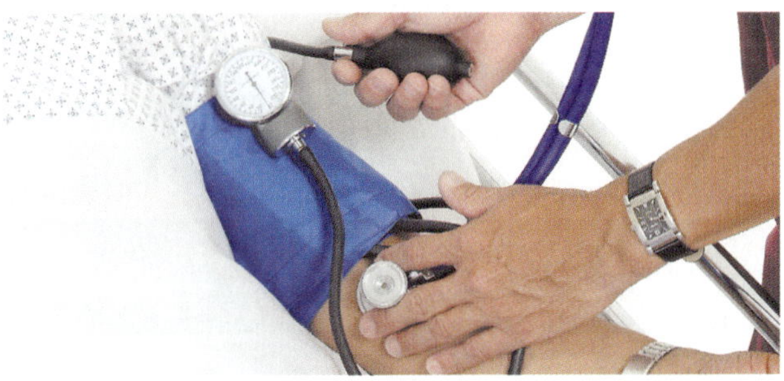

Fig. 10-16. *Close the valve by turning it clockwise until it stops. Do not overtighten it.*

16. Inflate the cuff to between 160 mm Hg and 180 mm Hg. If a beat is heard immediately upon cuff deflation, completely deflate the cuff. Reinflate the cuff to no more than 200 mm Hg.
17. Open the valve slightly with the thumb and index finger. Deflate the cuff slowly. Releasing the valve slowly allows you to hear beats accurately.
18. Watch the gauge and listen for the sound of the pulse.
19. Remember the reading at which the first pulse sound is heard. This is the systolic pressure.
20. Continue listening for a change or muffling of the pulse sound. The point of a change or the point at which the sound disappears is the diastolic pressure. Remember this reading.
21. Open the valve to deflate the cuff completely. Remove the cuff.
22. Wash your hands.
23. Clean the earpieces and diaphragm of the stethoscope with alcohol swabs. Store equipment.
24. Immediately record both the systolic and diastolic pressures. Record the numbers like a fraction, with the systolic reading on top and the diastolic reading on the bottom (for example: 110/70). Note which arm was used. Use *RA* for right arm and *LA* for left arm.
25. Return the bed to its lowest position. Remove privacy measures.
26. Place the call light within the patient's reach.
27. Wash your hands.
28. Report any changes in patient to the nurse.

Measuring and recording blood pressure electronically

Equipment: electronic blood pressure machine

1. Identify yourself by name. Identify the patient according to facility policy.
2. Wash your hands.
3. Explain the procedure to the patient. Speak clearly, slowly, and directly. Maintain face-to-face contact whenever possible.
4. Provide for the patient's privacy with a curtain, screen, or door.
5. Adjust the bed to a safe level, usually waist high. Lock the bed wheels.
6. Ask the patient to roll up his sleeve so that his upper arm is exposed. Do not measure blood pressure over clothing.
7. Position the patient's arm with his palm up. The arm should be level with the heart.

8. Make sure the cuff is completely deflated. Place the blood pressure cuff snugly on the patient's upper arm. The center of the cuff with the sensor/arrow is placed over the brachial artery (1–1½ inches above the elbow, toward the inside of the elbow).
9. Ask the patient to remain still and quiet during the measurement. Be sure the patient's legs or feet are not crossed.
10. Turn on the blood pressure machine and press the start button.
11. When the measurement is complete, the reading will be displayed on the screen and the machine may beep. The cuff should deflate.
12. Remove the cuff.
13. Wash your hands.
14. Immediately record both the systolic and diastolic pressures that are displayed on the screen. Note which arm was used.
15. Store equipment.
16. Return the bed to its lowest position. Remove privacy measures.
17. Place the call light within the patient's reach.
18. Wash your hands.
19. Report any changes in patient to the nurse.

Orthostatic Blood Pressures

PCTs may be asked by the nurse to take an orthostatic blood pressure measurement (also known as a *postural blood pressure*). To do this, the patient must first lie down. The PCT records the systolic and diastolic pressures. Next, the patient sits up. The PCT waits 2 minutes and measures blood pressure again, recording the systolic and diastolic pressures. Finally, the patient stands up. The PCT waits 2 minutes and measures blood pressure again, recording both pressures. Orthostatic blood pressures must be checked in this order: lying down, sitting, and standing up. All 3 blood pressure measurements should be reported to the nurse.

6. Describe guidelines for measuring height and weight

A patient's weight and height may be checked at admission. PCTs may also measure weight as part of regular care. Weight is measured in kilograms. A kilogram is a unit of mass equal to 1000 grams; 1 kilogram equals 2.2 pounds. Kilograms are the standard unit used in hospitals, but patients and family members may be unfamiliar with metric units. Multiplying a metric weight measurement by 2.2 gives the patient's weight in pounds. Digital scales may be able to display both units. Measurements in pounds, however, should never be entered in a patient's EHR. Medication doses are based on metric measurements. Entering weight in pounds can cause serious medication errors, especially in pediatric patients.

Measuring and recording weight of an ambulatory patient

Equipment: standing/upright scale

1. Identify yourself by name. Identify the patient according to facility policy.
2. Wash your hands.
3. Explain the procedure to the patient. Speak clearly, slowly, and directly. Maintain face-to-face contact whenever possible.
4. Provide for the patient's privacy with a curtain, screen, or door.
5. Make sure the patient is wearing nonskid footwear that is securely fastened before walking to the scale.
6. Start with the scale balanced at 0 before weighing the patient.
7. Help the patient to step onto the center of the scale. Be sure she is not holding, touching, or leaning against anything. This interferes with weight measurement. Do not force someone to let go. If you are unable to obtain a weight, notify the nurse.

8. Determine the patient's weight. Balance the scale by making the balance bar level. Move the small and large weight indicators until the bar balances. Read the 2 numbers shown (on the small and large weight indicators) when the bar is balanced. Add these 2 numbers together. This is the patient's weight (Fig. 10-17).

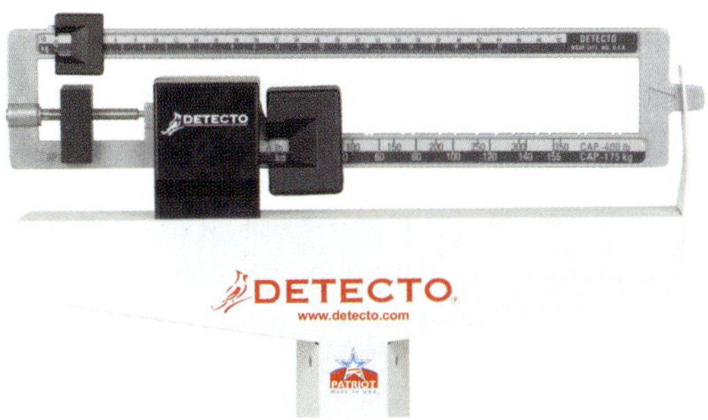

Fig. 10-17. *This scale is balanced at 0.* (PHOTO COURTESY OF DETECTO, WWW.DETECTO.COM)

9. Help the patient to safely step off the scale before recording the weight.
10. Wash your hands.
11. Immediately record the patient's weight in kilograms (kg).
12. Remove privacy measures.
13. Place the call light within the patient's reach.
14. Report any changes in the patient's weight (when weighing the patient after admission) to the nurse.

When patients are not able to get out of wheelchairs easily, they are weighed using a wheelchair scale. Wheelchairs are rolled directly onto this type of scale (Fig. 10-18). On some wheelchair scales, the PCT will need to subtract the weight of the wheelchair from a patient's weight. If the wheelchair's weight is not listed on the chair, the PCT should weigh the empty wheelchair first. The footrests should be attached if they will be attached when the patient is in the chair. Then the PCT should subtract the wheelchair's weight from the total.

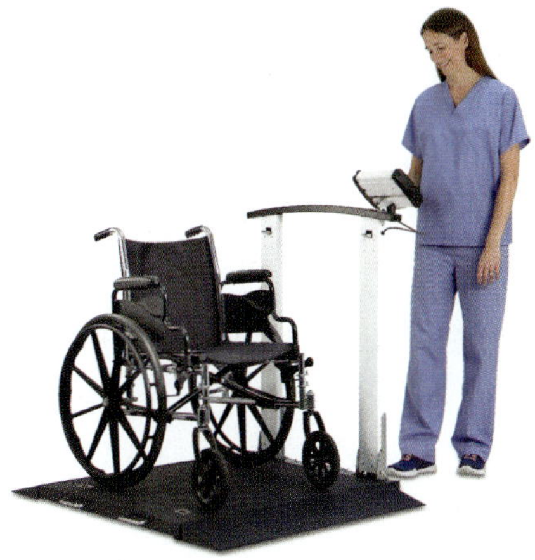

Fig. 10-18. *Wheelchairs can be rolled directly onto wheelchair scales to determine weight.* (PHOTO COURTESY OF DETECTO, WWW.DETECTO.COM)

When patients are not able to get out of bed, they may be weighed on special bed scales (Fig. 10-19). Before using a bed scale, the PCT should know how to use it properly and safely. Some beds have built-in scales so that patients do not have to be transferred out of bed to be weighed. These beds have displays and controls for use. The PCT should follow facility policy for using these scales.

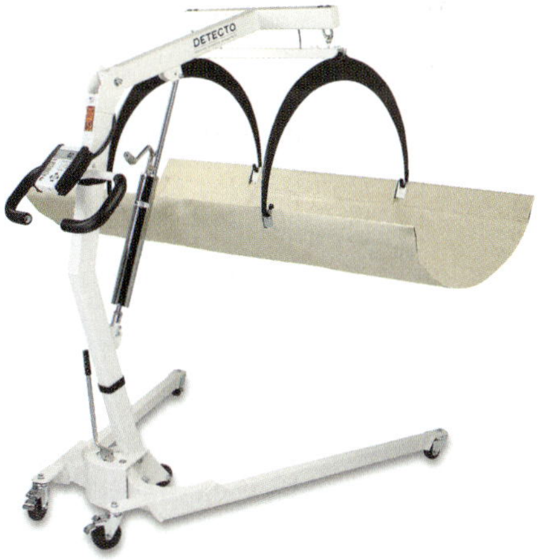

Fig. 10-19. *A type of bed scale.* (PHOTO COURTESY OF DETECTO, WWW.DETECTO.COM)

Scales for weighing infants may be either manual or digital (Fig. 10-20). A manual infant scale has weights that are moved to make a balance bar level. A digital scale registers the infant's weight on a digital readout. Some infant scales include sliding bars for measuring the baby's length.

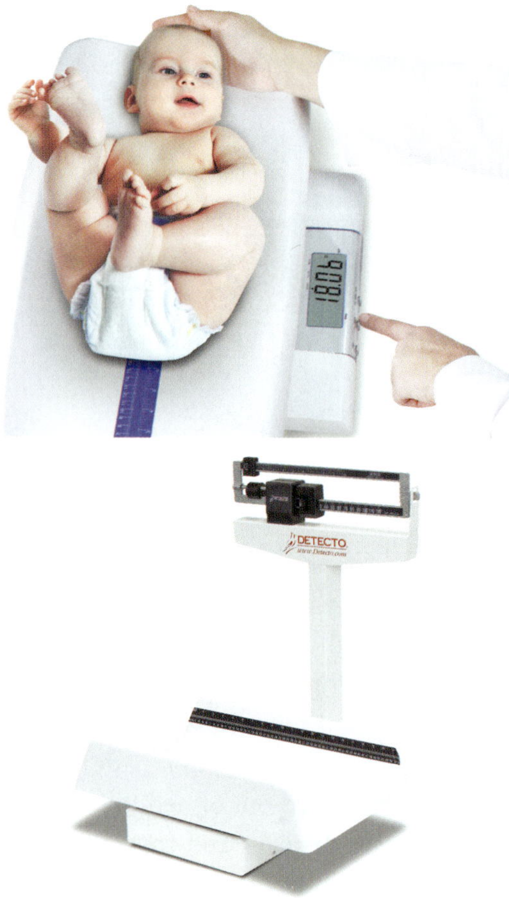

Fig. 10-20. *Infant scales allow the infant to be laid down for measurement. They may be manual or digital.* (PHOTOS COURTESY OF DETECTO, WWW.DETECTO.COM)

Measuring and recording weight of an infant

Equipment: infant scale

1. Identify yourself by name. Identify the patient according to facility policy.
2. Wash your hands.
3. Explain the procedure to the infant's parent or guardian, if present. Speak clearly, slowly, and directly. Maintain face-to-face contact whenever possible.
4. Start with the scale balanced at 0 (zero) before weighing the patient. If the infant is weighed while wearing a diaper, the diaper should be added to the scale before balancing.
5. Remove the infant's clothing.
6. Place the infant in the center of the scale, protecting the sides so he does not roll. Keep at least one hand very near the baby at all times.
7. Determine the patient's weight. Balance the scale by making the balance bar level. Move the small and large weight indicators until the bar balances. Read the 2 numbers shown on the small and large weight indicators when the bar is balanced. This is the infant's weight. (For a digital scale, the number on the readout indicates the weight.)
8. Remove the infant from the scale before recording the weight.
9. Wash your hands.
10. Immediately record the patient's weight in kilograms (kg).
11. Replace the infant's clothing.
12. Report any changes in the patient's weight (when weighing the patient after admission) to the nurse.

For measuring height, the rod measures in centimeters and may also measure in inches and fractions of inches. The PCT should record the height in centimeters. If the patient or family requests a measurement in feet and inches, the height in centimeters divided by 2.54 gives the height in inches. To convert inches to feet, the number of inches is divided by 12.

Measuring and recording height of an ambulatory patient

For patients who can get out of bed, measure height using a standing scale or *stadiometer*, which is similar to the height rod on a standing scale, but is usually mounted on a wall.

Equipment: standing scale or stadiometer

1. Identify yourself by name. Identify the patient according to facility policy.

2. Wash your hands.
3. Explain the procedure to the patient. Speak clearly, slowly, and directly. Maintain face-to-face contact whenever possible.
4. Provide for the patient's privacy with a curtain, screen, or door.
5. Make sure the patient is wearing nonskid shoes that are securely fastened before walking to the scale.
6. Help the patient to step onto the scale, facing away from the scale.
7. Ask the patient to stand straight if possible. Help as needed.
8. Pull up the measuring rod from the back of the scale and gently lower the rod until it rests flat on the patient's head (Fig. 10-21).

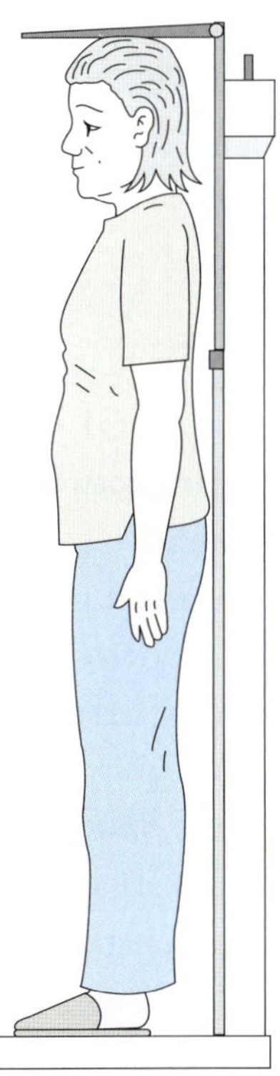

Fig. 10-21. *To determine height on a standing scale, gently lower the measuring rod until it rests flat on the patient's head.*

9. Determine the patient's height.
10. Help the patient to safely step off the scale before recording height. Make sure that the measuring rod does not hit the patient in the head while doing so.
11. Wash your hands.
12. Immediately record the patient's height in centimeters (cm).
13. Remove privacy measures.
14. Place the call light within the patient's reach.
15. Document the procedure using facility guidelines.

Some patients will be unable to get out of bed. Height can be measured by using a tape measure and making 2 pencil marks on the sheet that is underneath the patient. The PCT makes a mark at the top of the patient's head and one at his feet and measures the distance between the marks (Fig. 10-22). Height can also be measured in other ways. In some cases, one part of the arm or leg is measured and a chart is then used to estimate the patient's height. PCTs should follow the procedures used at their facilities.

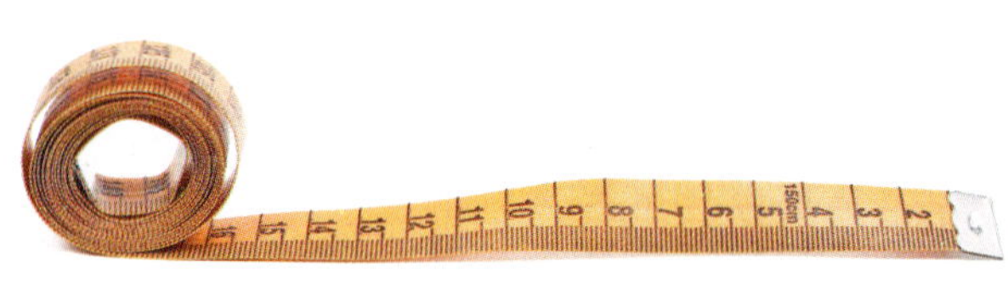

Fig. 10-22. *Height can be measured in bed using a tape measure.*

Since infants are unable to stand, infant height is usually called *length*. It can be measured by using a tape measure and making 2 pencil marks on a bassinet sheet or on exam table paper that is underneath the patient. The PCT makes a mark at the top of the infant's head and one at her feet. The PCT then uses a tape measure to measure the distance between the marks. Infant length may also be measured with an infant stadiometer. This device is adjusted so that one bar is at the top of the infant's head and the other at the bottom of the infant's feet. Then a measurement can be read. Some infant scales have built-in stadiometers (Fig. 10-23).

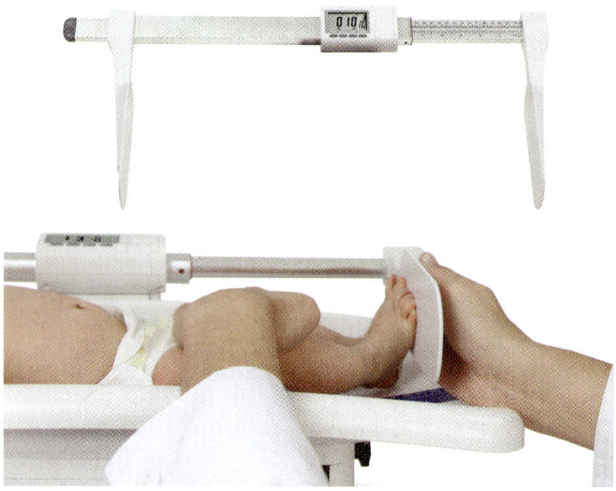

Fig. 10-23. *The length of an infant can be measured using a stadiometer, which may be a fixed part of an infant scale or may be a separate device.* *(PHOTOS COURTESY OF DETECTO, WWW.DETECTO.COM)*

The PCT may also measure an infant's head circumference, or the distance around the head. The measurement is used to screen for **hydrocephalus**. This is an abnormal accumulation of fluid in the head. Head circumference is measured by placing the tape measure right above the eyebrows and around the widest part of the back of the head. The result is recorded to the nearest 0.5 centimeters.

Height and weight determine a patient's **body mass index** (**BMI**). BMI is calculated by dividing a person's weight in kilograms by the square of their height in meters. (A *square* is a number multiplied by itself.) Some EHR systems calculate BMI automatically. Calculators are also available online. BMI is categorized as *underweight, normal weight, overweight,* or *obese*. However, BMI is a screening tool and does not give a reliable diagnosis. It does not directly measure body fat or health risk. BMI that does not fall into the *normal weight* category may show a need for further assessment. BMI categories are as follows:

- Below 18.5 = underweight
- 18.5–24.9 = normal weight
- 25–29.9 = overweight
- 30 or above = obese

Connected Care

BMI Is Not Diagnostic

While BMI is one of the oldest screening tools for obesity, it is imperfect. Athletic people may have a large amount of muscle mass, which weighs more than fat. This could lead to a falsely high BMI. A pregnant woman's weight could lead to the same result. Further, BMI standards were developed based mostly on measurements of white men. BMI may not be reliable for other populations.

Other measurements may be used along with or instead of BMI. Waist circumference, or distance around the waist, measures body fat distribution. Increased weight in the middle of the body has been associated with heart disease. The waist-to-hip ratio is another measurement used to calculate a person's risk for heart disease. Accurate measurement of body fat requires more complex assessments such as skinfold measurements or underwater weight measurement. These tools are better than BMI for assessing body composition, obesity, and disease risk.

7. Discuss pre- and postoperative patient care and related tasks

Depending on where a PCT works, their duties may include giving **preoperative**, or before-surgery, care. Preoperative care includes both physical and psychological preparation. Before a person has surgery, a doctor will explain the procedure, the risks and benefits, and what to expect after surgery. The person will be encouraged to ask questions and give opinions. This is part of informed consent, a process in which a person, with the help of a doctor, makes informed decisions about her health care. The person must sign a consent form for surgery or have one signed by a guardian or someone with medical power of attorney.

People who are going to have surgery often experience anxiety, fear, worry, sadness, and other emotions (Fig. 10-24). It is often helpful to express these concerns to members of the healthcare team. Being prepared psychologically may help the patient cope better after surgery. Part of a PCT's role in assisting with this preparation is listening to a patient's concerns. The PCT should report any concerns or questions, including requests for a visit from a religious leader, to the nurse.

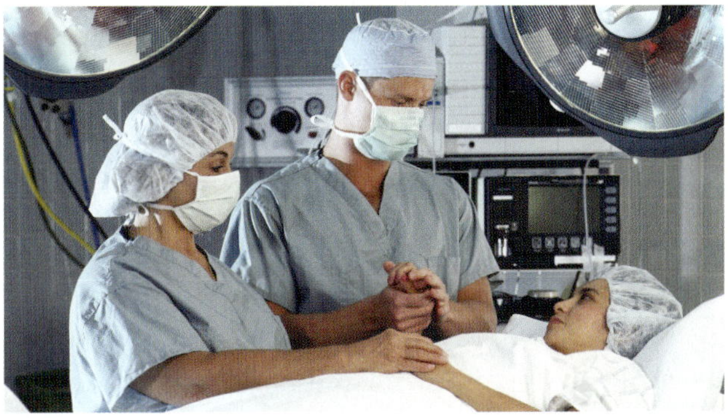

Fig. 10-24. *Patients often have many worries before surgery. A compassionate response by staff may help alleviate concerns.*

A person who is having surgery will require preoperative physical preparation as well. These general guidelines explain physical preparation for surgery:

Guidelines: Preoperative Care

G Before surgery, there will be an order for the patient to receive nothing by mouth (**NPO**) for a specific period of time. This time usually ranges from 2 to 8 hours. Having this medical order means that nothing is allowed by mouth, including water, ice chips, food, etc. Remove the water pitcher, glass, and any other food and fluids from the immediate area. Explain to the patient why you are doing this. Report any concerns to the nurse.

G Assist the patient with urinating before surgery.

G For some patients having surgery of the gastrointestinal tract, the bowels may need to be cleared. An enema or rectal suppository may be ordered. Assist as trained, ordered, and allowed. (Enemas are described in Chapter 18.) Be ready to bring the bedpan or portable commode when needed. Provide plenty of privacy.

G Assist with bathing as needed. Some facilities may require that patients bathe with a special soap that contains an antiseptic agent called *chlorhexidine gluconate* (*CHG*). This can help reduce the amount of bacteria on a patient's skin and may prevent HAIs. Follow facility policy when helping a patient to bathe with CHG or telling a patient how to use it. It must stay in contact with the skin for a certain amount of time to be effective.

G Make sure the call light is within reach every time you leave the room.

G Measure and record vital signs as ordered.

G Remove dentures, eyeglasses, contact lenses, hearing aids, jewelry, hairpieces, hairpins, and any other personal items. Store these safely according to policy. For local or regional anesthetic, the doctor may want the person to wear hearing aids and dentures so that communication will be easier.

G Put sequential compression devices (SCDs) and socks on the patient as ordered. SCDs are sleeve-like inflatable garments placed on a patient's lower legs (Fig. 10-25). They are connected to a machine that inflates and deflates the devices to promote circulation. This can help prevent blood clots from forming. Blood clots are a serious risk for patients having surgery.

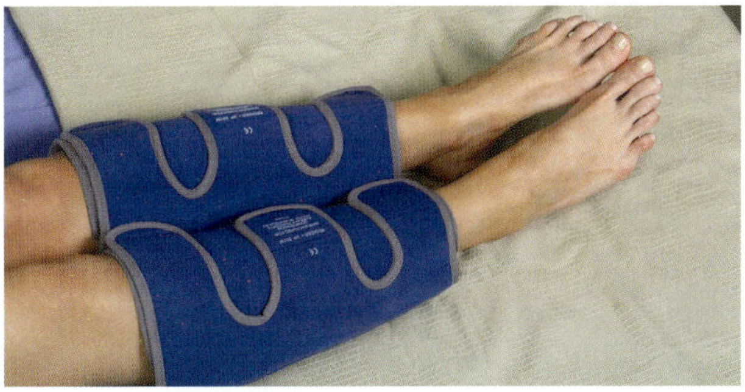

Fig. 10-25. *Sequential compression devices (SCDs) help promote blood circulation and prevent blood clots.*

- **G** Transfer the patient to a stretcher/gurney if necessary.
- **G** Make sure the patient's identification bracelet is accurate and on the wrist or ankle prior to transport. You may need to verify if the patient has any known allergies by asking this question and verifying what is written on an allergy bracelet.

Postoperative, or after-surgery, care begins immediately following surgery. The goal of postoperative care is to prevent infections, promote healing, and return the person to a state of health. Immediate postoperative concerns are problems with breathing, mental status, pain, and wound healing. Complications of surgery can also include urinary retention or infections, constipation, blood pressure variances, and blood clots. Careful postoperative monitoring is critical.

After surgery, the patient is taken to the recovery room and may remain there for some time. This depends on the type of surgery that the patient had, as well as how long the surgery lasted, what type and how much anesthetic was used, and the patient's level of consciousness. Some hospitals have a postanesthesia care unit (PACU) where patients may be monitored until they are either discharged or returned to a standard room.

While the patient is in recovery, the PCT's duties include changing bed linens and gathering equipment, which may include the following:

- Bed protector
- Towels and washcloths
- Vital signs equipment
- Emesis basin
- Pillows and other positioning devices
- Warming blankets
- IV pole
- Oxygen and suction equipment

When the patient returns to the room, the following guidelines are used:

Guidelines: Postoperative Care

- **G** Move furniture as needed to allow for the transfer back into bed from the stretcher.
- **G** Assist with transferring the patient back into bed.
- **G** Return dentures, eyeglasses, contact lenses, and hearing aids to the patient. Remember that without these items, patients may not be able to talk, eat, see, or hear.
- **G** Measure and record vital signs often after surgery as directed. The schedule may look like this: every 15 minutes for the first hour, every 30 minutes for the next hour to 2 hours, every hour for the next 4 hours, and then every 4 hours. Report any changes immediately.
- **G** Reposition the patient every 1 to 2 hours, or as ordered. Elevate the extremities as ordered.
- **G** Assist with deep breathing and coughing exercises as ordered. More information about these exercises is in Chapter 16.
- **G** Assist with compression stockings, SCDs, and leg exercises as instructed. The procedure for applying compression stockings is later in the chapter.
- **G** Binders are stretchable pieces of fabric that can be fastened. They hold dressings in place and give support to surgical wounds. Binders can also reduce swelling and ease discomfort. Apply binders as ordered.
- **G** Surgical drains may be placed near the incision (Fig. 10-26). These drains help prevent fluid buildup, which can lead to infection. Surgical drains are connected to a collection device such as a bulb, which is emptied regularly. Observe the amount and appearance of the drainage as directed. Report any increase in the amount, as well as any change in color. Sometimes PCTs are also responsible for measuring the amount of drainage. If this

is part of your responsibilities, you will be trained how to do it.

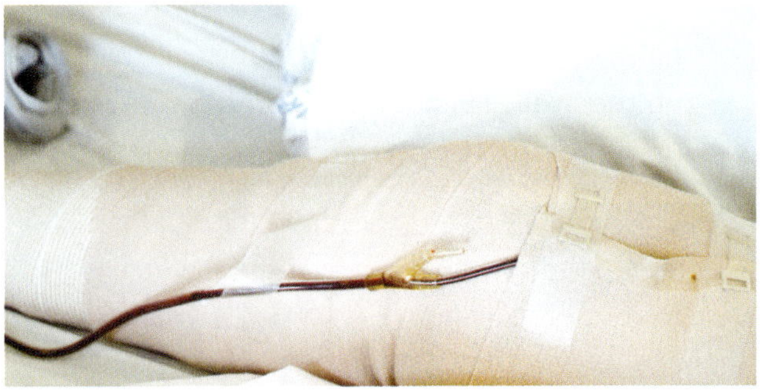

Fig. 10-26. This photo shows a postoperative knee with a drainage tube in it.

- **G** Be aware of any special diet orders. A postoperative patient may have a nothing by mouth (NPO) order or an order for a clear liquid diet. The patient may be on a high-protein diet to promote wound healing. Following diet orders can help speed recovery.
- **G** Assist with elimination (urination and bowel movements). Always provide plenty of privacy for elimination.
- **G** Help with bathing and grooming as requested and as ordered.
- **G** Assist with ambulation as needed and as ordered. Be encouraging and positive.

Observing and Reporting: Postoperative Care

Report the following signs and symptoms of complications to the nurse immediately:

- O/R Changes in vital signs
- O/R Difficulty breathing
- O/R Mental changes, such as confusion or disorientation
- O/R Changes in consciousness
- O/R Discolored, pale, or cyanotic (bluish) skin
- O/R Skin that is cold or clammy
- O/R Increase in amount of drainage
- O/R Swelling at IV site
- O/R IV that is not dripping
- O/R Nausea or vomiting
- O/R Numbness or tingling
- O/R Tenderness, swelling, or heat in the calves
- O/R Patient complaints of pain

Connected Care

Unbiased Pain Management

Every patient's pain management should be treated with equal importance. Every person experiences and reports pain in different ways. These differences may lead to patients not being treated equally. A care team member's biases, which may be unconscious, can also lead to incorrect judgments about a patient's pain. It is important that the care team give unbiased care to all patients. It is not the PCT's job to diagnose or interpret a patient's pain. PCTs can provide high-quality, unbiased care by listening without judgment to what patients say about their pain. PCTs should use the patient's own words to report pain whenever possible.

Compression stockings are applied to postoperative patients. These stockings help prevent swelling and promote blood circulation by gently squeezing the legs to increase blood flow. Compression stockings are also known as *antiembolic* or *elastic stockings*. They are sometimes referred to as *antiembolic* because they may help prevent an embolism. An **embolism** is an obstruction of a blood vessel, usually by a blood clot. The embolism can travel from where it was formed to another part of the body, blocking blood flow. It can cause serious damage and even death.

Compression stockings may be knee-high, thigh-high, or pantyhose style. When possible, it is best to put them on in the morning because legs are at their smallest size then. They are usually removed in the evening.

Applying knee-high compression stockings

Equipment: knee-high compression stockings

1. Identify yourself by name. Identify the patient according to facility policy.

2. Wash your hands.
3. Explain the procedure to the patient. Speak clearly, slowly, and directly. Maintain face-to-face contact whenever possible.
4. Provide for the patient's privacy with a curtain, screen, or door.
5. The patient should be in the supine position (on her back) in bed. With the patient lying down, remove any footwear, and expose one leg. Expose no more than one leg at a time.
6. Take one stocking and turn it inside out at least to the heel area (Fig. 10-27).

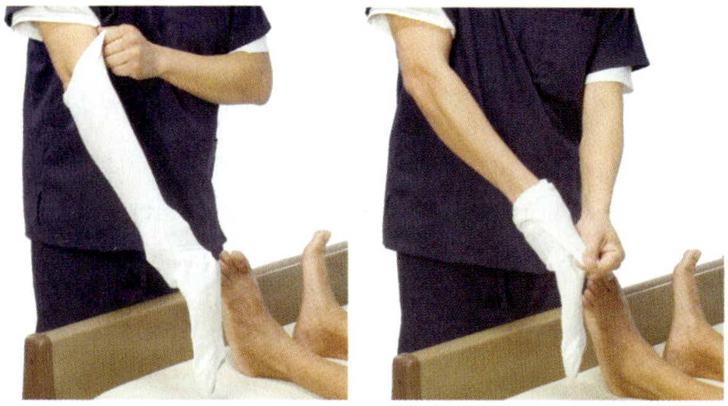

Fig. 10-27. *Turning the stocking inside out allows the stocking to roll on gently.*

7. Gently place the foot of the stocking over the toes, foot, and heel (Fig. 10-28). Make sure the heel is in the right place. The heel of the foot should be in the heel of the stocking.

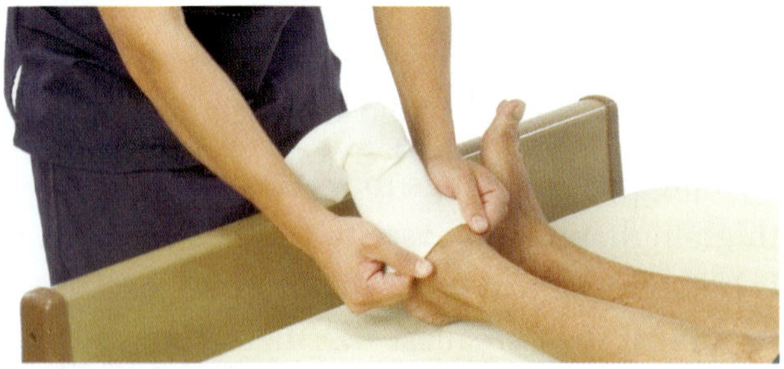

Fig. 10-28. *Gently place the foot of the stocking over the toes, foot, and heel. Promote the patient's comfort and safety. Avoid force and overextension of joints.*

8. Gently pull the top of the stocking over the foot, heel, and leg.
9. Make sure there are no twists or wrinkles in the stocking after it is on. It must fit smoothly (Fig. 10-29). Make sure the heel of the stocking is over the heel of the foot. If the stocking has an opening in the toe area, make sure the opening is either over or under the toe area. This depends on the manufacturer's instructions. Adjust if needed.

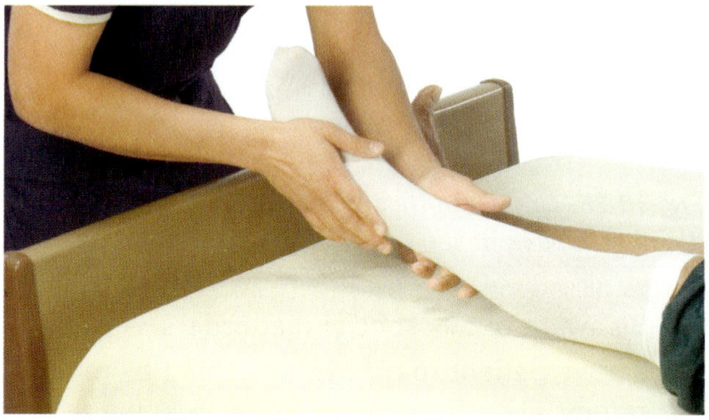

Fig. 10-29. *Make the stocking smooth. Twists or wrinkles cause the stocking to be too tight, which reduces circulation.*

10. Repeat steps 6 through 9 for the other leg.
11. Place the call light within the patient's reach.
12. Wash your hands.
13. Report any changes in the patient to the nurse.
14. Document the procedure using facility guidelines.

8. Discuss sterile technique

In some hospitals a PCT may assist with preparations for surgery or other procedures that require sterile technique. PCTs who work in the ED may assist doctors as they clean or repair wounds. PCTs who care for patients who have burns or other physical trauma may assist nurses with dressing changes or other care.

As described in Chapter 5, *surgical asepsis,* or *sterile technique,* makes an object or area completely free of all microorganisms (not just pathogens). This provides the sterile environment needed for surgical procedures. Surgical aseptic techniques include the following:

- Sanitizing and disinfecting the room and instruments using a disinfectant solution such as a 1:10 mixture of hypochlorite (bleach) and water; instruments that will be used in a procedure must also be sterilized.
- Sterilizing supplies that will be used in the procedure
- Applying sterile gloves after performing a special type of handwashing called a *surgical scrub*
- Preparing a **sterile field**. This involves setting up instruments and equipment for a procedure while maintaining a sterile environment.

If a PCT is assigned to disinfect surfaces before a procedure, she will be trained how to do so. It is very important to follow facility policy regarding contact time, or the amount of time the disinfectant is in contact with a surface.

When preparing to don sterile gloves, a PCT may need to first perform a surgical scrub. In addition to using special antibacterial soap, this type of hand hygiene is performed with a special scrub brush and a nail brush. Kits are available with these brushes already filled with soap (Fig. 10-30).

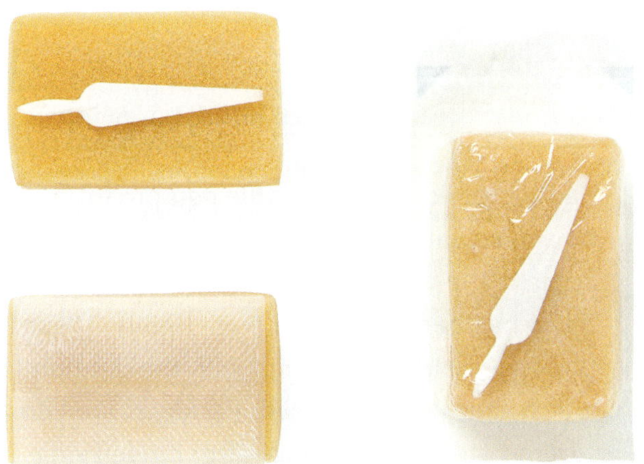

Fig. 10-30. *A surgical scrub brush is used for thorough cleaning of the hands and forearms.* (IMAGE COURTESY OF MEDLINE INDUSTRIES, LP. USED WITH PERMISSION.)

Performing a sterile hand scrub

Equipment: surgical soap, surgical scrub brush, sink (preferably with knee or foot faucet control), sterile towel

1. Remove all jewelry.
2. Open the surgical scrub brush package.
3. Turn on the faucet and adjust the water temperature to warm.
4. Apply a generous amount of surgical soap to your skin. Use the scrub brush to produce a lather.
5. Perform a scrub for 5 minutes, keeping fingers pointed upward. Scrub one hand thoroughly. Move from your fingernails and fingers to your thumb, between your fingers, the palm of your hand, the back of your hand, your wrist, and your forearm. Always move away from your fingertips (Fig. 10-31).

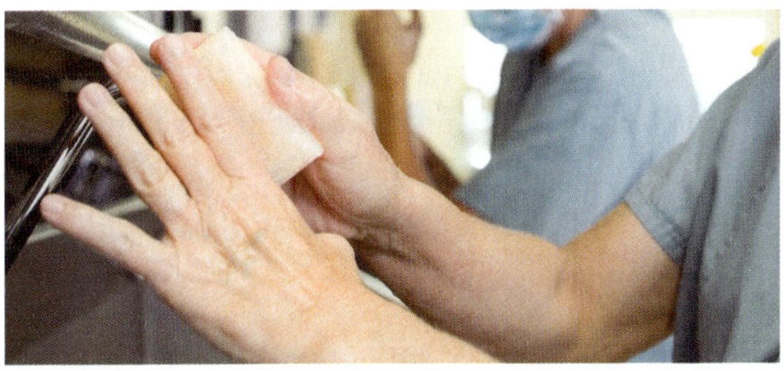

Fig. 10-31. *Fingertips must always point upward during a surgical hand scrub.*

6. Repeat this with your remaining hand for at least 5 minutes.
7. Rinse thoroughly from your fingers to your wrists with your fingers pointing upward.
8. Turn off the faucet. If a knee or foot control is not available, use a sterile towel and discard the towel after use.
9. Pat your hands dry with a sterile towel, moving from your fingertips to your forearms.
10. Keep your hands pointed upward, above the waist, and in front of your body.

After performing a surgical scrub, the PCT is ready to don sterile gloves. Sterile gloves are required to perform surgical procedures. They come in a variety of sizes. The PCT should choose the size that fits best. The outer surface of a sterile glove is considered sterile. The inside surface, which touches the skin, is nonsterile.

Donning sterile gloves

Equipment: sterile gloves, clean work surface

1. Perform a surgical scrub (see previous procedure).
2. Remove the outer packaging of the sterile gloves and place the inner package on a clean surface. Most packages have an illustration of the gloves to use as a guide.
3. Grasp the edges of the package and pull out each side to expose the gloves. Do not touch other surfaces of the package.
4. The bottom edges of surgical gloves are folded up to form a cuff. This cuff allows you to grasp the gloves without contaminating the outer surfaces. Grasp one glove at the fold along the bottom of the cuff with your nondominant hand.
5. Insert your dominant hand into the first glove. Do not touch the outside of the glove (Fig. 10-32).

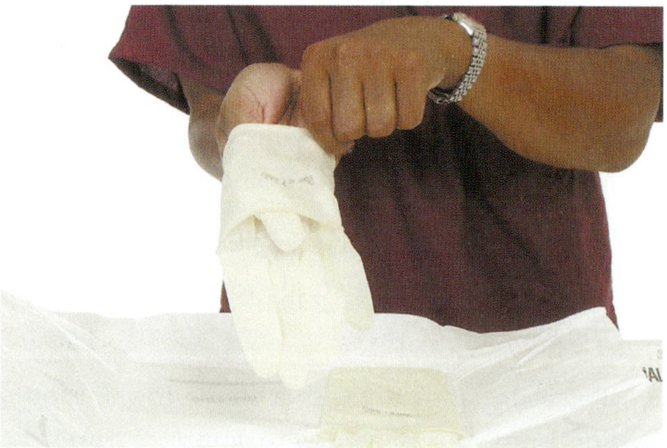

Fig. 10-32. *Insert your hand without touching the outside of the glove.*

6. Insert the fingers of your gloved hand under the folded cuff of the second glove. Touch only the outer surface of the glove. Take care not to touch the glove with your thumb.
7. Insert your ungloved hand into the second glove. Take care not to touch the outside of the glove (Fig. 10-33).

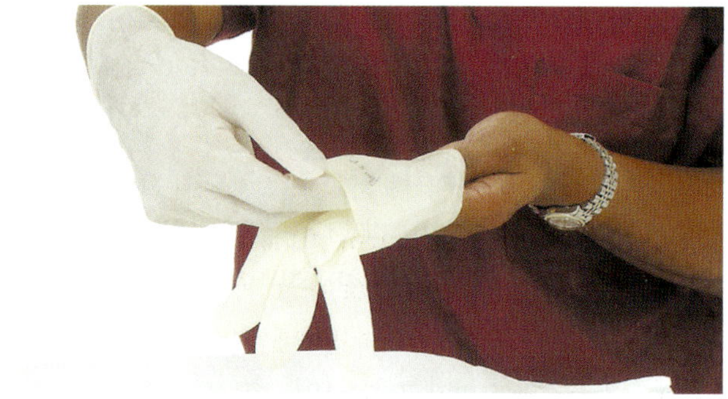

Fig. 10-33. *Insert your nondominant hand in the second glove, touching only the inside of the glove.*

8. Keep your gloved hands above the waist and in front of your body at all times.

Hospitals usually have sterile supplies and equipment ready for common procedures. Equipment may have been wrapped and sterilized in an autoclave at the facility, or it may be in a prepackaged, sealed tray from a medical supply company. Sterile supplies are in individual, sealed packages. All sterile items must be handled carefully.

Guidelines: Sterile Supplies and Equipment

- **G** Packets of autoclaved sterile equipment may be sealed with a special tape that changes color in the autoclave to show that the equipment has been sterilized (Fig. 10-34). These packets should be marked with the date on which they were sterilized. Packages are considered sterile for 30 days after autoclaving.
- **G** If a wrapper on a sterile supply or equipment is torn, it is no longer considered sterile and cannot be used.

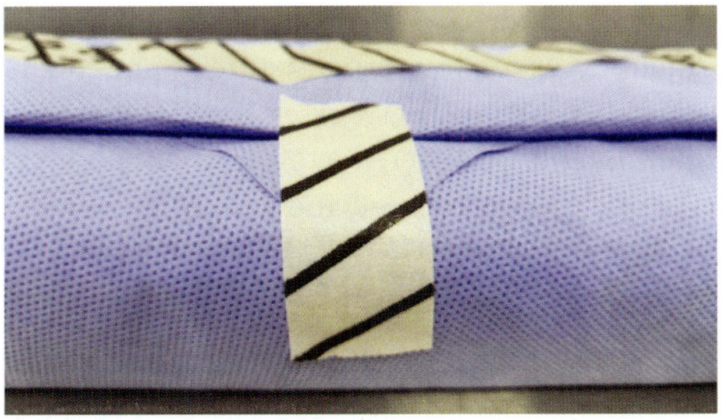

Fig. 10-34. A change in the autoclave tape verifies sterilization. Some tapes change color (e.g., from red stripes to black). Some have markings that appear or disappear.

- G The wrapper cannot be opened and closed again. Once a wrapper is opened, the contents inside are no longer sterile.
- G If a wrapper is wet or has wrinkles or marks that indicate it was once wet, it is no longer considered sterile.
- G If the date on a supply shows it has expired, it is no longer considered sterile. All commercially prepared supplies and equipment are dated. Sterile items that have expired should not be used.
- G If you are unsure whether an item is sterile or not, do not use it.

A sterile field provides a safe work surface during a sterile procedure. If a PCT is assigned to set up a sterile field, she arranges items in order of use. Facilities will train PCTs to do this. The outer 1-inch border of a sterile field is considered nonsterile. No equipment or supplies should be placed in this area. Sterile fields should be set up as close as possible to the time a procedure begins. They must be protected from contamination until the procedure begins.

Guidelines: Sterile Fields

- G Perform a surgical scrub and don sterile gloves before preparing the sterile field.
- G Know the following equipment and items needed to set up a sterile field:
  - A **Mayo stand** is a portable stainless-steel tray and holder (Fig. 10-35) often used to set up a sterile field.

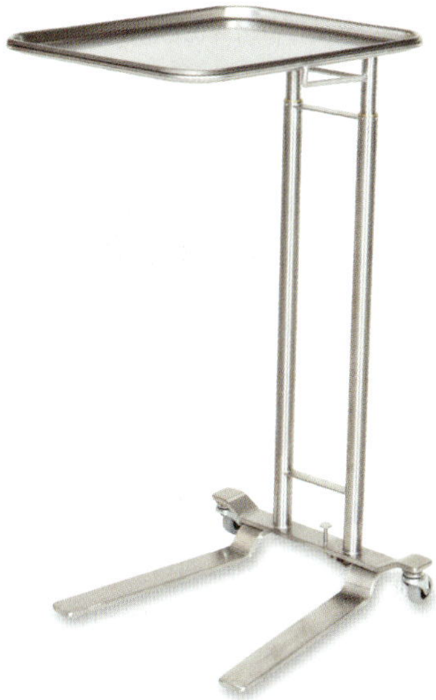

Fig. 10-35. A Mayo stand is the most common site to set up a sterile field. (IMAGE COURTESY OF MEDLINE INDUSTRIES, LP. USED WITH PERMISSION.)

  - **Solutions** are liquids used during the procedures and may include an anesthetic (numbing agent); an antiseptic such as povidone-iodine (antiseptics are cleaning agents used to reduce the spread of pathogens); and saline, which is a sterile salt and water solution used for rinsing or flushing.
  - **Bowls** are used to hold liquids. Place these near the edge of the sterile field. Before adding any liquid to a sterilized bowl, pour some of the solution down a drain or into another container to decontaminate the rim of the bottle.
  - **Sutures** are stitches used to repair a cut in the skin.
  - **Staples** are metal bands used to repair a cut in the skin.
  - A **sterile procedure tray** contains tools and other items needed to perform the procedure.

G Add small, soft items to the sterile field by the "drop method." This means opening an item (e.g., a package of gauze) and holding it downward, allowing it to fall on the sterile field. Add larger, heavier items using sterile transfer forceps. This is a gripping tool with scissor-like handles.

G Cover the sterile field with a sterile towel until the procedure begins.

9. Discuss medications and the importance of avoiding medication errors

In most hospitals, nurses are responsible for giving, or administering, medications to patients. PCTs do not usually handle or administer medications. However, PCTs need to know some things about medications to help keep patients safe.

PCTs should understand the difference between prescription and nonprescription (over-the-counter, or OTC) medication. Antibiotics (such as penicillin), heart medication (such as nitroglycerin), and strong pain medication (such as codeine) are examples of prescription drugs. These drugs must be ordered by a healthcare professional. Aspirin and cold medications, such as decongestants, are examples of over-the-counter drugs. In the community, a person can buy and take OTC drugs without a doctor's order. In the hospital, however, all medications must be approved by the provider caring for the patient and given to the patient by the nurse. If a PCT sees a patient taking any medication that was not given by the nurse, he should report this immediately. This includes vitamins, supplements, and herbal medications.

As medications work in the body their effects may be increased or decreased by **drug interactions**. Prescription or OTC drugs, vitamins, supplements, and herbal medications can all interact with a medication. Certain foods and health conditions can also interact with a medication (for example, a drug that treats one condition may make another worse). This is why it is so important for patients in a hospital to only take medications ordered and administered by the healthcare professionals caring for them.

The **route** is the path that gets a drug into the patient's body. PCTs do not administer medications by any route. They may assist with patient positioning or by providing the patient with water or food, as requested by the nurse. The oral route is the most common way to give medications. Oral drugs are administered by mouth as liquids, tablets, or capsules. Injection routes get medications into a patient's system quickly. Depending on the medication, it may be injected into a muscle, the fatty layer under the skin, or a vein (IV). Medications may also be dissolved in the mouth; inserted into the vagina or rectum; placed in the eye, ear, or nose; or inhaled. Topical medications may be rubbed or sprayed on the skin. Transdermal medications are absorbed through the skin from adhesive patches. PCTs should never touch or remove a medicated patch. Even used patches may still contain medication and should not be handled.

Every healthcare facility has the goal of never making a medication error. Unfortunately, medication errors do happen. At their worst, errors can cause death. Medication safety is a top priority for all healthcare workers. Part of promoting medication safety is knowing the "rights" of medication administration. All healthcare workers should know these "rights":

1. **The right patient**: The nurse must check the patient's identity before medications are administered.
2. **The right medication**: The medication must match the order in the patient's record.
3. **The right time**: Medications must be given at the correct time, and with the correct amount of time between doses.

4. **The right route**: The instructions for how a medication is taken should match the order in the patient's record.
5. **The right dose**: Medication orders state how much medicine a patient should take at once. The amount given to the patient must be exactly the amount ordered.
6. **The right documentation**: After a patient has taken a medication, it is immediately documented in the patient's record according to facility policy.

Many hospitals have systems to help prevent medication errors. Automatic dispensing cabinets (ADCs) are often used. These cabinets (Pyxis is a common brand) track medication use and release the proper dose of the correct medication based on orders in the patient's record. These cabinets also help prevent the misuse or **diversion** (stealing) of controlled medications. **Controlled medications** are drugs that are considered to have the potential for abuse. Many strong painkillers are controlled medications.

A PCT's main role in medication safety is thinking critically and making careful observations. PCTs can observe for signs and symptoms that may be caused by drug reactions or interactions. One very dangerous type of reaction is **anaphylaxis**. This is a type of allergic reaction and a medication can cause it. The body's immune system overreacts to the drug, causing potentially deadly signs and symptoms. It does not always occur the first time a patient takes a drug. It can happen at any time. Antibiotics such as penicillin are common causes of anaphylaxis. PCTs should always report the following signs and symptoms immediately:

- Difficulty breathing
- Hypotension (low blood pressure)
- Hives or itching
- Dizziness, nausea, vomiting, and/or diarrhea

Emergency treatment with a drug called *epinephrine*, administered with a pen-style injection, can reverse anaphylaxis. Reporting signs of anaphylaxis immediately can save a patient's life.

Helping with Self-Administered Medications

PCTs sometimes work in assisted living facilities or in home care. In these settings PCTs may help residents or clients who self-administer their medications. When helping with self-administered medications, the PCT should check the medication label for the right person, medication, time, route, and dose. He should also check to be sure the medication is not expired.

Tasks the PCT may perform include reminding the client/resident to take medication, providing food or water as needed, shaking liquid medications if ordered, and opening and closing containers. The PCT should never touch the inside of the medication container or lid. After observing the client/resident taking the medication, the PCT must document according to facility policy. The PCT should never pour or mix medication from one bottle into another, even if both contain the same medicine. Any questions about medications should be referred to a nurse or healthcare provider. A client/resident refusing to take an ordered medication should also be reported.

Chapter Review

1. List 4 benefits of a patient rounding schedule.
2. How often are patient vital signs usually measured?
3. List 4 vital signs that must be monitored.
4. How does a small child's normal pulse compare to an adult's?
5. What are the sites for measuring body temperature?
6. What is *diaphoresis*? Why should it be reported to a nurse?
7. What is the most common site for monitoring the pulse rate? Where is it located?

8. Why should respirations be counted immediately after measuring the pulse rate?
9. What is a normal pulse oximetry reading for an adult? What is a normal reading for a child?
10. List and define the 2 phases measured in a blood pressure reading.
11. Why is it important for PCTs to report any weight loss or gain that a patient has, no matter how small?
12. List 2 ways patients may be weighed other than a standing scale.
13. What does a stadiometer measure?
14. List 8 guidelines for assisting with preoperative care.
15. List 8 guidelines for assisting with postoperative care.
16. Describe 3 situations when a sterile supply should no longer be considered sterile and should not be used.
17. Give an example of a supply that may be added to a sterile field using the "drop method."

11
Nutrition and Hydration

1. Define *nutrition* and explain special diets

Proper nutrition is very important. **Nutrition** is how the body uses food to maintain health. Bodies need a well-balanced diet with nutrients and plenty of fluids. This helps the body grow new cells, maintain normal body function, and have energy. Proper nutrition in early life helps ensure health later in life. For people who are ill, a well-balanced diet helps maintain muscle and skin tissues and prevent pressure injuries. A healthy diet promotes the healing of wounds and it also helps a person cope with stress.

Patients who do not have any health problems that require a change in diet often eat a *regular diet*. However, patients who are ill may be placed on **special diets** (also called *therapeutic* or *modified* diets). With special diets, certain nutrients or fluids may need to be restricted or removed. A **nutrient** is a necessary substance that provides energy, promotes growth and health, and helps regulate metabolism. Some medications may also interact with certain foods, which then must be restricted. Patients who do not eat enough may be placed on supplementary diets. Diets are also used for weight control and food allergies.

Several types of diets may be ordered for different illnesses. Some patients may be on a combination of special diets. The care plan should specify any special diet the patient needs. Special diets can only be prescribed by providers and planned by dietitians. PCTs should report to the nurse if a patient on a special diet eats food not prepared by the dietary department.

Low-Sodium Diet: People are most familiar with sodium as a component of salt. Salt is restricted first in a low-sodium diet because it is high in sodium. Patients who have high blood pressure, heart disease, or kidney disease may be placed on a low-sodium diet. A modified fluid intake may also be required for people with these conditions. For patients on a low-sodium diet, salt will not be used. Salt will not be served with meals. Common abbreviations for this diet are *Low Na*, which means low sodium, or *NAS*, which stands for *No Added Salt*.

Fluid-Restricted Diet: The fluid taken into the body through food and fluids must equal the fluid that leaves the body through perspiration, stool, urine, and expiration (breathing out). This is fluid balance. When fluid intake is greater than fluid output, body tissue becomes swollen with fluid. People with severe heart disease or kidney disease may have trouble processing fluid. To prevent further damage, providers may restrict fluid intake. For patients on fluid restriction, the PCT will measure and document exact amounts of fluid intake and report excesses to the nurse. Additional fluids or foods that count as fluids, such as ice cream, puddings, gelatin, etc., should not be offered. If the patient mentions being thirsty or requests fluids, the PCT should tell the nurse. A common abbreviation for this diet is *RF*, which stands for *Restrict Fluids*.

High-Potassium Diet: Some people take certain blood pressure medications or diuretics, which are medications that reduce fluid volume. These people may be excreting so much fluid that their bodies could be depleted of potassium. Other people may be placed on a high-potassium diet for different reasons.

Foods high in potassium include bananas, grapefruit, oranges, orange juice, prune juice, prunes, cantaloupes, tomatoes, potatoes with skins, sweet potatoes and yams, winter squash, legumes (beans or lentils), and avocados. *K+* is the common abbreviation for this diet.

Low-Protein/Renal Diet: People who have kidney disease may be on low-protein diets. Protein is restricted because it breaks down into compounds that may lead to further kidney damage. The extent of the restrictions depends on the stage of the disease and if the person is on dialysis. **Dialysis** is an artificial means of removing the body's waste products. Vegetables and starches, such as breads and pasta, are encouraged.

Lowfat Diet: Eating a diet high in saturated fats may put a person at risk for heart disease. Eating unsaturated fat can reduce the risk of heart disease and improve HDL (good) cholesterol levels (Fig. 11-1). People who have heart disease or who have had heart attacks are often prescribed a diet that is low in saturated fat. People with gallbladder disease, diseases that interfere with fat digestion, and liver disease may be placed on a diet that restricts all fats. *Low-Fat/Lowfat* may be the abbreviation used for this diet. Sometimes *Cardiac Diet* is used, which means a diet that is low in sodium, fat, and cholesterol, as well as excess sugar.

Modified-Calorie Diet: Some patients may need to reduce calories to lose weight or prevent weight gain. Other patients may need to gain weight or increase calories because of malnutrition, surgery, illness, or fever. Common abbreviations for this diet are *Low-Cal* or *High-Cal*.

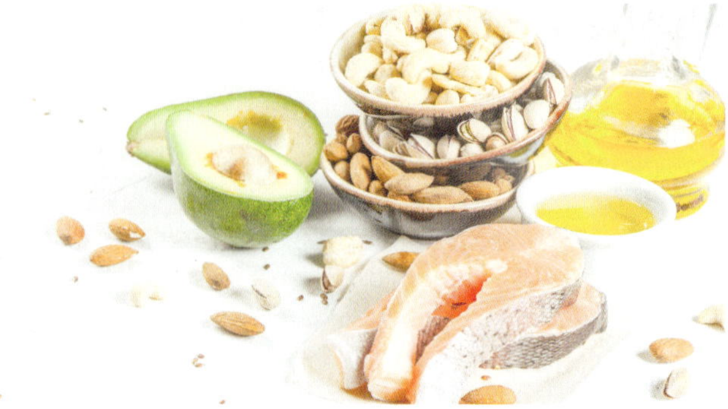

Fig. 11-1. *Foods that contain healthier fats include olive oil, nuts, avocado, and fatty fish like salmon.*

Bland Diet: Gastric and duodenal ulcers are sores in the digestive tract. They can be irritated by foods that produce or increase levels of acid in the stomach, so these foods are eliminated. The bland diet is also used for people who have intestinal disorders, such as Crohn's disease or irritable bowel syndrome (IBS). The following foods and drinks should be avoided: alcohol; beverages containing caffeine, such as coffee, tea, and soft drinks; citrus juices; spicy foods; and spicy seasonings, such as black pepper, cayenne, and chili pepper.

Diabetic Diet: Calories and carbohydrates are carefully controlled in the diets of people who have diabetes. Protein and fats are also regulated. The types and amounts of food are determined by nutritional and energy needs. A dietitian creates a meal plan that includes all the right types and amounts of food for each day. The patient may be able to choose between certain options. Meal plans for people with diabetes may use a carbohydrate-counting approach (often called *carb counting*). After the proper amount of carbohydrates is determined by the dietitian, they are counted in each meal or snack.

To keep their blood glucose levels near normal, people who have diabetes must eat the right amount of the right type of food at the right time. They must eat all that is served. PCTs should encourage them to do so. Any other foods must be approved by the nurse. If a patient will not eat what is recommended, does not finish meals, or is not following the diet, the PCT should tell the nurse.

People who have diabetes should avoid foods that are high in sugar. Sugary foods can cause problems with insulin balance. A meal tray for a patient with diabetes may have artificial sweetener, low-calorie jelly, and/or low-calorie maple syrup. Artificial sweeteners, rather than sugar, may be used in coffee or tea. Common abbreviations for this diet are *NCS* (*No Concentrated Sweets*) or *LCS* (*Low Concentrated Sweets*).

Low-Residue/Low-Fiber Diet: This diet decreases the amount of fiber, whole grains, raw fruits and vegetables, seeds, and other foods, such as dairy products and coffee, in a person's diet. The low-residue diet is used for people with bowel disorders such as diverticulitis.

High-Residue/High-Fiber Diet: This diet increases the intake of fiber and whole grains, such as whole grain cereals, breads, and raw fruits and vegetables. This diet helps with constipation and other bowel disorders.

Gluten-Free Diet: This diet is free of gluten, which is a protein found in wheat, rye, and barley. It is used for people with celiac disease, which is an autoimmune disease that can damage the intestines if gluten is consumed. Foods containing wheat flour, such as tortillas, crackers, breads, cakes, pastas, and cereals, are eliminated from the diet. Some sauces and dressings also have wheat in them. Other items that may contain gluten include beer, hot dogs, candy, broths, vitamins, and medications.

Gluten can cause abdominal pain, gas, or diarrhea for some people who do not have celiac disease. These people may choose not to eat foods containing gluten.

Vegetarian Diet: Health issues, such as diabetes or obesity, may cause a person to follow a vegetarian diet. A person may also choose to eat a vegetarian diet for religious or cultural reasons, or due to a dislike of meat, a compassion for animals, a belief in nonviolence, or financial issues. There are different types of vegetarian diets:

- A lacto-ovo vegetarian diet excludes all meats, fish, and poultry, but allows eggs and dairy products.
- A lacto-vegetarian diet eliminates poultry, meats, fish, and eggs, but allows dairy products.
- An ovo-vegetarian diet omits all meats, fish, poultry, and dairy products, but allows eggs.

Vegan Diet: A vegan diet consists of only plant-based foods and eliminates all poultry, meats, fish, eggs, and dairy products, along with foods that are derived from animals, such as gelatin and honey (Fig. 11-2). This may be ordered for people who have heart disease, diabetes, or other health issues, or a person may choose to eat a vegan diet for ethical or other reasons.

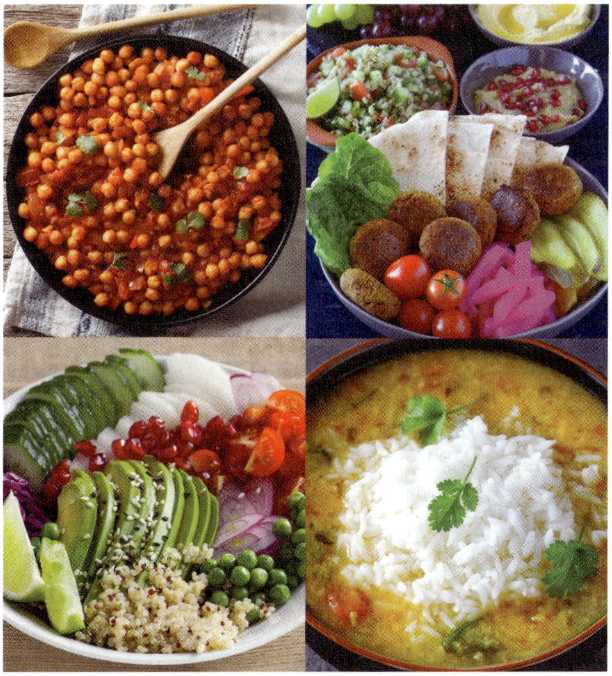

Fig. 11-2. *A person who eats a vegan diet only eats plant-based foods.*

Diets may also be modified by consistency:

Liquid Diet: A liquid diet is usually ordered for a short time due to a medical condition or before or after a test or surgery. It is ordered when a person needs to keep the intestinal tract free of food. A liquid diet consists of foods that are in a liquid state at body temperature. Liquid diets are usually ordered as *clear* or *full*. A clear liquid diet includes clear juices, broth, gelatin, and popsicles. A full liquid diet includes all the liquids served on a clear liquid diet, with the addition of cream soups, milk, and ice cream.

Soft Diet and Mechanical Soft Diet: The soft diet is soft in texture and consists of soft or chopped foods that are easier to chew and swallow. Foods that are hard to chew and swallow, such as raw fruits and vegetables and some meats, will be restricted. High-fiber foods, fried foods, and spicy foods may also be limited. Providers order this diet for people who have trouble chewing and swallowing due to dental problems or other medical conditions. It is also ordered for people who are going from a liquid diet to a regular diet.

The mechanical soft diet consists of chopped or blended foods that are easier to chew and swallow. Foods are prepared with blenders, food processors, or cutting utensils. Unlike the soft diet, the mechanical soft diet does not limit spices, fat, and fiber. Only the texture of foods is changed. This diet is used for people recovering from surgery or who have trouble chewing and swallowing.

Pureed Diet: To **puree** a food means to blend or grind it into a thick paste of baby food consistency. The food should be thick enough to hold its form in the mouth. This diet does not require a person to chew his food. A pureed diet is often used for people who have trouble chewing and/or swallowing more textured foods. Learning Objective 4 has more information on food texture and swallowing.

NPO: The abbreviation *NPO* stands for *nil per os*, the Latin term for *nothing by mouth*. This means that a patient is not allowed to have anything to eat or drink. Some patients have such a severe problem with swallowing that it is unsafe to give them anything by mouth. These patients will receive nutrition and hydration through a feeding tube or intravenously. Some patients may not be able to eat and drink for a short time before a medical test or surgery. PCTs need to know this abbreviation. They should never offer any food or drink, even water, to a patient with this order.

Connected Care

Menus

Many facilities provide menus for patients to choose what meals they want. Patients who eat special diets may receive menus that show options that meet their diet needs. PCTs may help patients complete their menu choices. If asked to help with a menu, the PCT should speak clearly and make the choices sound appealing. He should answer any questions the patient has and should mark the selection the patient wants. After completing each category, he should submit the menu according to facility policy. When food arrives, it must always be checked against what the patient requested and the diet ordered for the patient. The patient's identity must also be checked against the name on the tray.

2. Discuss fluid balance and explain intake and output (I&O)

To maintain health, the body must be properly **hydrated**, or have absorbed enough water or other fluid. Fluid comes in the form of liquids that a person drinks. It is also found in semiliquid foods like gelatin, soup, ice cream, pudding, and yogurt. The fluid a person consumes is called **intake**, or **input**.

Water is an essential nutrient for life. Proper fluid intake is important. Drinking enough water or other fluids can help prevent constipation and urinary incontinence. Without enough fluid, urine becomes concentrated. More concentrated urine creates a higher risk for infection. Proper fluid intake also helps to dilute wastes and flush out the urinary system. It may even help prevent confusion.

There is no single rule regarding fluid intake. The amount needed depends on factors such as activity level, overall health, and climate/temperature. The patient's provider or the dietitian may make recommendations based on the patient's specific needs.

All fluid taken in each day cannot stay in the body. It must be eliminated as **output**. Output includes urine, feces (including diarrhea), and vomitus. It also includes perspiration, moisture in the air that a person exhales, and wound drainage.

Fluid balance is maintaining equal input and output, or taking in and eliminating equal amounts of fluids. Most people do this naturally. Some patients must have their intake and output, or I&O, monitored and documented. To do this, all food and fluids the patient takes by mouth, IV, or tube feedings are measured, as well as all urine, vomitus, and liquid stool (diarrhea) produced. If wound drainage or respiratory secretions are removed by pump or suction, these may also be counted as output. IV pumps display the amount of fluid that has been administered. If assigned and allowed to measure IV intake, the PCT should follow manufacturer instructions to view the amount (in mL) that has been infused. After documenting how much has been infused, the PCT must then clear the IV pump reading. This means setting the reading to 0 (zero). All intake and output is recorded in the patient's medical record.

Conversions

Milliliters (mL) are units of measurement in the metric system. One milliliter is 1/1000 of a liter. Ounces (oz) are converted to milliliters. One ounce equals 30 milliliters. To convert ounces to milliliters, the number of ounces must be multiplied by 30.

1 oz = 30 mL
2 oz = 60 mL
3 oz = 90 mL
4 oz = 120 mL
5 oz = 150 mL
6 oz = 180 mL
7 oz = 210 mL
8 oz = 240 mL
¼ cup = 2 oz = 60 mL
½ cup = 4 oz = 120 mL
1 cup = 8 oz = 240 mL

Before beginning, the PCT should explain to the patient that she needs to keep track of their intake. The patient should be asked to let the PCT know when they drink something (if it is not something she served to them) and how much it was. If the patient is in isolation, full PPE may be required. The PCT should follow facility policy.

For measuring output, if the bedpan or urinal has measurement markings on it, the urine does not need to be poured into a measuring container. Chapter 16 contains information about suction canisters, which have volume markings on them. Chapter 17 contains information on measuring urine when emptying a urinary catheter drainage bag.

Measuring and recording intake and output

Equipment: I&O form in patient's record, measuring container, gloves (and any other required PPE)

Measure intake first.

1. Identify yourself by name. Identify the patient according to facility policy.
2. Wash your hands.
3. Explain the procedure to the patient. Speak clearly, slowly, and directly. Maintain face-to-face contact whenever possible.
4. Provide for the patient's privacy with a curtain, screen, or door.
5. Note the amount of fluid the patient is served. The amount of fluid is often marked on the container.
6. When the patient has finished a meal or snack, measure any leftover fluids with the measuring container. Note this amount. (If the amount is between measurement lines, you may need to round up to the nearest 25 mL. Follow policy.)
7. Subtract the leftover amount from the amount served. If you have measured

in ounces, convert to milliliters (mL) by multiplying by 30.

8. Wash your hands before recording intake.
9. Document the amount of fluid consumed (in mL) in the input column, as well as the time and the type of fluid consumed. Report anything unusual, such as the patient drinking little or nothing or feeling ill.

Measuring output is the other half of monitoring fluid balance.

Equipment: I&O form in patient's record, measuring container, gloves (and any other required PPE)

1. Wash your hands.
2. Put on gloves before handling the bedpan or urinal.
3. If the bedpan or urinal has volume markings on it, note the amount. If not, pour the contents into the measuring container. Do not spill or splash urine.
4. Place the container on a flat surface. Measure the amount of urine at eye level (Fig. 11-3). Keep the container level. Note the amount, converting to mL if necessary. (If the amount is between measurement lines, you may need to round up to the nearest 25 mL. Follow policy.)

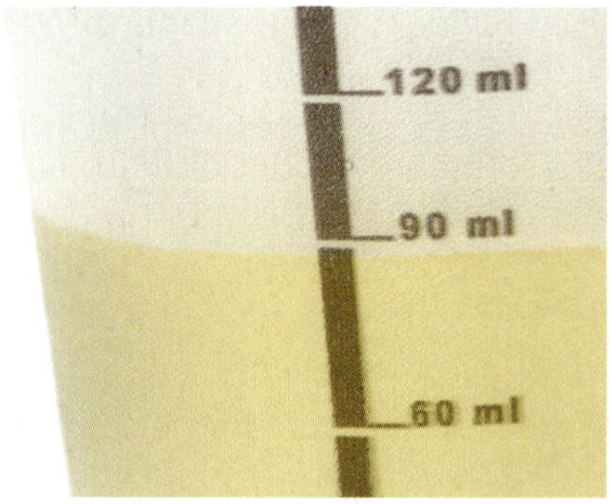

Fig. 11-3. *A container for measuring fluid, sometimes called a* graduated measuring cup *or* graduate, *shows the volume in milliliters.*

5. After measuring urine, empty the graduate into the toilet without splashing.
6. Turn on the faucet with a paper towel. Rinse the graduate with cold water and pour the rinse water into the toilet.
7. Rinse the bedpan/urinal with cold water and pour the rinse water into the toilet. Flush.
8. Place the graduate and bedpan in the area for cleaning or clean and store according to policy.
9. Remove and discard your gloves.
10. Wash your hands before recording output.
11. Document the time and amount of urine in the output column. For example: 1545 hours, 200 mL urine. To measure vomitus, pour it into the measuring container, then discard the vomitus in the toilet. If the patient vomits on the bed or floor, estimate the amount. Document emesis and the amount.
12. Return the bed to its lowest position. Remove privacy measures.
13. Place the call light within the patient's reach.
14. Report any changes in the patient to the nurse.

Dehydration is a serious condition that occurs when a person does not have enough fluid in the body. People can become dehydrated if they do not drink enough or if they have diarrhea or are vomiting. Prevention is very important.

Guidelines: Preventing Dehydration

- **G** Report observations and warning signs to the nurse immediately. Be especially alert to dehydration in infants and elderly patients. These patients can become dehydrated very quickly and the effects can be more severe.
- **G** Encourage patients to drink every time you see them.
- **G** Offer fresh water or other fluids often. Offer drinks that the patient enjoys. Some patients

may prefer water or sparkling water (seltzer water). Some may not like water and prefer other types of beverages, such as juice, soda, tea, or milk. Some patients do not want ice in their drinks. As always, it is important to provide person-centered care. Honor personal preferences. Report to the nurse if the patient tells you she does not like the fluids being served.

- G Ice chips, frozen flavored ice sticks, and gelatin are also forms of liquids. Offer them often. Do not offer ice chips or sticks if a patient has a swallowing problem.
- G If appropriate, offer sips of liquid between bites of food at meals and snacks if you are helping a patient eat.
- G Make sure a pitcher and cup are nearby and are light enough for the patient to lift. Follow the schedule for replacing with fresh water.
- G Offer assistance if the patient cannot drink without help. Use assistive cups as needed.
- G Record fluid intake and output as ordered.
- G IV fluids are sometimes given to prevent dehydration. Report if the tubing or needle falls out or if the fluid is not dripping or is leaking.

Observing and Reporting: Dehydration

Report any of these to the nurse:

- O/R Patient drinks fewer than six 8-ounce glasses of liquid per day if he is not receiving IV fluids
- O/R Patient drinks little or no fluids at meals
- O/R Patient needs help drinking from a cup
- O/R Patient has trouble swallowing liquids
- O/R Patient has an average output of less than 30 mL/hour during a shift
- O/R Patient has frequent vomiting, diarrhea, or a fever
- O/R Patient is easily confused or tired

Report any of these signs and symptoms:

- O/R Dry mouth, cracked lips
- O/R Sunken eyes
- O/R Dark urine, strong-smelling urine, or less frequent urination
- O/R Weight loss
- O/R Fatigue
- O/R Dizziness
- O/R Abdominal pain
- O/R Patient says he is very thirsty

Fluid overload occurs when the body cannot handle the fluid consumed. This often affects people with heart or kidney disease.

Observing and Reporting: Fluid Overload

Report any of these to the nurse:

- O/R Swelling/edema of extremities (ankles, feet, fingers, hands); **edema** is swelling caused by excess fluid in body tissues.
- O/R Weight gain (daily weight gain of 0.5 to 1 kilogram)
- O/R Decreased urine output
- O/R Shortness of breath
- O/R Increased heart rate
- O/R Anxiety
- O/R Skin that appears tight, smooth, or shiny

3. Demonstrate how to assist with eating

In some facilities, PCTs may be assigned to help patients with meals. Patients need different levels of help with eating. Many patients do not need any help, while others only need help setting up their meal. They may only need someone to open cartons and cut and season their food. Once that is done, they can feed themselves. The PCT should check with these patients from time to time to see if they need anything else.

Some patients will be completely unable to feed themselves. It may be the PCT's job to feed them. Patients who must be fed are often embarrassed and depressed about their dependence on another person. PCTs should be sensitive to this and give privacy while patients are eating. Patients should not be rushed through their meals. PCTs should only give assistance as specified, when necessary, or when patients request it.

Guidelines: Assisting a Patient with Eating

- **G** Ask if the patient needs to go to the bathroom before eating. Assist as needed.
- **G** Before you begin serving or helping patients, wash your hands. Help the patient wash their hands.
- **G** It is very important to identify patients before serving a meal tray. Feeding a patient the wrong food can cause serious problems, even death. Identify the patient using 2 unique identifiers (e.g., full name, date of birth). Check the meal to be sure it matches what is ordered for the patient you have identified. Follow facility policy.
- **G** Sit at a patient's eye level. The patient should be sitting upright, at a 90-degree angle. Make eye contact with the patient.
- **G** If the patient wishes, allow time for prayer.
- **G** Never treat an adult patient like a child. This is embarrassing and disrespectful. It is hard for many people to accept help with eating. Be supportive and encouraging.
- **G** Test the temperature of the food by putting your hand over the dish to sense the heat. Do not touch food to test its temperature. If you think the food is too hot, do not blow on it. Offer other food to give it time to cool.
- **G** Cut foods and pour liquids as needed. Season foods to the patient's preference.
- **G** Identify the foods and fluids that are in front of the patient. Call pureed foods by the correct name. For example, ask, "Would you like green beans?" rather than referring to it as "some green stuff."
- **G** Ask the patient which food he wants to eat first. Allow him to make the choice, even if he wants to eat dessert first.
- **G** Do not mix foods unless the patient requests it.
- **G** Do not rush the meal. Allow time for the patient to chew and swallow each bite. Be relaxed.
- **G** Be social and friendly. Make simple conversation if the patient wishes to do so. Use appropriate topics, such as the news, weather, and things the patient has said about their life or what they enjoy, including food preferences. Say positive things about the food being served, such as "This smells really good" and "This looks really fresh."
- **G** Give the patient your full attention while she is eating. Do not talk to other staff members while helping a patient eat.
- **G** Alternate food and drink. Alternating cold and hot foods or bland foods and sweets can help increase appetite.
- **G** If the patient wants a different food from what is being served, inform the nurse so that an alternative may be offered.

Assisting a patient with eating

Equipment: meal and beverage; eating utensils; clothing protector; washcloths, wipes, or towel

1. Identify yourself by name. Identify the patient according to facility policy.
2. Wash your hands.

3. Explain the procedure to the patient. Speak clearly, slowly, and directly. Maintain face-to-face contact whenever possible.
4. Provide for the patient's privacy with a curtain, screen, or door.
5. Follow facility policy to verify that the patient has received the right tray.
6. Raise the head of the bed. Make sure the patient is in an upright sitting position (at a 90-degree angle).
7. Adjust the bed height to sit at the patient's eye level. Lock the bed wheels.
8. Place the tray where it can be easily seen by the patient, such as on the overbed table.
9. Help the patient clean her hands if she cannot do it herself.
10. Help the patient put on a clothing protector if desired.
11. Sit facing the patient at the patient's eye level (Fig. 11-4). Sit on the stronger side if the patient has one-sided weakness.

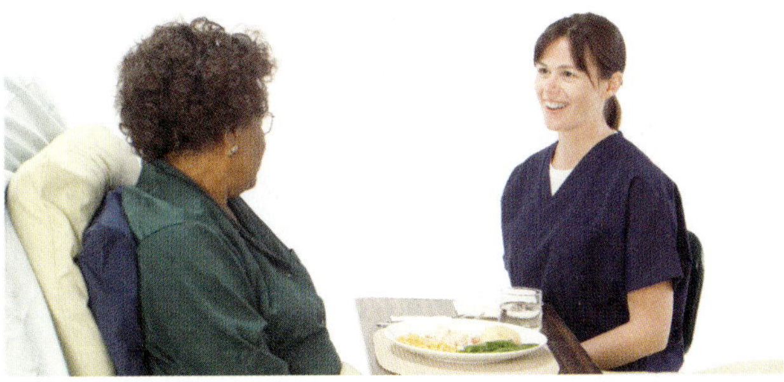

Fig. 11-4. *The patient should be sitting upright, and the PCT should be sitting at her eye level.*

12. Tell the patient what foods are on the tray. Offer a drink of beverage. Ask what the patient would like to eat first.
13. Check the temperature of the food. Using utensils, offer the food in bite-sized pieces. Tell the patient the content of each bite of food offered (Fig. 11-5). Alternate types of food, allowing for the patient's preferences. Do not feed all of one type before offering another type. Make sure the patient's mouth is empty before the next bite or sip. Report any swallowing problems immediately.

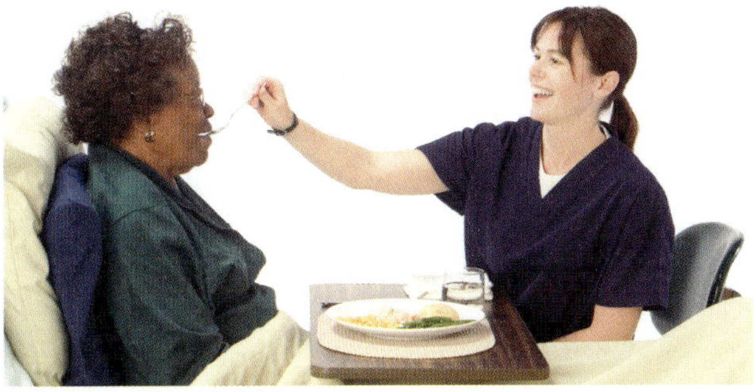

Fig. 11-5. *Offer the food in bite-sized pieces. Tell the patient the content of each bite of food.*

14. Offer sips of beverage throughout the meal. If you are holding the cup, touch it to the patient's lips before you tip it. Give small, frequent sips.
15. Talk with the patient during the meal (Fig. 11-6). Do not rush the patient.

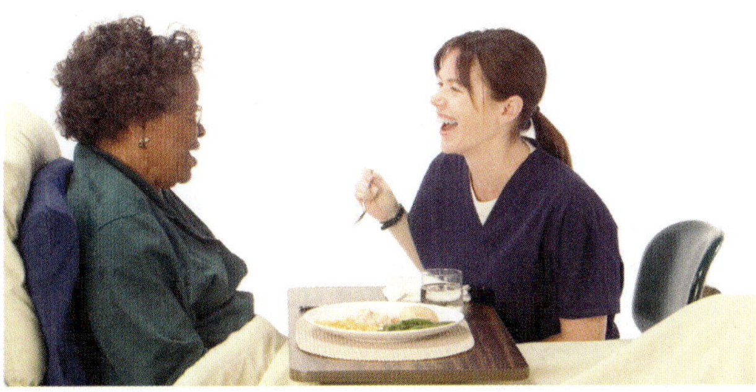

Fig. 11-6. *Socializing during mealtime makes eating more enjoyable. It may help promote a healthy appetite.*

16. Wipe food from the patient's mouth and hands as needed during the meal (Fig. 11-7). Wipe again at the end of the meal.

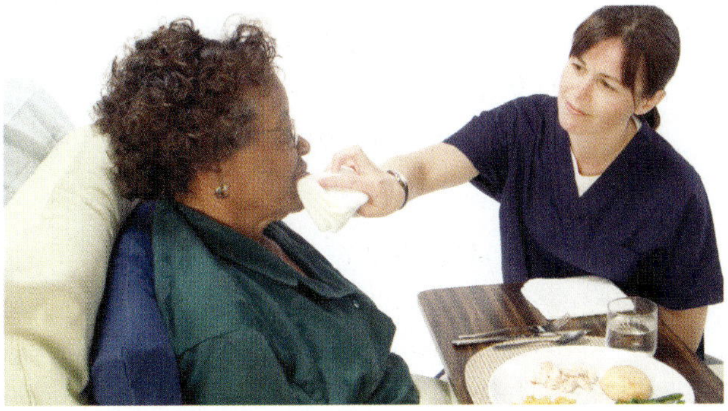

Fig. 11-7. *Wiping food from the mouth during the meal helps to maintain the patient's dignity.*

17. Remove the clothing protector if used. Place it and used washcloths or wipes in the proper containers.
18. Remove the food tray. Check for eyeglasses, dentures, or any personal items before removing the tray. Place it in the proper area.
19. Make the patient comfortable. Keep the patient in the upright position for at least 30 minutes. Make sure the bed is free from crumbs.
20. Return the bed to its lowest position. Remove privacy measures.
21. Place the call light within the patient's reach.
22. Wash your hands.
23. Report any changes in the patient to the nurse.
24. Document the procedure using facility guidelines.

Most facilities keep track of how much food and fluid a patient consumes. PCTs should follow their facility's policies for documenting intake.

Connected Care

Food Choices

Patients have the legal right to make choices about their food. They can choose what kind of food they want to eat. They can refuse the food and drink being offered. PCTs must honor a patient's personal beliefs and preferences about selecting and avoiding specific foods. Although patients have the right to refuse, it is best to ask questions when they do. For example, if a patient refuses dinner, the PCT can ask if there is something wrong with the food. The patient may say he is Jewish and cannot eat a pork chop because it is not kosher. PCTs should respond to requests for different food in a pleasant way. The PCT can explain that she will get him another meal as quickly as possible. She can take the tray and follow facility policy to make sure the patient is offered an alternative meal.

4. Identify signs and symptoms of swallowing problems

Patients may have conditions that make eating or swallowing difficult. **Dysphagia** means difficulty in swallowing. A stroke, or CVA, can cause weakness and paralysis on one side of the body. Nerve and muscle damage from head and neck cancer, multiple sclerosis, Parkinson's disease, or Alzheimer's disease may also cause dysphagia.

PCTs need to be able to recognize and report signs that a patient has a swallowing problem. Signs and symptoms of swallowing problems include the following:

- Coughing during or after meals
- Choking during meals
- Dribbling saliva, food, or fluid from the mouth
- Having food residue inside the mouth or cheeks during or after meals
- Gurgling during or after meals or losing one's voice
- Eating slowly
- Avoiding eating
- Spitting out pieces of food
- Swallowing several times per mouthful
- Clearing the throat frequently during and after meals
- Watering eyes when eating or drinking
- Food or fluid coming up into the nose
- Making a visible effort to swallow
- Breathing rapidly or with shorter breaths while eating or drinking
- Difficulty chewing food
- Difficulty swallowing medications

Patients with swallowing problems may need to consume only thickened liquids and foods that have a modified texture. Thickened liquids have a thickening powder or agent added to them. This improves the ability to control fluid in the mouth and throat. A provider orders the necessary thickness after the patient has been evaluated by a speech-language pathologist.

Some beverages arrive already thickened and ready to drink. Other beverages must have the thickening agent added before serving. If thickening is ordered, it must be used with all liquids. This means that regular liquids, such as water or other beverages, should not be offered to patients who must have thickened liquids.

There are 3 basic thickened consistencies: nectar thick, honey thick, and pudding thick. Nectar thick is thicker than water. It is the thickness of a thick juice, such as a tomato juice. A patient can drink this from a cup. Honey thick has the thickness of honey and pours very slowly. A patient uses a spoon to consume it. With pudding thick, the liquid has become semisolid, much like pudding. A spoon should stand up straight when put into the middle of the drink. A patient uses a spoon to consume it.

In 2016 the International Dysphagia Diet Standardisation Initiative (IDDSI) developed different levels to identify food textures and drink thicknesses, and in 2019 they updated their framework (Fig. 11-8). The goal of this is to make descriptions standard, so that they can be used internationally, across all care settings. There are 8 levels (0–7) listed for drinks and foods, but not all facilities use all of these levels.

Swallowing problems put patients at high risk for choking on food or drink. Inhaling food, fluid, or foreign material into the lungs is called *aspiration*. Aspiration can cause pneumonia or death. A PCT should alert the nurse immediately if any problems occur while eating.

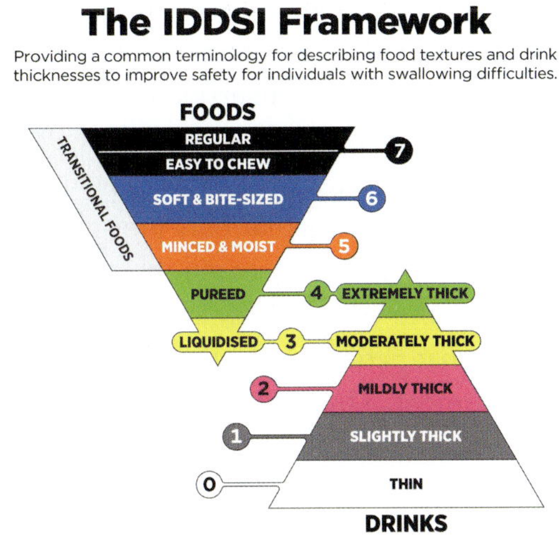

***Fig. 11-8.** The IDDSI framework to describe thickened liquids and food textures.* (© THE INTERNATIONAL DYSPHAGIA DIET STANDARDISATION INITIATIVE 2019 @ HTTPS://IDDSI.ORG/FRAMEWORK. LICENSED UNDER THE CREATIVECOMMONS ATTRIBUTION SHAREALIKE 4.0 LICENSE HTTPS://CREATIVECOMMONS.ORG/LICENSES/BY-SA/4.0/LEGALCODE. DERIVATIVE WORKS EXTENDING BEYOND LANGUAGE TRANSLATION ARE NOT PERMITTED.)

Guidelines: Preventing Aspiration

- **G** Position patients in an upright position (90-degree angle) for eating and drinking. Do not feed patients in a reclined position.
- **G** Offer small pieces of food or small spoonfuls of pureed food.
- **G** Feed patients slowly. Do not rush them.
- **G** Place food in the unaffected, or stronger, side of the mouth.
- **G** Make sure the mouth is empty before offering another bite of food or sip of drink.
- **G** Keep patients in the upright position for at least 30 minutes after eating and drinking.

5. Describe feeding tubes and related care

When a person is unable to swallow, he may be fed through a tube. A **nasogastric (NG) tube** is inserted into the nose and goes to the stomach. A tube can also be placed into the stomach through the abdominal wall. This is called a

percutaneous endoscopic gastrostomy (PEG) tube. The surgically created opening into the stomach that allows the insertion of a tube is called a **gastrostomy** (Fig. 11-9). Tube feedings are used when patients cannot swallow but can digest food. Conditions that may prevent swallowing include coma, cancer, stroke, refusal to eat, and extreme weakness. It is important to remember that patients have the legal right to refuse treatment. This includes the insertion of tubes.

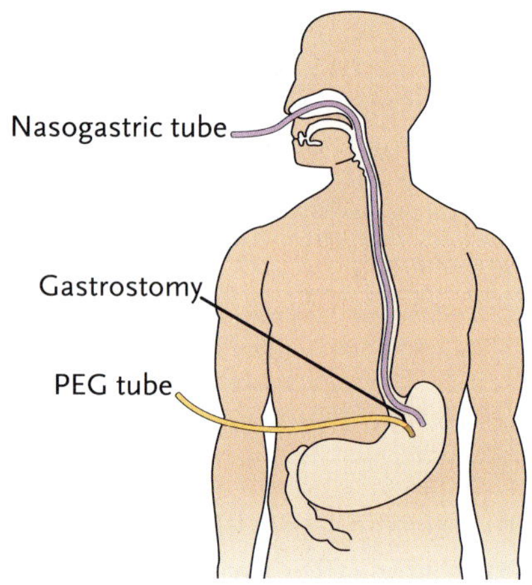

Fig. 11-9. *Nasogastric tubes are inserted through the nose. PEG tubes are inserted through the abdominal wall into the stomach.*

PCTs never insert or remove tubes, do the feeding, or irrigate (clean) the tubes. They may assemble equipment and supplies and hand them to the nurse. PCTs may position patients in a sitting position for feeding. They may also discard or clean and store used equipment and supplies. In addition, PCTs may observe, report, and document any changes in the patient or problems with the feeding.

Guidelines: Tube Feedings

- G Wash your hands before assisting with any aspect of tube feedings.
- G Make sure the tubing is not coiled, kinked, or resting underneath the patient.
- G Be aware if the patient has an order for *nothing by mouth* or *NPO*.
- G The tube is only inserted and removed by a provider or nurse. If it comes out, report it immediately.
- G A provider will prescribe the type and amount of feeding. The feedings should be at room temperature and in liquid form.
- G A patient with a feeding tube should always have the head of the bed elevated 30 degrees. However, during a feeding, the patient should remain in a sitting position with the head of the bed elevated at least 45 degrees. This helps prevent serious problems, such as aspiration. The elderly can develop pneumonia or even die from improper positioning during tube feedings. After the feeding, keep the patient upright for as long as ordered, at least 30 minutes.
- G Give regular oral care.
- G If the patient must remain in bed for long periods during feedings, give careful skin care. This helps to prevent pressure injuries on the hips and sacral area.

Observing and Reporting: Tube Feedings

Report any of these to the nurse immediately:

- O/R Discoloration or drainage around the opening
- O/R Skin sores or bruises
- O/R Cyanotic or discolored skin
- O/R Patient reports pain or nausea
- O/R Choking or coughing
- O/R Vomiting
- O/R Diarrhea
- O/R Swollen abdomen
- O/R Fever
- O/R Tube falls out
- O/R Tubing is kinked
- O/R Problems with the equipment

O/R Feeding pump alarm sounds

O/R Change of patient's inclined position

When the digestive system does not function properly, **parenteral nutrition** (**PN**) (sometimes referred to as *total parenteral nutrition* or *TPN*) may be needed. With parenteral nutrition, a solution of nutrients goes directly into the bloodstream. It bypasses the digestive system. PCTs are not responsible for parenteral nutrition. They may be assigned to measure the patient's temperature or assemble supplies. In addition, duties include observing, reporting, and documenting any changes in the patient or problems with the feeding.

6. Describe how to assist patients with special needs

Patients with specific diseases or conditions, such as Parkinson's disease, Alzheimer's disease or other dementias, head trauma, blindness, confusion, or those recovering from a stroke, may need special assistance when eating.

Guidelines: Dining Techniques

G Use assistive devices such as utensils with built-up handle grips and plate guards. Assistive devices for eating help people feed themselves. These devices should be included on the meal tray.

G Patients may benefit from physical and verbal cues. These promote independence. A *cue* is something that signals that a person should do something. The hand-over-hand approach is an example of a physical cue. The patient lifts a utensil if he is able. You put your hand over his to help with eating. With your hand placed over the patient's hand, help him get food on the utensil. Steer the utensil from the plate to the mouth and back. Repeat this until the patient is finished.

G Verbal cues must be short and clear. The cues should prompt the patient to do something. Give verbal cues one at a time. Wait until the patient has finished one task before asking him to do another. Repeat the cues until the patient is done eating. Examples of verbal cues include the following:

- "Pick up your spoon."
- "Put some carrots on your spoon."
- "Raise the spoon to your lips."
- "Open your mouth."
- "Place the spoon in your mouth."
- "Close your mouth."
- "Take the spoon out of your mouth."
- "Chew."
- "Swallow."
- "Drink some water."

G As needed, read menus to patients who are visually impaired. Place the plate or tray directly in front of patients. Use the face of an imaginary clock to explain the position of what is in front of them (Fig. 11-10).

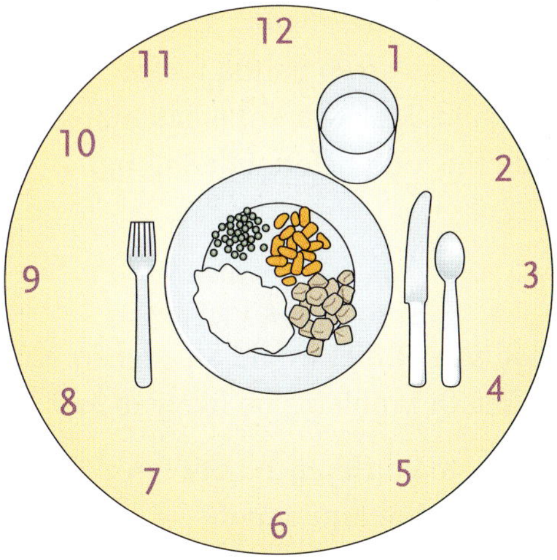

Fig. 11-10. *Use the face of an imaginary clock to explain the position of food to patients who are visually impaired.*

- **G** For patients who have had a stroke and have a paralyzed or weaker side, place food in the stronger side of the mouth. Make sure food is swallowed before offering another bite.
- **G** Place food in the patient's field of vision. The nurse will determine a patient's field of vision.
- **G** For patients who have Parkinson's disease, tremors or shaking can make it difficult to eat. Help by using physical cues. Place food and drinks close so that the patient can easily reach them. Use assistive devices as needed.
- **G** If a patient has poor neck control, a neck brace may be used to stabilize the head. Use assistive devices as needed.
- **G** If the patient bites down on utensils, ask him to open his mouth. Do not pull the utensil out of his mouth. Wait until his jaw relaxes.
- **G** If the patient pockets food in his cheeks, ask him to chew and swallow the food. Touch the side of his cheek. Ask him to use his tongue to get the food. Using your fingers on the cheek (near the lower jaw), gently push the food toward his teeth.
- **G** If the patient holds food in his mouth, ask him to chew and swallow the food. You may need to trigger swallowing. To do this, gently press down on the tongue when taking the spoon out of the mouth. You can also try to gently press down on the top of his head with your hand. Make sure the patient has swallowed the food before offering more.

Chapter Review

1. What type of diet would a patient without any health problems be likely to eat?
2. What is the difference between a clear liquid diet and a full liquid diet?
3. How is the mechanical soft diet different from the soft diet?
4. List 5 reasons that a person may choose to be a vegetarian.
5. What is the first item to be restricted in a low-sodium diet?
6. What does the abbreviation *NPO* mean?
7. What is fluid balance?
8. How many milliliters (mL) equal 1 ounce (oz)?
9. What counts as output when measuring intake and output?
10. Describe 6 ways that a PCT can help prevent dehydration.
11. List 4 signs of fluid overload that a PCT should report.
12. What is the proper position to place a patient in for eating?
13. How might being cheerful and positive during mealtimes affect the amount of food a patient consumes?
14. How can a PCT verify that she has the correct patient for the meal tray that she is serving?
15. How should a PCT test the temperature of food?
16. What should the PCT do if a patient wants a different food than what is being served?
17. When feeding a patient, how should the bed height be adjusted?
18. How can thickened liquids help a person with swallowing problems?
19. What is the medical term for difficulty swallowing?
20. Describe 5 guidelines to help prevent aspiration.
21. What are 2 ways a patient may be fed if he has a digestive system that does not function properly or if he cannot swallow?

22. At what angle should a patient with a feeding tube have the head of the bed during a feeding? At what angle should the head of the bed be at other times? Why is this important?
23. How do verbal cues assist a patient with eating?
24. When assisting a patient who has a visual impairment, how should the PCT explain the position of food and objects to the patient?
25. To which side of the mouth should food be directed if a patient has a weaker side—the weaker (affected) or stronger (unaffected) side?

12 The Integumentary System and Related Care

1. Describe body systems and define key anatomical terms

The human body can be organized into 10 body systems. These systems are often described in terms of **anatomy**, or the parts of the system, and **physiology**, or how the system functions. Body systems are made up of organs. **Organs** are organized groups of **tissues** with specific functions. Tissues are composed of **cells**, which are the basic units of the body. Living cells divide, grow, and die, renewing the tissues and organs of the body. In this book, the human body is divided into 10 systems:

1. Integumentary (skin)
2. Musculoskeletal
3. Nervous
4. Circulatory
5. Respiratory
6. Urinary
7. Gastrointestinal
8. Endocrine
9. Reproductive
10. Immune and lymphatic

Each system in the body has a condition under which it works best. **Homeostasis** is the name for the condition in which all the body's systems are balanced and are working together to maintain internal stability. To be in homeostasis, the body's **metabolism**, or physical and chemical processes, must be working at a steady level. When disease or injury occurs, the body's metabolism is disturbed, and homeostasis is lost.

Changes in metabolic processes are called *signs* (objective information) and *symptoms* (subjective information). For instance, changes in body temperature could indicate that the body is fighting an infection. Noticing and reporting changes in patients is a very important part of a PCT's job. The changes noted could be signs of significant problems.

PCTs must know anatomical terms to communicate properly. Medical professionals use these terms to describe parts of the body. They also use anatomical terms to communicate about medical diagnosis and treatment (Fig. 12-1).

Anatomical terms that describe location or direction include the following:

- Anterior or ventral: the front of the body or body part
- Posterior or dorsal: the back of the body or body part
- Superior or cephalic: toward the head. The term *cephalic* means relating to the head.
- Inferior or caudal: away from the head. The term *caudal* means relating to the tail.
- Medial: toward the midline of the body
- Lateral: to the side, away from the midline of the body

- Proximal: closer to the torso
- Distal: farther away from the torso

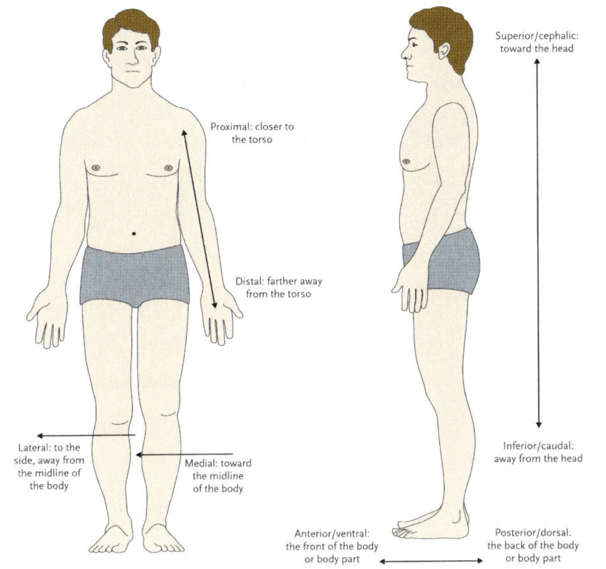

Fig. 12-1. *Documentation in medical records may include terms of location or direction. Providers and nurses may also use these terms when talking to PCTs.*

2. Describe the structure and function of the integumentary system

The largest organ and system in the body is the skin, a natural protective covering, or **integument**. Skin prevents injury to internal organs, and protects the body against entry of bacteria. Skin also prevents the loss of too much water, which is essential to life. Skin is made up of layers of tissues. Within these layers are sweat glands, which secrete sweat to help cool the body when needed, and sebaceous glands, which secrete oil (sebum) to keep the skin lubricated. There are also hair follicles, many tiny blood vessels (capillaries), and tiny nerve endings (Fig. 12-2).

The skin is also a *sense organ*. It feels heat, cold, pain, touch, and pressure. It then tells the brain what it is feeling. Body temperature is regulated in the skin. Blood vessels **dilate**, or widen, when the outside temperature is too high. This brings more blood to the body's surface to cool it off. The same blood vessels **constrict**, or narrow, when the outside temperature is too cold. By restricting the amount of blood reaching the skin, the blood vessels help the body retain heat.

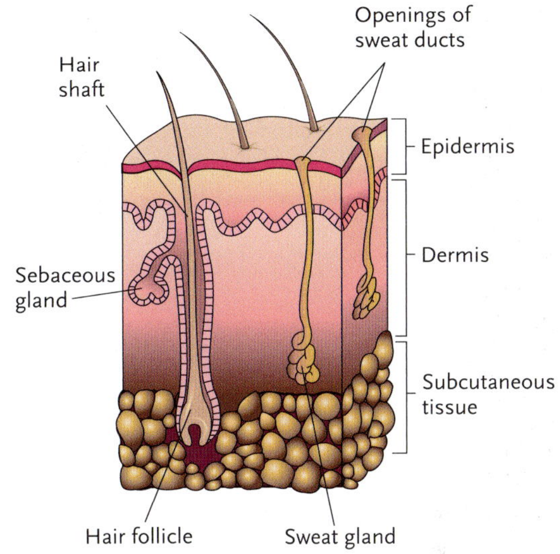

Fig. 12-2. *Cross-section showing details of the integumentary system.*

The blood vessels, called **capillaries**, are located in the dermis, which is the inner layer of skin. The dermis also contains nerves, sweat glands, sebaceous (oil) glands, and hair roots. Sweat glands help control body temperature by secreting sweat. Sweat is made up of mostly water, but it also contains salt and a small amount of waste products. Sweat comes to the body's surface through pores, or tiny openings in the skin. It cools the body as it evaporates. Sebaceous glands in the dermis secrete sebum (oil). Sebum comes to the skin surface through hair follicles, or roots. Sebum keeps the skin and hair lubricated.

No blood vessels and only a few nerve endings are located in the epidermis, which is the outer layer of skin. Thinner than the dermis, the epidermis contains both dead and living cells. The dead cells begin deeper in the epidermis. They are pushed to the surface as other cells divide. They are eventually worn off. The epidermis also contains pigment cells that give skin its color.

Hair grows from roots located in the dermis. It grows through hair follicles that extend through the epidermis to the outside of the body. Hair protects the body from heat and cold. Hair inside the nose and ears keeps out particles and bacteria trying to enter the body.

The functions of the integumentary system are to protect internal organs from injury, protect the body against bacteria, and prevent the loss of too much water. It also responds to heat, cold, pain, touch, and pressure, and it regulates body temperature.

Observing and Reporting: Integumentary System

During care, a patient's skin should be observed for changes that may indicate injury or disease:

- O/R Any discolored areas (for example, pale, white, reddened, or purple)
- O/R Blisters, bruises, or rashes
- O/R Complaints of tingling, warmth, or burning
- O/R Dry or flaking skin
- O/R Itchy skin
- O/R Swelling
- O/R Cuts, boils, sores, wounds, or abrasions
- O/R Fluid or blood draining from the skin
- O/R Broken skin
- O/R Changes in moistness or dryness
- O/R Changes in an injury or wound (size, depth, drainage, color, or odor)
- O/R Discolored or broken skin between toes or around toenails
- O/R Scalp or hair changes
- O/R Skin that appears different from normal or that has changed
- O/R In dark skin tones, also look for changes in skin tone, skin temperature, and the feel or appearance of the tissue as compared to the skin nearby

3. List common conditions of the integumentary system and discuss related care

Pressure Injuries

Immobility reduces the amount of blood that circulates to the skin. Patients who have restricted mobility are at an increased risk of skin deterioration at pressure points. **Pressure points** are areas of the body that bear much of the body's weight. Pressure points are mainly located at bony prominences. **Bony prominences** are areas of the body where the bone lies close to the skin. The skin here is at a much higher risk for skin breakdown. These areas include the elbows, shoulder blades, sacrum (tailbone), hips and knees (inner and outer parts), ankles, heels, toes, and the back of the head. Other areas at risk are the ears, the area under the breasts or scrotum, the area between the folds of the buttocks or abdomen, and skin between the legs (Fig. 12-3). Medical devices such as oxygen tubing or feeding tubes can also cause skin breakdown.

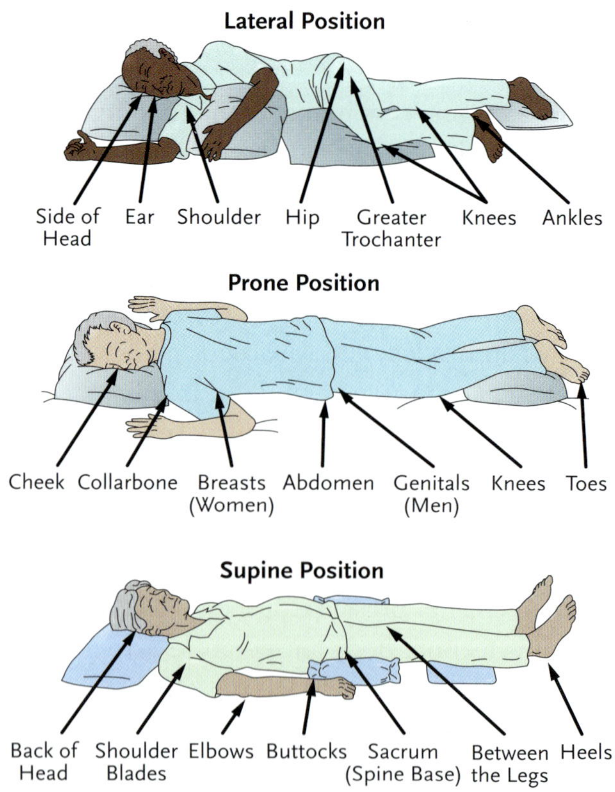

Fig. 12-3. Pressure injury danger zones.

The pressure on these areas reduces circulation, decreasing the amount of oxygen the cells receive. Warmth and moisture also contribute to skin breakdown. Once the surface of the skin has broken down and is weakened, injuries can occur and may become infected, causing damage to the underlying tissue. When infection occurs, the healing process slows down. The injuries or wounds that result from skin deterioration and shearing are called **pressure injuries** (formerly known as *pressure ulcers, pressure sores, decubitus ulcers,* or *bed sores*). Shearing is rubbing or friction resulting from the skin moving one way and the bone underneath it remaining fixed or moving in the opposite direction.

If caught early, a break or tear in the skin can heal fairly quickly without other complications. However, if not caught early, a pressure injury can get bigger, deeper, and infected. Pressure injuries are painful and are difficult to heal. They can lead to life-threatening infections. Hospital-associated pressure injuries (HAPI) are a danger to patients. They are considered a sign of poor care. Serious cases may cause a hospital to be reported to state authorities. Medicare and private insurance may not pay for the patient's care, leaving the hospital to cover the cost. Prevention of these injuries is very important and is the key to skin health. Pressure injuries are categorized by stages, which are as follows (Fig. 12-4):

- **Stage 1**: Skin is intact, but light skin tones may look red, and the redness is not relieved after removing pressure. Dark skin tones may not look red, but may appear to be a different color than the surrounding area. The area may be swollen, painful, firmer, softer, and warmer or cooler when compared to the area around it.
- **Stage 2**: There is partial-thickness skin loss involving the outer and/or inner layers of skin. The injury may be moist and a different color than the surrounding area or pink or red. It may also look like a blister.

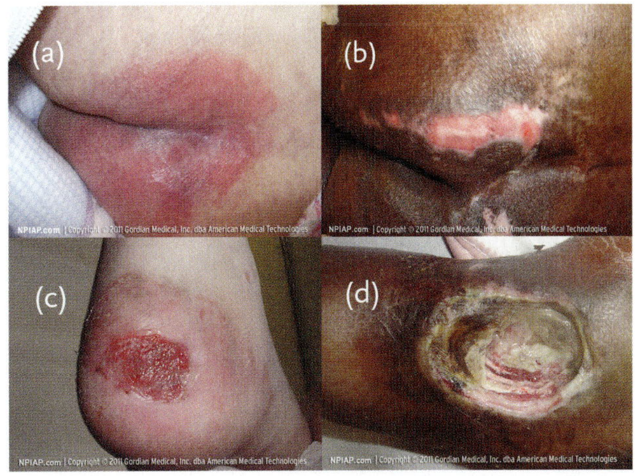

Fig. 12-4. *Pressure injury stages in photos as described by the National Pressure Injury Advisory Panel (NPIAP): (a) Photo of a Stage 1 pressure injury on the buttocks. (b) Photo of a Stage 2 pressure injury on the buttocks. (c) Photo of a Stage 3 pressure injury on the heel. (d) Photo of a Stage 4 pressure injury on the foot.* (ALL PHOTOS ARE REPRINTED WITH PERMISSION OF THE COPYRIGHT HOLDER, GORDIAN MEDICAL, INC. DBA AMERICAN MEDICAL TECHNOLOGIES.)

- **Stage 3**: There is full-thickness skin loss in which fat is visible in the injury. Slough and/or eschar may be present. *Slough* is yellow, tan, gray, green, or brown tissue that is usually moist. *Eschar* is dead tissue that is hard or soft in texture and black, brown, or tan, and may be similar to a scab. The damage may extend down to, but not through, the tissue that covers muscle.
- **Stage 4**: There is full-thickness skin loss extending through all layers of the skin, tissue, muscle, bone, and other structures, such as tendons. The injury will look like a deep crater, and slough and/or eschar may be visible.
- **Unstageable Pressure Injury**: There is full-thickness skin and tissue loss but the extent of the damage cannot be determined because it is covered with slough or eschar. Once the slough and/or eschar is removed, the injury can then be staged (either Stage 3 or Stage 4).
- **Deep Tissue Pressure Injury**: The skin area is intact or nonintact and in light skin tones is deep red, purple, or maroon. In dark skin tones, the skin may appear to be a different

color than the surrounding area. The wound may appear as a blood-filled blister. The area may be painful and may be warmer or cooler than the surrounding tissue.

Breaks in the skin can cause serious, even life-threatening, complications. It is much better to prevent skin problems and keep the skin healthy than to treat skin problems after they occur.

Guidelines: Basic Skin Care

- **G** Report any changes you observe in a patient's skin. When documenting changes, use the terms *left* or *right* in reference to the left or right side of the patient's body (not your own left or right).
- **G** Provide regular, daily care for skin to keep it clean and dry. Check the skin daily, even when complete baths are not given or taken every day.
- **G** Reposition immobile patients often (at least every 2 hours).
- **G** Give frequent, thorough skin care as often as needed for patients who are incontinent. Change clothing and linens often as well. Check on patients at least every 2 hours.
- **G** Massage the skin as ordered. Use light, circular strokes to increase circulation. Use little or no pressure on bony areas. Do not massage a white, red, or purple area or put any pressure on it. Massage the healthy skin and tissue around the area.
- **G** Elderly patients may have very fragile, thin skin. This makes the skin more susceptible to injury. Be gentle during transfers. Avoid pulling or tearing fragile skin.
- **G** Patients who are overweight may have poor circulation and extra folds of skin. The skin under the folds may be difficult to clean and to keep dry. Pay careful attention to these areas and give regular skin care. Report signs of skin irritation.
- **G** Encourage patients to eat well-balanced meals. Proper nutrition is important for keeping skin healthy. Nutrition affects the color and texture of the skin. Very thin patients may be malnourished, which puts them at risk for skin injuries and poor wound healing. Be gentle when moving and positioning them.
- **G** Keep plastic or rubber materials from coming into contact with the patient's skin. These materials prevent air from circulating, which causes the skin to sweat.
- **G** Use barrier creams as ordered for patients who are incontinent. Barrier creams are applied to the perineal area to protect the skin from contact with urine.
- **G** The care plan may include instructions on giving special skin care for dry, closed wounds or other conditions. The skin may have to be washed with a special soap or a brush may have to be used on the skin. Follow the care plan and nurse's instructions.

Here are guidelines for patients who are immobile or who cannot change positions easily:

- **G** Keep the bottom sheet tight and free from wrinkles. Keep the bed free from crumbs. Keep clothing or gowns free of wrinkles, too.
- **G** Do not pull the patient across sheets during transfers or repositioning. This causes shearing, which can lead to skin breakdown.
- **G** Place an absorbent bed pad under the back and buttocks to absorb moisture or perspiration that may build up. This also protects the skin from irritating bed linens. Absorbent pads are also available for wheelchairs.
- **G** Relieve pressure under bony prominences. Use pillows and other positioning devices to keep elbows and heels from resting on the surface of the bed (Fig. 12-5).

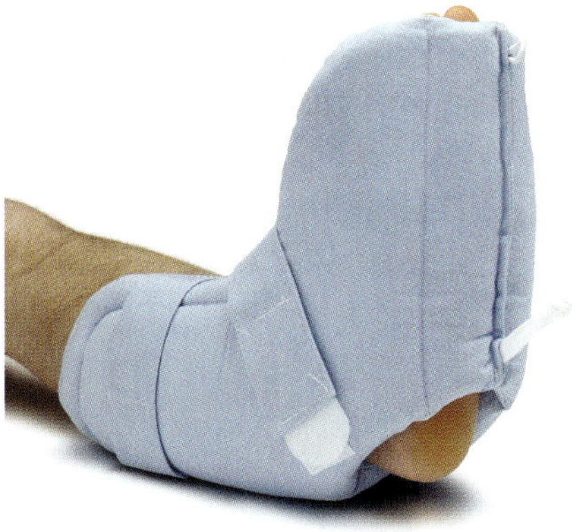

Fig. 12-5. This heel protector raises the heel to help reduce pressure. (IMAGE COURTESY OF MEDLINE INDUSTRIES, LP. USED WITH PERMISSION.)

- **G** Special mattresses such as an alternating pressure or low air loss mattress may be used to help prevent pressure injuries.
- **G** A bed or chair can be made softer with flotation cushions or special foam overlays.
- **G** Use a bed cradle to keep top sheets from rubbing the patient's skin.
- **G** Patients seated in chairs or wheelchairs need to be repositioned often. Reposition patients at least every hour if they are in a wheelchair or chair and cannot change positions easily.

Applying Nonprescription Ointments, Lotions, or Powders

If allowed and instructed to do so, a PCT may apply ointments, lotions, or powders to a patient's skin (Fig. 12-6). The PCT should follow these rules and ask questions if anything is unclear:

- Read the directions.
- Know exactly where it is to be applied.
- Know if it should be rubbed in or left on the top of the skin.
- Wash her hands before and after application.
- Wear gloves.
- Avoid getting any on the patient's gown or bedding or on the PCT's uniform, as it may stain.

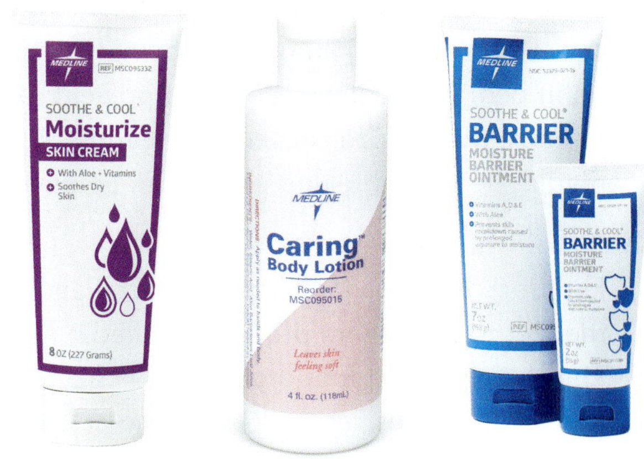

Fig. 12-6. There are many types of ointments, creams, and lotions that are used to treat, soften, and protect the skin. (IMAGES COURTESY OF MEDLINE INDUSTRIES, LP. USED WITH PERMISSION.)

Many positioning devices are available to help make patients safer and more comfortable.

Guidelines: Positioning Devices

- **G** Backrests provide support and comfort for the back. They can be regular pillows or special wedge-shaped foam pillows.
- **G** Bed cradles or foot cradles are used to keep the bed covers from resting on patients' legs and feet (Fig. 12-7). Sometimes even the light pressure of a sheet draped over the toes can eventually lead to pressure injuries.

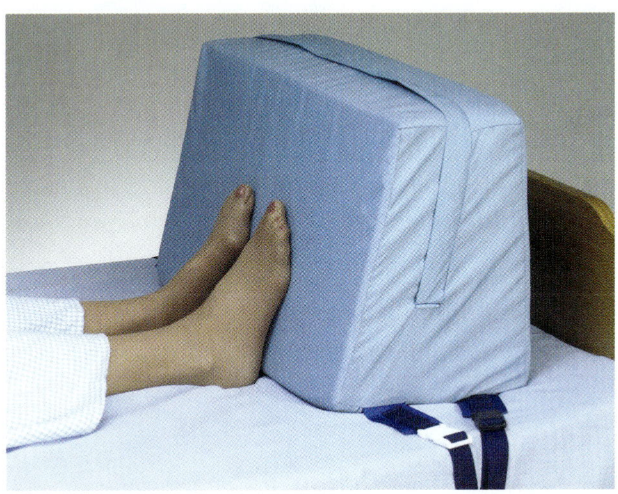

Fig. 12-7. This is one type of bed-foot support that helps prevent bed covers from resting on the legs and feet. (PHOTO COURTESY OF SKIL-CARE CORPORATION, WWW.SKIL-CARE.COM)

- **G** Draw sheets may be placed under patients to assist with turning, lifting, or moving patients up in bed. Draw sheets also help prevent skin damage that can be caused by shearing. A regular bed sheet folded in half can be used as a draw sheet.
- **G** Footboards are padded boards placed against the feet to keep them properly aligned. They help prevent foot drop. **Foot drop** is a weakness of muscles in the feet and ankles that causes difficulty with the ability to flex the ankles and walk normally. Foot splints may also be used to help prevent foot drop. Footboards are also used to keep bed covers off the feet. Rolled blankets or pillows can also be used as footboards.
- **G** Handrolls are cloth-covered or rubber items that keep the hand and/or fingers in a normal, natural position (Fig. 12-8). A rolled washcloth, gauze bandage, or a rubber cone placed inside the palm may be used to keep the hand in a natural position. Handrolls can help prevent finger, hand, or wrist contractures.

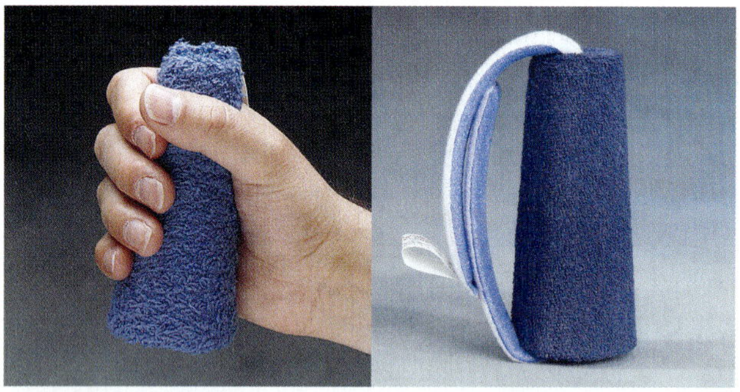

Fig. 12-8. *Handrolls keep the fingers and hand in a natural position, helping to prevent contractures.* (PHOTOS COURTESY OF NORTH COAST MEDICAL, INC., WWW.NCMEDICAL.COM)

- **G** Trochanter rolls are rolled towels or blankets used to keep a patient's hips and legs from turning outward (Fig. 12-9).

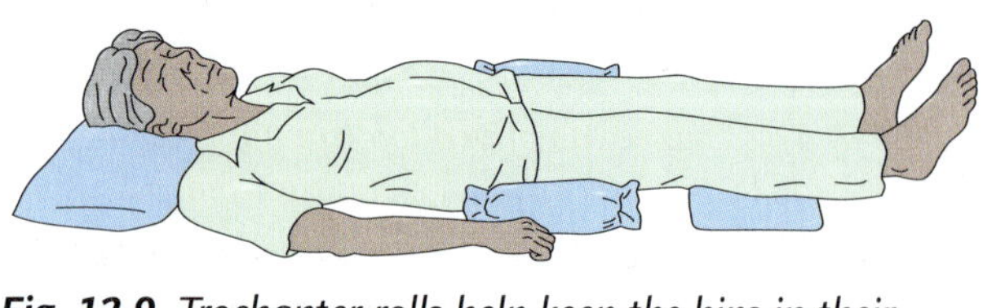

Fig. 12-9. *Trochanter rolls help keep the hips in their proper position.*

- **G** Abduction pillows/wedges/splints/pads or hip wedges keep hips in the proper position after hip surgery. Pillows between the legs from knees to ankles, while in the lateral position, can help keep the spine, hips, and knees in the proper position.

Scabies

Scabies is a skin infection caused by a mite called *Sarcoptes scabiei*. The mite burrows under the outer layer of the skin, where it lays eggs, which causes intense itching and a skin rash that may look like thin burrow tracks. These tracks typically appear in the folds of the skin.

Scabies is contagious and is spread through direct contact with an infected person. It can spread quickly in crowded places, such as hospitals, long-term care facilities, and childcare facilities. Treatment of scabies involves medications, often in the form of prescription creams and lotions. Oral medications may be used if the person does not respond to the creams and/or lotions. Contact Precautions should be in place for patients with scabies.

Shingles

Shingles, also called *herpes zoster*, is a rash caused by the varicella-zoster virus (VZV), which is the same virus that causes chickenpox. (Herpes zoster is not the same virus that causes the sexually transmitted infection.) Any person who has had chickenpox is at risk for developing shingles. After having chickenpox, the virus remains in the body, where it usually does not cause problems. However, it can reappear later in life and cause shingles.

Initial signs and symptoms of shingles include pain, tingling, or itching in an area, which later develops into a rash of fluid-filled blisters that is similar to chickenpox (Fig. 12-10). The rash usually goes away within 2 to 4 weeks.

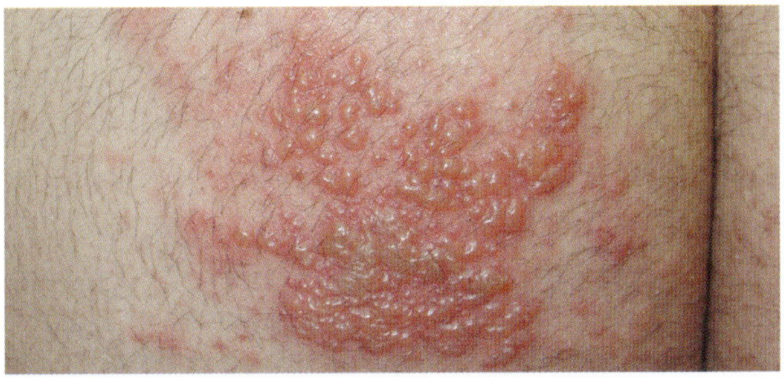

Fig. 12-10. Shingles in blister form. (PHOTO COURTESY OF DR. JERE MAMMINO, DO)

Shingles cannot be transmitted to other people. However, if a person has never had chickenpox, he may acquire chickenpox from a person who has active shingles (when the rash is in the blister phase). The risk of getting shingles increases as a person ages. People with immune systems weakened by diseases such as cancer and HIV are at greater risk of getting shingles.

Keeping the rash covered, especially while it is in blister form, is important. Infected people should wash their hands often and should not scratch or touch the rash. Contact Precautions and, in some cases, Airborne Precautions, should be in place.

Shingles is treated with medication, which should be started as soon as possible. Starting medication immediately can help reduce the severity of the disease and can shorten the length of the illness. There is a vaccine for shingles that is recommended for all people 50 years or older. The vaccine can help reduce the risk of contracting shingles.

Fungal Infections

A **fungus** (plural fungi) is a type of living organism. Mushrooms, mold, and yeasts (Candida) are all examples of fungi. Some types of fungi normally live in and on the body, in such places as the skin, the vagina, and the intestines. However, sometimes normal balances of fungi can change, resulting in fungal infections.

Fungal infections of the skin can occur when moisture is trapped on the skin. They can also be caused by certain medications. Fungi that do not cause infection in healthy people may be very dangerous to people whose immune systems are compromised.

Fungi can be difficult to kill. Treatment generally consists of applying antifungal agents directly on the area of the body where the infection is located. Medication may also need to be taken orally or injected if the infection is more serious.

Cellulitis

Cellulitis is a common condition that affects the skin and soft tissue. It can develop when sores, cuts, or open wounds let bacteria through the skin. Bacteria may also enter through hair follicles. The 2 bacteria most likely to cause cellulitis are streptococci and staphylococci. MRSA can cause cellulitis. It is especially hard to treat.

Signs of cellulitis are skin discoloration, swelling, and warmth (Fig. 12-11). PCTs should report any new swelling or discoloration they see during care. Cellulitis can also cause fever and **malaise**, or a general sense of feeling unwell. Pressure injuries, obesity, and other skin conditions put a person at a higher risk for cellulitis. Diabetes is also a risk factor. Oral or injected (IV or intramuscular) antibiotics are used to treat cellulitis.

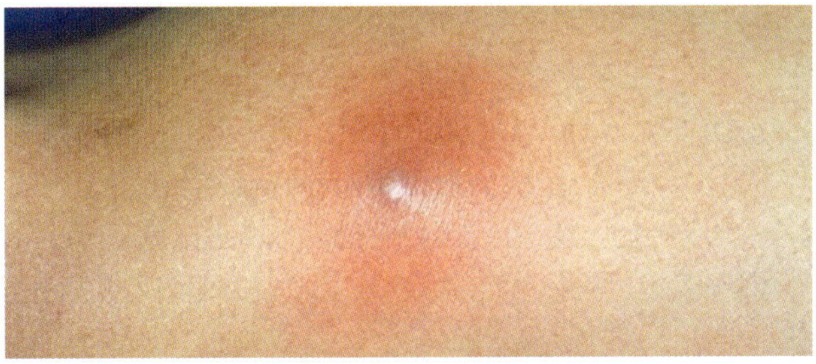

Fig. 12-11. Signs of cellulitis include skin redness, swelling, and warmth. (PHOTO COURTESY OF DR. JERE MAMMINO, DO)

Wounds

A **wound** is a type of injury to the skin. Wounds are classified as either *closed* or *open*. In a closed wound, the skin's surface has not been broken. Closed wounds can be contusions (bruises) or hematomas. A contusion is caused by blunt force trauma that damages tissue under the skin (Fig. 12-12). A hematoma is caused by damage to a blood vessel that causes blood to collect under the skin.

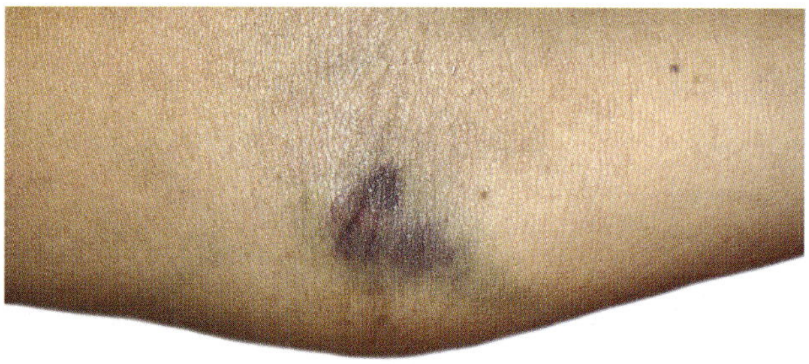

Fig. 12-12. A contusion/bruise appears on the skin due to blunt force trauma.

An open wound has skin that is not intact. An open wound can be categorized in the following ways: incision, laceration, abrasion, and puncture wound.

- An incision is caused by a sharp-edged object, such as a knife or razor. An example of this type of open wound is a cut made during surgery with a surgical instrument. This type of wound may also be seen in the emergency department (ED) as a result of violence or accidental injury.
- A laceration is an irregular wound caused by ripping or blunt trauma, such as tearing of skin during childbirth.
- An abrasion is a wound in which the top layer of skin is scraped or worn off, often by coming into moving contact with a rough surface.
- A puncture wound is a break in the skin caused by a sharp object, such as a nail or a needle.

Damage caused by trauma, such as gunshot wounds and wounds from accidents, is often seen in the ED. It usually involves several types of open and closed wounds.

Open wounds are examined and cleaned with various liquids, such as saline or antiseptic solution. Bleeding may need to be stopped. Any foreign objects or materials must be removed. Dressings, bandages, sutures, staples, or special strips or glue may need to be applied. Transparent dressings are sometimes used to improve visibility of the wound. Doctors or other licensed healthcare providers perform this care.

Several factors can affect wound healing. Some conditions, such as diabetes or poor circulation, can slow or prevent healing. Proper nutrition speeds healing. So does a good supply of blood and oxygen to the tissue around the wound. Wound infection is a serious concern, especially as the risk of multidrug-resistant organisms (MDROs) continues to increase. Infection prevents healing and can also become systemic (affecting the whole body).

As wounds heal, it is normal for them to leak fluid. Wound drainage is often absorbed by dressings. If there is a large amount of drainage, different systems (vacuum or pump-based) may be used to remove the fluid. This fluid must be included in a patient's I&O measurements. Changes in wound drainage are a sign of possible infection. PCTs should know the difference between normal and abnormal wound drainage. There are 4 types of wound drainage:

- **Sanguineous drainage** is bright red blood from a new cut. It is part of the normal process of wound healing, but it should not continue for very long. If a wound that had stopped bleeding shows this type of drainage, it should be reported right away.
- **Serous drainage** is yellow or transparent. It contains white blood cells and is also part of the normal healing process, especially in the first 2–3 days. An increase in this type of drainage should be reported.
- **Serosanguineous drainage** is pink drainage that is similar to serous drainage but contains some red blood cells. It is often

part of normal healing, but any changes or increase in this type of drainage should be reported right away.

- **Purulent drainage** (pus) is yellow, green, brown, or white drainage that may have an odor. It may appear milky or thick. It is not part of the normal healing process. This type of drainage usually contains bacteria and should be reported right away.

Infected wounds and wounds that are not healing properly must be treated carefully. A provider will remove infected or necrotic (dead) tissue in a process called **debridement**. This may be done surgically or with medications called debriding agents. Oral or injected (IV or intramuscular) antibiotics are used to treat the infection.

When observing wounds, PCTs should be sensitive to a patient's comfort and dignity. The patient may be embarrassed to have others see the wound or the area around it. PCTs must always behave professionally. They should not show discomfort, even if they are bothered by the appearance of the wound.

Observing and Reporting: Wounds

Signs and symptoms that should be reported to the nurse include the following:

- O/R Odors from the wound site
- O/R Increased pain
- O/R Discoloration or swelling around the wound
- O/R Change in the color, amount, or type of wound drainage
- O/R Wound dressing that is soiled or wet
- O/R Signs of cellulitis in the tissue around the wound
- O/R Fever, chills, fatigue, and malaise, which may mean the infection has become systemic

Burns

Chapter 6 has basic information about burns and first aid for minor burns. Patients who are hospitalized with burns may have been injured in a fire, explosion, or chemical accident. They may have been in a car or motorcycle accident. Care for severe burns is complex, and many situations that cause severe burns can cause other injuries that must be treated as well. Many body systems are affected.

PCTs must follow any instructions they are given for care. They should always report pain, change in consciousness, and change in appearance of the burns or any drainage from wounds immediately.

Psoriasis

Psoriasis is a condition that causes the body to create too many skin cells. These extra cells die and build up, causing white or red scaly patches that may be very itchy and painful. Common sites are the scalp, knees, elbows, and trunk. Psoriasis is an autoimmune condition. This means that it involves the body attacking itself. Psoriasis is treated with anti-inflammatory medications and topical creams such as hydrocortisone. Severe cases may be treated with light therapy (phototherapy) and medications that suppress the immune system.

Cancer

Cancer is a general term to describe a disease in which abnormal cells grow in an uncontrolled way. Skin cancer is one of the most common forms of cancer in the United States. It develops when abnormal cells in the epidermis grow rapidly and form lesions on the skin. Sun exposure is the primary cause. There are 3 types of skin cancer: basal cell carcinoma, squamous cell carcinoma, and malignant melanoma, which is the most dangerous type. This form of skin cancer is very aggressive and can spread quickly to surrounding tissues and organs. Cancer treatment is discussed in Chapter 21.

4. Discuss sterile and nonsterile dressings

Sterile dressings cover new, open, or draining wounds. They help protect from infection and injury. Preassembled kits contain all of the items needed to apply a sterile dressing. This includes sterile gloves, antiseptic wipes, sterile gauze pads, and tape. Nurses or other licensed healthcare providers change these dressings, but PCTs may assist. The procedure for performing a sterile hand scrub and guidelines for setting up a sterile field are in Chapter 10. These steps must be followed before assisting to apply or change a sterile dressing.

PCTs may be assigned to gather and store equipment and supplies and observe and report about a sterile dressing site. They may be assigned to clean the equipment. (Chapter 10 includes more information about sterile technique.) Duties may also include properly positioning the patient, cutting the tape, and disposing of the soiled dressing. Supplies that may be needed for sterile dressings include the following:

- Special gauze has one side with a shiny, nonstick surface, which will not stick to wounds when removed.
- Abdominal pads (ABDs) are large, heavy gauze dressings that cover smaller gauze dressings and help keep them in place and provide absorbency.
- Cotton bandages (sometimes called *Kerlix* or *Kling* bandages) can stretch and mold to a body part and help hold it in place; these are often used on bony areas, such as the knees and elbows.
- Binders are stretchable pieces of fabric that can be fastened. They hold dressings in place and give support to surgical wounds. Binders can also reduce swelling and ease discomfort.
- Medical-grade adhesive tape panels (sometimes called *Montgomery Straps*) help keep frequently changed dressings in place. The adhesive is not removed with each dressing change so that the skin is less likely to become irritated.

Nonsterile dressings are applied to dry, closed wounds that have less chance of infection. PCTs may change nonsterile dressings.

Changing a dry dressing using nonsterile technique

Equipment: package of square gauze dressings, adhesive tape, scissors, 2 pairs of gloves, plastic bag

1. Identify yourself by name. Identify the patient according to facility policy.
2. Wash your hands.
3. Explain the procedure to the patient. Speak clearly, slowly, and directly. Maintain face-to-face contact whenever possible.
4. Provide for the patient's privacy with a curtain, screen, or door.
5. Open the gauze package without touching the gauze. Place the opened package on a flat surface.
6. Put on gloves.
7. Remove the soiled dressing by gently peeling the tape toward the wound. Lift the dressing off the wound, angling it so that the patient cannot see the soiled side. Do not drag it over the wound. Observe the dressing for odor or drainage. Notice the color and size of the wound. Discard the used dressing in the plastic bag.
8. Remove and discard your gloves in the plastic bag. Wash your hands.

9. Put on clean gloves. Touching only the outer edges of the new gauze, remove it from the package. Apply it to the wound. Tape the gauze in place. Secure it firmly (Fig. 12-13). Follow facility policy to record the time and date of the change on the dressing. Many facilities use stickers that are applied to the dressing. Some may note the time and date on the dressing tape. This should be done before it is applied to the patient.

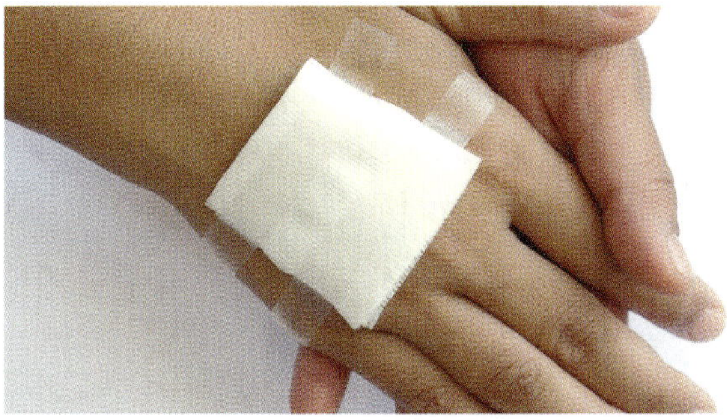

Fig. 12-13. *Tape gauze in place to secure the dressing. Do not completely cover all areas of the dressing with tape.*

10. Discard supplies in the proper container.
11. Remove and discard your gloves. Wash your hands.
12. Make the patient comfortable. Remove privacy measures.
13. Place the call light within the patient's reach.
14. Report any changes in the patient to the nurse.
15. Document the procedure using facility guidelines.

Chapter Review

1. What is homeostasis?
2. What direction does the word *medial* indicate?
3. What are 3 functions of the skin, or integument?
4. What are the common terms for objective and subjective changes in metabolic processes?
5. Why is preventing pressure injuries extremely important?
6. At a minimum, how often should patients who are immobile or have very limited mobility be repositioned?
7. List 4 examples of positioning devices and explain how they can help.
8. What are signs and symptoms of scabies? How is scabies spread?
9. What causes shingles?
10. What is an open wound? List 4 examples of open wounds.
11. What is a closed wound? Give 1 example.
12. What are signs that a wound infection may be systemic and should be reported immediately?
13. What are the 3 types of skin cancer? Which type is the most dangerous?
14. When are nonsterile dressings usually used?
15. What duties might a PCT have regarding the application of sterile dressings?

13 The Musculoskeletal System and Related Care

1. Describe the structure and function of the musculoskeletal system

Muscles, bones, ligaments, tendons, and cartilage give the body shape and structure. They work together to move the body. The skeleton, or framework, of the human body has 206 bones (Fig. 13-1). In addition to allowing the body to move, **bones** also protect organs. For example, the skull protects the brain and the vertebrae protect the spinal cord. Bones are hard and rigid, but are made up of living cells. Blood vessels supply oxygen and nutrients to the bones as well as to other tissues of the body.

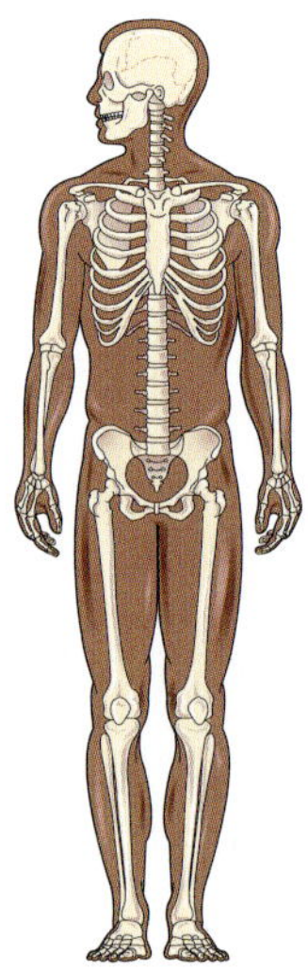

Fig. 13-1. *The skeleton is composed of 206 bones that aid movement and protect organs.*

Two bones meet at a **joint**. Some joints, such as the ball-and-socket joint, make movement possible in all directions. This joint is a type of synovial joint. In this joint, the round end of one bone fits into the hollow end of the other bone, which allows it to move in all directions. The hip and shoulder joints are examples.

Other joints permit movement in one direction only. The hinge joint is another example of a synovial joint. Like the hinge of a door, a hinge joint permits movement in one direction only. The elbow and knee are hinge joints. They bend in one direction only (Fig. 13-2).

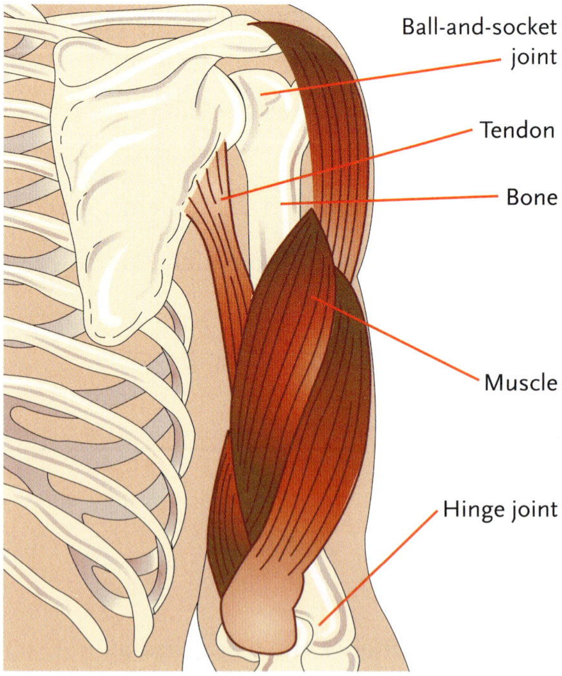

Fig. 13-2. *Muscles are connected to bones by tendons. Bones meet at different types of joints. The ball-and-socket joint and the hinge joint are shown here.*

Muscles provide movement of body parts to maintain posture and to produce heat. Muscles can be voluntary or involuntary. Voluntary muscles are also called skeletal muscles. They are attached to bones and can be moved when a person wants them to move. Examples of voluntary muscles are the arm and leg muscles, which are consciously controlled. Involuntary muscles cannot be consciously controlled. They automatically regulate the movement of organs and blood vessels. An example of an involuntary muscle is the heart.

Exercise is important for improving and maintaining physical and mental health. Inactivity and immobility can result in a loss of self-esteem, depression, pneumonia, and urinary tract infections. They can also lead to constipation, blood clots, dulling of the senses, and muscle atrophy or contractures. When **atrophy** occurs, the muscle wastes away, decreases in size, and becomes weak. When a **contracture** develops, the muscle or tendon shortens, becomes inflexible, and "freezes" in position. This causes permanent disability of the limb.

Range of motion (ROM) exercises can help prevent these conditions. With these exercises, the joints are extended and flexed in the measured degrees of a circle. Exercise increases circulation of blood, oxygen, and nutrients and improves muscle tone. There is more information about range of motion exercises later in this chapter.

The functions of the musculoskeletal system are to give the body shape and structure, to allow the body to move, to protect body organs, to maintain posture, and to produce heat.

Observing and Reporting: Musculoskeletal System

Observe and report these signs and symptoms:

- O/R Changes in ability to move or ambulate or to do routine activities
- O/R Changes in ability to perform range of motion exercises
- O/R Pain during movement
- O/R Loss of strength
- O/R Unsteadiness or loss of balance
- O/R Falls
- O/R New or increased swelling of joints
- O/R White, shiny, discolored, or warm areas over a joint
- O/R Bruising
- O/R Aches and pains reported

2. List common conditions of the musculoskeletal system and discuss related care

Arthritis

Arthritis is a general term that refers to inflammation, or swelling, of the joints. It causes stiffness, pain, and decreased mobility. Arthritis may be the result of aging, injury, or an **autoimmune illness**. An autoimmune illness causes the body's immune system to attack normal tissue in the body. Two common types of arthritis are osteoarthritis and rheumatoid arthritis.

Osteoarthritis, also called *degenerative arthritis* or *degenerative joint disease* (*DJD*), is a common type of arthritis that affects the elderly. It may occur with aging or as the result of joint injury. Hips and knees, which are weight-bearing joints, are usually affected. Joints in the fingers, thumbs, and spine can also be affected. Pain and stiffness seem to increase in cold, damp weather.

Rheumatoid arthritis (**RA**) can affect people of any age. Joints become red, swollen, and very painful (Fig. 13-3). Deformities can result and may be severe and disabling. Movement is eventually restricted. Fever, fatigue, and weight loss are also symptoms. Rheumatoid arthritis usually affects the smaller joints first, then progresses to larger ones. Other parts of the body that may be affected are the heart, lungs, eyes, kidneys, and skin. Rheumatoid arthritis is considered an autoimmune disease.

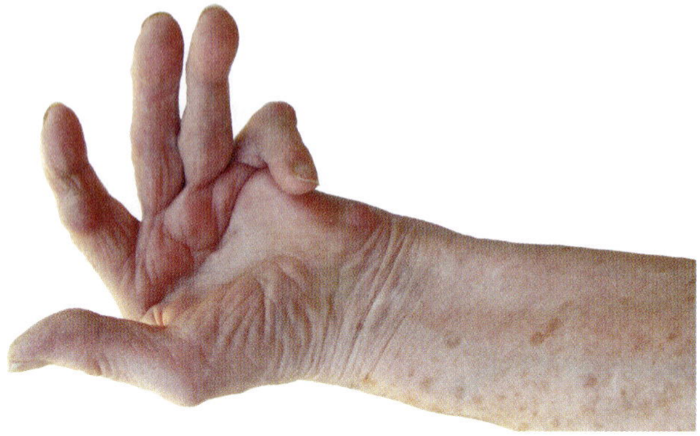

Fig. 13-3. Rheumatoid arthritis.

Arthritis is generally treated with the following:

- Anti-inflammatory medication such as aspirin or ibuprofen, as well as other medication
- Local applications of heat to reduce swelling and pain
- Range of motion exercises (later in this chapter)
- Regular exercise and/or activity routine
- Diet to reduce weight or maintain strength

Patients with arthritis should be encouraged to use handrails and safety bars in the bathroom. They may need assistive devices for bathing, dressing, or eating (Fig. 13-4). Occupational therapists (OTs) decide if patients need devices like this. PCTs should report to the nurse if a patient is having a difficult time with activities of daily living.

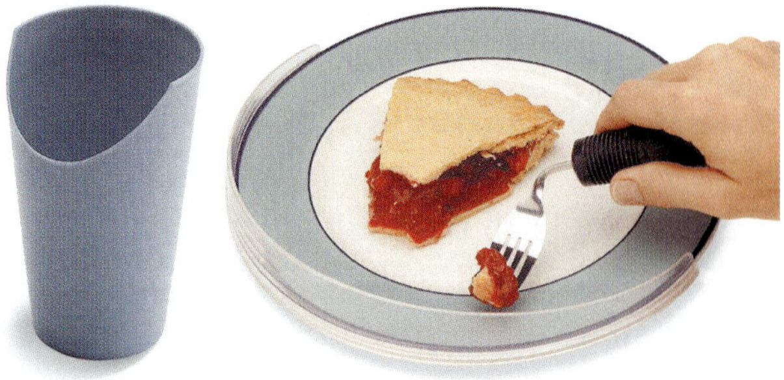

Fig. 13-4. Special equipment, such as this plate, fork, and cup, can help a person with arthritis remain independent. (PHOTOS COURTESY OF NORTH COAST MEDICAL, INC., WWW.NCMEDICAL.COM)

Osteoporosis

Osteoporosis is a condition in which bones lose density, which causes them to become porous and brittle. Brittle bones can break easily. Osteoporosis may be caused by a lack of calcium in the diet, a loss of estrogen after menopause, a lack of exercise, reduced mobility, or age. Low back pain, stooped posture, becoming shorter over time, and fractures are signs and symptoms of osteoporosis.

PCTs should encourage patients to walk and do other light exercise as ordered. Exercise can strengthen bones as well as muscles. PCTs must move patients with osteoporosis very carefully. They may fall more easily than other patients, and falls can cause more severe injury. Medication and supplements are also used to treat osteoporosis.

Imaging Tests

Imaging and other tests are valuable tools for diagnosing many diseases and conditions. Here are some common tests:

An *ultrasound* uses sound waves to produce images of the body's organs, tissues, and other structures.

An *X-ray* produces images of the body's structures using a type of radiation called electromagnetic waves.

A *computerized tomography (CT) scan* produces horizontal (cross-section) images of the body. These images are much more detailed than traditional X-rays.

Magnetic resonance imaging (MRI) uses magnets and radio waves to produce detailed images of the body.

A *positron emission tomography (PET)* scan uses a radioactive substance injected into a patient's vein to view body organs and tissues.

Fractures

A fracture is a broken bone caused by an accident or by osteoporosis. A **closed fracture** is a broken bone that does not break the skin. An **open fracture**, also known as a *compound* *fracture,* is a broken bone that penetrates the skin. An open fracture carries a high risk of infection and usually requires immediate surgery.

Preventing falls, which can lead to fractures, is very important. Fractures of arms, wrists, elbows, legs, and hips are the most common. Signs and symptoms of a fracture are pain, swelling, bruising, changes in skin color at the site, and limited movement.

When bones are fractured, the sections of broken bone must be placed back into alignment so the body can heal. The body can grow new bone tissue and fuse the sections of fractured bone together. The bone must be unable to move to allow this healing to occur. This is often, although not always, accomplished by the use of a cast.

Casts are generally made of fiberglass. A fiberglass cast is lightweight and dries quickly after it is made. A cast must be completely dry before a person can bear weight on it.

Pain management is important for patients with fractured bones. Medication therapy to improve bone strength starts after the bone is set properly for healing. Supplements may be used as well. Surgery is needed to treat some fractures.

Guidelines: Cast Care

- **G** The extremity in a cast is usually elevated. This helps stop swelling (Fig. 13-5). Follow instructions for positioning and assisting the patient with mobility.

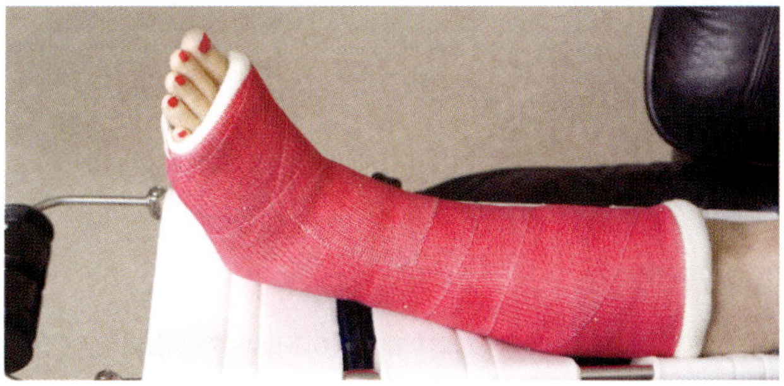

Fig. 13-5. *Elevating the extremity can help stop swelling.*

- **G** Observe the affected extremity for swelling, skin discoloration, cast tightness or pressure, sores, skin that feels hot or cold, pain, burning, numbness or tingling, drainage, bleeding, or odor. Compare to the extremity that does not have a cast. Report any of these signs or symptoms to the nurse, along with any signs of infection, such as fever or chills.
- **G** Protect the patient's skin from the rough edges of the cast. The stocking that lines the inside of the cast can be pulled up and over the edges and secured with tape. Tell the nurse if cast edges irritate the patient's skin.
- **G** Keep the cast dry at all times. Although fiberglass is waterproof, the padding inside the cast is not. Some fiberglass casts may have a waterproof lining, but unless instructed otherwise, keep the cast dry. Keep the cast clean. If you are assigned to assist a patient with bathing, a waterproof cover may be used to keep the cast dry (Fig. 13-6).

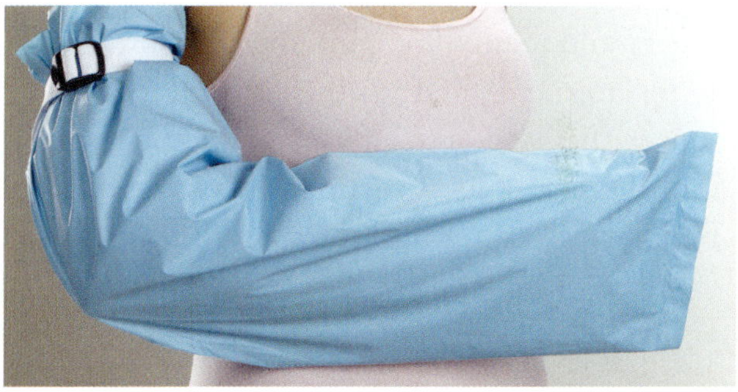

Fig. 13-6. *Cast covers can make it easier to assist with bathing for patients with fractures.* (IMAGE COURTESY OF ENCOMPASS GROUP, LLC)

- **G** Do not insert or allow the patient to insert anything inside the cast, even when the skin itches. Pointed or blunt objects may injure the skin, which is already dry and fragile. Skin can become infected under the cast.
- **G** Tell the nurse prior to moving the patient or before the patient exercises if pain medication is needed. Help with range of motion exercises as ordered. Allow plenty of time for movement. Assist the patient with a cane, walker, or crutches as needed.

G Use bed cradles as assigned to reduce pressure from bed linens.

Hip Fractures

Weakened bones make hip fractures more common. A sudden fall can result in a fractured hip that takes months to heal. Preventing falls is very important. Hip fractures can also occur because of weakened bones that fracture and then cause a fall. A hip fracture is a serious condition. For an elderly person, the healing process takes longer, and they are at risk for secondary illnesses and disabilities.

Most fractured hips require surgery. The type of hip replacement surgery performed is determined by various factors, such as the person's age, weight, and fitness level. One type is a minimally invasive hip replacement. This surgery generally results in a shorter hospital stay, a faster recovery time, and less pain for the patient. There is also lower risk of muscle damage; however, some people are not candidates for this surgery and require total hip replacement. Total hip replacement (THR) is the surgical replacement of the head of the long bone of the leg (femur) where it joins the hip. This surgery is often performed for the following reasons:

- Fractured hip from an injury or fall that does not heal properly
- Weakened hip due to aging
- Hip is painful and stiff because the joint is weak and the bones are no longer strong enough to bear the person's weight

After surgery, the person may not be able to bear full weight on that leg while the hip heals. A physical therapist will assist after surgery. The goals of care include surgical incision healing, slowly strengthening the hip muscles, mobility and gait improvement, and increased endurance.

The patient's care plan will state when the patient may begin putting weight on the leg. It will also give instructions on how much the patient is able to do. It is important for PCTs to help with personal care and using assistive devices, such as walkers or canes.

Guidelines: Hip Replacement

G Keep often used items, such as medications, phone, tissues, call lights, and water, within reach. Avoid placing items in high places.

G Dress the affected (weaker) side first.

G Never rush the patient. Use praise and encouragement often, even for small tasks.

G The nurse may give pain medication prior to moving and positioning if needed. Report patient complaints of pain to the nurse.

G After surgery, there may be a provider's order for *non-weight-bearing* (*NWB*), *toe-touch weight-bearing* (*TTWB*)/*touch-down weight-bearing* (*TDWB*), or *partial weight-bearing* (*PWB*). Another possible order is *weight-bearing as tolerated*. Non-weight-bearing means the patient is unable to touch the floor or support any weight on one or both legs. Toe-touch weight-bearing means the foot or the toes may touch the floor but only to maintain balance; no weight should be placed on the toes. Partial weight-bearing means the patient is able to support some body weight on one or both legs. An order for weight-bearing as tolerated allows the patient to bear as much weight as they are able. Help as needed with a cane, walker, or crutches. After recovering from hip replacement surgery a patient will be allowed *full weight-bearing*. This means both legs can bear 100% of the body weight on a step.

G Never perform range of motion exercises on the operative leg unless directed by the nurse.

G Caution the patient not to sit with their legs crossed in bed or in a chair or turn the toes inward or outward (Fig. 13-7). The hip cannot be bent or flexed more than 90 degrees. It also cannot be turned inward or outward.

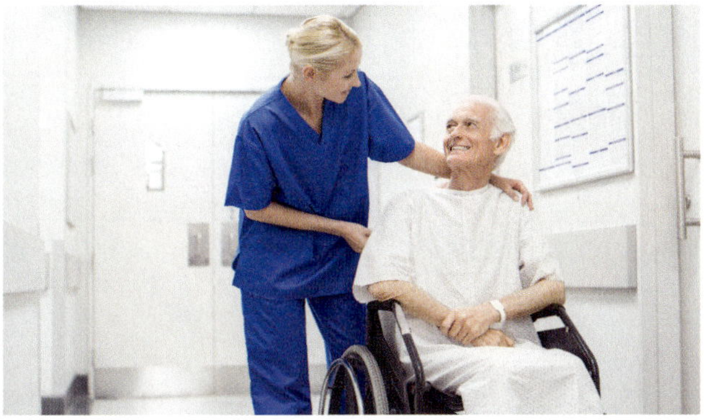

Fig. 13-7. The patient should sit with his legs uncrossed.

- **G** An abduction pillow may be used after surgery while the patient is sleeping. The abduction pillow immobilizes and positions the hips and lower extremities (Fig. 13-8). Follow the nurse's and the care plan's instructions for application and positioning.

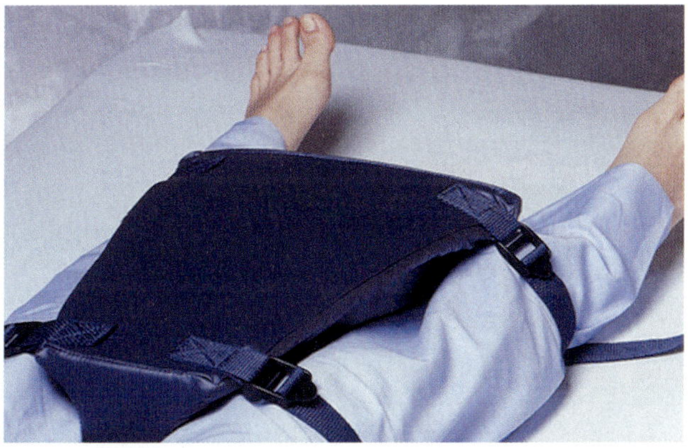

Fig. 13-8. An abduction pillow is placed between the legs to immobilize and position the hips and lower extremities. (IMAGE COURTESY OF MEDLINE INDUSTRIES, LP. USED WITH PERMISSION.)

- **G** When transferring from the bed, use a pillow between the thighs to keep the legs separated. Raise the head of the bed to allow the patient to move their legs over the side of the bed with the thighs still separated. Stand on the side of the unaffected hip so that the strong side leads in standing, pivoting, and sitting.
- **G** With chair or toilet transfers, the operative leg should be straightened. The stronger leg should stand first (with a walker or crutches) before bringing the foot of the affected leg back to the walking position.

Observing and Reporting: Hip Replacement

Report any of these to the nurse:

- O/R Discoloration, drainage, bleeding, or warmth in the incision area
- O/R An increase in pain
- O/R Numbness or tingling
- O/R Tenderness or swelling in the calf of the affected leg
- O/R Shortening and/or external rotation of the affected leg
- O/R Abnormal vital signs, especially a change in temperature
- O/R Any problems with appetite

A cast or traction may also be used to immobilize the hip. Traction helps to immobilize a fractured bone, relieve pressure, and lessen muscle spasms due to injury. A patient in traction will require special care that will be included in the care plan. The traction assembly must never be disconnected, and PCTs should keep the weights off the floor and not add or remove weights. Proper skin care and repositioning are essential for all patients who are immobilized. Skin will rapidly deteriorate over pressure points. Range of motion exercises should be performed as directed. PCTs should report complaints of pain, numbness, tingling, or burning, as well as the presence of swelling, redness, bleeding, or sores.

Trapeze

A trapeze is a triangular piece of equipment that hangs over the head of the bed. It may be mounted to the bed or freestanding. People in bed can grasp the trapeze with their hands, which enables them to lift themselves. The trapeze assists with repositioning and exercise activities.

Knee Replacement

Total knee replacement (TKR) is the surgical replacement of the knee with a prosthetic knee. A **prosthesis** is a device that replaces a body part that is missing or deformed because of an accident, injury, illness, or birth defect. It is used to improve a person's ability to function and/or to improve appearance. Total knee replacement surgery is performed to relieve pain and to restore motion to a knee damaged by injury or arthritis. It can help stabilize a knee that buckles or gives out repeatedly. After the surgery, care is similar to that for a hip replacement, but the recovery time is longer and may be more painful.

Guidelines: Knee Replacement

- **G** To prevent blood clots, apply an SCD or compression stockings as ordered. (Chapter 10 contains more information.)
- **G** Encourage the patient to perform ankle pumps as ordered. These are simple exercises that promote circulation to the legs. Ankle pumps are done by raising the toes and feet toward the ceiling and lowering them again.
- **G** Encourage fluids to prevent urinary tract infections (UTIs).
- **G** Assist with deep breathing exercises as ordered. (Chapter 16 contains more information.)
- **G** A continuous passive motion (CPM) machine may be used after a knee replacement. This machine constantly moves the knee through its normal range of motion (Fig. 13-9). The person does not have to actively help; the machine does the work. Using a CPM machine can help speed recovery. The goal is to decrease stiffness, increase range of motion, and promote healing. The nurse or physical therapist will set the rate and position the patient. You may be asked to stay with the patient while the machine is on.

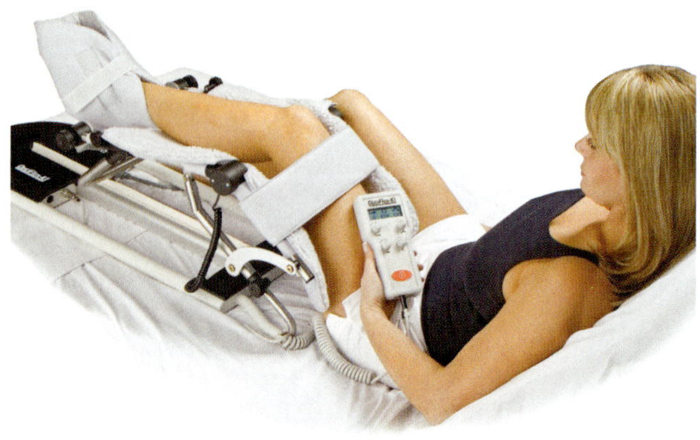

Fig. 13-9. *One type of CPM machine.* (PHOTO COURTESY OF THE MEDCOM GROUP, LTD., 800-231-4276, WWW.MEDCOMGROUP.COM)

- **G** Ask the nurse to give pain medication prior to moving and positioning if needed.
- **G** Report to the nurse if you notice discoloration, swelling, heat, or deep tenderness in one or both calves. Other symptoms to report are chest pain, shortness of breath, and anxiety.

Muscular Dystrophy (MD)

Muscular dystrophy (**MD**) refers to a number of progressive diseases that cause a variety of physical disabilities due to muscle weakness. Progressive means the disease gets worse with time. MD is an inherited disease; it causes a gradual wasting away of muscle, weakness, and deformity. The muscles of the hands are impaired, and there may be twitching of the hand and arm muscles. Legs may be weak and stiff. The person may be in a wheelchair.

Most forms of MD are present at birth or become apparent during childhood. Many forms of MD are very slow to progress. Often people with MD can live to middle or even late adulthood.

Treatment of MD includes medications, physical and occupational therapy, and surgery. Regular monitoring is important.

Amyotrophic Lateral Sclerosis (ALS)

Amyotrophic lateral sclerosis, or **ALS**, often called *Lou Gehrig's disease,* is a progressive disease that causes muscle atrophy (weakening or wasting away) and eventually leads to death. A person may be diagnosed with ALS at any age. The average time a person lives with this disease is between 2 and 5 years, though some people can live longer. Physical disabilities may begin with muscle weakness in the limbs or throat. Because ALS is progressive, disabilities get worse. Eventually, people who have this disease may have to breathe and be fed with the assistance of ventilators and tubes.

Treatment of ALS includes medications; physical, occupational, speech, and respiratory therapy; and nutritional support. PCTs caring for patients who have MD or ALS may assist with range of motion exercises. They need to observe carefully for swallowing problems and report them to the nurse. PCTs may need to assist with skin care and positioning and perform ADLs for patients in more advanced stages.

Amputation

Amputation is the surgical removal of some or all of a body part, usually an arm, hand, leg, or foot. Amputation may be the result of an injury or disease. After amputation, some people feel that the amputated limb is still there, or they feel pain in the part that has been amputated. **Phantom sensation** is the term used when a person feels that the body part is still there. The person may experience warmth, tingling, or itching in the area where the limb existed. **Phantom limb pain** occurs when the person feels pain in a limb (or extremity) that has been amputated. It may persist for a short time or for several years. The pain or sensation, which has various possible causes, including remaining damaged nerve endings, is real. It should not be ignored. Medication and physical therapy may be used to treat these conditions.

Guidelines: Amputation

- **G** Patients who have had a body part amputated must make many physical, psychological, social, and occupational adjustments due to their disability. Be supportive.
- **G** Assist patients in performing their ADLs as needed/as assigned.
- **G** Assist with changes of position as ordered to prevent pressure injuries.
- **G** Perform range of motion exercises as instructed. These exercises will help prevent contractures and other complications.
- **G** Phantom limb pain is real pain and should be treated that way. Report pain to the nurse.

3. Describe prosthetic and orthotic devices

Prostheses may replace a missing limb. Hearing aids, artificial eyes, dentures, and artificial breasts are also considered prostheses.

Artificial limbs, such as artificial hands, arms, feet, and legs, are made to resemble the body part that they are replacing (Fig. 13-10). Many advances have been made and continue to be made in the field of prosthetic limbs. Today's artificial limbs are usually made of strong and lightweight plastics and other materials, such as carbon fiber. Most artificial limbs are attached by belts, cuffs, or suction. Direct bone attachment is a newer method of attaching the limb to the body.

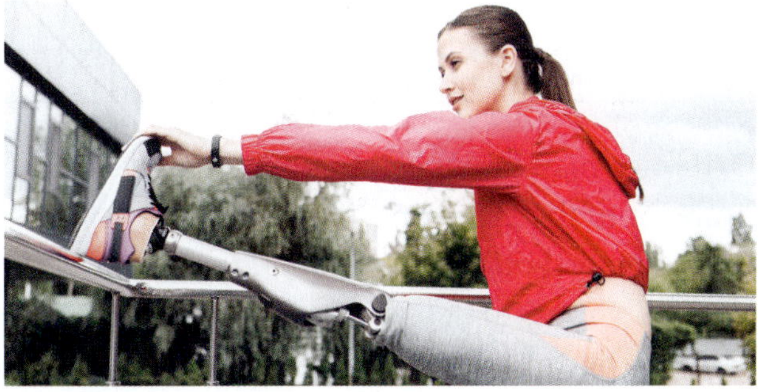

Fig. 13-10. *A woman with one type of prosthetic leg.*

Guidelines: Prosthetic Devices

- **G** Because prostheses are specially fitted, expensive pieces of equipment (some cost tens of thousands of dollars), only care for them if you are assigned and trained to do so. If you have questions, talk to the nurse.
- **G** Respect a patient's decision not to wear a prosthetic limb. Some patients may find the limb uncomfortable and only wish to wear it at certain times.
- **G** Keep the prosthesis and the skin under it dry and clean. The socket of the prosthesis must be cleaned at least daily. Follow the care plan and the nurse's instructions.
- **G** If assisting with putting on a prosthesis, apply a stump sock first as ordered.
- **G** Observe the skin on the stump for signs of skin breakdown caused by pressure and abrasion. Report discoloration or broken skin.
- **G** Never try to fix a prosthesis. Report any problems to the nurse.
- **G** Do not show negative feelings about a patient's stump during care.

An **orthotic device**, or *orthosis,* is a device that helps support and align a limb and improve its functioning (Fig. 13-11). Orthoses also help prevent or correct deformities. Splints are a type of orthotic device.

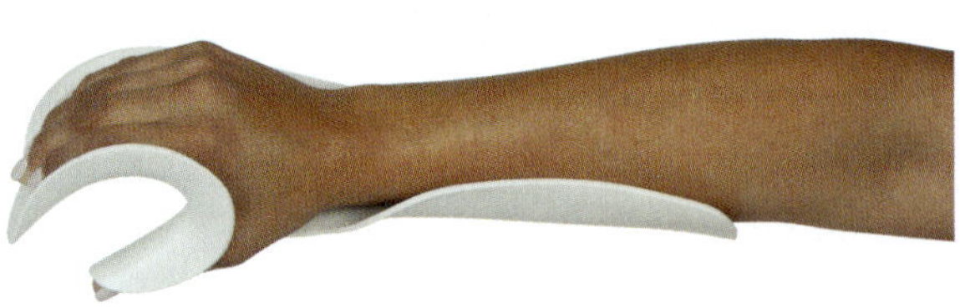

Fig. 13-11. This is one type of orthotic splint. (PHOTO COURTESY OF NORTH COAST MEDICAL, INC., WWW.NCMEDICAL.COM)

Orthotics may be applied to upper or lower limbs or to the spine and/or neck. In some cases, the orthotic device is intended to prevent motion. For example, when a part of the body needs to be kept in place to heal, an orthotic device such as a splint may be used. In other cases, the orthotic device helps to improve motion. An ankle foot orthosis (AFO) is an example of this type of orthosis. It may be placed on the lower limbs to help stabilize the joints, improve functioning, and assist with ambulation. An AFO may help improve balance and prevent falls.

Guidelines: Orthotic Devices

- **G** Only apply a splint or orthotic device as ordered. If you are assigned to apply a device you have never used before or do not understand, ask the nurse for help.
- **G** If the device has straps or buckles, do not overtighten them.
- **G** After applying an orthosis, check for patient comfort. If the device is applied properly and the patient still reports pain or discomfort, report to the nurse.
- **G** Splints and orthoses and the skin area around them should be cleaned at least once daily and as needed. Assist as instructed.

4. Discuss guidelines for elastic bandages

Elastic bandages, also called *nonsterile bandages, ACE bandages,* or *ACE wraps,* are stretchy bandages that are used to hold dressings in place, secure splints, and support and protect body parts. In addition, these bandages may decrease swelling that occurs from an injury. PCTs may be assigned to assist with these bandages.

Guidelines: Elastic Bandages

- **G** Ensure that the area to be wrapped is clean and dry.
- **G** Apply elastic bandages snugly enough to control bleeding and prevent movement of dressings. However, make sure that the body part is not wrapped too tightly. This can decrease circulation.
- **G** Wrap the bandage evenly, in a figure-eight pattern, so that no part of the wrapped area is

pinched. Wrap from distal to proximal. This means to wrap starting at the point farthest from the center of the body and moving toward the center of the body.

- **G** Do not tie the bandage because this cuts off circulation to the body part. Use special clips or tape to hold the end in place.
- **G** Remove the bandage as often as indicated in the care plan.
- **G** Check the patient 10 to 15 minutes after the bandage is applied. Loosen the bandage and report to the nurse immediately if you note these signs of poor circulation:
  - Swelling
  - Discolored skin
  - Shiny, tight skin
  - Skin that is cold to the touch
  - Sores
  - Numbness
  - Tingling
  - Pain or discomfort

5. Describe how to assist with range of motion exercises

Range of motion (**ROM**) exercises put a particular joint through its full arc of motion. The goals of range of motion exercises are to decrease or prevent contractures or atrophy, improve strength, and increase circulation. Types of range of motion exercises are as follows:

Active range of motion (**AROM**) exercises are performed by a patient himself, without help. The PCT's role in AROM exercises is to encourage the patient.

Active assisted range of motion (**AAROM**) exercises are done by the patient with some assistance and support from the PCT or other healthcare worker.

Passive range of motion (**PROM**) exercises are used when patients are not able to move on their own. PROM exercises are performed by healthcare workers, without the patient's help. When assisting with PROM exercises, the PCT should support the patient's joints while moving them through the range of motion.

Range of motion exercises are specific for each body area. They include the following movements (Fig. 13-12):

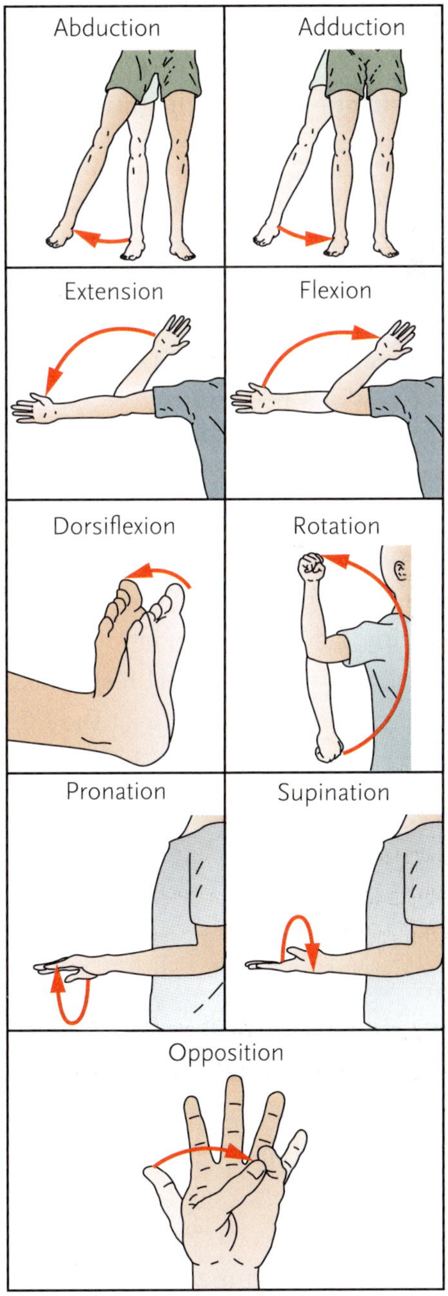

Fig. 13-12. The different range of motion body movements.

- **Abduction**: moving a body part away from the midline of the body
- **Adduction**: moving a body part toward the midline of the body
- **Extension**: straightening a body part
- **Flexion**: bending a body part
- **Dorsiflexion**: bending backward
- **Rotation**: turning the joint
- **Pronation**: turning downward
- **Supination**: turning upward
- **Opposition**: touching the thumb to any other finger

Range of motion exercises are not performed without a specific order from a provider, nurse, or physical therapist. Depending on the care plan, the PCT will repeat each exercise 3 to 5 times, once or twice a day, working on both sides of the body. When performing PROM exercises, the PCT should begin at the patient's shoulders and work down the body. The upper extremities (arms) should be exercised before the lower extremities (legs). The PCT should give support above and below the joints. The joints should be moved gently, slowly, and smoothly through the range of motion to the point of resistance. The patient should be instructed to let the PCT know if she experiences pain during PROM exercises. The PCT should also watch for nonverbal signs that the patient is in pain. Pain must be reported to the nurse and the exercises stopped immediately.

Assisting with passive range of motion exercises

1. Identify yourself by name. Identify the patient according to facility policy.
2. Wash your hands.
3. Explain the procedure to the patient. Speak clearly, slowly, and directly. Maintain face-to-face contact whenever possible.
4. Provide for the patient's privacy with a curtain, screen, or door.
5. Adjust the bed to a safe level, usually waist high. Lock the bed wheels.
6. Position the patient lying supine—flat on her back—on the bed. Use proper alignment. Ask the patient to let you know if she has any pain during the procedure.
7. While supporting the limbs, move all joints gently, slowly, and smoothly through the range of motion to the point of resistance. Repeat each exercise at least 3 times. Ask the patient if an exercise is causing pain. Watch for signs of pain and stop performing exercises if the patient appears to be in pain or reports pain. Report pain to the nurse.
8. **Shoulder**. Support the patient's arm at the elbow and wrist while performing ROM for the shoulder. Place one hand under the elbow and the other hand under the wrist. Raise the straightened arm from the side position upward toward the head to ear level and return the arm down to the side of the body (extension) (Fig. 13-13).

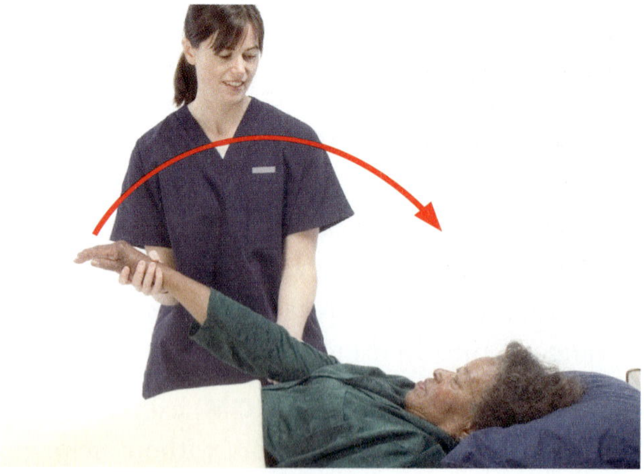

Fig. 13-13. *Raise the straightened arm upward toward the head to ear level, and return it to the side of the body.*

Keep one hand under the elbow and one under the wrist. Move the straightened arm away from the side of the body to the shoulder level and return the arm to the side of the body (abduction/adduction) (Fig. 13-14).

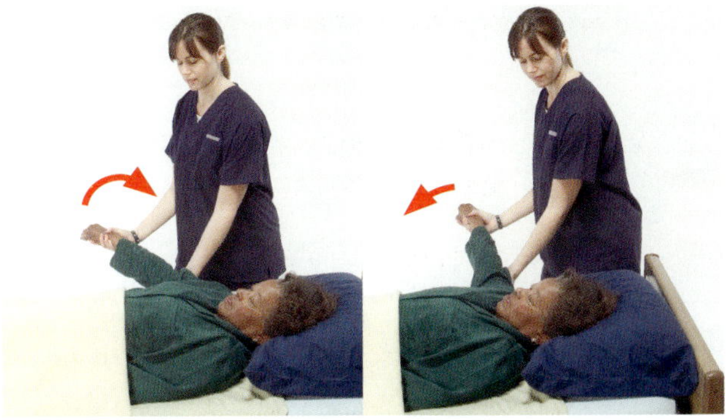

Fig. 13-14. Move the straightened arm away from the side of the body to the shoulder level and return the arm to the side.

9. **Elbow**. Hold the patient's wrist with one hand and the elbow with the other hand. Bend the elbow so that the hand touches the shoulder on that same side (flexion). Straighten the arm (extension) (Fig. 13-15).

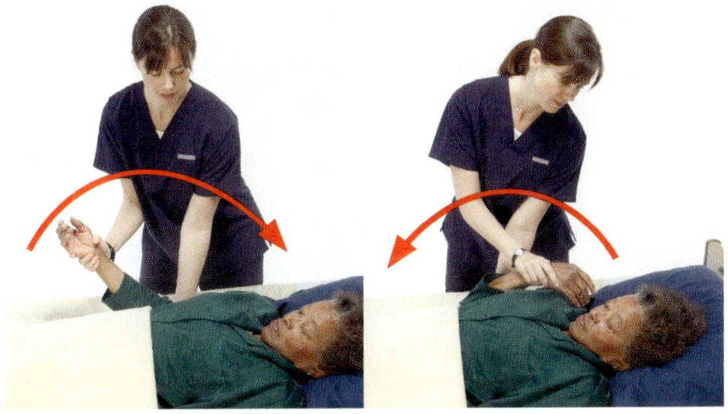

Fig. 13-15. Bend the elbow so that the hand touches the shoulder on the same side, and then straighten the arm.

Exercise the forearm by moving it so the palm is facing downward (pronation) and then the palm is facing upward (supination) (Fig. 13-16).

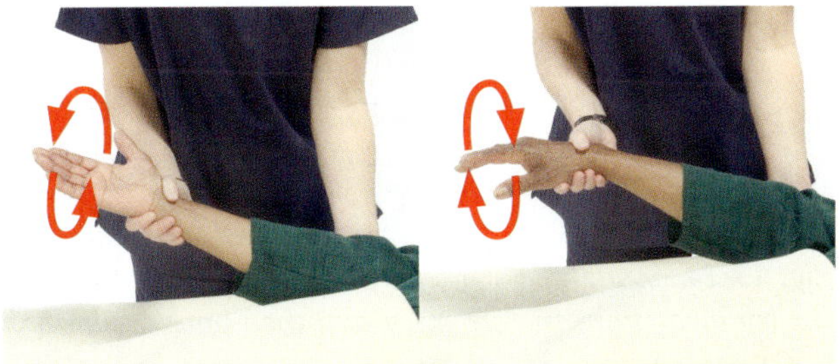

Fig. 13-16. Exercise the forearm so that the palm is facing downward and then upward.

10. **Wrist**. Hold the wrist with one hand and use the fingers of your other hand to move the joint through the motions. Bend the hand down (flexion). Bend the hand backward (dorsiflexion) (Fig. 13-17).

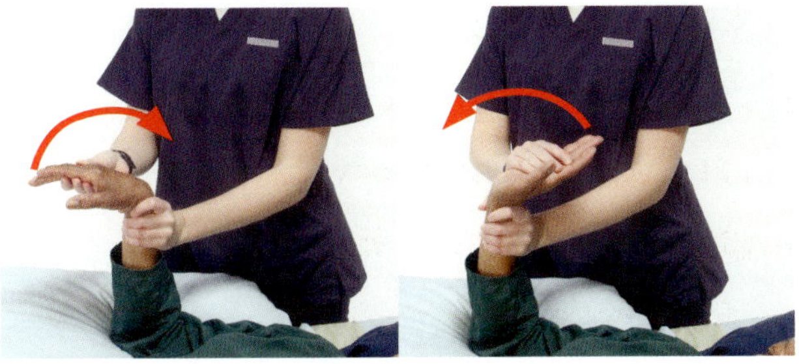

Fig. 13-17. While supporting the wrist, gently bend the hand down and then backward.

Turn the hand in the direction of the thumb (radial flexion). Then turn the hand in the direction of the little finger (ulnar flexion) (Fig. 13-18).

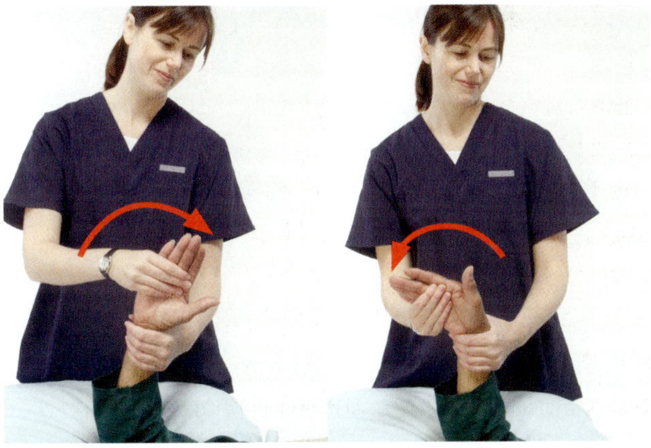

Fig. 13-18. Turn the hand in the direction of the thumb, then turn it in the direction of the little finger.

11. **Thumb**. Move the thumb away from the index finger (abduction). Move the thumb back next to the index finger (adduction) (Fig. 13-19).

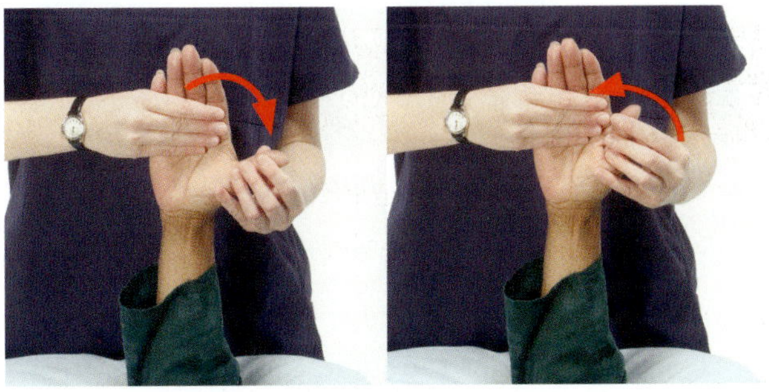

Fig. 13-19. Move the thumb away from the index finger and then back to the index finger.

Touch each fingertip with the thumb (opposition) (Fig. 13-20).

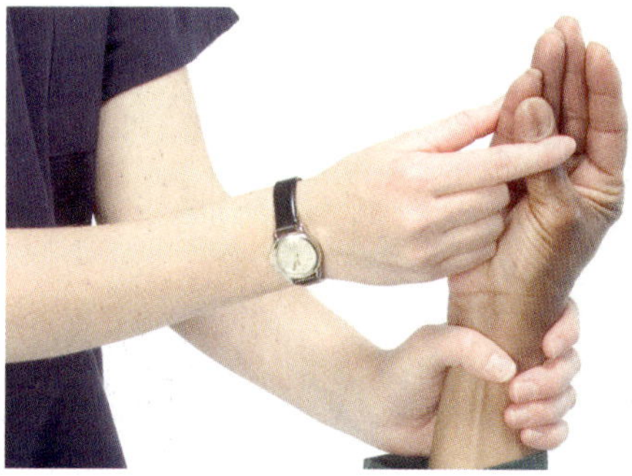

Fig. 13-20. *Touch each fingertip with the thumb.*

Bend the thumb into the palm (flexion) and out to the side (extension) (Fig. 13-21).

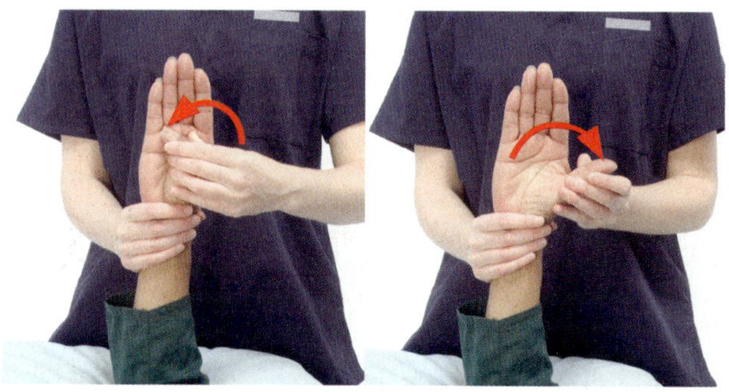

Fig. 13-21. *Bend the thumb into the palm and then out to the side.*

12. **Fingers**. Make the hand into a fist (flexion). Gently straighten out the fist (extension) (Fig. 13-22).

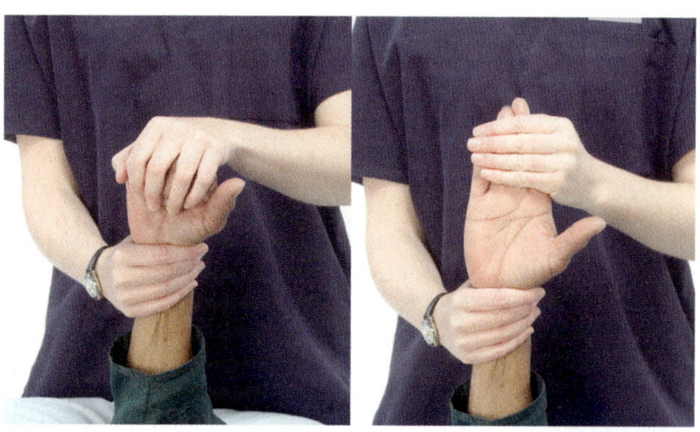

Fig. 13-22. *Make the fingers into a fist and then gently straighten out the fist.*

Spread the fingers and the thumb far apart from each other (abduction). Bring the fingers back next to each other (adduction) (Fig. 13-23).

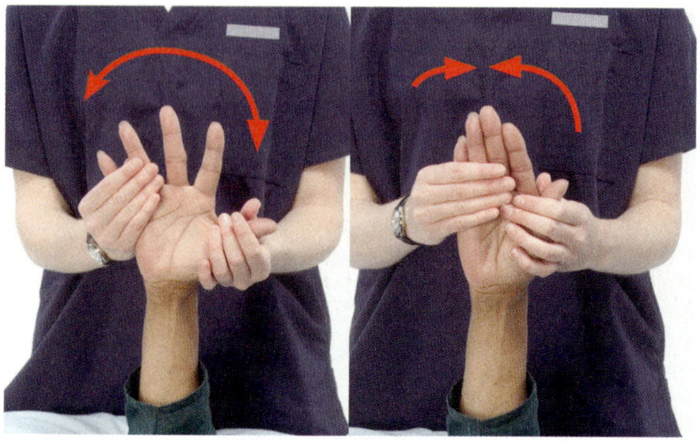

Fig. 13-23. *Spread the fingers and thumb far apart from each other and then bring them back next to each other.*

13. **Hip**. Support the leg by placing one hand under the knee and one under the ankle. Straighten the leg and gently raise it upward. Move the leg away from the other leg (abduction). Move the leg toward the other leg (adduction) (Fig. 13-24).

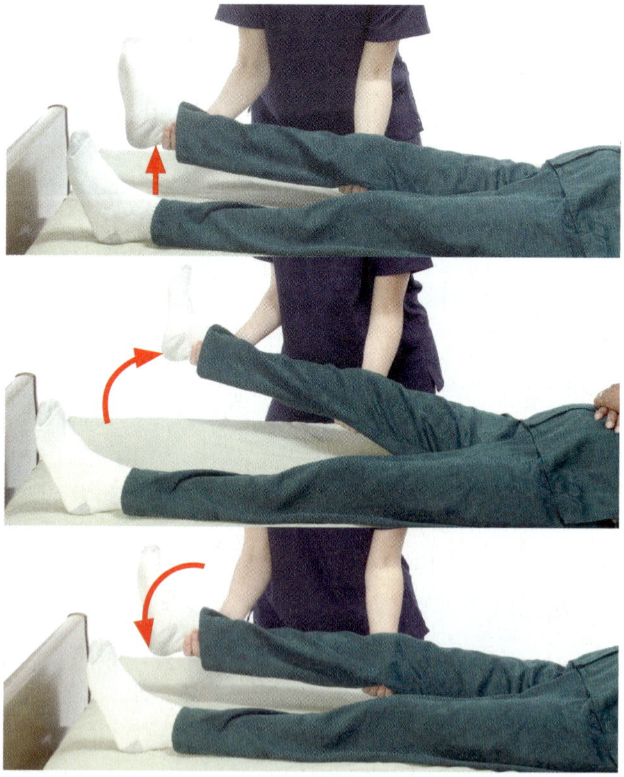

Fig. 13-24. *Straighten the leg and gently raise it. Move the leg away from the other leg and then back toward the other leg.*

Gently turn the leg inward (internal rotation), then turn the leg outward (external rotation) (Fig. 13-25).

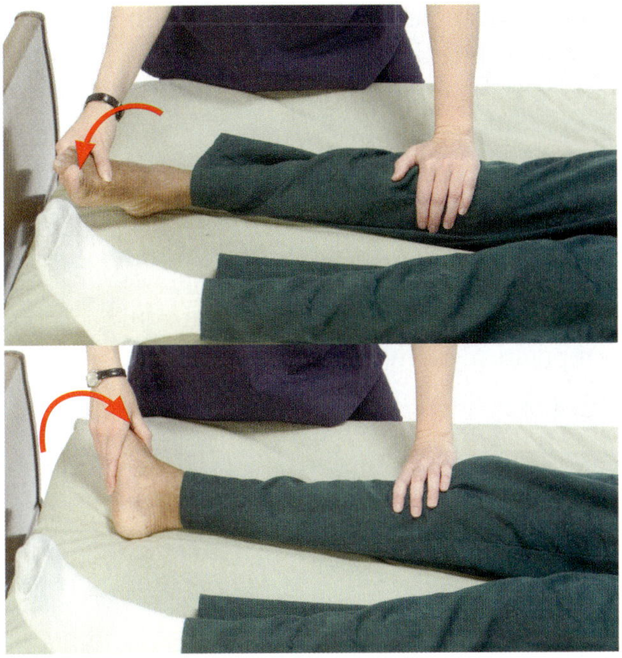

Fig. 13-25. *Gently turn the leg inward and then outward.*

14. **Knee**. Support the leg under the knee and under the ankle while performing ROM for the knee. Bend the knee to the point of resistance (flexion). Return the leg to the patient's normal position (extension) (Fig. 13-26).

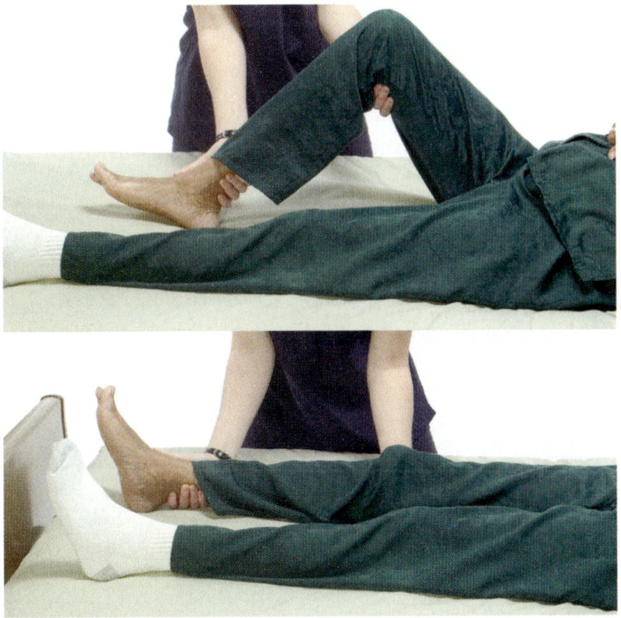

Fig. 13-26. *Gently bend the knee to the point of resistance and return the leg to its normal position.*

15. **Ankle**. Support the foot and under the ankle close to the bed. Push/pull the foot up toward the head (dorsiflexion). Push/pull the foot down, with the toes pointed down (plantar flexion) (Fig. 13-27).

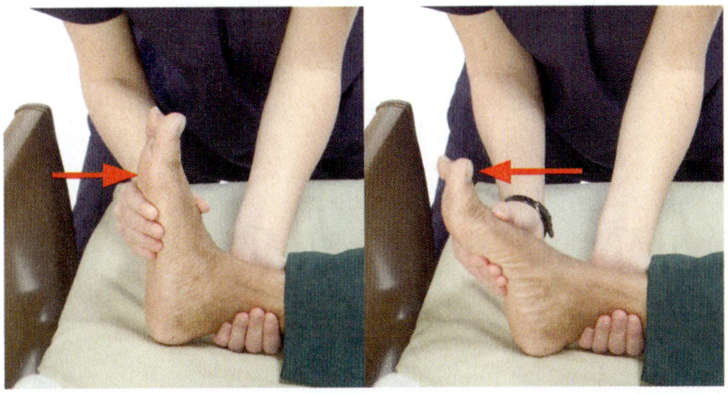

Fig. 13-27. *Push the foot up toward the head and then push it back down.*

Turn the inside of the foot inward toward the body (supination). Bend the sole of the foot so that it faces away from the body (pronation) (Fig. 13-28).

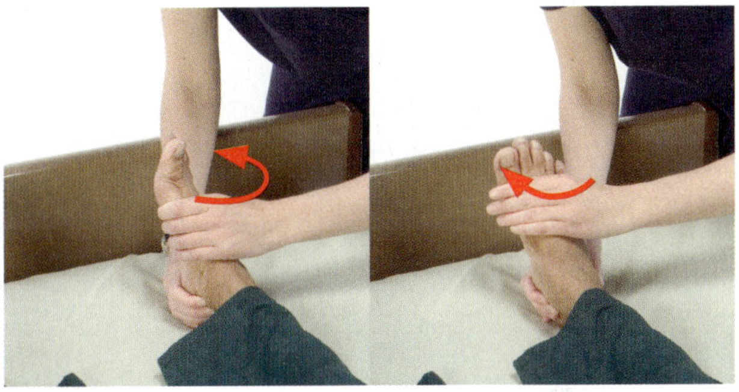

Fig. 13-28. *Turn the inside of the foot inward, toward the body, and then bend it to face away from the body.*

16. **Toes**. Curl and straighten the toes (flexion and extension) (Fig. 13-29).

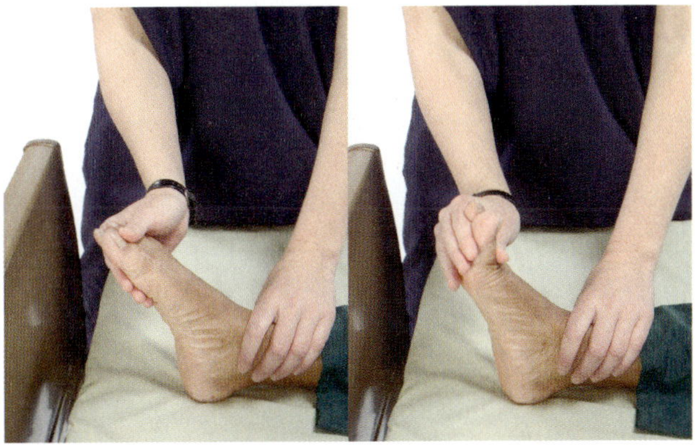

Fig. 13-29. *Curl and straighten the toes.*

Gently spread the toes apart (abduction) (Fig. 13-30).

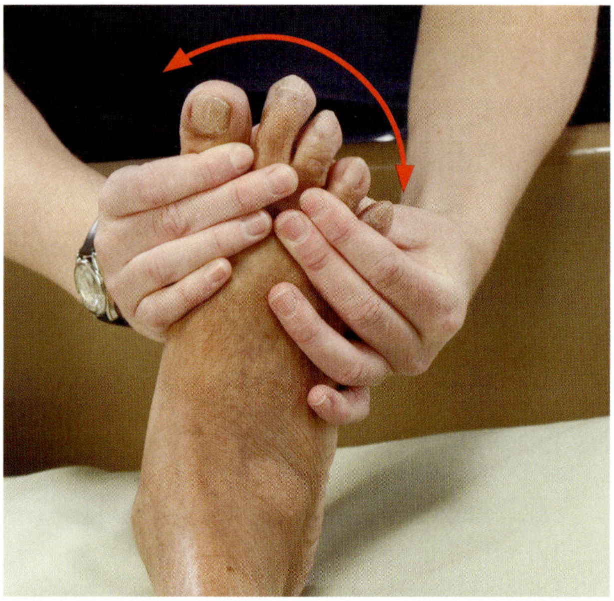

Fig. 13-30. *Gently spread the toes apart.*

17. Return the patient to a comfortable position. Return the bed to its lowest position. Remove privacy measures.
18. Place the call light within the patient's reach.
19. Wash your hands.
20. Report any changes in the patient to the nurse.
21. Document the procedure using facility guidelines. Note any decrease in range of motion or any pain experienced by the patient. Notify the nurse or the physical therapist if you find increased stiffness or physical resistance. Resistance may be a sign that a contracture is developing.

6. Explain the benefits of warm and cold applications

Applying heat or cold to injured areas can have several positive effects. Heat relieves pain and muscular tension. It reduces swelling, elevates the temperature in the tissues, and increases blood flow. Increased blood flow brings more oxygen and nutrients to the tissues for healing.

Cold applications can help stop bleeding. They help prevent swelling, reduce pain, and bring down high fevers. Applying ice bags or cold compresses immediately after an injury can stop bleeding and prevent swelling.

PCTs may be assigned to use these applications. They should know how long the application should be performed and should use the correct temperature as given in the care plan. Using warm and cold applications for too long can cause the opposite effect of what is intended. Patients receiving warm or cold applications should be checked often, especially those who have conditions that may make them unaware of possible injury.

Warm and cold applications may be dry or moist. Moisture strengthens the effect of heat and cold. This means that moist applications are more likely to cause injury. Paralysis, numbness, disorientation, confusion, dementia, and other conditions may make a person unable to feel, notice, or understand damage that is occurring from a warm or cold application. For example, a patient recovering from a stroke who has paralysis on one side may not be able to feel if a warm pack is burning his skin. A patient who has a cognitive impairment may not understand that he is being burned and/or be able to communicate pain clearly.

Moist applications include the following:

- Compresses (warm or cold)
- Soaks (warm or cold)
- Tub baths (warm)
- Sponge baths (warm or cold)
- Sitz baths (warm)
- Ice packs (cold)

Dry applications include the following:

- Electric heating pads (warm)
- Disposable warm packs (warm)

- Ice bags (cold)
- Disposable cold packs (cold)

PCTs should only perform procedures that are assigned to them and that they are trained to do.

Observing and Reporting: Warm and Cold Applications

These signs indicate that the application may be causing tissue damage and should be reported:

O/R Excessive discoloration

O/R Pain

O/R Blisters

O/R Numbness

Connected Care

Warm and Cold Applications

When applying warm or cold applications, the PCT should keep the patient's body covered and only expose the area that needs treatment. Doing this promotes dignity and honors a patient's legal right to privacy.

A washcloth or a commercial warm or cold compress may be used as a compress. In a hospital setting, a commercial compress is most likely used. There are different types of commercial compresses available (Fig. 13-31). If these are provided, the PCT should follow the package directions and the nurse's instructions.

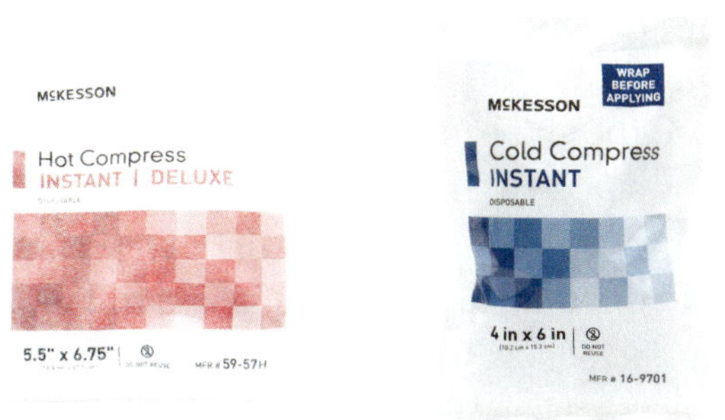

Fig. 13-31. *Disposable compresses are used only once and then discarded. Often these compresses must be squeezed to activate before being applied.* (PHOTOS COURTESY OF MCKESSON MEDICAL-SURGICAL, MMS.MCKESSON.COM)

Applying a warm or cold compress

Equipment: compress

1. Identify yourself by name. Identify the patient according to facility policy.
2. Wash your hands.
3. Explain the procedure to the patient. Speak clearly, slowly, and directly. Maintain face-to-face contact whenever possible.
4. Provide for the patient's privacy with a curtain, screen, or door.
5. Follow manufacturer instructions for activating the compress. In most cases, the compress must be squeezed and kneaded to activate the chemicals inside. This causes the pack to become hot or cold.
6. Immediately apply the compress to the affected area. Most compresses can be placed directly on the patient's skin. Follow instructions.
7. Check the area every 5 minutes. Remove the compress if the area is discolored or numb or if the patient complains of pain or discomfort. Remove the compress after 20 minutes.
8. Make the patient comfortable. Remove privacy measures.
9. Discard the compress.
10. Place the call light within the patient's reach.
11. Wash your hands.
12. Report any changes in the patient to the nurse.
13. Document the procedure using facility guidelines.

Administering warm soaks

Equipment: towel, basin, bath blanket, disposable absorbent pad

1. Identify yourself by name. Identify the patient according to facility policy.
2. Wash your hands.
3. Explain the procedure to the patient. Speak clearly, slowly, and directly. Maintain face-to-face contact whenever possible.
4. Provide for the patient's privacy with a curtain, screen, or door.
5. Fill the basin half full of warm water. Test the water temperature against the inside of your wrist to ensure it is safe. Have the patient check the water temperature. Adjust if necessary.
6. Place the basin on a disposable absorbent pad (protective barrier) in a comfortable position for the patient.
7. Immerse the body part in the basin. Pad the edge of the basin with a towel (Fig. 13-32). Use a bath blanket to cover the rest of the patient, if needed, for extra warmth.

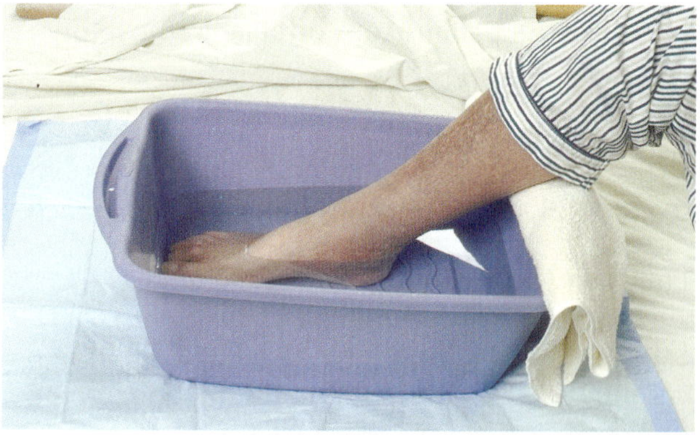

Fig. 13-32. *Pad the edge of the basin with a towel to make the patient more comfortable.*

8. Check the water temperature every 5 minutes. Add hot water as needed to maintain the temperature. Always test the water by touch and do not add uncomfortably hot water. To prevent burns, ask the patient not to add hot water. Observe the area for discoloration. Discontinue the soak if the patient has pain or discomfort.
9. Soak for 15 to 20 minutes or as ordered.
10. Remove the basin. Use the towel to dry the patient.
11. Make the patient comfortable. Remove privacy measures.
12. Discard the disposable pad. Empty, rinse, and dry the bath basin. Place the basin in the designated dirty supply area or return to storage, depending on facility policy.
13. Place the soiled towel in the proper container.
14. Place the call light within the patient's reach.
15. Wash your hands.
16. Report any changes in the patient to the nurse.
17. Document the procedure using facility guidelines.

Another type of heat application is a **sitz bath**, or a warm soak of the perineal area. Sitz baths clean perineal wounds and reduce inflammation and pain. Sitz baths cause circulation to be increased to the perineal area. Patients with perineal swelling (such as hemorrhoids) or perineal wounds (such as those that occur during childbirth) may be ordered to take sitz baths. Because the sitz bath causes increased blood flow to the pelvic area, blood flow to other parts of the body is decreased. Patients may feel weak, faint, or dizzy after a sitz bath. Urinating may be stimulated by a sitz bath. PCTs must always wear gloves when helping with a sitz bath.

A disposable sitz bath fits on the toilet seat and is attached to a rubber bag containing warm water (Fig. 13-33).

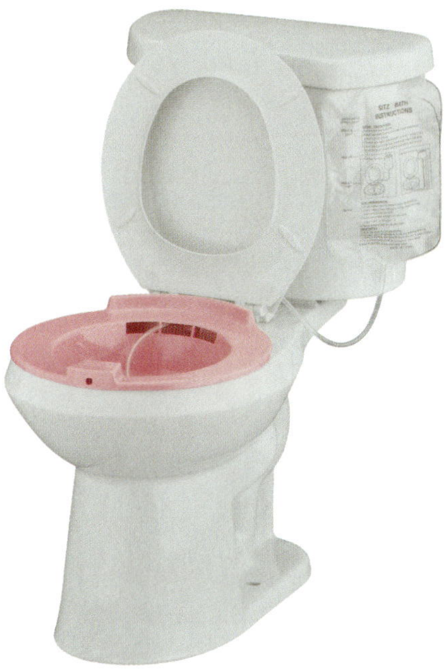

Fig. 13-33. *A disposable sitz bath.* (PHOTO COURTESY OF NOVA MEDICAL PRODUCTS, WWW.NOVAJOY.COM)

Assisting with a sitz bath

Equipment: disposable sitz bath, towels, gloves

1. Identify yourself by name. Identify the patient according to facility policy.
2. Wash your hands.
3. Explain the procedure to the patient. Speak clearly, slowly, and directly. Maintain face-to-face contact whenever possible.
4. Provide for the patient's privacy with a curtain, screen, or door.
5. Put on gloves.
6. Fill the sitz bath 2/3 full with warm water. Place the sitz bath on the toilet seat. Test the water temperature against the inside of your wrist to ensure it is safe. If the sitz bath is being used to help relieve pain and to stimulate circulation, the water may need to be hotter than for other uses. The water should never be uncomfortable to touch. This can cause burns. Follow instructions in the care plan.
7. Help the patient remove underwear, lift her gown, and sit on the sitz bath. A valve on the tubing connected to the bag allows the patient or you to refill the sitz bath with warm water. Show the patient how to use this valve if you will not be staying with her during the sitz bath.
8. You may be required to stay with the patient for safety reasons. If you leave the room, check on the patient every 5 minutes to make sure she is not dizzy or weak. Stay with a patient who seems unsteady.
9. Help the patient off the sitz bath after 20 minutes. Provide towels and help with dressing if needed.
10. Make the patient comfortable. Remove privacy measures.
11. Clean and store supplies. Discard disposable supplies as indicated in the care plan. Place soiled towels in the proper container.
12. Remove and discard your gloves.
13. Wash your hands.
14. Place the call light within the patient's reach.
15. Report any changes in the patient to the nurse.
16. Document the procedure using facility guidelines.

Chapter Review

1. How many bones make up the skeleton of the human body?
2. What type of exercises can help prevent contractures and muscle atrophy?
3. What causes arthritis?
4. What can happen to bones when they are brittle?

5. What type of fracture carries a higher risk of infection and usually requires immediate surgery?
6. Why should extremities in casts be elevated?
7. When dressing a person who has just had a hip replacement, which side should be dressed first: the affected/weaker side or the unaffected/stronger side?
8. What is the difference between partial weight-bearing (PWB), touch-down weight-bearing (TDWB), and non-weight-bearing (NWB)?
9. What are 2 possible reasons for knee replacement surgery?
10. List 3 physical problems that muscular dystrophy can cause.
11. At what age is a person likely to be diagnosed with ALS?
12. What is phantom limb pain? What is phantom sensation?
13. What is a prosthesis?
14. What should be observed about the skin on the stump of an amputated body part?
15. What is the purpose of an orthotic device?
16. List 6 signs of poor circulation that a PCT should observe for when an elastic bandage is applied.
17. When performing PROM exercises, where should the PCT begin? Which parts of the body should be exercised first?
18. Describe the difference between passive, active, and active assisted range of motion exercises.
19. What are the benefits of warm applications? What are the benefits of cold applications?
20. What are 2 conditions for which a sitz bath may be ordered?

14 The Nervous System and Sense Organs and Related Care

1. Describe the structure and function of the nervous system

The nervous system is the control and message center of the body. It controls and coordinates all body functions. The nervous system also senses and interprets information from outside the human body.

The neuron, or nerve cell, is the basic unit of the nervous system. Neurons send messages or sensations from the receptors in different parts of the body, through the spinal cord, to the brain.

The nervous system has 2 main parts: the **central nervous system** (**CNS**) and the **peripheral nervous system** (**PNS**). The central nervous system is composed of the brain and spinal cord. The peripheral nervous system deals with the periphery, or outer part, of the body via the nerves that extend throughout the body (Fig. 14-1).

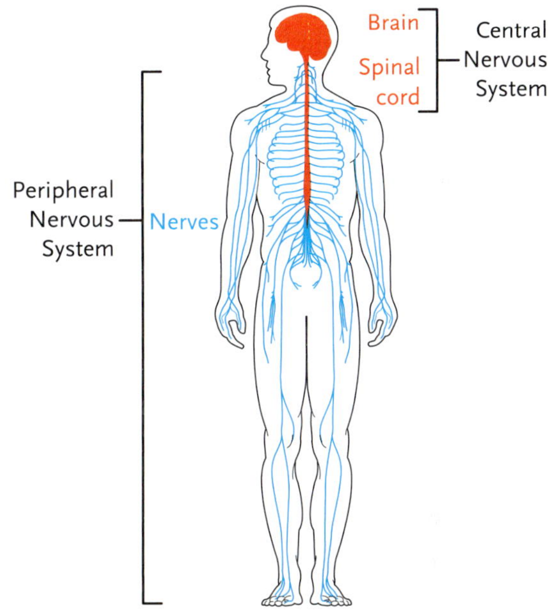

Fig. 14-1. *The nervous system includes the brain, spinal cord, and nerves throughout the body.*

The Central Nervous System

The brain is housed within the skull. The spinal cord is housed within the spinal column. The spinal column extends from the brain into the trunk of the body. Both the brain and the spinal cord are covered by a protective membrane made up of 3 layers. Between 2 of these layers is the cerebrospinal fluid. This fluid circulates around the brain and spinal cord. It provides a cushion against injuries.

The brain has 3 main sections: the cerebrum, the cerebellum, and the brainstem (Fig. 14-2). The largest section of the human brain is the cerebrum. The outside layer of the cerebrum is the cerebral cortex. The cerebral cortex is the part of the brain in which thinking, analysis, association of ideas, judgment, emotions, and memory occur. The cerebral cortex also

- Directs speech and emotions
- Interprets messages from the eyes, ears, nose, tongue, and skin
- Controls voluntary muscle movement

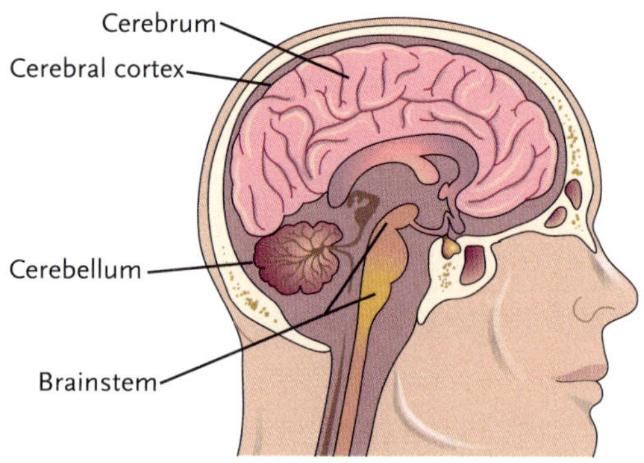

***Fig. 14-2.** The 3 main sections of the brain are the cerebrum, cerebellum, and brainstem.*

The cerebrum is divided into right and left hemispheres. The right hemisphere controls movement and function in the left side of the body. The left hemisphere controls movement and function in the right side of the body (Fig. 14-3). Illness or injury in the right hemisphere affects functions on the left side of the body. Illness or injury in the left hemisphere disrupts function on the right side.

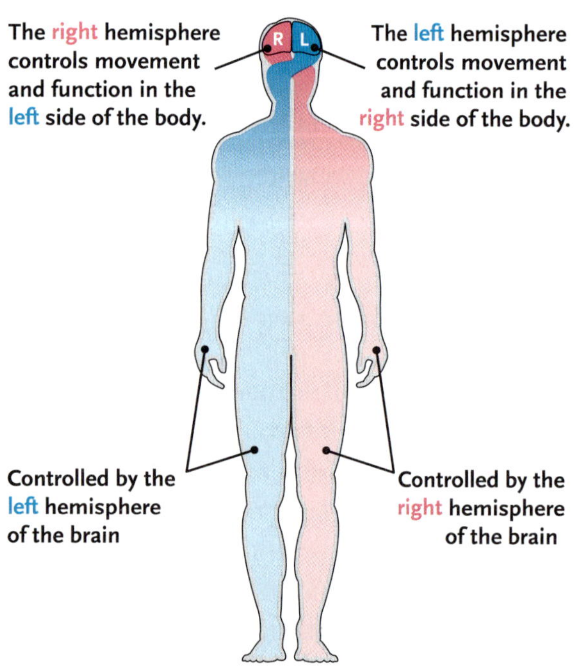

***Fig. 14-3.** The right hemisphere controls movement and function in the left side of the body. The left hemisphere controls movement and function in the right side of the body.*

The cerebellum controls balance and regulates the body's voluntary muscles. It produces and coordinates smooth movements. Someone who has a problem in the cerebellum will be uncoordinated and have jerky movements and muscle weakness.

The cerebrum and cerebellum are connected to the spinal cord by the brainstem. The brainstem contains a kind of regulatory center. It controls heart rate, breathing, swallowing, coughing, vomiting, and closing or opening of blood vessels.

The spinal cord is connected to the brain. It is protected by the bones of the spinal column. Nerve pathways run through the spinal cord. They conduct messages between the brain and the body. Cranial nerves attach to the brain and brainstem. Some of these nerves bring information from the sense organs to the brain. Some control muscles and others are connected to glands or organs, such as the lungs. There are 12 pairs of cranial nerves. Nerves that are attached to the spinal cord and connect the spinal cord to other parts of the body are called spinal nerves. The brain communicates with most of the body through the spinal nerves. There are 31 pairs of spinal nerves.

The functions of the nervous system are to control and coordinate all body functions and to sense, interpret, and respond to changes occurring both inside and outside the human body.

Observing and Reporting: Nervous System

Observe and report these signs and symptoms:

- O/R Fatigue or pain with movement or exercise
- O/R Shaking or trembling
- O/R Drooping of one side of the face
- O/R Inability to move one side of the body
- O/R Difficulty speaking or slurring of speech
- O/R Numbness or tingling
- O/R Disturbance or changes in vision or hearing
- O/R Dizziness or loss of balance

- Changes in eating patterns and/or fluid intake
- Difficulty swallowing
- Bowel and bladder changes
- Depression or mood changes
- Memory loss or confusion
- Violent behavior
- Any unusual or unexplained change in behavior
- Decreased ability to perform ADLs

The Nervous System: Sense Organs

The eyes, ears, nose, tongue, and skin are the body's major sense organs. They are considered part of the nervous system because they contain receptors that receive impulses from the environment. They relay these impulses to the nerves.

The eye, which is about an inch in diameter, is located in a bony socket in the skull (Fig. 14-4). The bony socket protects the eye, which is surrounded by muscles that control its movements.

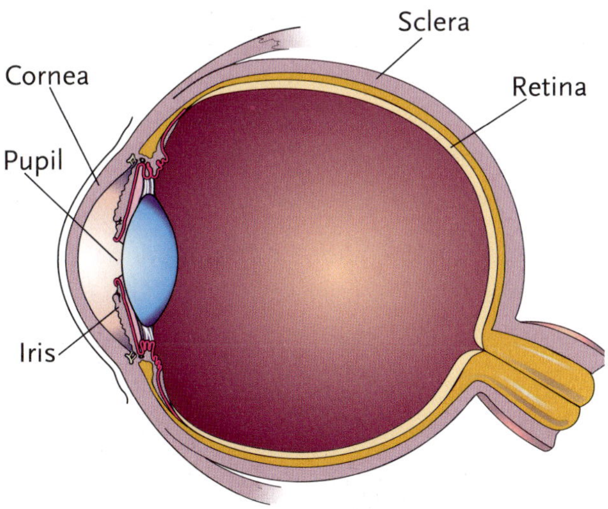

***Fig. 14-4.** The parts of the eye.*

The outer part of the eye is called the sclera. The sclera appears white, except in front, where it is called the cornea. The cornea is actually clear, but it appears colored because it lies over the iris, or the colored part of the eye. The pupil, or black circle in the center of the iris, widens or narrows to adjust the amount of light that enters the eye. Inside the back of the eye is the retina. The retina contains cells that respond to light and send a message to the brain, where the picture is interpreted so a person can see.

The ear is a sense organ that provides balance and hearing. It is divided into 3 parts: the outer, middle, and inner ear (Fig. 14-5). The outer ear is the funnel-shaped outer part, sometimes called the auricle or pinna. It guides sound waves into the auditory canal. This canal is about 1 inch long and contains many glands that secrete earwax. Earwax and hair in the ear protect the ear from foreign objects. The eardrum, or tympanic membrane, separates the outer ear from the middle ear.

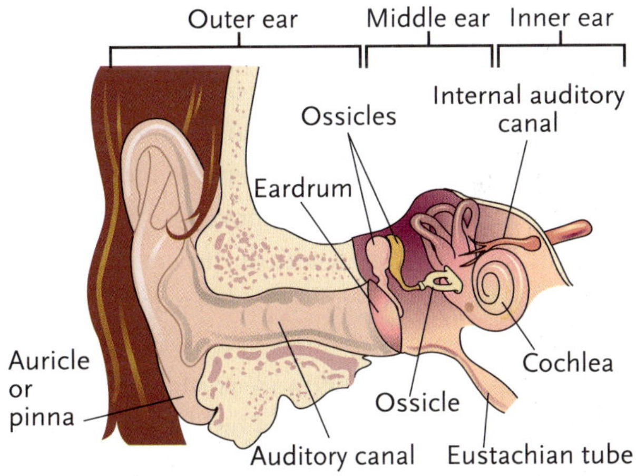

***Fig. 14-5.** The outer ear, middle ear, and inner ear are the 3 main divisions of the ear.*

The middle ear consists of the eustachian tube and 3 ossicles, small bones that amplify sound. The ossicles transmit sound to the inner ear. The eustachian tube connects the middle ear to the throat. It functions to allow air into the middle ear to equalize pressure on the tympanic membrane. The inner ear contains fluid that carries sound waves from the middle ear to the auditory nerve. The auditory nerve then transmits the impulse to the brain. The inner ear also contains structures that help in maintaining balance.

Observing and Reporting: Eyes and Ears

Observe and report these signs and symptoms:

- O/R Changes in vision or hearing
- O/R Dizziness
- O/R Complaints of pain in the eyes or ears
- O/R Discharge from the eyes, red/bloodshot eyes, or eyes that appear yellow

2. List common conditions of the nervous system and discuss related care

Information about mental health and mental health disorders is located in Chapter 4.

CVA or Stroke

The medical term for a stroke is a cerebrovascular accident (CVA). CVA, or stroke (sometimes called *brain attack*), occurs when the blood supply to a part of the brain is blocked or a blood vessel leaks or ruptures within the brain. A stroke can be mild or severe. Afterward, a patient may experience paralysis, weakness, inability to speak or understand words, trouble swallowing, and loss of bowel or bladder control.

Strokes occur on either the right or left side of the brain. Symptoms resulting from a stroke differ; they depend on which side of the brain is affected. Strokes that occur on the right side of the brain affect functioning on the left side of the body. Strokes that occur on the left side of the brain affect functioning on the right side of the body.

If the stroke was mild, the patient may experience few, if any, complications. Physical therapy may help restore physical abilities. Speech and occupational therapy can also help with communication and performing activities of daily living.

Guidelines: CVA/Stroke

- G Patients with paralysis (hemiplegia), weakness (hemiparesis), or loss of movement will usually receive physical or occupational therapy. Range of motion exercises will help strengthen muscles and keep joints mobile. Patients may also need to perform leg exercises to improve circulation. Safety is important when patients are exercising. Assist carefully with exercises as ordered.
- G Never refer to the weaker side as the "bad side," or talk about the "bad" leg or arm. Use the terms *weaker* or *involved* to refer to the side with paralysis.
- G Patients with speech loss or communication problems may receive speech therapy. You may be asked to help. This includes helping patients recognize written or spoken words. Speech-language pathologists will also evaluate a patient's swallowing ability. They will decide whether swallowing therapy or thickened liquids and texture-modified foods are needed. (Chapter 11 has more information.)
- G Use verbal and nonverbal communication to express your positive attitude. Let the patient know you have confidence in his abilities through smiles, touches, and gestures. Gestures and pointing can also help give information or allow the patient to communicate with you.
- G Use communication boards or special cards to make communication easier (Fig. 14-6).
- G Experiencing confusion or memory loss is upsetting. People often cry for no apparent reason after suffering a stroke. Be patient and understanding. Your positive attitude will be important. Keeping a routine may help patients feel more secure.
- G Encourage independence and self-esteem. Let the patient do things for himself whenever possible, even if you could do a better or faster job. Make tasks less difficult for the

patient to do. Appreciate and acknowledge patients' efforts to do things for themselves, even when they are unsuccessful. Praise even the smallest successes to build confidence.

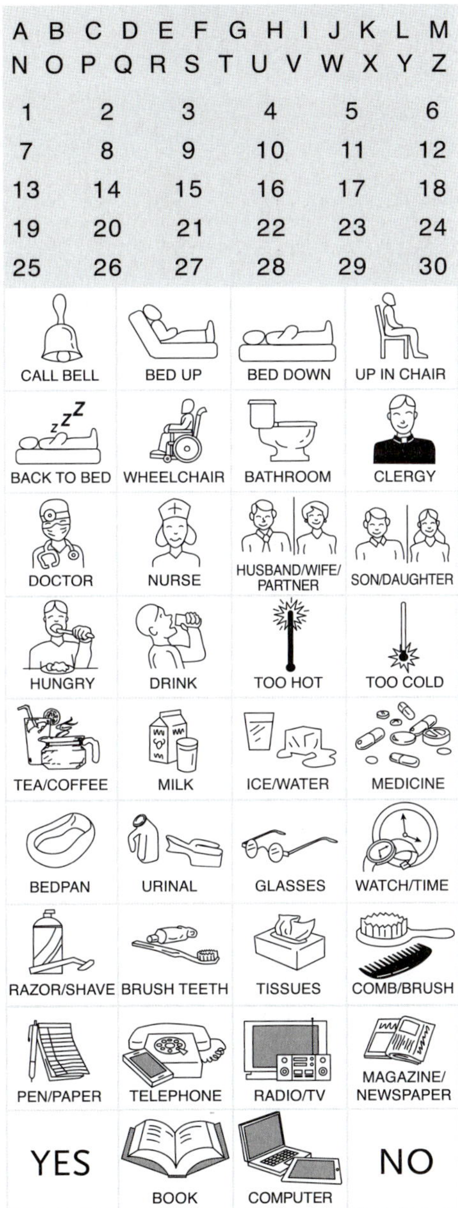

Fig. 14-6. *A sample communication board.*

- **G** Always check on the patient's body alignment. Sometimes an arm or leg can be caught on something and the patient is unaware.
- **G** Pay special attention to skin care and observe for changes in the skin if a patient is unable to move.
- **G** If patients have a loss of touch or sensation, check for potentially harmful situations. Diminished sensation or paralysis causes a lack of awareness about such things as water temperature and sharpness of razors. If patients are unable to sense or move a part of the body, check and change positioning often to prevent pressure injuries.
- **G** Adapt procedures when caring for patients with one-sided paralysis or weakness. Carefully assist with grooming and bathing.
- **G** When assisting with transfers or walking, always use a transfer belt for safety. Stand on the weaker side. Support the weaker side. Lead with the stronger side (Fig. 14-7).

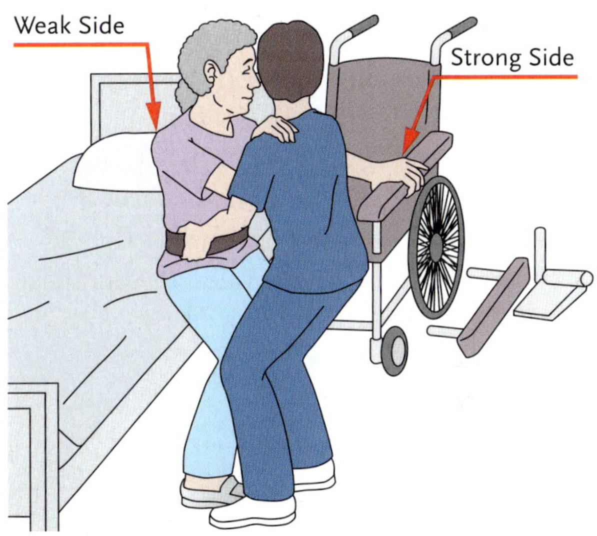

Fig. 14-7. *When helping a patient transfer, support the weaker side while leading with the stronger side.*

When assisting with dressing, remember to

- **G** Dress the weaker side first. Place the weaker arm or leg into the clothing/gown first. This prevents unnecessary bending and stretching of the limb. Undress the stronger side first, then remove the weaker arm or leg from the clothing/gown to prevent the limb from being stretched and twisted.
- **G** Use assistive equipment to help the patient dress himself if it is available and needed. Encourage self-care.

Chapter 6 contains information about recognizing and responding to CVAs. Chapter 11 contains information about how a PCT can assist a patient who has had a CVA with eating.

Parkinson's Disease

Parkinson's disease is a progressive, incurable disease that causes a section of the brain to degenerate. Neurons in the brain that produce the substance called *dopamine,* a neurotransmitter, begin to break down and die. Parkinson's disease affects the muscles, causing them to become stiff, and movement may slow. In addition, it causes stooped posture and a shuffling gait, or walk. It can also cause pill-rolling. Pill-rolling is a circular movement of the tips of the thumb and the index finger when brought together, which looks like rolling a pill. Tremors or shaking make it very difficult for a person to perform ADLs such as eating and bathing. A person with Parkinson's disease may have a mask-like facial expression. Other symptoms are slurred speech and a soft, monotone voice. Medications are commonly used to treat this disease. Surgery may be an option for some people.

Guidelines: Parkinson's Disease

- **G** Patients are at a high risk for falls. This may be noted in the medical record or on the patient's door or whiteboard. The patient may have a wristband warning of fall risk. Visual and spatial impairments may occur, causing problems with bumping into doorways and navigating around obstacles. Protect patients from any unsafe areas and conditions. Assist with ambulation as necessary.
- **G** Help with ADLs as needed.
- **G** Assist with range of motion exercises exactly as ordered to prevent contractures and to help strengthen muscles (Fig. 14-8).
- **G** Observe for any swallowing problems and report them to the nurse.

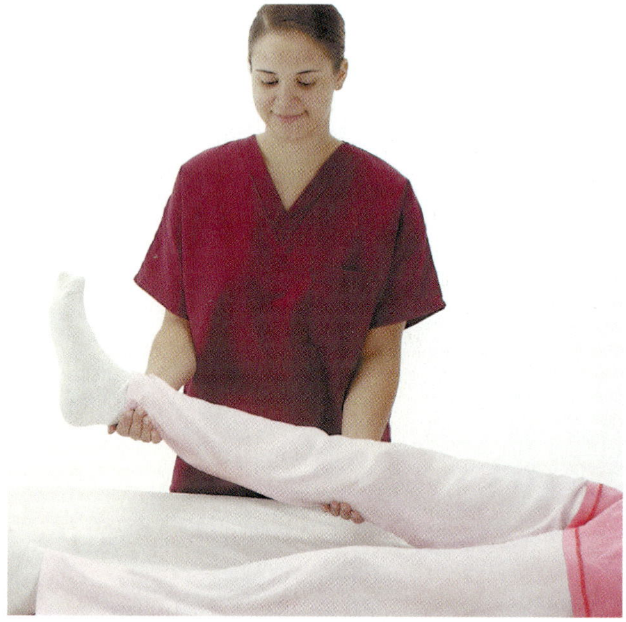

Fig. 14-8. *Range of motion exercises help prevent contractures, strengthen muscles, and increase circulation.*

- **G** Encourage self-care. Be patient with self-care and communication.
- **G** Depression and anxiety may accompany Parkinson's disease. Listen to patients when they want to talk. Offer relaxation techniques such as massage and listening to music. Report signs of depression to the nurse.

Multiple Sclerosis (MS)

Multiple sclerosis (MS) is a progressive disease that affects the central nervous system. When a person has MS, the myelin sheath that covers the nerves, spinal cord, and white matter of the brain breaks down over time. Without this covering, or sheath, nerves cannot send messages to and from the brain in a normal way.

MS progresses slowly and unpredictably. Patients who have this disease will have widely varying abilities. Symptoms will vary as well and may include blurred vision, fatigue, tremors, poor balance, and trouble walking. Weakness, numbness, tingling, incontinence, and behavior changes are also symptoms. MS can eventually cause blindness, contractures, and loss of function in the arms and legs (Fig. 14-9).

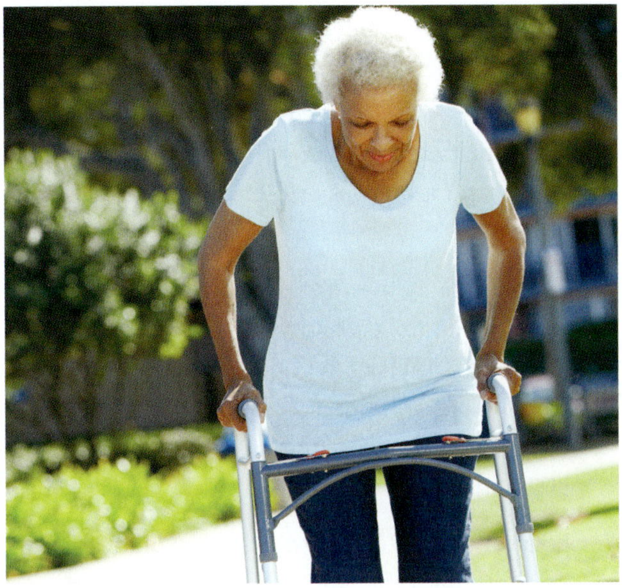

Fig. 14-9. Multiple sclerosis is an unpredictable disease that causes varying symptoms and abilities. MS can cause a range of problems, including fatigue, poor balance, and trouble walking.

Multiple sclerosis is often diagnosed in early adulthood. The exact cause is not known, but it may be an autoimmune disease. There is no cure for this disease; it is mostly treated with medication.

Guidelines: Multiple Sclerosis

- **G** Assist with ADLs as needed. Be patient with self-care and movement. Allow enough time for tasks. Offer rest periods as necessary.
- **G** Give the patient plenty of time to communicate. People with MS may have trouble forming their thoughts. Be patient. Do not rush them.
- **G** Prevent falls, which may be due to a lack of coordination, fatigue, or vision problems. Patients with MS may have extra precautions for preventing falls. Follow these carefully.
- **G** Stress can worsen the effects of MS. Be calm and listen to patients when they want to talk.
- **G** Symptoms of MS can sometimes change daily; offer support and encouragement, and adapt care to the symptoms reported.
- **G** Encourage a healthy diet with plenty of fluids.
- **G** Give regular skin care to prevent pressure injuries.
- **G** Assist with range of motion exercises as assigned to prevent contractures and strengthen muscles.

Head and Spinal Cord Injuries

Diving, sports injuries, falls, car and motorcycle accidents, industrial accidents, war, and criminal violence are common causes of head and spinal cord injuries. Problems from these injuries range from mild confusion or memory loss to coma, paralysis, and death.

There are different types of head injuries, including a bruise (contusion), bleeding in the brain that collects and forms a clot (hematoma), a skull fracture, scalp wound, or concussion (a banging movement of the brain against the skull). The effects a person experiences from a head injury vary, depending on what caused the injury and how severe it is. Patients who have had a head injury may have the following problems: permanent brain damage, intellectual disabilities, personality changes, breathing problems, seizures, coma, memory loss, loss of consciousness, paresis, and paralysis. *Paresis* is paralysis, or loss of muscle function, that affects only part of the body. This term is often used to describe a weakness or loss of ability on one side of the body.

The effects of spinal cord injuries depend on the force of impact and the location of the injury. The higher the injury on the spinal cord, the greater the loss of function. People with head and spinal cord injuries may have **paraplegia**, or loss of function of the lower body and legs. These injuries may also cause **quadriplegia**, which is loss of function in the legs, trunk, and arms (Fig. 14-10).

Rehabilitation is necessary for patients with spinal cord injuries. It will help them maintain the muscle function that remains and to live as independently as possible. Patients will need emotional support as they adjust to their disability. Their specific needs will vary.

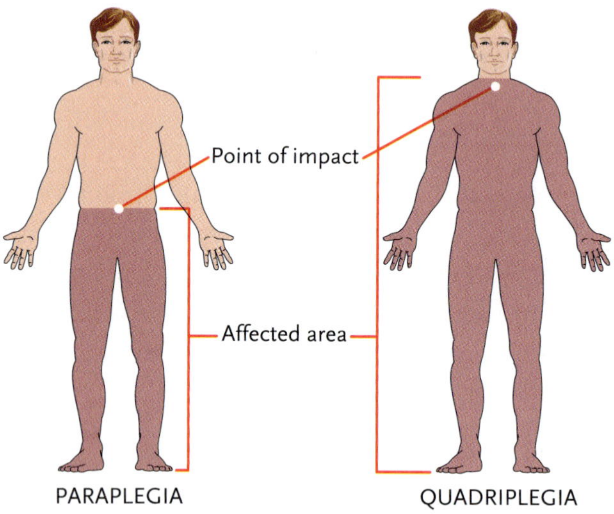

Fig. 14-10. *Loss of function depends on where the spine is injured.*

Guidelines: Head or Spinal Cord Injury

- **G** Give emotional support, as well as physical help. Frustration and anger may surface as patients attempt to deal with the reality of their lives. Try not to take it personally.
- **G** Safety is very important. Be very careful that patients do not fall or burn themselves. Because patients who are paralyzed have no sensation, they are unable to feel a burn. Check water temperature carefully when bathing or providing other personal care.
- **G** Be patient with self-care. Allow as much independence as possible with ADLs.
- **G** Give careful skin care. It is essential to prevent pressure injuries when mobility is limited.
- **G** Assist patients to change positions at least every 2 hours to prevent pressure injuries. Be gentle when repositioning.
- **G** Perform range of motion exercises exactly as ordered to prevent contractures and strengthen muscles.
- **G** Immobility leads to constipation. Encourage fluids and a high-fiber diet if ordered in the care plan.
- **G** Loss of ability to empty the bladder may lead to the need for a urinary catheter. Urinary tract infections (UTIs) are common. Encourage high intake of fluids. Give extra catheter care as needed. There is more information about UTIs and about catheters in Chapter 17.
- **G** Lack of activity leads to poor circulation and fatigue. Offer rest periods as needed. Compression stockings to help increase circulation may be ordered.
- **G** Difficulty coughing and shallow breathing can lead to pneumonia. Encourage deep breathing exercises as ordered. There is more information about these exercises in Chapter 16.
- **G** Male patients may have involuntary erections. Provide for privacy and be sensitive if this happens. Professional behavior helps put patients at ease.
- **G** Assist with bowel and bladder training as directed.

Dementia

Dementia is a general term that refers to a serious loss of mental abilities such as thinking, remembering, reasoning, and communicating. As dementia advances, these losses make it difficult to perform activities of daily living such as eating, bathing, dressing, and eliminating. Dementia is not a normal part of aging.

The following are a few of the common causes of dementia:

- Alzheimer's disease
- Multi-infarct or vascular dementia (a series of strokes causing damage to the brain)

- Lewy body dementia (abnormal structures, called *Lewy bodies*, develop in areas of the brain, causing a variety of symptoms)
- Parkinson's disease
- Huntington's disease (an inherited disease that causes certain nerve cells in the brain to waste away)

Alzheimer's disease (**AD**) is the most common cause of dementia in elderly patients. Although the risk of getting AD increases with age, it is not a normal part of aging. Alzheimer's disease is a progressive, degenerative, and irreversible disease. It causes tangled nerve fibers and protein deposits to form in the brain, eventually causing dementia. The brain of a patient with AD shrinks and the folds of the brain become less organized. There is no known cause of AD, and there is no cure. Diagnosis is difficult. It involves many physical and mental tests to rule out other causes. However, the only sure way to confirm an AD diagnosis at this time is by autopsy.

Symptoms of AD appear gradually. It generally begins with memory loss. As the disease progresses, it causes greater and greater loss of health and abilities. People with AD may get disoriented. They may be confused about time and place. Communication problems are common. They may lose their ability to read, write, speak, or understand. Skills that a person has used often over a lifetime are usually kept longer. Mood and behavior change. Aggressiveness, wandering, suspiciousness, and withdrawal are all part of AD. A patient with AD or other forms of dementia may be more likely to wander and be agitated in the late afternoon and evening. This is called **sundowning**. A patient who has dementia may repeat words, phrases, questions, or activities over and over again. This is called **perseverating**. Alzheimer's disease generally progresses in stages. In each stage, the symptoms become worse. Most people who have AD are eventually completely dependent on others for care.

Maintaining as much independence as possible for as long as possible can help slow the progress of the disease. Patients may be treated with medications to slow cognitive decline and improve behavioral health symptoms.

Guidelines: Dementia

- **G** Always approach from the front, and do not startle the patient.
- **G** Smile and look happy to see the patient. Be friendly.
- **G** Try to minimize background noise and distraction.
- **G** Always identify yourself and use the patient's name. Continue to use the patient's name as you provide care.
- **G** Speak slowly, using a lower tone of voice than normal. This is calming and easier to understand.
- **G** Repeat yourself, using the same words and phrases, as often as needed.
- **G** Use signs, pictures, gestures, or written words to help communicate as needed.
- **G** PCTs must touch patients in order to do their job, but be aware that patients may prefer more personal space when needed.
- **G** Check your body language; make sure you are not tense or hurried.
- **G** Watch for nonverbal cues from the patient. Observe body language—eyes, hands, and face.
- **G** Encourage normal sleep/wake cycles.
- **G** Encourage family members to bring items and pictures from home.

Elopement

Patients with Alzheimer's disease or other forms of dementia might try to elope, or leave a facility unsupervised and unnoticed. It is very important that patients who elope are located and returned to the facility as quickly as possible. The longer a patient is gone, the greater danger he may encounter. PCTs may be assigned to check often on patients with dementia. If a PCT believes a patient may have eloped, she must alert the nurse immediately. The facility may use a code green notification when a patient has eloped. Patients who elope are often found near where they were last seen, and the earlier a search is begun, the more likely the patient is to be found nearby and safe.

Vision Impairment

Vision impairment can affect people of all ages. Some vision impairment causes people to wear corrective lenses, such as eyeglasses or contact lenses. Some people need to wear eyeglasses all the time. Others only need them to read or for activities that require seeing distant objects, such as when driving (Fig. 14-11).

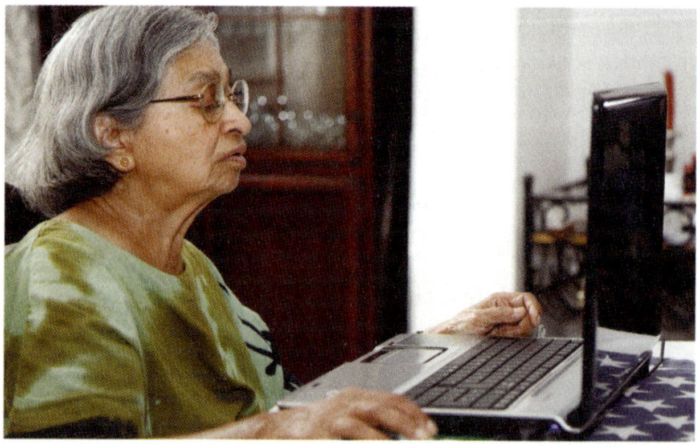

Fig. 14-11. *Some people wear eyeglasses all of the time, while others only need them for certain activities that require seeing distant objects.*

People over the age of 40 are at risk for developing certain serious vision problems. These include cataracts, glaucoma, and blindness. When a **cataract** develops, the lens of the eye, which is normally clear, becomes cloudy. This prevents light from entering the eye. Vision blurs and dims initially. Vision is eventually lost entirely. This disease process can occur in one or both eyes. It is corrected with surgery, in which a permanent lens implant is usually performed. After cataract surgery a patient will likely be prescribed eye drops or ointment to prevent inflammation.

Glaucoma is the leading cause of blindness in the United States. With glaucoma, the pressure in the eye (intraocular pressure) increases. This eventually damages the retina and the optic nerve. It causes loss of vision and blindness. Glaucoma can occur suddenly, causing severe pain, nausea, and vomiting. It can also occur gradually, with symptoms that include blurred vision, tunnel vision, and blue-green halos around lights. Glaucoma is treated with medicated eye drops and other medications and sometimes with surgery.

Diabetic retinopathy is a complication of diabetes caused by damage to the retina. Symptoms include seeing spots, blurred vision, and difficulty seeing well at night. Diabetic retinopathy can lead to blindness. The longer a person has diabetes, the greater the risk for developing this condition. Other risk factors include diabetes that is not managed well, high blood pressure, high cholesterol, and tobacco use. Diabetic retinopathy is treated with laser treatment, surgery, or injection of medication into the eye.

Age-related macular degeneration (AMD) is a condition that usually affects older adults (50 and over). It occurs when the macula, which is part of the retina, gradually deteriorates, eventually causing vision loss and such problems as the inability to recognize faces, drive, read, and write. Peripheral (side) vision is not affected.

This condition may evolve slowly, and symptoms may not be apparent in the early stages. A person may experience dark or blurred areas in the center of vision, or objects may appear less bright. The 2 forms of this condition are wet and dry age-related macular degeneration. The dry form is more common.

Risk factors include age, smoking, gender, race (white people are more likely to develop it), and family history of the disease. There is no cure for AMD, but zinc and antioxidants may slow the progression of dry AMD. Wet AMD may be treated with injections and laser surgery.

Guidelines: Vision Impairment

- **G** Identify yourself immediately when you approach the patient.
- **G** Do not touch the patient until you have said your name.
- **G** Let the patient know if you need to step away at any time. Do not simply walk away.
- **G** Make sure there is proper lighting in the room. Face the patient when speaking.
- **G** Always tell the patient what you are doing as you provide care. Give specific directions, such as "on your right" or "in front of you."

Chapter 11 has more information about how a PCT can assist a patient who has a visual impairment with eating.

Hearing Impairment

Hearing impairment can happen at any age but commonly occurs with aging. **Presbycusis** is age-related hearing loss. It happens gradually as the bones of the middle ear harden. This lessens their ability to conduct sound waves. This is known as *conductive hearing loss.*

Exposure to loud noises over time, which can damage the cells of the cochlea, can also be a factor. When the cochlea is damaged it cannot transmit sensory input to the brain. This causes *sensorineural hearing loss.*

The most common treatment for most hearing loss is a hearing aid, which amplifies sound waves. Some types of hearing loss require surgery. Conductive hearing loss may be treated by inserting tympanostomy tubes. These small tubes are placed in the tympanic membrane to improve air flow in the ear. A cochlear implant is a procedure used to treat sensorineural hearing loss.

Guidelines: Hearing Impairment

- **G** If the patient has a hearing aid, make sure that it is turned on and working properly.
- **G** Reduce background noise as much as possible.
- **G** Get the patient's attention before speaking.
- **G** Speak clearly, slowly, and in good lighting. Directly face the patient. Ask if she can hear what you are saying.
- **G** Do not shout or mouth words in an exaggerated way.
- **G** Keep the pitch of your voice low.
- **G** Patients may read lips, so keep your hands away from your face while talking.
- **G** If the patient hears better out of one ear, try to speak and stand on that side.
- **G** Use short sentences and simple words. Avoid sudden topic changes.
- **G** Use picture cards or a notepad as needed.
- **G** Some patients have speech problems and may be difficult to understand. Do not pretend you understand if you do not. Ask the patient to repeat what was said.

Hearing Aids and Ocular Prosthetics

A hearing aid is a small device placed in the ear to amplify sound for persons with hearing loss. Many elderly people have hearing aids. Hearing aids are expensive and must be treated with care. Make sure that it is stored safely, according to facility policy, if it must be removed for testing or procedures.

An artificial eye, or ocular prosthetic, replaces an eye that has been lost to disease or injury. It is usually made of plastic. It is held in place by suction. An ocular prosthetic does not provide vision; it can, however, improve appearance. Some artificial eyes do not require frequent removal. Others need daily removal and cleaning. PCTs should tell the nurse if a patient needs help caring for an artificial eye.

Chapter Review

1. What are 2 functions of the nervous system?
2. What does the cerebral cortex control?
3. How many pairs of cranial nerves are there? What is their function?
4. What are the body's sense organs?
5. What are the 2 main functions of the ear?
6. What causes a CVA (stroke)?
7. What terms should a healthcare worker use to refer to the weaker side of a person who has had a stroke?
8. When helping a patient who has had a stroke with transfers or walking, on which side should the PCT stand—the weaker or stronger?
9. When dressing a patient with a one-sided weakness, which side should a PCT dress first?
10. Why may people with Parkinson's disease have trouble eating and bathing themselves?
11. When a person has multiple sclerosis, what covering breaks down over time?
12. What is paraplegia? What is quadriplegia?
13. What is dementia?
14. List 3 behavioral changes that may happen as a result of Alzheimer's disease.
15. What does the term *elopement* refer to in health care?
16. What are conditions that can cause vision impairment?
17. List 5 guidelines for communicating with a patient who has a hearing impairment.

15 The Circulatory System and Related Care

1. Describe the structure and function of the circulatory system

The circulatory, or cardiovascular, system is made up of the heart, blood vessels, and blood (Fig. 15-1). The heart pumps blood through the blood vessels to the cells. The blood carries food, oxygen, and other substances cells need to function properly. A healthy circulatory system is essential for life. Cells, tissues, and organs need proper circulation to function well. If circulation is reduced, cells do not receive enough oxygen and nutrients. Waste products of cell metabolism are not removed, and organs become diseased.

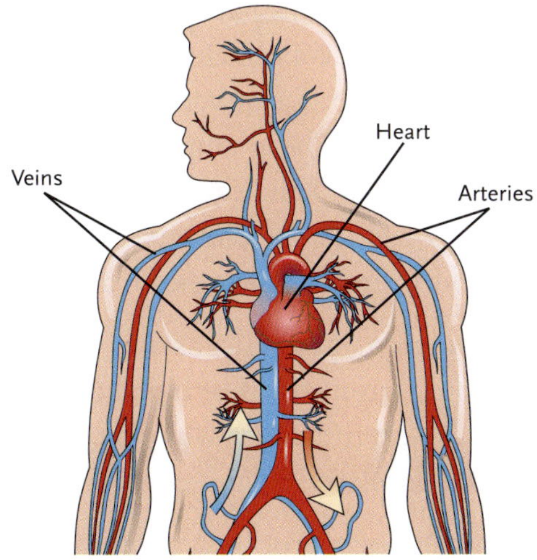

Fig. 15-1. The heart, blood vessels, and blood are the main parts of the circulatory system.

The Heart

The heart is the pump of the circulatory system (Fig. 15-2). The heart is a muscle. It is located in the middle lower chest, on the left side. The heart muscle is made up of 3 layers: the pericardium, the myocardium, and the endocardium.

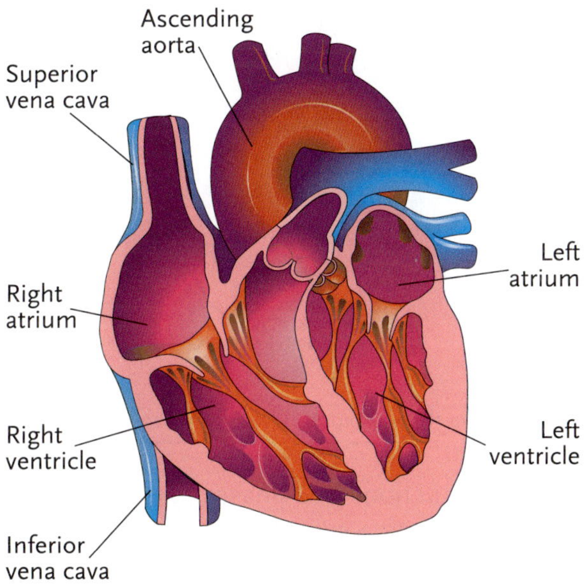

Fig. 15-2. The 4 chambers of the heart connect to the body's largest blood vessels.

The interior of the heart is divided into 4 chambers. The 2 upper chambers are called the left atrium and right atrium. They receive blood. The 2 lower chambers, or ventricles, pump blood. The right atrium receives blood from the veins. This blood, containing carbon dioxide, then flows into the right ventricle. It is pumped to the blood vessels in the lungs. Carbon dioxide is exchanged for oxygen. The heart's left atrium receives the oxygen-saturated blood. It then flows into the left ventricle. There it is pumped through the arteries to all parts of the body (Fig. 15-3). A series of valves makes sure that blood flows in the correct direction as it is pumped through the heart. The 4 major valves of the heart are the tricuspid valve, the pulmonary valve, the bicuspid valve (also called the *mitral valve*), and the aortic valve.

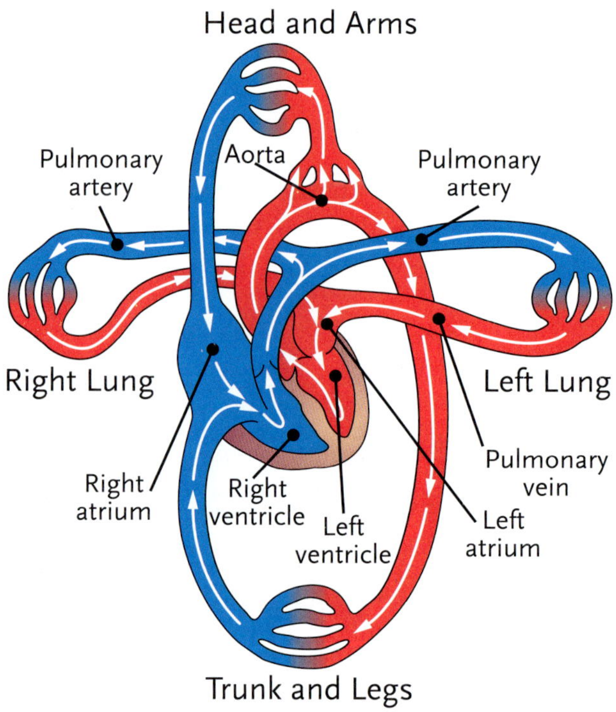

Fig. 15-3. *The flow of blood through the heart.*

The heart functions in 2 phases: the contracting phase, or **systole**, when the ventricles pump blood through the blood vessels, and the resting phase, or **diastole**, when the chambers fill with blood. When a person's blood pressure is checked, the numbers measure these 2 phases.

The pumping of the heart is triggered by a system of tissue that can create electrical signals. This tissue begins, or *initiates*, electrical impulses. It then *conducts*, or carries, them through the heart. These impulses are the "spark" that triggers heart muscle to contract. This network of tissue is called the **cardiac conduction system**.

The cardiac conduction system begins in the upper part of the right atrium. It continues through the heart to the walls of the ventricles. The timing of the electrical signals allows contractions to happen in an organized way. First the atria contract and then the ventricles. This delay allows the atria to empty of blood and the ventricles to fill before they contract. There is more information about the cardiac conduction system in Chapter 23.

Blood and Blood Vessels

There are 3 types of blood vessels found in the body: arteries, capillaries, and veins. Arteries carry oxygen-rich blood away from the heart. The blood is pumped from the left ventricle through the aorta, the largest artery. Blood is then pumped through other arteries that branch off from it. The coronary arteries carry blood to the heart itself.

Capillaries are tiny blood vessels that receive blood from the arteries. Nutrients, oxygen, and other substances in the blood pass from the capillaries to the cells. Waste products, including carbon dioxide, pass from the cells into the capillaries.

Veins carry the blood containing waste products from the capillaries back to the heart. Near the heart, the veins come together to form the 2 largest veins, the inferior vena cava and the superior vena cava. These empty into the right atrium. The inferior vena cava carries blood from the legs and trunk. The superior vena cava carries blood from the arms, head, and neck.

Blood is made up of blood cells and plasma. There are 3 different types of blood cells: red blood cells, or erythrocytes; white blood cells, or leukocytes; and platelets, or thrombocytes.

Red blood cells (erythrocytes) carry oxygen from the lungs to all parts of the body. Red blood cells are produced by bone marrow, a substance found inside hollow bones. Iron, found in bone marrow and red blood cells, is essential to blood. It gives it its red color. Red blood cells function for a short time, then die. They are filtered out of the blood by the liver and spleen. Iron in the diet allows the body to produce new red blood cells.

White blood cells (leukocytes) defend the body against foreign substances, such as bacteria and viruses. When the body becomes aware of these invaders, white blood cells rush to the site of infection. They multiply rapidly. The bone marrow, spleen, and thymus gland produce white blood cells.

Platelets (thrombocytes) are also carried by the blood. They cause the blood to clot, preventing excess bleeding. Platelets are also produced by bone marrow.

Plasma is the liquid portion of the blood. It is made up of mostly water and carries many substances, including blood cells, nutrients, and waste products.

The functions of the circulatory system are to supply food, oxygen, and hormones to cells and to supply the body with infection-fighting blood cells. The circulatory system removes waste products from cells and also helps control body temperature.

Observing and Reporting: Circulatory System

Observe and report these signs and symptoms:

- O/R Changes in pulse rate
- O/R Weakness, fatigue
- O/R Loss of ability to perform activities of daily living
- O/R Swelling (edema) of ankles, feet, fingers, or hands
- O/R Discolored hands, feet, or lips
- O/R Chest pain
- O/R Weight gain
- O/R Shortness of breath, changes in breathing patterns, or an inability to catch breath
- O/R Severe headache
- O/R Inactivity (which can lead to circulatory problems)

2. List common conditions of the circulatory system and discuss related care

Hypertension (HTN) or High Blood Pressure

When blood pressure consistently measures 130/80 or higher, a person is diagnosed as having hypertension (HTN), or high blood pressure. The major cause of hypertension is **atherosclerosis**, or a hardening and narrowing of the blood vessels (Fig. 15-4). It can also result from kidney disease, tumors of the adrenal gland, pregnancy, and certain medications. Hypertension can develop in people of any age. Signs and symptoms of hypertension are not always obvious, especially in the early stages. Often it is only discovered when a blood pressure measurement is taken by a healthcare provider. People with the disease may complain of headaches, blurred vision, and dizziness. Hypertension may be treated with medication.

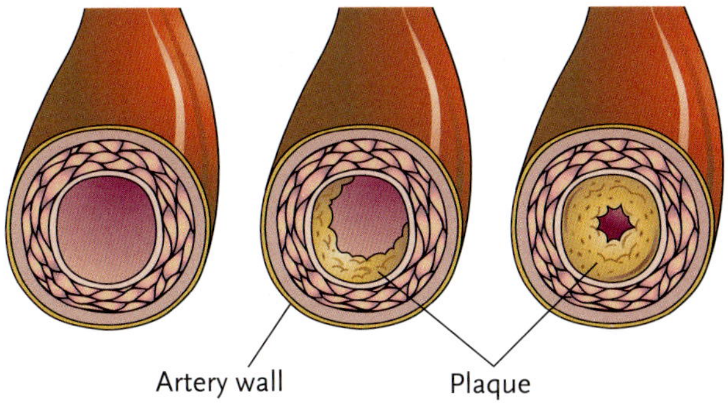

Fig. 15-4. *Arteries may harden or narrow because of a buildup of plaque. Hardened arteries are one cause of high blood pressure.*

Guidelines: Hypertension

- G Because it can lead to serious conditions such as CVA, heart attack, kidney disease, and blindness, treatment to control hypertension is vital. Patients may take medication that lowers blood pressure. They may take diuretics. Diuretics (sometimes called *water pills*) are medications that reduce the amount of fluid in the body and increase the need to urinate. Offer trips to the bathroom regularly. Answer call lights promptly.

- G You may be required to measure blood pressure frequently. Monitor blood pressure and pulse rate as directed.
- G Patients may have prescribed exercise programs and special diets, such as lowfat or low-sodium diets. Reducing the amount of sodium in the diet can help reduce extra fluid in the body.

Coronary Artery Disease (CAD)

Coronary artery disease occurs when the blood vessels in the coronary arteries narrow. This reduces the supply of blood to the heart muscle and deprives it of oxygen and nutrients. Over time, as fatty deposits block the arteries, the muscles that are supplied by the blood vessels die. CAD can lead to heart attack or stroke.

In CAD, narrow blood vessels prevent the extra blood with oxygen from getting to the heart (Fig. 15-5). The heart muscle that is not getting enough oxygen causes chest pain, pressure, or discomfort, called **angina**. The heart needs more oxygen during exercise, stress, and excitement, as well as to digest a heavy meal. These situations can cause angina.

The pain of angina is usually described as pressure or tightness in the left side or the center of the chest, behind the sternum or breastbone. Some people have pain moving down the inside of the left arm or to the neck and left side of the jaw. A person suffering from angina may sweat or appear pale and may feel dizzy and have trouble breathing. This type of angina can be a sign of a heart attack.

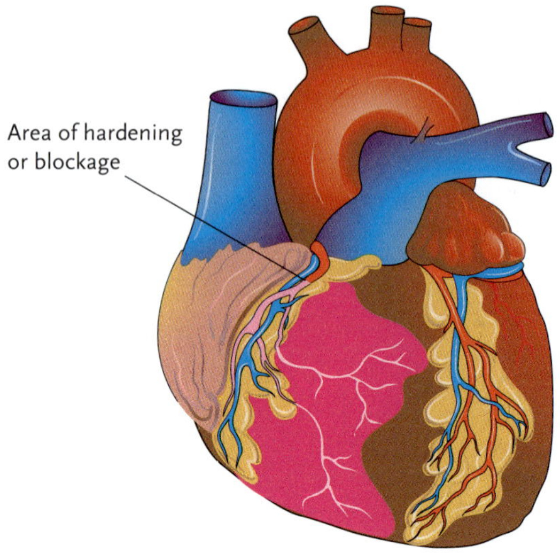

Fig. 15-5. *Angina is chest pain or pressure that results from the heart not getting enough oxygen.*

Risk factors for coronary artery disease include aging, gender (men are more likely to get CAD than women), family history of heart disease, tobacco use, high cholesterol, hypertension, lack of activity, obesity, and diabetes.

Guidelines: Angina

- G Encourage patients to rest. Rest is extremely important. Rest reduces the heart's need for extra oxygen. It helps the blood flow return to normal, often within 3 to 15 minutes.
- G Medication is also needed to relax the walls of the coronary arteries. This allows them to open and get more blood to the heart. This medication, **nitroglycerin**, is a small tablet that the patient places under the tongue. There it dissolves and is rapidly absorbed. PCTs are not allowed to give medication. Tell the nurse if a patient says she needs medication or is having chest pain. Nitroglycerin is also available as a patch. Do not remove any medicated patch and do not touch it with your bare hands, as it is absorbed through intact skin. Tell the nurse immediately if the patch comes off. Nitroglycerin may also come in the form of a spray that is sprayed on or under the tongue.

G Patients may also need to avoid heavy meals, overeating, intense exercise, and exposure to cold or hot and humid weather.

Myocardial Infarction (MI) or Heart Attack

When all or part of the blood flow to the heart muscle is blocked, oxygen and nutrients fail to reach the cells in that area (Fig. 15-6). Waste products are not removed, and the muscle cell dies. This is called a *myocardial infarction (MI)*, or a heart attack. The area of dead tissue may be large or small, depending on the artery involved. Someone having a myocardial infarction must receive emergency treatment from medical personnel. This helps minimize damage and may prevent further illness or death. Chapter 6 has a list of warning signs of an MI.

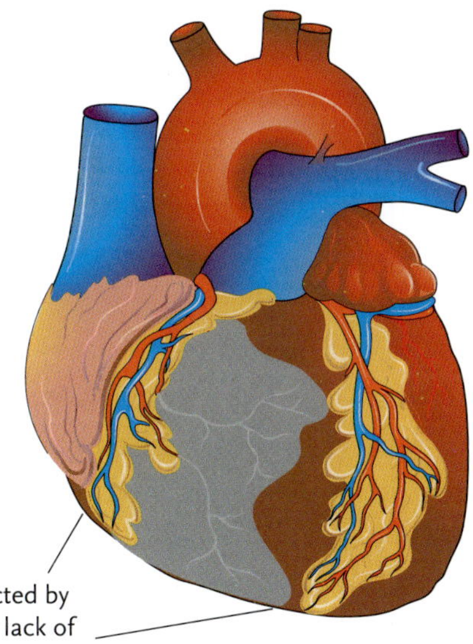

Fig. 15-6. *A heart attack occurs when all or part of the blood flow to the heart is blocked.*

After an MI, cardiac rehabilitation is usually ordered. This ongoing program is comprehensive and consists of regular exercise, medications, blood testing, stopping smoking, and a diet low in saturated fats and sodium and rich in fruits, vegetables, and whole grains. A stress management program and mental health care to help deal with anxiety and depression are parts of the program too. While the patient is in the hospital the PCT should monitor vital signs as instructed and perform blood draws as trained and directed.

Congestive Heart Failure (CHF)

Coronary artery disease, myocardial infarction, hypertension, and other disorders may all damage the heart. When the heart muscle has been severely damaged, it fails to pump effectively. When the left side of the heart is affected, blood backs up into the lungs. When the right side of the heart is affected, blood backs up into the legs, feet, or abdomen. When one or both sides of the heart stop pumping blood properly, it is called **congestive heart failure** (**CHF**).

Signs and symptoms of congestive heart failure include the following:

- Fatigue
- Rapid or irregular heartbeat
- Shortness of breath
- Dizziness
- Weakness
- Edema of the feet and ankles
- Increased urination at night
- Weight gain

Although congestive heart failure is a serious illness, it can be treated and controlled. Medications can strengthen the heart muscle and improve its pumping.

Guidelines: Congestive Heart Failure

G Assist the patient as needed with getting to the toilet or commode. Because diuretics help eliminate excess fluids, the patient will need more frequent trips to the bathroom. Answer call lights promptly. If the patient has trouble getting out of bed and walking to the bathroom, a portable commode may be placed by the bed.

- A low-sodium diet or fluid restrictions may be ordered.
- A weakened heart may make activity difficult for patients. Limited activity or bedrest may be prescribed. Allow for a period of rest after an activity.
- Measure intake of fluids and output of urine as ordered.
- Weigh patients as instructed. The patient may need to be weighed daily at the same time to note weight gain from fluid retention.
- Apply compression stockings as ordered to reduce swelling in feet and ankles.
- Assist with range of motion exercises as ordered. These exercises improve muscle tone when activity and exercise are limited.
- Extra pillows may help patients who have trouble breathing. Keeping the head of the bed elevated may also help with breathing.
- Assist with personal care and activities of daily living as needed.
- A common side effect of medications for congestive heart failure is dizziness. This may result from a lack of potassium, although not all medications for CHF deplete potassium. A patient with CHF may be on a high-potassium diet.

Dysrhythmias

Dysrhythmias, sometimes called *arrhythmias*, are abnormal heart rhythms. There are many different types. They range from harmless to life-threatening and are caused by problems with the cardiac conduction system. In the most life-threatening rhythms, atrial fibrillation and ventricular fibrillation, the heart is *fibrillating*, or quivering. These rhythms are medical emergencies. They may require CPR and *defibrillation*. A defibrillator delivers a shock to the heart to restore the normal heart rhythm.

Atrial fibrillation is especially common in elderly patients. It can cause blood to pool in the heart. This increases the risk of blood clots and stroke (more about this later in the learning objective). Dysrhythmias that may be dangerous are treated with medications and sometimes surgery. Most hospital patients have cardiac monitoring in place that will alert the nurse to any changes in heart rhythm. PCTs should tell the nurse if a patient reports feeling a fluttering or thumping sensation in his chest.

Peripheral Vascular Disease (PVD)

Peripheral vascular disease (**PVD**) is a disease in which the legs, feet, arms, or hands do not have enough blood circulation. This is often due to fatty deposits in the blood vessels that harden over time. This form of PVD may cause the legs, feet, arms, and hands to feel cool or cold. Nail beds and/or feet may be ashen or blue.

PVD may also be caused by damage to the valves in the veins. These valves help keep blood moving toward the heart. When they are damaged, blood may pool in the legs. Swelling occurs in the hands and feet. Ulcers of the legs and feet may develop and can become infected. Pain may be very severe when walking; however, it is usually relieved with rest. Risk factors for peripheral vascular disease include smoking, diabetes, high cholesterol, hypertension, inactivity, and obesity. Treatment includes quitting smoking, medications, exercise, and surgery. The PCT may need to apply compression stockings to increase circulation to the legs and feet. Information about compression stockings is located in Chapter 10.

Deep Vein Thrombosis (DVT)

Blood clots can develop in the veins or arteries. Some blood disorders cause blood to clot more easily. Inactivity and damage to blood vessels can also increase the risk of blood clots. **Deep vein thrombosis** (**DVT**) occurs when a blood clot forms in the deep veins of the legs, pelvis, or arms. DVT happens most often in the veins of the calf. Symptoms include pain, swelling, discoloration, and warmth. The greatest danger of DVT is that a clot may travel to the lungs.

Because they can interrupt breathing and circulation, clots in the lungs have a higher risk of death. This condition is called **pulmonary embolism** (**PE**). It is most often caused by clots originally formed in the legs. Signs and symptoms include chest pain, shortness of breath, cyanosis, and anxiety.

Patients who have had surgery are at risk for developing DVT. PCTs should apply sequential compression devices or compression stockings as ordered and report any signs or symptoms of DVT to the nurse (Fig. 15-7). Following instructions for ambulation and/or range of motion exercises can also help prevent DVT.

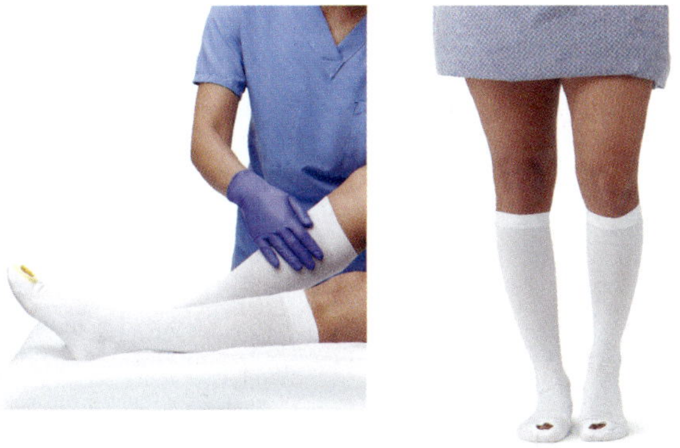

Fig. 15-7. *Compression stockings promote blood circulation and may need to be applied after surgery.* (IMAGES COURTESY OF MEDLINE INDUSTRIES, LP. USED WITH PERMISSION.)

Clots formed in the arteries can also be very dangerous. Clots that block blood flow through the coronary arteries can cause MI. Clots that block the arteries leading to the brain, or that travel to the brain, can cause a cerebrovascular accident (CVA)/stroke (Chapter 14). Some forms of dysrhythmia can cause blood to pool in the heart. This increases the risk of a clot forming. Artificial heart valves can also increase this risk. Signs and symptoms of CVA or MI must be reported immediately.

Sickle Cell Disease (SCD)

Sickle cell disease (**SCD**) is a condition that can cause anemia and many other health problems. **Anemia** is a condition in which the blood has an inadequate supply of red blood cells to supply oxygen to body tissues. SCD is the most common inherited blood condition in the US. It affects Black people at higher rates than other groups. As many as 1 in 365 Black Americans is born with SCD. In patients with SCD, unusual hemoglobin molecules cause red blood cells to become deformed. Instead of being disc-shaped, the cells are shaped like a sickle. A sickle is a C-shaped tool. These cells can get stuck in blood vessels. This causes extreme pain and can damage organs.

There are several forms of SCD. The severity can vary widely. SCD is usually diagnosed through screening tests done on all newborn infants. Medications and blood transfusions can help manage the disease. Bone marrow transplant can cure SCD, but it is a complicated process that cannot be used for every patient. New gene editing technologies may also be able to cure SCD. These treatments are still in the process of being developed and approved. It is very important for patients with SCD to get all routine vaccinations. This includes yearly flu shots.

Cancer

Leukemia is a type of cancer in which the bone marrow produces defective white blood cells. These abnormal white blood cells cannot defend the body against pathogens. Risk of developing leukemia can be increased by heredity or exposure to certain toxins. People who have had previous chemotherapy and radiation (common treatments for cancer) also have an increased risk for developing leukemia. In addition to standard cancer treatments (described in Chapter 21), bone marrow transplant may be used to treat leukemia. There are several different types of leukemia. Some forms mostly affect young children.

More information about the circulatory system and EKGs is located in Chapter 23.

Chapter Review

1. How many chambers does the human heart have? What are they called?
2. What are 4 functions of the circulatory system?
3. What is the function of the capillaries?
4. What are the 3 types of blood cells? What is the basic function of each cell type?
5. What blood pressure measurement, if it is consistent, is classified as hypertension?
6. What is the medical term for chest pain, pressure, or discomfort?
7. What are some parts of a cardiac rehabilitation plan?
8. List 7 care guidelines for a patient who has congestive heart failure.
9. The PCT should always report to the nurse when a patient is feeling either of these changes to their heart rhythm.
10. Which patients in the hospital may be at higher risk for developing a deep vein thrombosis (DVT)?
11. How is sickle cell disease usually detected? Which people have a higher risk of SCD?

16
The Respiratory System and Related Care

1. Describe the structure and function of the respiratory system

Respiration, the body taking in oxygen and removing carbon dioxide, involves breathing in, or *inspiration*, and breathing out, or *expiration*. The lungs accomplish this process (Fig. 16-1).

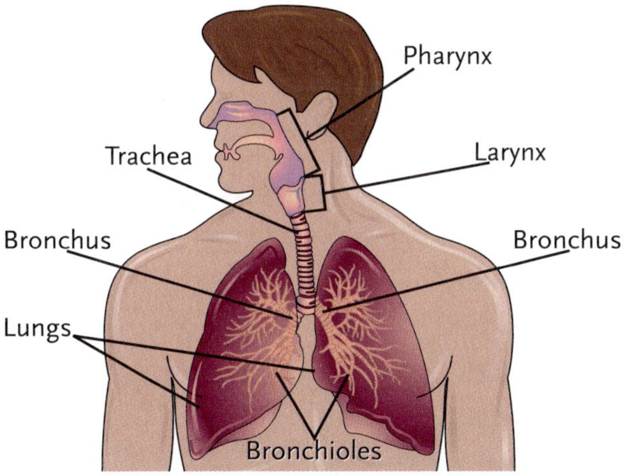

Fig. 16-1. *The respiratory process begins with inspiration through the nose or mouth. The air travels through the trachea and into the lungs via the bronchi, which then branch into bronchioles.*

As the lungs inhale, the air is pulled in through the nose and into the pharynx, a tubular passageway for both food and air. From the pharynx, air passes into the larynx, or voice box. The larynx is located at the beginning of the trachea, or windpipe. The trachea divides into 2 branches at its lower portion, the right bronchus and the left bronchus, or bronchi. Each bronchus leads into a lung and then subdivides into bronchioles. These smaller airways subdivide further. They end in alveoli: tiny sacs that appear in grape-like clusters. Blood is supplied to the alveoli by capillaries. Oxygen and carbon dioxide are exchanged between the alveoli and capillaries.

Oxygen-saturated blood then circulates through the capillaries and venules (small veins) of the lungs into the pulmonary vein and left side of the heart. The carbon dioxide is exhaled through the alveoli into the bronchioles and bronchi of the lungs, the trachea, through the larynx, the pharynx, and out the nose and mouth.

Each lung is covered by the pleura, a membrane with 2 layers. One is attached to the chest wall. The other is attached to the surface of the lung. The space between the layers is filled with a thin fluid that lubricates the layers, preventing them from rubbing together during breathing.

The functions of the respiratory system are to bring oxygen into the body and to eliminate carbon dioxide produced as the body uses oxygen.

Observing and Reporting: Respiratory System

Observe and report these signs and symptoms:

- O/R Change in respiratory rate
- O/R Shallow breathing or breathing through pursed lips; shortness of breath
- O/R Low oxygen saturation (below 95%)
- O/R Coughing or wheezing

- Nasal congestion or discharge
- Sore throat, difficulty swallowing, or swollen tonsils
- The need to sit after mild exertion
- Pale, bluish, or gray color of the lips, arms, and/or legs
- Pain in the chest area
- Discolored **sputum**, or mucus a person coughs up from the lungs (green, yellow, blood-tinged, or gray)

2. List common conditions of the respiratory system and discuss related care

Chronic Obstructive Pulmonary Disease (COPD)

Chronic obstructive pulmonary disease (**COPD**) is a chronic, progressive disease. This means a person may live for years with it but never be cured. Patients with COPD have trouble breathing, especially with getting air out of their lungs. There are 2 chronic lung diseases that are grouped under COPD: chronic bronchitis and emphysema.

Bronchitis is an irritation and inflammation of the lining of the bronchi. Chronic bronchitis is a form of bronchitis that is usually caused by cigarette smoking. Symptoms include coughing that brings up sputum (phlegm) and mucus. Breathlessness and wheezing may be present. Treatment includes stopping smoking and possibly medications.

Emphysema is a chronic disease of the lungs and also usually results from cigarette smoking. People with emphysema have trouble breathing. Other symptoms are coughing, breathlessness, and a rapid heartbeat. There is no cure for emphysema. Treatment includes managing symptoms, including pain. Oxygen therapy, as well as medications, may be prescribed. Quitting smoking is very important.

Over time, a patient with either of these lung disorders becomes chronically ill and weakened. There is a high risk of acute lung infections, such as pneumonia. **Pneumonia** is an illness that can be caused by a bacterial, viral, or fungal infection. Acute inflammation occurs in lung tissue. The affected person develops a high fever, chills, cough, greenish or yellow sputum, chest pains, and rapid pulse. Treatment includes antibiotics, along with plenty of fluids. Recovery may take longer for older adults and people with chronic illnesses. Pneumonia acquired in a hospital setting (*hospital-acquired pneumonia* [*HAP*], or *nosocomial pneumonia*) is a serious risk to these patients. PCTs should report signs and symptoms right away.

When the lungs and brain do not get enough oxygen, all body systems are affected. Patients may live with a constant fear of not being able to breathe. This can cause them to sit upright in an attempt to improve their ability to expand the lungs. These patients can have poor appetites. They usually do not get enough sleep. All of this can add to feelings of weakness and poor health. They may feel they have lost control of their bodies, particularly of their breathing. They may fear suffocation.

Patients with COPD may experience the following symptoms:

- Chronic cough or wheeze
- Difficulty breathing, especially when inhaling and exhaling deeply
- Shortness of breath, especially during physical effort
- Discolored, cyanotic, or reddish-purple skin
- Confusion
- General state of weakness
- Difficulty completing meals due to shortness of breath
- Fear and anxiety

Guidelines: COPD

- **G** Encourage patients who are trying to quit smoking. Quitting smoking helps improve symptoms of COPD.
- **G** Colds or viruses can make COPD worse. Always observe and report signs and symptoms of colds or illness.
- **G** Help patients sit upright or lean forward. Offer pillows for support (Fig. 16-2).

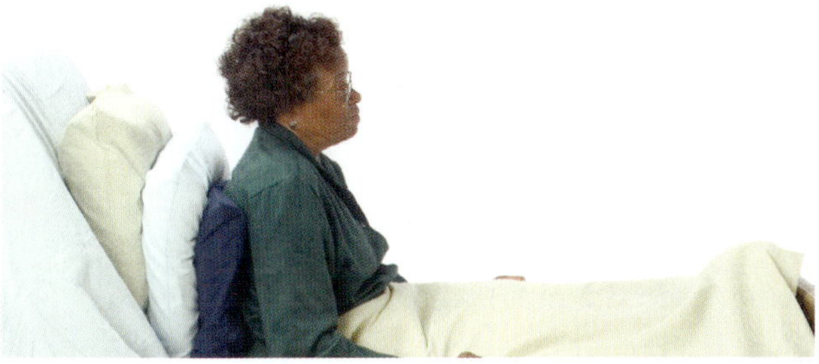

Fig. 16-2. *It helps patients with COPD to sit upright and lean forward slightly.*

- **G** Encourage the patient to drink plenty of fluids.
- **G** Encourage a well-balanced diet.
- **G** Keep an oxygen supply available as ordered. There is more information about supplemental oxygen later in this chapter.
- **G** Being unable to breathe or fearing suffocation can be very frightening. Be calm and supportive.
- **G** Use proper infection prevention practices. Wash your hands often and encourage the patient and visitors to do the same. Discard used tissues immediately.
- **G** Remind patients that respiratory infections can worsen their condition. Family and friends with respiratory illnesses (including colds, flu, and COVID-19) should not visit.
- **G** Encourage pursed-lip breathing. Pursed-lip breathing involves inhaling slowly through the nose and exhaling slowly through pursed lips (as if about to whistle). A nurse or respiratory therapist should teach patients how to do this.
- **G** Encourage patients to rest and save energy for important tasks.

Observing and Reporting: COPD

Report any of the following to the nurse:

- **O/R** Temperature over 101°F
- **O/R** Changes in breathing patterns, including shortness of breath
- **O/R** Changes in color or consistency of lung secretions
- **O/R** Changes in mental state or personality
- **O/R** Signs that the patient is not taking medications (e.g., pills pocketed in the patient's cheek or placed under a pillow)
- **O/R** Weight loss
- **O/R** Increasing need for help with ADLs

Asthma

Asthma is a chronic, episodic disorder. It occurs when the respiratory system is hyperreactive (that is, it reacts quickly and strongly) to irritants, infection, cold air, or allergens such as pollen and dust. Exercise and stress can also worsen asthma. When the bronchi become irritated due to any of these triggers, they constrict, making it difficult to breathe. As a response to irritation and inflammation, the mucous membrane produces thick mucus. This further inhibits respiration. As a result, air is trapped in the lungs, causing coughing and wheezing.

The exact cause of asthma is unknown. It may be caused by a combination of factors, such as family history and certain environmental exposures. Treatment for asthma includes medications that are given directly into the lungs using sprays or inhalers (Fig. 16-3). Patients with asthma should avoid triggers that bring on asthma attacks, such as allergens, smoke, strong odors, and strenuous exercise.

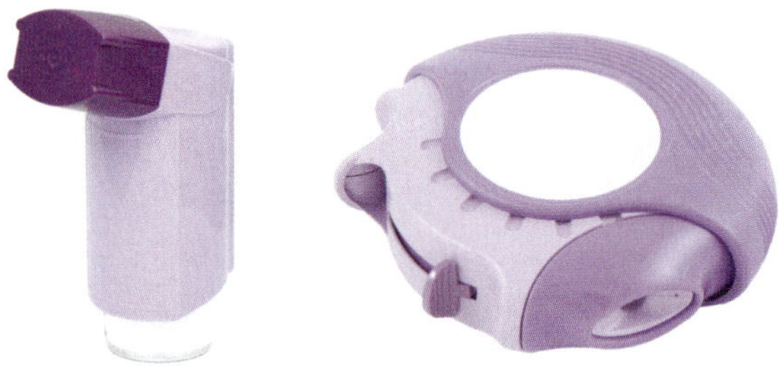

Fig. 16-3. Two types of asthma inhalers.

Bronchiectasis

Bronchiectasis is a condition in which the bronchial tubes are abnormally enlarged. A person may have it in childhood or may acquire it later in life as a result of chronic infections and inflammation. Cystic fibrosis is a common cause of bronchiectasis. This abnormal state of the bronchial tubes is permanent. Bronchiectasis causes chronic coughing, which produces thick white or green sputum. A person with this disorder may have recurrent pneumonia and weight loss.

Treatment of bronchiectasis includes controlling infections and preventing complications. Antibiotics may be prescribed. Postural drainage may be ordered to eliminate fluid from the lungs. Postural drainage involves using different body positions to drain mucus from the lungs or to loosen it so that it can be coughed up.

Influenza

Influenza, often called the flu, is a respiratory illness caused by a virus. Different strains of the flu virus spread each year. Flu is especially common in the fall and winter. Influenza usually begins suddenly with a fever and/or chills. Muscle aches and fatigue are common. Congestion, headache, sore throat, and cough may also occur. Some people have nausea, vomiting, or diarrhea. These symptoms are more often seen in children.

Influenza can cause serious problems. It may lead to pneumonia, or to inflammation in the tissues of the heart or the brain. Treatment includes antiviral medications to reduce the severity of illness.

Cancer

Lung cancer is the growth of abnormal cells or tumors in the lungs. Symptoms of lung cancer include chronic cough, shortness of breath, and bloody sputum. Cancer can also affect the pharynx (throat) or larynx (voice box). More information about cancer is located in Chapter 21.

Tuberculosis (TB)

Tuberculosis, or **TB**, is a highly contagious disease caused by a bacterium, *Mycobacterium tuberculosis*, that is carried on mucous droplets suspended in the air. The bacteria usually affect the lungs, which is known as *pulmonary tuberculosis*. TB is an airborne disease. People can be exposed to TB when they spend time with a person who is infected with TB. When the infected person talks, coughs, breathes, sings, laughs, or sneezes, he may spread the disease. Pulmonary tuberculosis causes coughing, trouble breathing, fever, weight loss, and fatigue (Fig. 16-4). Usually it can be cured by taking all prescribed medication. However, if left untreated, TB may cause death.

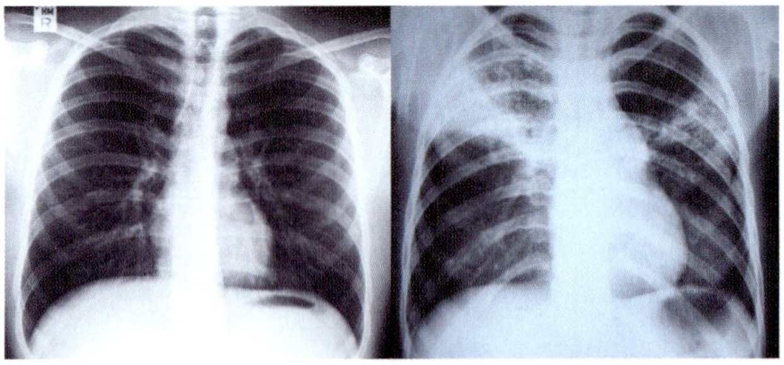

Fig. 16-4. A normal lung X-ray on the left, and an X-ray of a lung with tuberculosis on the right.

There are 2 types of tuberculosis: **latent TB infection (LTBI)** and **TB disease**. Someone with latent TB infection carries the disease but does not show symptoms and cannot infect others. A person with TB disease shows symptoms of the disease and can spread TB to others. Latent TB infection can progress to TB disease. These are some signs and symptoms of TB:

- Fatigue
- Loss of appetite
- Weight loss
- Slight fever and chills
- Night sweats
- Prolonged coughing
- Coughing up blood
- Chest pain
- Shortness of breath
- Trouble breathing

Tuberculosis is more likely to be spread in areas with poor ventilation or in small, confined spaces. People are more likely to get TB disease if their immune systems are weakened by illness, malnutrition, cancer, HIV/AIDS, alcoholism, or substance use disorder.

Multidrug-resistant TB (**MDR-TB**) is a form of tuberculosis that is caused by an organism that is resistant to medication that is used to treat TB. **Resistant** means that drugs no longer work to kill the specific bacteria. It may develop when a person infected with TB does not take all of his prescribed medication. When the full course of medication is not taken, bacteria remain in the body and are less likely to be killed by the medication. The disease becomes more difficult to cure. Drug resistance may also result if TB medication is used or stored incorrectly or the medication is of poor quality.

Hospital employees are generally required to be tested for tuberculosis before they can begin working, and they may be tested again annually. PCTs must follow their facility's policy.

Guidelines: Tuberculosis

G Follow Standard Precautions and Airborne Precautions.

G Wear personal protective equipment as instructed during care. Special masks (respirators), such as N95 or high efficiency particulate air (HEPA) masks, are required. These masks help prevent a person from inhaling droplets. You must be fitted for these respirators and will be trained how to use them.

G Use special care when handling sputum or phlegm. **Phlegm** is thick mucus from the respiratory passage.

G Patients with TB will be placed in an airborne infection isolation room (AIIR). These rooms have a controlled flow of air. All of the air inside the room will be exhausted directly to the outside, or all air will first be recirculated through a special HEPA filter before returning to circulation. The room will be marked with a sign identifying it as a special respiratory isolation room. Keep doors to these rooms closed except when entering or exiting the room. When entering this room, do not open or close the door quickly. This pulls contaminated room air into the hallway.

G Follow isolation procedures for airborne diseases if directed.

G Failure to take all medication is a major factor in the spread of TB. Report to the nurse if you see signs that a patient may not be taking all of her medications.

COVID-19

In late 2019 a new human coronavirus was identified in Wuhan, China. Although there are many types of coronaviruses (some of which cause mild respiratory illnesses like the common cold), this virus had not previously been seen in humans. This virus, called *severe acute respiratory syndrome coronavirus 2* (*SARS-CoV-2*), causes coronavirus disease, or COVID-19. COVID-19 was declared a pandemic in March 2020 by the World Health Organization. (SARS-CoV-2 is not the same virus that caused the SARS outbreak in 2003.)

COVID-19 (coronavirus disease) is classified as both a droplet and airborne disease. It is transmitted through respiratory droplets produced when the infected person breathes, sneezes, coughs, sings, or talks. It is also carried on mucous droplets suspended in the air. It can spread easily among people who are in close contact, within 6 feet of one another. However, inhalation of the virus in the air can also occur at distances greater than 6 feet. Aerosol particles can move through an indoor space and can linger for some time even after an infected person has left the area. Enclosed/indoor spaces with poor ventilation increase the risk of infection, as do crowded spaces and prolonged exposure. In addition, the CDC states it may be possible for a person to become infected by touching a surface or an object that has the virus on it and then touching his nose or mouth, but this is not considered the main method of transmission.

Signs and symptoms of COVID-19 often appear within 3–5 days of exposure to the virus. They include fever, chills, cough, congestion, fatigue, and shortness of breath. Muscle aches, sore throat, loss of taste or smell, nausea or vomiting, diarrhea, and headache are also signs and symptoms. Some people experience mild symptoms, while others have severe symptoms that require hospitalization, medication, and the use of a ventilator (a machine that assists with or replaces breathing when a person cannot breathe on his own). The disease can also result in death.

People who are at a higher risk for serious complications and death from this disease include older adults and people of any age with certain underlying conditions.

Some people develop *long COVID* or *post-COVID conditions* (*PCC*) after having the disease, which has been defined as signs, symptoms, and conditions lasting 3 months or more after having the virus that were not present before the person had SARS-CoV-2 infection or COVID-19. Long COVID can happen even in patients who had a mild infection.

Treatment for COVID-19 includes antiviral medications and monoclonal antibodies. Some treatments need to be started immediately in order to be effective in reducing the risk of serious illness or death.

Several vaccines have been approved for preventing or reducing the severity of COVID-19. The recommended vaccine may be a single dose or multiple doses, depending on a person's age and health condition. The CDC encourages everyone to remain up to date with all recommended COVID-19 vaccine doses.

If possible, a patient with this infection will be placed in a single-person room or in a room with another patient who has COVID-19. The door should be kept closed. Ideally certain staff members will be assigned to care for certain patients. This helps build relationships with patients, and it decreases the number of staff members interacting with each patient.

A patient with COVID-19 will be asked to stay in his room as much as possible. Leaving the room should be limited to what is considered medically necessary.

Guidelines: Caring for Patients with Suspected or Confirmed COVID-19

Healthcare facilities must follow federal and state guidelines, so policies may change as new information becomes available.

G Follow Standard Precautions and Transmission-Based Precautions.

G Wash your hands often. Use soap and running water and scrub for at least 20 seconds. If soap and water is not available, use a hand sanitizer that contains at least 60% alcohol.

- **G** Wear the proper mask—usually an N95 or other respirator—that covers your nose and mouth when caring for the patient (Fig. 16-5). Wear additional PPE (gown, gloves, and eye protection) as required.

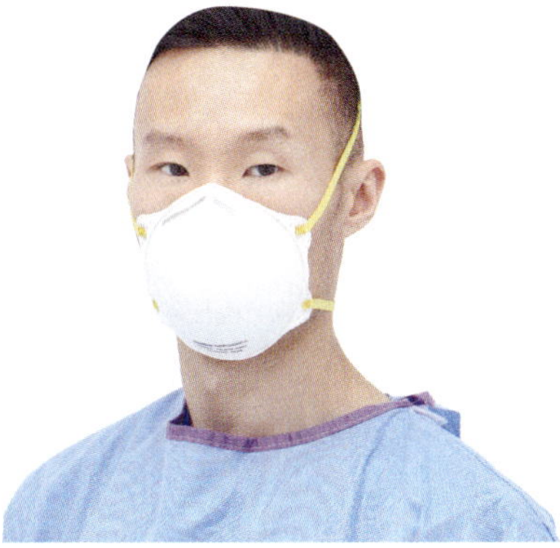

Fig. 16-5. *Healthcare workers should wear an N95 or other respirator that covers their nose and mouth when caring for patients with COVID-19.* (IMAGE COURTESY OF MEDLINE INDUSTRIES, LP. USED WITH PERMISSION.)

- **G** When you are in the patient's room, maintain a distance of at least 6 feet when possible. Keep the door closed.
- **G** Visitors should also wear a high-quality mask and maintain a distance of 6 feet when possible.
- **G** Because enclosed spaces with poor ventilation increase the risk of infection, help improve room ventilation as directed, such as by opening windows.
- **G** The patient will need to be monitored more frequently. Measure vital signs as ordered and report changes to the supervisor immediately. Report anything that the patient tells you about his symptoms.
- **G** Do not share any personal items among patients.
- **G** Clean frequently touched surfaces with the proper cleaning spray or wipes.
- **G** Encourage patients to rest and drink fluids to maintain hydration.
- **G** Do not touch your eyes, nose, or mouth. Wash your hands after coughing or sneezing.
- **G** Do not go to work if you feel sick or have a fever. Follow your facility's policies regarding testing, quarantine, and isolation.
- **G** For many people, symptoms improve within a week, but it is important to report any signs and symptoms that indicate the illness is getting worse:
    - Difficulty breathing or shortness of breath
    - Chest pain or pressure
    - Confusion
    - Difficulty waking or remaining alert
    - Prolonged elevated temperature
    - Discolored or cyanotic skin

3. Describe how to assist with breathing exercises

Deep breathing exercises help expand the lungs, clearing them of mucus and preventing infections such as pneumonia. Patients who have had surgery or who are paralyzed are often instructed to do deep breathing exercises regularly to expand the lungs. There may also be orders for the patient to be turned regularly. This protects the patient's skin, preventing pressure injuries. It also makes it easier to clear mucus from the lungs.

Guidelines: Breathing and Coughing Exercises

- **G** Know what exercises are ordered. If you are not familiar with an exercise, ask the nurse for help. *Diaphragmatic breathing*, also called *abdominal breathing*, is a common form of therapeutic breathing. (One method is described below; follow instructions for exercises done at your facility.)
- **G** Position the patient as ordered. Breathing exercises may be done with the patient in the supine, Fowler's, or semi-Fowler's position. This depends on the patient's condition.

- **G** Follow the care plan or nurse's instructions to protect surgical incisions. If there is a surgical incision on the patient's torso, a pillow or other protective covering may be held over it during the exercises.
- **G** Have tissues and/or an emesis basin ready in case the patient needs to spit out respiratory mucus during the exercises. Use PPE as ordered (e.g., gloves, high-quality mask/respirator).
- **G** For diaphragmatic breathing, follow instructions for where to place the patient's hands. One way is to have the patient place both hands just below the rib cage with fingers barely touching. The patient then tries to breathe in deeply so that the touching fingers separate. Patients may also be asked to place one hand just below the rib cage and one hand on the chest. The patient then breathes in so that the hand below the rib cage rises and the hand on the chest does not.
- **G** Ask the patient to breathe in deeply through the nose, hold the breath for a count of 3, then breathe out through pursed lips.
- **G** Have the patient rest and then repeat this as many times and as often as ordered (usually 10 deep breaths once an hour).
- **G** At the end of the exercises, ask the patient to breathe in deeply one last time and then cough 2–3 times.

A patient's care plan may include using a deep breathing device called an incentive spirometer (Fig. 16-6). Incentive spirometry helps the patient to take long, slow, deep breaths. The device has an air chamber with a ball or other indicator that rises as the patient inhales through the connected tube. A marker can be set to show the goal height for the indicator. A licensed healthcare provider determines the patient's spirometry goal. An incentive spirometer is used for only one patient and is either sent home with the patient at discharge or discarded.

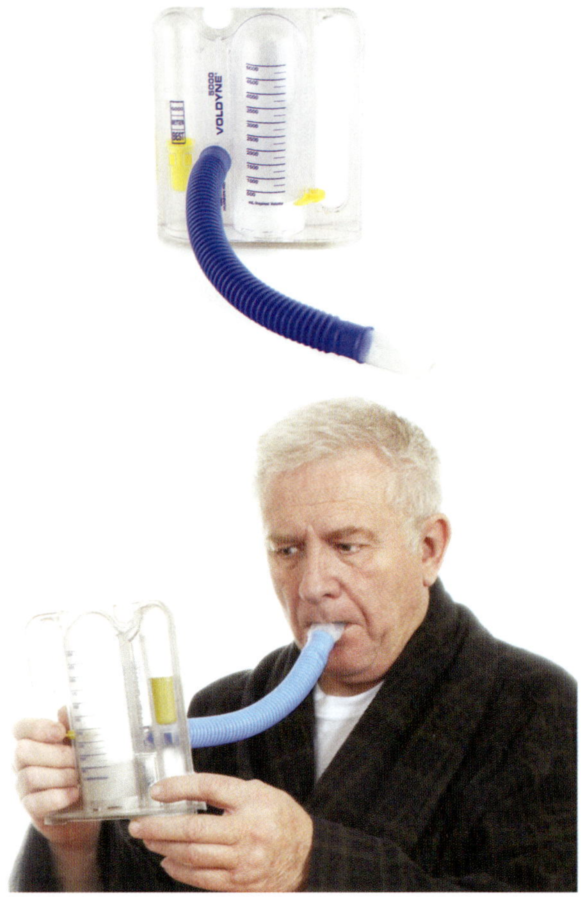

Fig. 16-6. *Incentive spirometers are used for deep breathing exercises.*

Assisting with an incentive spirometer

Equipment: incentive spirometer, gloves (and other PPE as required), pillow (if needed), tissues

1. Identify yourself by name. Identify the patient according to facility policy.
2. Wash your hands.
3. Explain the procedure to the patient. Speak clearly, slowly, and directly. Maintain face-to-face contact whenever possible.
4. Provide for the patient's privacy with a curtain, screen, or door.
5. Adjust the bed to a safe level, usually waist high. Lock the bed wheels.
6. Position the patient according to the nurse's instructions. The patient should be sitting as upright as possible. It is better if the patient

can sit on the edge of the bed. If there is a surgical incision on the patient's torso, a pillow or other protective covering may be held over it during the exercises.

7. Put on gloves and other PPE as required. Using an incentive spirometer may cause the patient to cough. If the patient has a known or suspected respiratory illness, wear a high-quality mask or respirator.
8. Remove any packaging from the incentive spirometer. Set the goal marker to the level indicated in the care plan.
9. Show the incentive spirometer to the patient and tell the patient he will follow these steps to use it:
   - Breathe out normally
   - Place the mouthpiece in his mouth and seal his lips around it
   - Breathe in as slowly and as deeply as possible, trying to raise the ball/indicator at least as high as the goal marker
   - Hold his breath for 3–5 seconds
   - Remove the mouthpiece and breathe out slowly
10. Hand the spirometer to the patient. Coach the patient to complete the steps listed above.
11. Allow the patient to rest for several seconds. Repeat the steps as ordered in the care plan. Spirometry may need to be done every 1–2 hours. The steps may be repeated, anywhere from 3–15 times.
12. Stop the exercise and report to the nurse if the patient reports dizziness or chest pain or has difficulty breathing. If the patient coughs out mucus during the exercise, offer tissues. Ask the patient to discard any used tissues in the trash.
13. Clean and store the patient's incentive spirometer according to facility policy. The patient will use the same device every time the exercises are performed.
14. Remove and discard your PPE.
15. Wash your hands.
16. Return the bed to its lowest position. Remove privacy measures.
17. Place the call light within the patient's reach.
18. Report any changes in the patient to the nurse.
19. Document the procedure using facility guidelines.

4. Discuss oral suctioning

Some patients may be unable to remove respiratory secretions from their mouths. Paralysis from a CVA or other condition may cause this situation. Patients who have dysphagia or who are unconscious may also have secretions build up. Oral suctioning is ordered when a patient cannot clear secretions from his mouth on his own for any reason. PCTs may be assigned to perform oral suctioning. Suctioning may be performed using a bulb syringe or using a device called a **Yankauer suction catheter** (Fig. 16-7). A Yankauer suction catheter is a rigid, hollow tube with a bend that makes it easier to maneuver. Different styles have tips with different shapes. In a hospital, Yankauer suctioning is much more common than bulb suctioning.

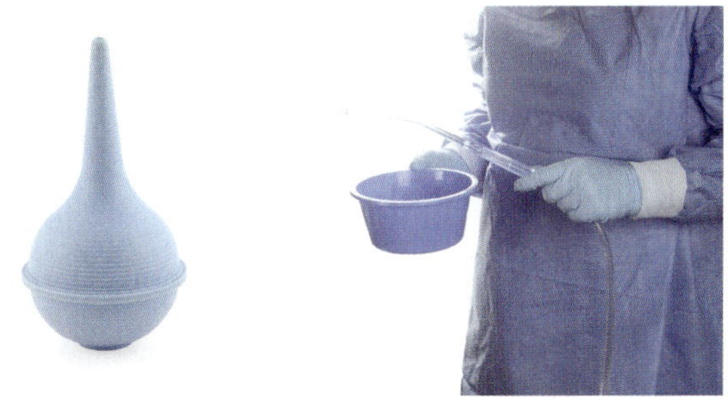

Fig. 16-7. *A bulb syringe or Yankauer suction catheter may be used to remove oral secretions or mucus from a patient's mouth.*

Most hospitals have a vacuum attachment, often called wall suction, in the wall near every patient bed. Suction devices are connected to the vacuum attachment (Fig. 16-8). The level of suction can be adjusted based on the age and condition of the patient. The canister that collects suctioned materials has volume markings. The volume is measured as output. Flexible tubing connects the vacuum to the Yankauer suction catheter. With many systems, suction is started and stopped when a healthcare worker plugs or unplugs a vent hole on the Yankauer with their thumb. Suction levels are measured in millimeters of mercury (mm Hg), like blood pressure. Levels for newborn babies are lower than levels for older children and adults. PCTs do not decide what level of suction to use. They must use the setting determined by a licensed healthcare provider.

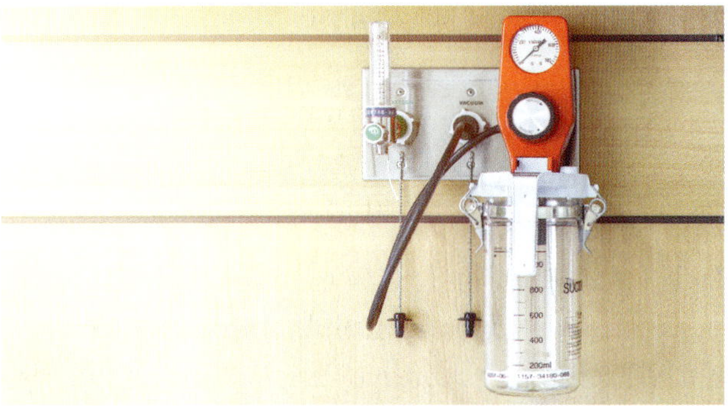

Fig. 16-8. *Vacuum attachments in hospitals make it possible to perform suction at a patient's bedside without bringing in a separate vacuum device.*

Performing oral suctioning using a Yankauer suction catheter

Equipment: Yankauer suction catheter of the ordered size/type, connective tubing, gloves (and other PPE as required), sterile water or saline for rinsing (follow facility policy), basin for rinsing liquid

1. Identify yourself by name. Identify the patient according to facility policy.
2. Wash your hands.
3. Explain the procedure to the patient. Speak clearly, slowly, and directly. Maintain face-to-face contact whenever possible. It is important to explain the procedure even if the patient is unconscious.
4. Provide for the patient's privacy with a curtain, screen, or door.
5. Adjust the bed to a safe level, usually waist high. Lock the bed wheels.
6. Assist the patient to semi-Fowler's position with her head turned toward you. If the patient must stay in supine position, the head should still be turned toward you.
7. Put on gloves and other PPE as required.
8. Pour sterile water or saline into the basin.
9. Use the tubing to connect the Yankauer suction catheter to the wall suction unit. The nurse usually sets the suction level. Check to be sure the suction is set to the ordered level.
10. Test the suction. This is often done by plugging the vent hole on the Yankauer catheter with your thumb. With the hole plugged, place the tip in the basin of rinsing liquid and suction a small amount. Remove your thumb to stop suction.
11. Place the end of the Yankauer catheter in the patient's mouth. Start suction according to device instructions. (Often this involves placing your thumb over a vent hole.)
12. Gently move the tip of the Yankauer catheter to suction any visible secretions in the patient's mouth. Do not use suction for more than 10 seconds at a time. As needed, stop suction by removing your thumb from the vent hole (or other action, based on the device). Remove the Yankauer suction catheter from the patient's mouth, and suction liquid from the basin to rinse the catheter.
13. Before finishing, move the Yankauer catheter all around the patient's mouth, including between the teeth/gums and cheeks and under the tongue. Rinse frequently.

14. Oral care may be ordered for some patients after suctioning (see Chapter 9).
15. Catheters and tubing are usually discarded and replaced on a schedule (e.g., every 48 hours). Store Yankauer catheter and tubing according to facility policy or discard in a biohazard waste bag if assigned to do so.
16. Remove and discard your PPE.
17. Wash your hands.
18. Return the bed to its lowest position. Remove privacy measures.
19. Place the call light within the patient's reach.
20. Report any changes in the patient to the nurse, including changes in the patient's secretions.
21. Document the procedure using facility guidelines. This may include documenting the amount of suctioned secretions in the patient's I&O record.

5. Discuss artificial airways, mechanical ventilation, chest tubes, and related care

An **artificial airway** is any tube inserted into the respiratory tract to maintain or promote breathing. Artificial airways keep the airway open. This is necessary when the airway is obstructed due to illness, injury, secretions, or aspiration. Some patients who are unconscious need an artificial airway.

The artificial airway is inserted using a method called **intubation**. Intubation involves the passage of a plastic tube through the mouth, nose, or an opening in the neck and into the trachea (windpipe). There are different types of artificial airways. One common type is a **tracheostomy**, which is a surgically created opening through the neck into the trachea. A hollow tube, called a *tracheostomy tube* or *trach tube*, is inserted through this opening into the trachea. More information on this type of artificial airway may be found later in this learning objective.

Guidelines: Artificial Airways

G Check the patient regularly. If the tubing falls out, tell the nurse immediately.

G Monitor vital signs as ordered. Report changes to the nurse.

G Perform oral care often, as directed.

G Watch for biting and tugging on the tube. If a patient is doing this, tell the nurse.

G Use other methods of communication if the patient cannot speak. Try writing notes, drawing pictures, and using communication boards. Watch for hand and eye signals.

G Be supportive and reassuring. It can be frightening and uncomfortable to have an artificial airway. Some patients may choke or gag. Be empathetic. Imagine how it might feel to have a tube in your nose, mouth, or throat.

A tracheostomy is a common type of artificial airway (Fig. 16-9). Tracheostomies may be necessary for many reasons, including the following:

- Tumors/cancer
- Infection
- Severe neck or mouth injuries
- Facial surgery and facial burns
- Long-term unconsciousness or coma
- Obstruction in the airway
- Paralysis of muscles related to breathing
- Aspiration as a result of muscle or sensory problems in the throat
- Severe allergic reaction
- Gunshot wound

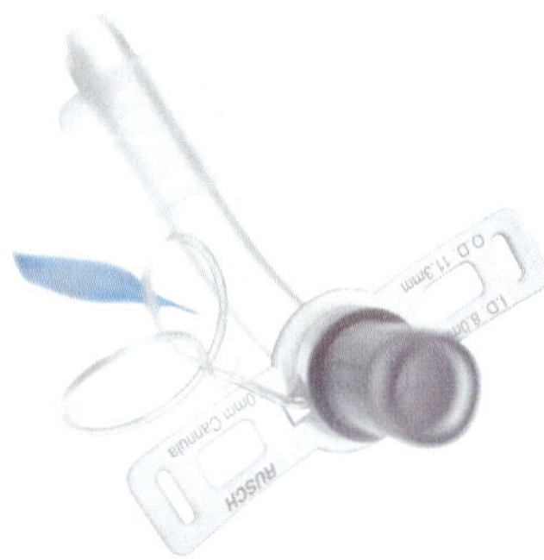

Fig. 16-9. *A tracheostomy tube is inserted into the trachea through a surgically created opening in the neck.* (IMAGE COURTESY OF TELEFLEX INCORPORATED.)

This procedure is usually temporary, but it can be permanent. It is easier to suction and attach respiratory equipment with a tracheostomy than with other artificial airways.

When the tracheostomy is first placed, it may be difficult for the patient to adapt to breathing through the tube. This can cause anxiety and frustration. It may be impossible for the patient to talk or make sounds at first, which also causes anxiety. During this time, PCTs should be especially supportive and encouraging. They can use other methods of communication, such as writing notes, drawing pictures, using communication boards, and using hand and eye signals. Checking on the patient often and answering call lights immediately may help lessen anxiety. People can usually learn to talk through a trach tube using a device called a speaking valve.

General tracheostomy care includes keeping the skin around the opening clean, helping with dressing changes, and cleaning the device. PCT responsibilities related to tracheostomies mostly involve observing and reporting.

Observing and Reporting: Tracheostomies

Report any of the following to the nurse:

O/R Shortness of breath

O/R Trouble breathing

O/R Gurgling sounds

O/R Any signs of skin breakdown around the opening, such as irritation, rash, cracks, breaks, sores, or bleeding on the skin

O/R The type and amount of discharge that the patient coughs up through the tracheostomy (normal discharge looks like white mucus or saliva)

O/R Any increase in the amount of discharge

O/R Discharge that is thick, yellow, green, bloody, or has an odor (this may indicate an infection or other problem in the lungs)

O/R Mouth sores or discomfort

O/R Disconnected tubing

Suctioning of the airway may be required for patients with tracheostomies. PCTs do not perform tracheostomy suctioning, but they may assist the nurse. They may also report signs that indicate suctioning is needed.

Guidelines: Airway Suctioning

G A patient who needs frequent suctioning may show signs of respiratory distress. Report signs of respiratory distress to the nurse immediately:

- Gurgling sounds
- Difficulty breathing
- Elevated respiratory rate
- Pale, cyanotic, or gray skin around the eyes, mouth, fingernails, or toenails
- Nostrils flaring (nostrils opening wider when breathing in may show that a person is having to work harder to breathe)
- Retracting (chest appears to sink in below the neck with each breath)
- Sweating
- Wheezing

G Monitor vital signs closely, especially respiratory rate. Report changes. Monitor oxygen saturation and report levels below 95%.

- **G** Follow Standard Precautions. Don gloves, gown, mask, or goggles as directed.
- **G** Assist the nurse with suctioning as needed. You may be asked to have a towel or washcloth ready to clean the patient after suctioning. Give oral care as ordered.
- **G** Report patient complaints of pain or difficulty breathing.

It is very important to prevent respiratory infections when caring for patients with tracheostomies. PCTs must wash their hands often and wear gloves when indicated. PCTs should wear masks if patients are coughing. It is vital that equipment be kept clean. Anything that is dropped on the floor must be sterilized before it can come in contact with the tubes. Great care must be taken so that nothing gets into the tube, which can cause an infection in the lungs.

Patients who cannot breathe on their own may be on a mechanical ventilator. **Mechanical ventilation** uses a machine to inflate and deflate the lungs. A person may require mechanical ventilation due to cardiac or respiratory arrest, lung injuries and diseases, or head and spinal cord injuries.

A patient will not be able to speak while on the mechanical ventilator. This is because air will no longer reach the larynx (vocal cords). Not being able to speak may increase anxiety. The patient may think that no one will know if they are having trouble breathing. Being on a ventilator has been compared to breathing through a straw. PCTs should be empathetic and think about how that might feel. The patient will need a lot of support while connected to the ventilator. The PCT should enter the room often so that the patient can see her. This helps to reassure the patient that they are being carefully observed. Clipboards, notepads, and communication boards will help with communication.

Patients on ventilators are often heavily sedated (Fig. 16-10). A **sedative** is an agent or drug that helps calm and soothe a person and may cause sleep. For a patient on a ventilator, being sedated helps lessen discomfort and anxiety. Even if a patient seems unaware of what is happening, the PCT must continue to speak to them and explain what she is doing.

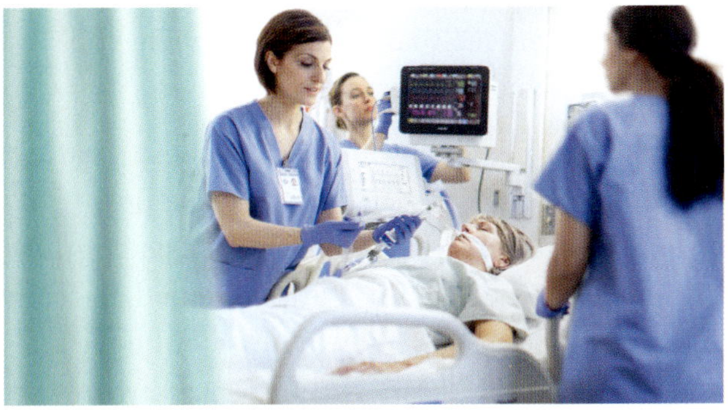

Fig. 16-10. *A patient on a mechanical ventilator is often heavily sedated to lessen discomfort and anxiety. Being on a ventilator has been compared to breathing through a straw.*

Guidelines: Mechanical Ventilator

- **G** Ventilators cause an increased risk for a special type of pneumonia. Wash your hands often when working with patients on mechanical ventilators.
- **G** Report to the nurse if the alarm sounds.
- **G** If you notice tubing that is disconnected or loose, report it immediately.
- **G** Answer the call light promptly.
- **G** Follow the care plan for repositioning instructions. The head of the bed may need to remain elevated.
- **G** Give regular, careful skin care to prevent pressure injuries. Check the skin around the intubation site often, as well as on the rest of the body. Report any of the following:
  - Swelling
  - Sores, redness, irritation
  - Fluid or blood draining from skin
  - Broken skin

- **G** Report if the patient is pulling on or biting the tube. Report if the patient is anxious, fearful, or upset.
- **G** Be patient during communication. Observe body language. Watch for hand or eye signals.
- **G** Check on the patient often, so that the patient can see that you are there. Be supportive, kind, and empathetic.

Chest tubes are hollow drainage tubes that are inserted into the chest during a sterile procedure. They can be inserted at the bedside or during surgery. Chest tubes drain air, blood or other fluid, or pus that has collected inside the pleural cavity. The *pleural cavity* is the space between the layers of the pleura, the thin membrane that covers and protects the lungs. Chest tubes are also inserted to allow a full expansion of the lungs. Some conditions that require chest tube insertion include the following:

- Air or gas in the pleural space (pneumothorax)
- Blood in the pleural space (hemothorax)
- Pus in the pleural space (empyema)
- Certain types of surgery
- Chest trauma or injuries

A provider normally inserts chest tubes. The chest tube is connected to a drainage system. When X-rays show that the air, blood, or fluid has been drained, the tube is removed.

Guidelines: Chest Tubes

- **G** Be aware of the number and location of chest tubes. Tubes may be in the front, back, or on the side of the body.
- **G** Check vital signs as directed. Report any changes immediately to the nurse.
- **G** Report signs of respiratory distress to the nurse immediately. Report complaints of pain.
- **G** Make sure drainage containers remain upright, level, and lower than the patient's chest at all times.
- **G** Make sure that tubing is not kinked or disconnected. Report problems with tubing to the nurse right away.
- **G** Certain equipment is kept nearby in case tubes are pulled out. Do not remove these items from the area.
- **G** Follow the repositioning schedule. Be very gentle with turning and repositioning. You must move the patient and the tubes at the same time to prevent the tubes from coming out. Always get enough help.
- **G** Provide rest periods as needed.
- **G** Follow fluid intake orders. Measure intake and output carefully, as ordered.
- **G** If asked to help with coughing and deep breathing exercises, be encouraging and patient.
- **G** Observe for and report the following:
    - Changes in color or amount of chest drainage
    - Increase or decrease in bubbling in the drainage system
    - Clots in the tubing
    - Odor in the chest tube area

6. Explain oxygen therapy and related care

Oxygen therapy is the administration of oxygen to increase the supply of oxygen to the lungs. This increases the availability of oxygen to the body tissues. Oxygen therapy is used to treat breathing difficulties and is prescribed by a provider. Nurses and respiratory therapists may administer oxygen therapy. PCTs should not stop, adjust, or administer oxygen for a patient.

In a hospital, oxygen is piped into a patient's room through a central system. In other settings, it may be in tanks or produced by an oxygen concentrator. Compressed oxygen and liquid oxygen are stored in tanks of varying sizes (Fig. 16-11). An oxygen concentrator produces and distributes oxygen, but it does not store oxygen.

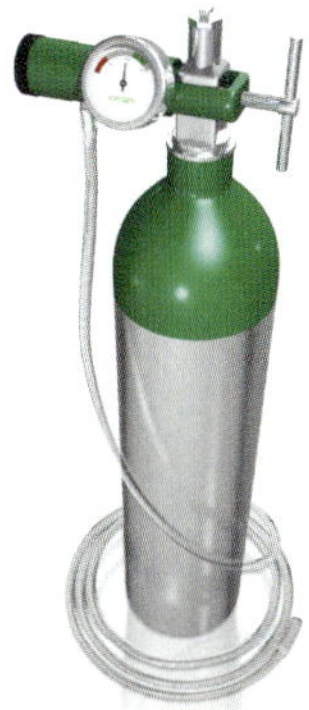

Fig. 16-11. *This is one type of oxygen tank.*

Some patients receive oxygen through a nasal cannula. A **nasal cannula** is a piece of plastic tubing that fits around the face and over the ears. The face piece has 2 short prongs made of tubing. These prongs fit inside the nose, and oxygen is delivered through them. A respiratory therapist or nurse fits the cannula. The length of the prongs (usually no more than 1/2 an inch) is adjusted for the patient's comfort. The patient can talk and eat while wearing the cannula (Fig. 16-12).

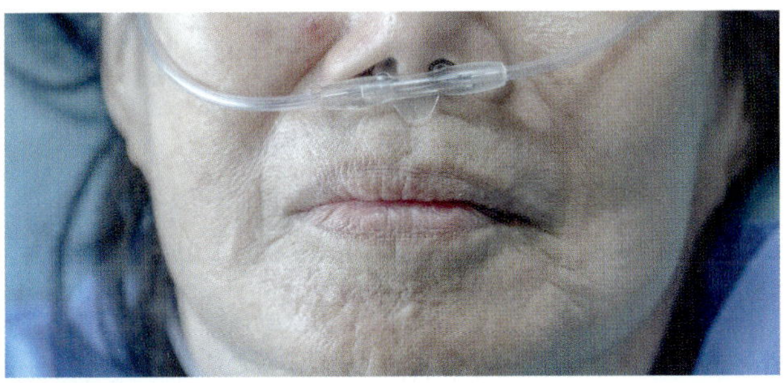

Fig. 16-12. *A nasal cannula.*

Patients who do not need concentrated oxygen all the time may use a face mask when they need oxygen (Fig. 16-13). The face mask fits over the nose and mouth. It is secured by a strap that goes over the ears and around the back of the head. Plastic tubing connects the mask to the oxygen source. The mask should be checked to see that it fits snugly on the patient's face, but it should not pinch the face. It is difficult for a patient to talk when wearing an oxygen face mask. The mask must be removed to eat or drink anything.

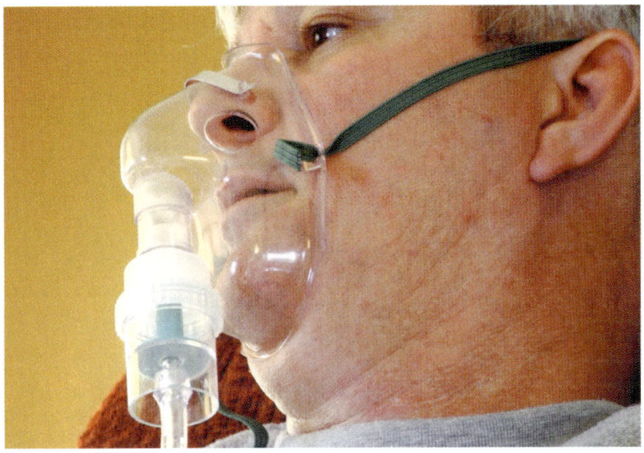

Fig. 16-13. *Patients who need oxygen only occasionally may use a face mask.*

Oxygen can be irritating to the nose and mouth. The nasal cannula or strap on a face mask can also cause irritation around the ears. PCTs should wash and dry skin carefully and provide frequent mouth care. They should offer the patient plenty of fluids and report any irritation observed.

Oxygen is a very dangerous fire hazard because it makes other things burn (supports combustion).

Guidelines: Oxygen Delivery Devices

- **G** A flow meter shows how much oxygen is flowing out to the patient at any time. It should be set at the amount stated in the care plan. If it is not, report this to the nurse. Do not adjust the oxygen level.
- **G** Oxygen is drying. Because of this, a humidifying bottle adds moisture to the oxygen administered to patients. Make sure the humidifying bottle has distilled water in it

and is attached correctly. Wash the humidifying bottle according to the care plan or equipment supplier's instructions.

- G Oxygen can be irritating to the nose and mouth. The strap of the nasal cannula or face mask can also cause irritation around the ears. Check the nasal area and behind the ears for signs of irritation. Report and document any irritation you observe.
- G Change the nasal cannula when ordered. It must be changed when it is hard or cracked. It should also be changed after the patient has had a cold or the flu.
- G If oxygen is ordered only for a certain period, you may be assigned to count and record pulse rate and respirations before and after the patient uses the oxygen to see if there are any changes.

Understand that oxygen is a very dangerous fire hazard because it makes other things burn (supports combustion). Combustion means the process of burning. Follow these safety precautions when working around oxygen:

- G Remove all fire hazards from the room or area. Fire hazards include electrical equipment, such as electric razors. Other fire hazards are cigarettes, matches, and flammable liquids. **Flammable** means easily ignited and capable of burning quickly. Examples of flammable liquids are alcohol and nail polish remover. Read the labels on liquids if you are unsure. If they say *flammable*, remove them from the area. Notify the nurse if a patient does not want a fire hazard removed.
- G Do not use an extension cord with an oxygen concentrator.
- G Do not place oxygen tubing under furniture.
- G If an oxygen tank is used, it must be secured and prevented from falling over. A falling oxygen tank may release oxygen at a dangerous rate.
- G Be aware that fabrics such as nylon and wool can cause static electricity discharges. Report any concerns to the nurse.
- G Do not use any petroleum-based products, such as Vaseline or ChapStick, on the patient or on any part of the cannula or mask. Oil-based lubricants can be a fire hazard.
- G Learn how to turn oxygen off in case of fire. Never adjust the oxygen setting or dose.

Bag Valve Masks

When a patient suddenly stops breathing, a bag valve mask (BVM) may be used by the code team. This mask covers the mouth and nose. Tubing connects it to an oxygen source. It has a one-way valve and an inflatable bag that allows oxygen to be squeezed into the patient's airway. The healthcare worker operating the BVM squeezes the bag at a regular rate to "breathe" for the patient. A BVM is used only during medical emergencies. It does not provide supplemental oxygen.

7. Discuss how to collect respiratory tract specimens

PCTs may need to collect a sputum specimen from patients who have tuberculosis or other respiratory conditions. A **specimen** is a sample that is used for analysis in order to try to make a diagnosis. *Sputum* is thick mucus coughed up from the lungs. It is not the same as saliva, which comes from the mouth. People with respiratory illnesses may cough up large amounts of sputum. Sputum specimens may be used to diagnose respiratory illness or to evaluate the effects of medication.

Early morning is the best time to collect sputum. The patient should cough up the sputum and spit it directly into the specimen container. Because sputum may be infectious, the PCT should not let the patient cough on him. Standing behind the patient during the collection process may prevent sputum from coming into contact with the PCT. Proper personal protective equipment (PPE) must be worn when collecting sputum. Gloves and a respirator are required. The PCT's hands and the specimen container must be clean before beginning this procedure.

A **requisition** is a paper or electronic order for testing. It lists the patient's name, hospital, date and time of collection, specimen type, and the tests that will be done on the specimen. A requisition needs to accompany each specimen.

Collecting a sputum specimen

Equipment: specimen container and lid; completed label (labeled with patient's name, date of birth, room number, date, and time); specimen bag; tissues; gloves; N95 or other respirator; requisition

1. Identify yourself by name. Identify the patient according to facility policy.
2. Wash your hands.
3. Explain the procedure to the patient. Speak clearly, slowly, and directly. Maintain face-to-face contact whenever possible.
4. Provide for the patient's privacy with a curtain, screen, or door.
5. Adjust the bed to a safe level, usually waist high. Lock the bed wheels.
6. Position the patient according to the nurse's instructions. The patient should be standing or sitting as upright as possible. If the patient is sitting, it is better if he can sit on the edge of the bed.
7. Put on the mask and gloves. Coughing is one way that respiratory pathogens can enter the air. Stand behind or some distance away from the patient if the patient can hold the specimen container by himself.
8. Ask the patient to cough deeply, so that sputum comes up from the lungs. To prevent the spread of infectious material, give the patient tissues to cover his mouth while coughing. Ask the patient to spit the sputum into the specimen container.
9. When you have obtained a good sample (at least 1 teaspoon, or the amount directed), cover the container tightly. Wipe any sputum off the outside of the container with tissues. Discard the tissues. Apply the label, place the container in a clean specimen bag, and seal the bag.
10. Remove and discard your gloves and mask.
11. Wash your hands.
12. Return the bed to its lowest position. Remove privacy measures.
13. Place the call light within the patient's reach.
14. Report any changes in the patient to the nurse.
15. Follow facility policy for getting the specimen and requisition to the laboratory. Document the procedure using facility guidelines.

Specimens are also taken from the nose or mouth to diagnose respiratory illnesses caused by viruses or bacteria. Swabs taken from the mouth may be from the inside of the cheek (a buccal swab) or from the throat. This includes the tonsils and the area around the tonsils.

Three types of specimens may be collected by inserting a swab in the nose:

1. An anterior nasal specimen is collected just inside the nostril, at a depth of ½–¾ of an inch (1–1.5 cm).
2. A mid-turbinate nasal specimen is collected at a depth of less than 1 inch (2 cm).
3. A nasopharyngeal specimen is collected at the back of the nasal cavity. The location is called the *posterior nasopharyngeal wall.* This is where the nasal cavity and throat cavity meet. It can be as far as 3–4 inches (8–10 cm) into the nose.

In some states and facilities, PCTs may be trained to collect buccal, throat, and/or nasal specimens. Nurses and other licensed healthcare professionals usually collect nasopharyngeal specimens. All of these specimens are taken using a swab. Most swabs have a soft, absorbent tip at the end of a rigid plastic shaft. Shafts for some specimens may be flexible. Buccal specimens are used for genetic tests (traits passed down from parent to child). Throat specimens are often cultured, or tested for pathogens. Nasal specimens are tested for viruses such as SARS-CoV-2 (the virus that causes COVID-19) or influenza. After specimen collection the swab is often placed tip-down in a tube with a chemical agent. This agent prepares the specimen for testing.

If assigned to collect a swab-based specimen, the PCT should follow the nurse's instructions. The following are general guidelines for collecting these specimens:

Guidelines: Nasal, Buccal, and Throat Swabs

- **G** Wash your hands and put on gloves (and any other PPE ordered).
- **G** These tests can be frightening or uncomfortable. Be reassuring. Use language that matches the patient's age. Let patients ask questions and answer them within your scope of practice.
- **G** Collecting specimens from the throat can cause a patient to gag or cough. Collecting nasal specimens can cause a patient to cough or sneeze. Be as gentle as possible.
- **G** Prepare for the procedure. This may include adding fluid to a specimen tube or preparing a card to receive the swab after collection. Follow manufacturer instructions.
- **G** Gently support the back of the patient's head. This can help steady the patient until the procedure is over.

Collecting a specimen using a swab

Equipment: kit including swab and test vial, tongue depressor (for throat swab), gloves (and other PPE as required), specimen label

1. Identify yourself by name. Identify the patient according to facility policy.
2. Wash your hands.
3. Explain the procedure to the patient. Speak clearly, slowly, and directly. Maintain face-to-face contact whenever possible.
4. Provide for the patient's privacy with a curtain, screen, or door.
5. Adjust the bed to a safe level, usually waist high. Lock the bed wheels.
6. Put on PPE as required.
7. Remove the swab from its packaging.
8. Collect the specimen:

- To collect a buccal specimen, ask the patient to open his mouth. Rub the swab up and down the inside of one cheek. Avoid the teeth, tongue, and gums. Use your other hand to put gentle pressure on the outside of the cheek. Repeat this on the other side of the mouth, using the same swab.
- To collect a specimen from the throat, ask the patient to tilt his head back slightly, open his mouth, and say "Ahhhh." It may help to use a tongue depressor to hold the tongue down and out of the way. Insert the swab in the patient's mouth and rub it along both of the patient's tonsils and the back of the throat. Avoid the uvula (the structure hanging down in the back of the throat). Be sure to swab any areas of the throat or tonsils that are white or blistered.
- To collect an anterior nasal specimen, insert the tip of the swab ½ to ¾ of an inch (1–1.5 cm) into the patient's nostril. Move

the swab in a circle around the nasal wall while rotating (spinning) the swab. Repeat this motion several times, following instructions. Repeat in the second nostril.

- To collect a mid-turbinate nasal specimen, insert the swab less than 1 inch (2 cm) into the patient's nostril. Move the swab in a circle around the nasal wall while rotating (spinning) the swab. Repeat this motion several times, following instructions. Repeat in the second nostril.

9. Place the swab in the required vial/tube. You may need to break off the swab stick and/or squeeze to break open a pocket of testing liquid before sealing the tube.
10. Apply the label, place the container in a clean specimen bag, and seal the bag.
11. Remove and discard your gloves and any other PPE. Wash your hands.
12. Return the bed to its lowest position. Remove privacy measures.
13. Place the call light within the patient's reach.
14. Report any changes in the patient to the nurse.

Chapter Review

1. What does respiration mean? What are the 2 processes involved in respiration?
2. What types of infections might cause pneumonia?
3. What usually causes emphysema and chronic bronchitis?
4. What position might a patient with chronic obstructive pulmonary disease (COPD) prefer to be in?
5. How is asthma treated?
6. How is bronchiectasis treated?
7. In which people is tuberculosis more likely to develop?
8. How is COVID-19 transmitted?
9. What are signs of worsening COVID-19 infection that should be reported immediately?
10. Why are deep breathing exercises performed?
11. When might oral suctioning be performed on a patient?
12. What are alternate methods of communication that PCTs can use with patients who have artificial airways?
13. What are a PCT's responsibilities with tracheostomy care?
14. In what ways can a PCT show support for a patient who is on a ventilator?
15. Is it the responsibility of a PCT to administer and adjust a patient's oxygen?
16. What is a nasal cannula?
17. Why is oxygen a dangerous fire hazard?
18. When is the best time of day to collect a sputum specimen?
19. What are the 3 types of specimens that can be collected from a patient's nose?
20. What are 2 other locations from which a respiratory specimen collection may be taken by swab?

17
The Urinary System and Related Care

1. Describe the structure and function of the urinary system

The urinary system is composed of 2 kidneys, 2 ureters, 1 urinary bladder, a single urethra, and a meatus (Figs. 17-1 and 17-2).

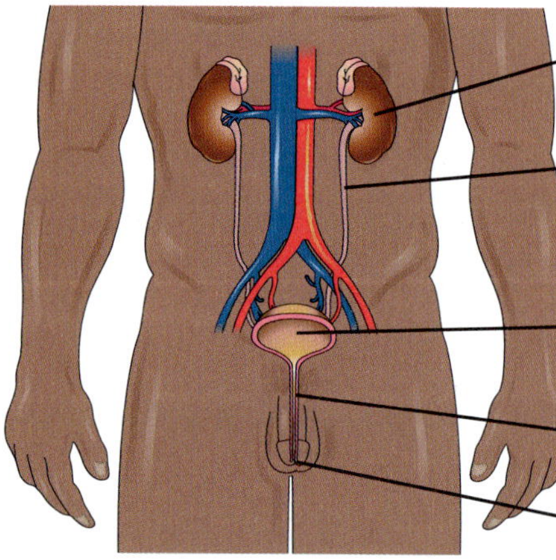

***Fig. 17-1.** The urinary system consists of 2 kidneys and 2 ureters, the bladder, the urethra, and the meatus. This is an illustration of the male urinary system.*

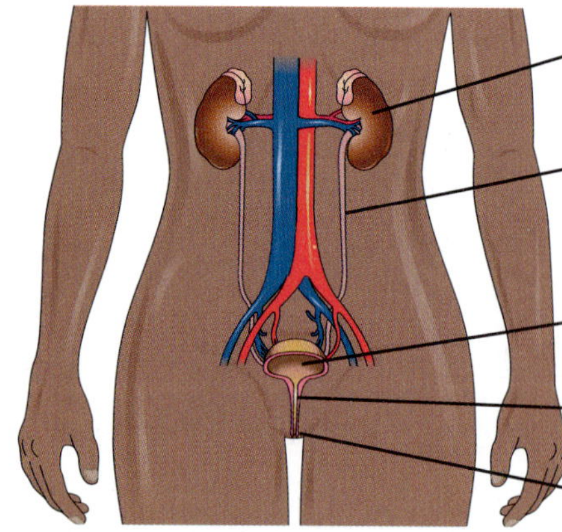

***Fig. 17-2.** The female urethra is shorter than the male urethra. This is one reason why the female bladder is more likely to become infected by bacteria.*

The kidneys are located in the upper part of the abdominal cavity on each side of the spine. These 2 bean-shaped organs are protected by the muscles of the back and the lower part of the rib cage. When blood flows through the kidneys, waste products and excess water are filtered out. Necessary water and substances are reabsorbed into the bloodstream. Waste and the remaining fluid form urine. The body must maintain a proper balance between water absorbed in the body and waste fluids that are released from the body.

Each kidney has a ureter, which is attached to the bladder. Urine flows through the ureters to the bladder, a muscular sac in the lower part of the abdomen. Urine flows from the bladder through the urethra. It then passes out of the body through the meatus, the opening at the end of the urethra. In the female, the meatus is located in the genital area just in front of the opening of the vagina. In the male, the meatus is located at the end of the penis.

The urinary system has 2 important functions. Through urine, the urinary system eliminates waste products created by the cells and it also maintains the water balance in the body.

Observing and Reporting: Urinary System

Observe and report these signs and symptoms:

O/R Weight loss or gain (patients who are taking medications that affect fluid balance may be weighed often)

O/R Swelling in the upper or lower extremities

O/R Pain or burning during urination

O/R Changes in urine, such as cloudiness, odor, or color

O/R Changes in frequency and amount of urination

O/R Inability to urinate or no urinary output for 8 hours

O/R Swelling in the abdominal/bladder area

O/R Complaints that bladder feels full or painful

O/R Urinary incontinence/dribbling

O/R Pain in the kidney or back/flank region

O/R Reduced fluid intake

O/R Confusion

2. List common conditions of the urinary system and discuss related care

Urinary Incontinence

Urinary incontinence is the inability to control the bladder, which leads to an involuntary loss of urine. Incontinence can occur in patients who are confined to bed, ill, elderly, paralyzed, or who have circulatory or nervous system diseases or injuries. There are different types of incontinence:

- Stress incontinence is the loss of urine due to an increase in intra-abdominal pressure, for example, when sneezing or coughing.
- Urge incontinence is involuntary voiding from a sudden urge to void.
- Mixed incontinence is a combination of both urge incontinence and stress incontinence.
- Functional incontinence is urine loss caused by environmental, cognitive, or physical reasons.
- Overflow incontinence is loss of urine due to overflow or overdistention of the bladder.

Incontinence is *not* a normal part of aging. PCTs should always report incontinence. It may be a sign or symptom of illness.

Guidelines: Urinary Incontinence

G Offer a bedpan, urinal, commode, or trip to the bathroom often. Follow elimination schedules in the care plan.

G Answer call lights and requests for help immediately.

G Urinary incontinence is a major risk factor for pressure injuries. Document all episodes of incontinence carefully and accurately.

G Cleanliness and careful skin care are important for patients who are incontinent. Urine is very irritating to the skin. It should be washed off immediately and completely. Keep patients clean, dry, and free from odor. Observe the skin carefully when bathing and giving perineal care.

G Change wet or soiled clothing immediately. Change bed linen any time it is wet or soiled. Use absorbent pads under bed linen for patients who are incontinent.

G Some patients wear disposable incontinence pads or briefs. They keep body wastes away from the skin (Fig. 17-3). As needed, assist patients with changing wet briefs immediately. Do not refer to an incontinence brief as a diaper. Patients are not infants, and using that term is disrespectful. Make sure incontinence briefs/products are not visible in the patient's room.

G Encourage patients to drink plenty of fluids.

G Patients who are incontinent need reassurance and understanding. Be professional and kind when dealing with incontinence. Doing so may help put patients at ease.

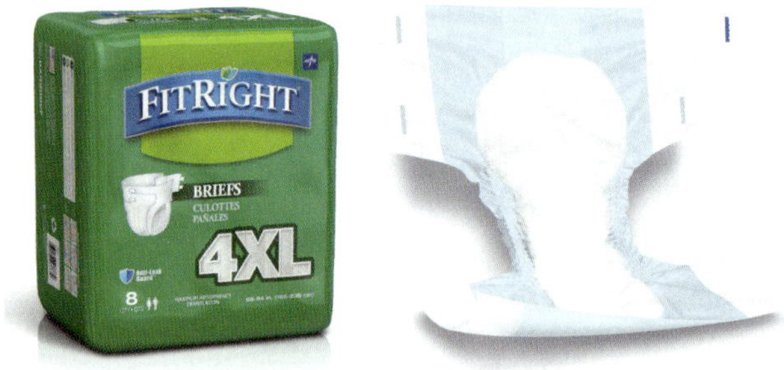

Fig. 17-3. A type of incontinence brief. (IMAGES COURTESY OF MEDLINE INDUSTRIES, LP. USED WITH PERMISSION.)

Changing Incontinence Briefs

When changing an incontinence brief, the PCT should assemble all needed items beforehand, including a protective pad, perineal care supplies, disposable wipes, gloves, and a clean brief. She should wash her hands and put on gloves before handling the brief. When removing the soiled brief, the PCT should roll it inward, soiled side inside, without spilling its contents. Working from front to back, she should carefully remove all urine and/or feces from the skin. After cleaning the area thoroughly, she should blot it dry, and apply the clean brief.

Urinary Tract Infection (UTI)

A **urinary tract infection** (**UTI**) is a bacterial infection of the urethra, bladder, ureter, or kidney. This results in pain or burning during urination and the frequent feeling of needing to urinate. The infection is commonly caused by *Escherichia coli* (*E. coli*), which is a type of bacteria usually found in the gastrointestinal tract. If it moves from the anus into the urethra and then the bladder, it can cause a urinary tract infection.

UTIs are more common in women. This is due, in part, to the female urethra being shorter (1 to 1 1/2 inches/2.5 to 3.8 centimeters) than the male urethra (7 to 8 inches/17.8 to 20.3 centimeters). In addition, because the female urethra is located directly in front of the vagina and anus, it is closer to potential sources of bacteria. Bacteria can reach a woman's bladder more easily.

Guidelines: Preventing UTIs

G Encourage patients to wipe from front to back after elimination (Fig. 17-4). When you give perineal care, make sure you do this too.

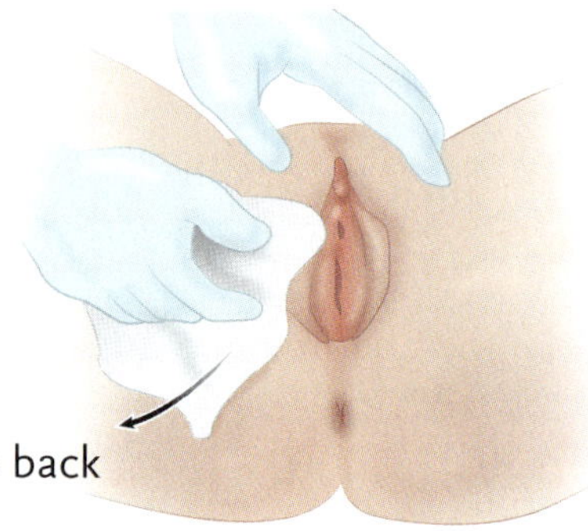

Fig. 17-4. After elimination, wipe from front to back to prevent infection.

G Give careful perineal care when changing incontinence briefs.

G Encourage plenty of fluids. Drinking water and other fluids helps prevent UTIs.

G Offer a bedpan or a trip to the toilet at least every 2 hours. Answer call lights promptly.

G Taking showers, rather than baths, helps prevent urinary tract infections.

G Report cloudy, dark, or foul-smelling urine, or if a patient urinates often and in small amounts.

G Report if the patient has a fever. Report new or worsening confusion. This is a common symptom of UTI, especially in older adults.

Kidney Stones

Kidney stones, also called *renal calculi,* form when urine crystallizes in the kidneys. The stones can block the kidneys and ureters, causing severe pain. Kidney stones often have no single cause, but may be the result of lack of fluid intake, diet, infection, disorders, or certain genetic factors.

Signs and symptoms of kidney stones may not be noticeable until they begin to move down the ureter, causing pain. Signs and symptoms include the following:

- Abdominal pain
- Flank or back pain
- Groin pain
- Burning during urination, painful urination
- Frequent urination
- Blood in the urine
- Nausea or vomiting
- Chills or fever

Kidney stones are treated with increased water intake, as well as pain relievers and other medications. Larger stones may need to be treated with surgery or a procedure that uses sound waves to break up the stones.

Renovascular Hypertension

Renovascular hypertension is a condition in which a blockage of arteries in the kidneys causes high blood pressure. Treatment of this condition includes medications to help control blood pressure and sometimes surgery. More information about hypertension and its symptoms, treatment, and related care is in Chapter 15.

Chronic Renal Failure

Chronic renal failure (**CRF**), also called *chronic kidney failure*, occurs because the kidneys become unable to eliminate certain waste products from the body. This disease can develop as the result of chronic urinary tract infections, high blood pressure, inflammation of the kidneys (nephritis), or diabetes. Excessive salt in the diet can also cause damage to the kidneys. Over time, the disease becomes worse. Signs and symptoms include the following:

- High blood pressure
- Decreased urine output or no urine output
- Dark urine
- Anemia
- Nausea, vomiting
- Loss of appetite
- Weight changes
- Fatigue and weakness
- Headaches
- Difficulty sleeping
- Back pain
- Edema
- Stool that is bloody or black

Kidney dialysis, an artificial means of removing the body's waste products, can improve and extend life for several years. Patients will be on fluid restrictions of different degrees. Chronic renal failure can progress to end-stage renal disease (ESRD), which is fatal without kidney dialysis or a kidney transplant.

Cancer

Renal cell cancer is the most common type of kidney cancer. People who are overweight, smoke, or have high blood pressure or kidney disease are at higher risk of developing kidney cancer. Symptoms may not appear until late in the disease. They include hematuria (blood in the urine), back pain, swelling in the abdomen, fatigue, weight loss, and fever.

In **bladder cancer** the cells of the bladder all mutate and grow rapidly. Bladder cancer affects men more often than women. Smoking and exposure to chemicals and radiation increase risk. There is more about cancer and cancer treatment in Chapter 21.

3. Describe how to assist patients with elimination

Patients who are unable to get out of bed to use the toilet may be given a standard bedpan, a fracture pan, or a urinal. A **fracture pan** is a bedpan that is flatter than a regular bedpan. It is used for patients who cannot assist with raising their hips onto a regular bedpan (Fig. 17-5). Women will generally use a bedpan for urination and bowel movements. Men will generally use a bedpan for bowel movements and a urinal for urination (Fig. 17-6).

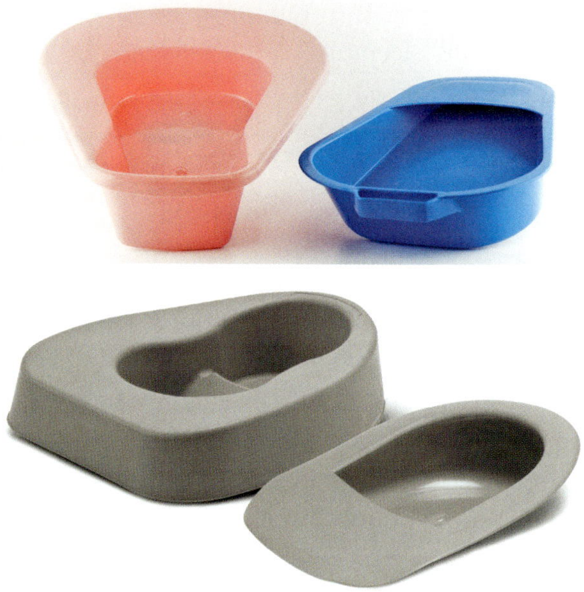

Fig. 17-5. In the top photo, a standard bedpan is on the left side, and a fracture pan is on the right. In the bottom photo, a bariatric standard bedpan is in back, and a bariatric fracture pan is in front. Bariatric bedpans can be used for people who are overweight or obese. (BOTTOM IMAGE COURTESY OF MEDLINE INDUSTRIES, LP. USED WITH PERMISSION.)

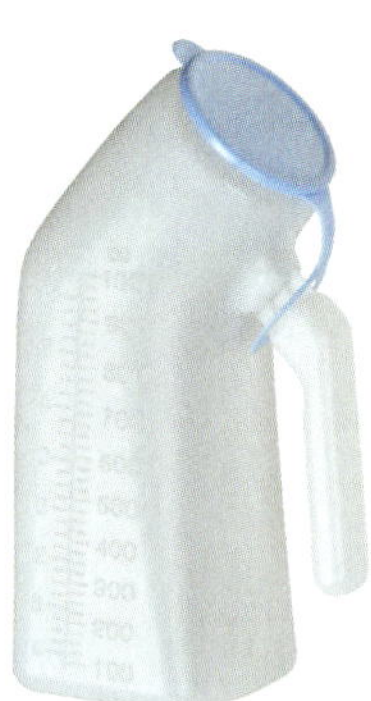

Fig. 17-6. A urinal. (PHOTO COURTESY OF NOVA MEDICAL PRODUCTS, WWW.NOVAJOY.COM)

Urinals are usually kept at the patient's bedside. Bedpans are kept in the bathroom between uses or are wrapped and kept in a bedside cabinet. Patients who share bathrooms may need to have bedpans labeled. PCTs should never place this equipment on overbed tables or on top of side tables.

Urine and feces are considered infectious wastes. PCTs must always wear gloves when handling bedpans, urinals, or basins that contain wastes, including dirty bath water. PCTs should be careful not to spill or splash wastes, and wastes should be discarded in the toilet. Immediately after use, containers used for elimination should be placed in the proper area for cleaning, or they should be cleaned and stored according to facility policy.

Connected Care

Rights with Elimination

Patients may be embarrassed about needing help with elimination. PCTs should be professional when giving assistance and provide as much privacy as possible. To help promote dignity, PCTs should treat patients as adults. When assisting with elimination needs, proper terms for bodily functions should be used; childish words should not be used.

Assisting a patient with the use of a bedpan

Equipment: bedpan, bedpan cover (towel), disposable bed protector, bath blanket, toilet paper, disposable wipes, 2 towels, supplies for perineal care, 2 pairs of gloves

1. Identify yourself by name. Identify the patient according to facility policy.
2. Wash your hands.
3. Explain the procedure to the patient. Speak clearly, slowly, and directly. Maintain face-to-face contact whenever possible.
4. Provide for the patient's privacy with a curtain, screen, or door.
5. Adjust the bed to a safe level, usually waist high. Raise the far side rail for safety. Before placing the bedpan, lower the head of the bed. Lock the bed wheels.
6. Put on gloves.

7. Cover the patient with the bath blanket and ask him to hold it while you pull down the top covers underneath. Do not expose more of the patient than you need to. Keep the patient covered from the chest down except when placing or removing the bedpan.
8. Place the bed protector under the patient's buttocks and hips. To do this, have the patient turn toward the raised side rail. If the patient cannot do this, you must turn him. Be sure the patient cannot roll off the bed. Place the bed protector on the empty side of the bed, on the area where the patient will lie on his back. The side of the protector nearest the patient should be fanfolded (folded several times into pleats) and tucked under the patient.

   Ask the patient to turn onto his back, or turn him as you did before. Unfold the rest of the bed protector so it completely covers the area under and around the patient's buttocks and hips.
9. Keeping him covered, ask the patient to remove his undergarments or help him do so.
10. Place the bedpan near his hips in the correct position. A **standard bedpan** should be positioned with the wider end aligned with the patient's buttocks. A **fracture pan** should be positioned with the handle toward the foot of the bed.
11. If the patient is able, ask him to raise his hips by pushing with his feet and hands at the count of 3 (Fig. 17-7). Slide the bedpan under his hips.

    If the patient cannot assist in getting on the bedpan, keep the bed flat and turn the patient away from you toward the raised side rail. Place the protective pad on the area where the patient will lie on his back. Place the bedpan firmly against the patient's buttocks (Fig. 17-8). Holding the bedpan securely, gently roll the patient back onto the bedpan. Keep the bedpan centered underneath.

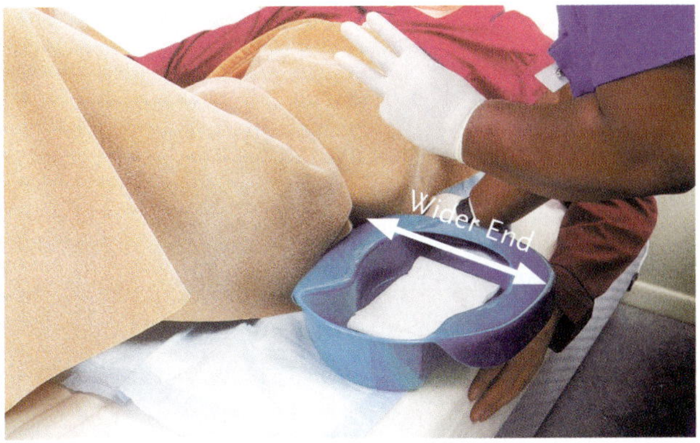

Fig. 17-7. *On the count of 3, slide the bedpan under the patient's hips. The wider end of the bedpan should be aligned with the patient's buttocks.*

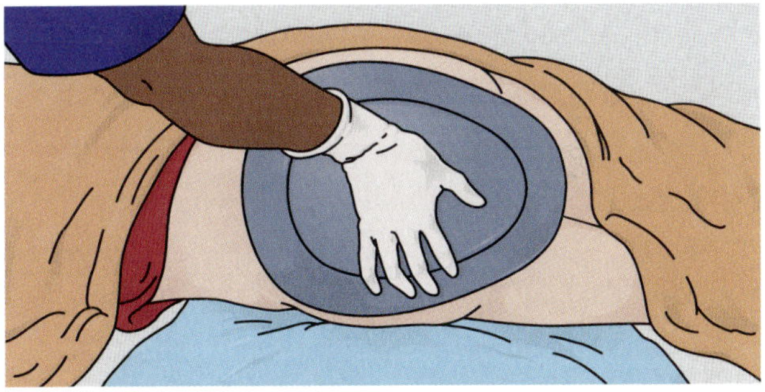

Fig. 17-8. *Placing the bedpan firmly against the patient's buttocks, gently roll him back onto the bedpan.*

12. Remove and discard your gloves. Wash your hands.
13. Raise the head of the bed. Prop the patient into a semisitting position using pillows. Raise the near side rail and leave the far rail up. Return the bed to its lowest position.
14. Make sure the bath blanket is still covering the patient. Place toilet paper and disposable wipes within the patient's reach. Ask the patient to clean his hands with a wipe when finished if he is able.
15. Place the call light within the patient's reach. Ask the patient to signal when done. Leave the room and close the door.
16. When called by the patient, return and wash your hands. Put on clean gloves.
17. Raise the bed to a safe level, and lower the head of the bed. Make sure the patient is

still covered. Lower the side rail on the near/working side.

18. Remove the bedpan carefully and cover it with a bedpan cover or towel.
19. Give perineal care if help is needed. Wipe from front to back. Dry the perineal area with a towel. Remove and discard the bed protector. Help the patient put on his undergarment. Cover the patient and remove the bath blanket.
20. Discard disposable supplies. Place the towel and bath blanket in a hamper or bag.
21. Return the bed to its lowest position. Leave the side rails in the ordered position.
22. Take the bedpan to the bathroom. Note the color, odor, and consistency of contents. Empty contents into the toilet unless a specimen is needed or urine is being measured for intake/output monitoring. Flush the toilet. If you notice anything unusual about the stool or urine (for example, the presence of blood), do not discard it. You will need to inform the nurse.
23. Rinse the bedpan if part of facility policy. Place it in the proper area for cleaning or clean and disinfect it according to facility policy.
24. Remove and discard your gloves. Wash your hands.
25. Make the patient comfortable.
26. Leave the bed in its lowest position. Remove privacy measures.
27. Place the call light within the patient's reach.
28. Report any changes in the patient to the nurse.
29. Document the procedure using facility guidelines.

Assisting a patient with a urinal

Equipment: urinal, disposable bed protector, disposable wipes, 2 pairs of gloves

1. Identify yourself by name. Identify the patient according to facility policy.
2. Wash your hands.
3. Explain the procedure to the patient. Speak clearly, slowly, and directly. Maintain face-to-face contact whenever possible.
4. Provide for the patient's privacy with a curtain, screen, or door.
5. Adjust the bed to a safe level, usually waist high. Raise the far side rail for safety. Lock the bed wheels.
6. Put on gloves.
7. Place the bed protector under the patient's buttocks and hips, as in step 8 of the previous procedure.
8. Hand the urinal to the patient. If the patient is not able to do this himself, place the urinal between his legs and position the penis inside the urinal (Fig. 17-9). Replace the covers.

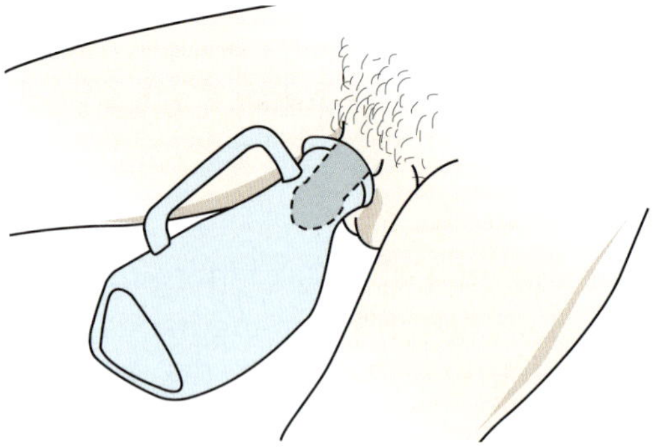

Fig. 17-9. *Position the penis inside the urinal if the patient cannot do it himself.*

9. Remove and discard your gloves. Wash your hands.
10. Raise the near side rail and leave the far rail up. Return the bed to its lowest position.

Place disposable wipes within the patient's reach. Ask the patient to clean his hands with a hand wipe when finished if he is able.

11. Place the call light within the patient's reach. Ask the patient to signal when done. Leave the room and close the door.
12. When called by the patient, return and wash your hands. Put on clean gloves.
13. Raise the bed to a safe level. Lower the side rail on the near/working side. Remove the urinal or have the patient hand it to you. Remove and discard the bed protector. Discard the disposable wipes.
14. Return the bed to its lowest position. Leave the side rails in the ordered position.
15. Take the urinal to the bathroom. Note the color, odor, and qualities (for example, cloudiness) of contents. Empty contents into the toilet unless a specimen is needed or the urine is being measured for intake/output monitoring. Flush the toilet.
16. Rinse the urinal if part of facility policy. Place the urinal in the proper area for cleaning or clean and disinfect it according to facility policy.
17. Remove and discard your gloves. Wash your hands.
18. Make the patient comfortable.
19. Leave the bed in its lowest position. Remove privacy measures.
20. Place the call light within the patient's reach.
21. Report any changes in the patient to the nurse.
22. Document the procedure using facility guidelines.

Some patients are able to get out of bed, but may still need help walking to the bathroom and using the toilet. Toilets may be fitted with raised seats to make it easier for patients to get up and down. Many bathrooms in patient rooms have handrails by the toilet. Those who are able to get out of bed but cannot walk to the bathroom may use a portable commode (also called a *bedside commode* [*BSC*]). A **portable commode** is a chair with a toilet seat and a removable container underneath (Fig. 17-10). The removable container must be cleaned after each use. The PCT should offer to help patients get to the bathroom or commode often. This can avoid accidents and embarrassment. It is also an important part of preventing falls.

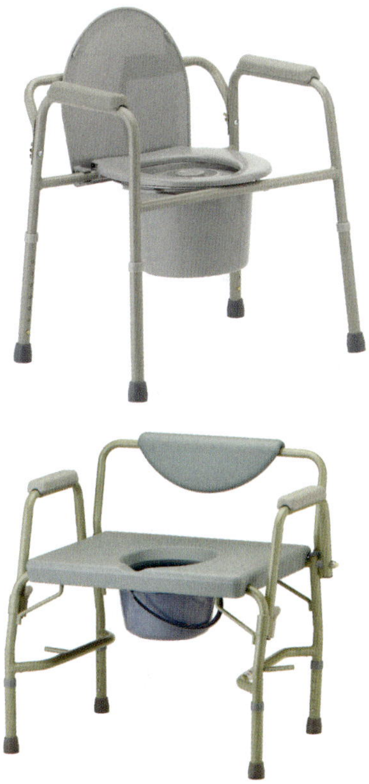

Fig. 17-10. *The top photo shows a regular portable commode and the bottom photo shows a bariatric portable commode, which can be used for people who are overweight or obese.* (PHOTOS COURTESY OF NOVA MEDICAL PRODUCTS, WWW.NOVAJOY.COM)

Assisting a patient to use a portable commode or toilet

Equipment: portable commode with basin, transfer belt (if needed), toilet paper, disposable wipes, towel, supplies for perineal care, 3 pairs of gloves

1. Identify yourself by name. Identify the patient according to facility policy.
2. Wash your hands.
3. Explain the procedure to the patient. Speak clearly, slowly, and directly. Maintain face-to-face contact whenever possible.
4. Provide for the patient's privacy with a curtain, screen, or door.
5. Lock the commode wheels. Adjust the bed to its lowest position. Lock the bed wheels. Assist the patient into a sitting position.
6. Put nonskid footwear on the patient if he is not already wearing it.
7. If needed, place the transfer belt around the patient's waist over his gown (not on bare skin). Help the patient out of bed and to the portable commode or bathroom.
8. Put on gloves.
9. If needed, help the patient pull down underwear and sit comfortably on the toilet seat. Put toilet paper and disposable wipes within reach. Ask the patient to wash his hands or clean them with a wipe when finished if he is able.
10. Remove and discard your gloves. Wash your hands.
11. Provide privacy. Place the call light within the patient's reach. Ask the patient to signal when done. Leave the room and close the door.
12. When called by the patient, return and wash your hands. Put on clean gloves. Provide perineal care if help is needed. Remember to wipe from front to back. Dry the perineal area. Help the patient pull up underwear.
13. Place the towel in a hamper or bag, and discard disposable supplies.
14. Remove and discard your gloves. Wash your hands.
15. Help the patient back to bed. Remove the transfer belt (if used). Make the patient comfortable.
16. Put on clean gloves.
17. When using a portable commode, remove the waste container. Note the color, odor, and consistency of contents. Empty it into the toilet unless a specimen is needed or the urine is being measured for intake/output monitoring. Flush the toilet.
18. Rinse the container if part of facility policy. Place it in the proper area for cleaning or clean and disinfect it according to facility policy.
19. Remove and discard your gloves. Wash your hands.
20. Leave the bed in its lowest position. Remove privacy measures.
21. Place the call light within the patient's reach.
22. Report any changes in the patient to the nurse.
23. Document the procedure using facility guidelines.

4. Discuss urinary catheters and bladder scanning

Some patients may have a urinary catheter. A **straight catheter** is a type of urinary catheter that is inserted to drain urine from the bladder and is removed after urine is drained. It does not remain inside the person. An **indwelling catheter** (also called a *Foley catheter*) remains inside the bladder for a period of time (Fig. 17-11). The urine drains into a bag.

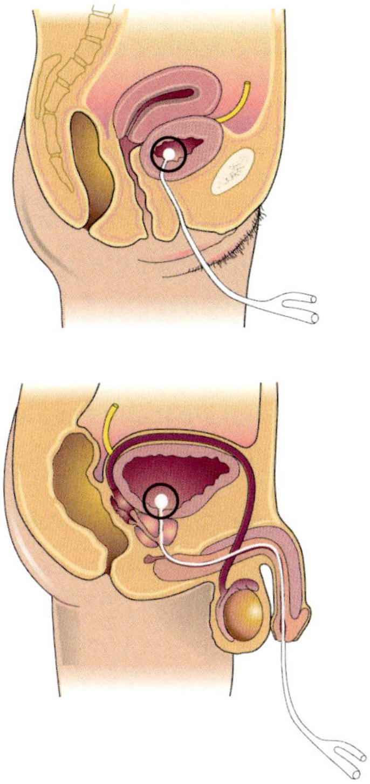

Fig. 17-11. *An illustration of female and male indwelling catheters. This type of catheter is held in place by a small, fluid-filled balloon in the bladder (circled in the illustrations).*

Another type of catheter that is used for males is an external catheter, or **condom catheter** (also called a *Texas catheter*). It has an attachment on the end that fits onto the penis and is fastened with special tape. Urine drains through the catheter into the tubing, then into the drainage bag. A smaller bag, called a *leg bag*, attaches to the leg and collects the urine (Fig. 17-12). The condom catheter is changed daily or as needed. External catheters for females are used less commonly. They are applied to the area around the urethra and drain or wick urine into a collection bag.

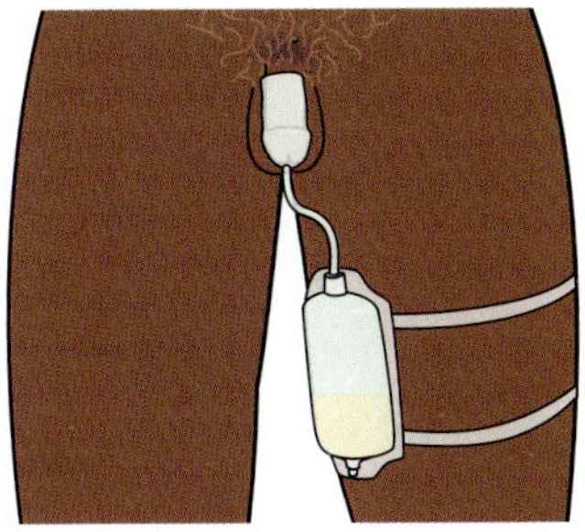

Fig. 17-12. *An illustration of a condom catheter with a leg bag.*

Nurses or providers usually insert urinary catheters, though in some states PCTs may be allowed to do this task with special training. PCTs may also be allowed to remove urinary catheters in some states. PCTs may be asked to give daily catheter care, clean the area around the urethral opening, and empty the drainage bag. The bag is emptied into a measuring container (a graduate).

Guidelines: Urinary Catheters

- **G** Thoroughly wash your hands before giving catheter care.
- **G** Keep the genital area clean to prevent infection. Because the catheter goes all the way into the bladder, bacteria can enter the bladder more easily. Daily care of the genital area (perineal care) is especially important.
- **G** Make sure that the drainage bag always hangs lower than the hips or bladder. Urine must never flow from the bag or tubing back into the bladder. This can cause infection.
- **G** Keep the drainage bag off the floor. Make sure the catheter tubing does not touch the floor.
- **G** To help keep urine draining properly, keep the tubing as straight as possible. Make sure there are no kinks in the tubing and that the patient is not sitting or lying on the tubing.
- **G** Make sure there are no *dependent loops* in the tubing. A dependent loop is an area where tubing falls below the drainage bag. Urine collects there and can create pressure that stops proper emptying of the bladder. This is a UTI risk.

Observing and Reporting: Urinary Catheters

Report any of the following to the nurse:

- **O/R** Blood in the urine or urine that looks unusual in any way
- **O/R** Catheter bag does not fill after several hours

O/R Catheter bag fills suddenly

O/R Catheter is not in place

O/R Urine leaks from the catheter

O/R Patient reports pain or pressure

O/R Odor is present

Providing urinary catheter care

Equipment: bath blanket, disposable bed protector, bath basin with warm water, soap, 2–4 washcloths or bath wipes for body and perineal care, 2 towels, gloves

1. Identify yourself by name. Identify the patient according to facility policy.
2. Wash your hands.
3. Explain the procedure to the patient. Speak clearly, slowly, and directly. Maintain face-to-face contact whenever possible.
4. Provide for the patient's privacy with a curtain, screen, or door.
5. Adjust the bed to a safe level, usually waist high. Lock the bed wheels.
6. Lower the head of the bed. Position the patient lying flat on her back.
7. Remove or fold back the top bedding, keeping the patient covered with the bath blanket.
8. Test the water temperature against the inside of your wrist. Have the patient check the water temperature to see if it is comfortable. Adjust if necessary.
9. Put on gloves.
10. Ask the patient to flex her knees and raise her buttocks off the bed by pushing against the mattress with her feet. If she needs help, place your arm under the small of her back and tell her to push with her heels and hands on your signal as you raise her hips. Place a clean bed protector under her perineal area, including her buttocks.
11. Expose only the area necessary to clean the catheter. Avoid overexposing the patient.
12. Place a towel under the catheter tubing before washing.
13. Wet a washcloth in the basin and apply soap to the washcloth. Clean the area around the meatus. Use a clean area of the washcloth for each stroke.
14. Hold the catheter near the meatus. Avoid tugging the catheter throughout the procedure.
15. Clean at least 4 inches of the catheter nearest the meatus. Move in only one direction, away from the meatus (Fig. 17-13). Use a clean area of the cloth for each stroke.

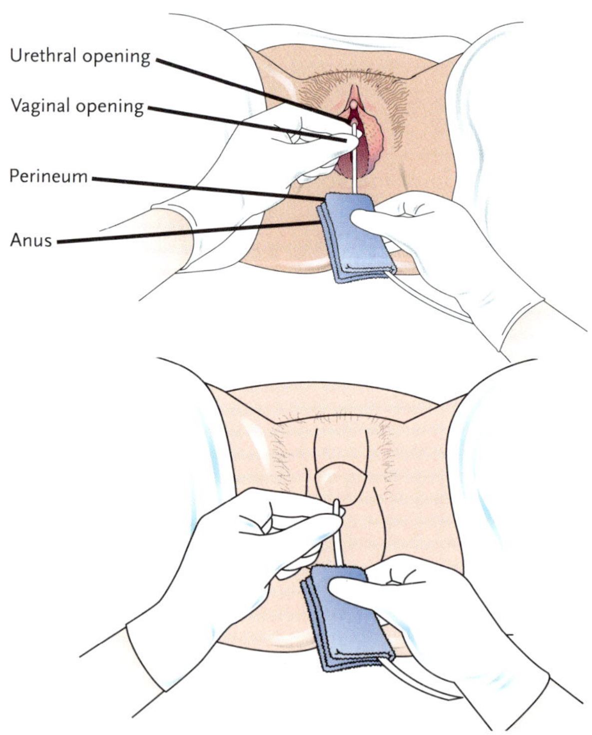

Fig. 17-13. *Hold the catheter near the meatus to avoid tugging the catheter. Moving in only one direction, away from the meatus, helps prevent infection. Use a clean area of the washcloth for each stroke.*

16. Dip a clean washcloth in the water. Rinse the area around the meatus, using a clean area of the washcloth for each stroke. With a clean, dry towel, dry the area around the meatus.

17. Dip a clean washcloth in the water. Rinse at least 4 inches of the catheter nearest the meatus. Move in only one direction, away from the meatus. Use a clean area of the washcloth for each stroke.
18. With a clean, dry towel, dry at least 4 inches of the catheter nearest the meatus. Move in only one direction, away from the meatus. Do not tug the catheter.
19. Remove and discard the bed protector. Remove the towel from under the catheter tubing and place it in the proper container.
20. Place linen and used washcloths in the proper containers.
21. Empty the basin into the toilet and flush the toilet. Place the basin in the proper area for cleaning or clean and store it according to facility policy.
22. Remove and discard your gloves. Wash your hands.
23. Remove the bath blanket and replace the top covers. Make the patient comfortable. Check that the catheter tubing is free from kinks and twists and that it is securely fastened to the leg.
24. Return the bed to its lowest position. Remove privacy measures.
25. Place the call light within the patient's reach.
26. Report any changes in the patient to the nurse.
27. Document the procedure using facility guidelines.

Connected Care

Urinary Catheters

The PCT can protect the patient's right to privacy by keeping the tubing and bag covered and by closing the door and pulling the privacy screen when providing catheter care.

Emptying the urinary catheter drainage bag

Equipment: measuring container (graduate), alcohol wipes, paper towels, gloves

1. Identify yourself by name. Identify the patient according to facility policy.
2. Wash your hands.
3. Explain the procedure to the patient. Speak clearly, slowly, and directly. Maintain face-to-face contact whenever possible.
4. Provide for the patient's privacy with a curtain, screen, or door.
5. Put on gloves.
6. Place a paper towel on the floor under the drainage bag. Place the graduate on the paper towel.
7. Open the clamp on the drainage bag so that the urine flows out of the bag and into the graduate (Fig. 17-14). Do not let the spout or clamp touch the graduate.

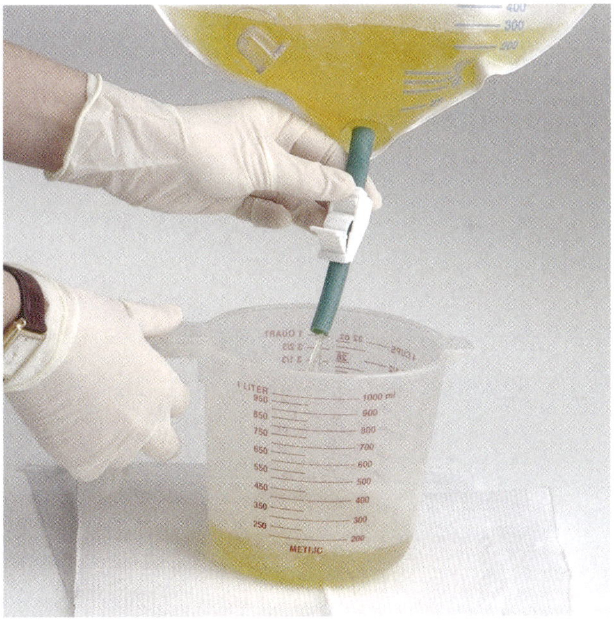

Fig. 17-14. *Keep the spout and clamp from touching the graduate while draining urine.*

8. When the urine has drained out of the bag, close the clamp. Using alcohol wipes, clean the drain spout. Replace the drain spout in its holder on the bag.

9. Go into the bathroom. Place the graduate on a flat surface and measure at eye level. Note the amount and characteristics of the urine. Empty the urine into the toilet and flush the toilet.
10. Clean and store the graduate. Discard paper towels.
11. Remove privacy measures.
12. Place the call light within the patient's reach.
13. Remove and discard your gloves. Wash your hands.
14. Report any changes in the patient to the nurse.
15. Document the procedure and the amount of urine.

A nurse or provider may decide that a patient's indwelling (Foley) catheter should be removed. This may be a step in preparing the patient for discharge. A catheter may also be removed from a patient who will still be in the hospital, but who no longer needs it. This is a decision that can only be made by a licensed healthcare professional. In some states, however, a trained PCT may be assigned to remove a catheter.

Before an indwelling catheter is removed, the drainage bag should be emptied and urine measured (as described in the last procedure). An indwelling catheter is kept in place by a water-filled balloon in the bladder (as seen in Fig. 17-11). This balloon must be drained before the catheter is removed. A syringe is inserted into a port near the catheter drainage tube. Pulling back on the plunger empties water from the balloon into the syringe. This allows the catheter to be removed.

It is very important to document the time of catheter removal. After a catheter is removed, the nurse must monitor the patient carefully. The nurse needs to know when the catheter was removed because the patient must void within a certain amount of time afterward.

Removing an indwelling urinary catheter

Equipment: bath blanket; disposable bed protector; syringe for balloon port; disposable wipes or bath basin with warm water, soap, and 2–4 washcloths; gloves

1. Identify yourself by name. Identify the patient according to facility policy.
2. Wash your hands.
3. Explain the procedure to the patient. Speak clearly, slowly, and directly. Maintain face-to-face contact whenever possible.
4. Provide for the patient's privacy with a curtain, screen, or door.
5. Adjust the bed to a safe level, usually waist high. Lock the bed wheels.
6. Lower the head of the bed. Position the patient lying flat on their back (supine).
7. Remove or fold back the top bedding, keeping the patient covered with the bath blanket.
8. Put on gloves.
9. Ask the patient to flex their knees and raise their buttocks off the bed by pushing against the mattress with their feet. If they need help, place your arm under the small of their back and ask them to push with their heels and hands on your signal to raise their hips. Place a clean bed protector under their perineal area, including the buttocks.
10. Tubing from the catheter branches into the tube that carries urine to the drainage bag and the balloon port. Insert the syringe into the balloon port. Draw back the plunger to drain the balloon (Fig. 17-15). When the plunger cannot be pulled further and/or the tubing collapses, the water is removed.

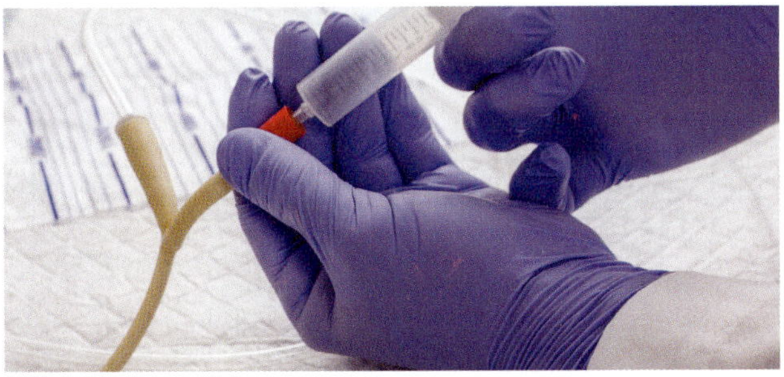

Fig. 17-15. Once the syringe has been inserted into the balloon port, draw back the plunger.

11. Uncovering the patient only as much as necessary, hold the catheter close to the meatus and pull gently to remove the catheter. Pull until it is removed completely. Catheters for male patients are longer than catheters for female patients and take slightly longer to remove. Stop pulling immediately if the catheter does not move easily or if the patient reports pain. Report this to the nurse.
12. Discard the syringe, catheter, tubing, and drainage bag according to facility policy.
13. Provide perineal care if help is needed.
14. Remove and discard the bed protector.
15. Remove and discard your gloves. Wash your hands.
16. Remove the bath blanket and replace the top covers. Make the patient comfortable.
17. Place linen and used washcloths in the proper containers.
18. Return the bed to its lowest position. Remove privacy measures.
19. Place the call light within the patient's reach.
20. Report any changes in the patient to the nurse.
21. Document the procedure using facility guidelines. Be sure to note the time.

Catheter use can increase a patient's risk of infection of the urethra, bladder, ureters, or kidneys. **Catheter-associated urinary tract infection (CAUTI)** can be a serious, life-threatening problem for hospitalized patients.

Because indwelling catheters can pose such a risk, many facilities try to reduce their use. **Bladder scanning** is one tool that can reduce unnecessary catheterization. A bladder scanner is a handheld ultrasound device. It is placed on the patient's abdomen and uses sound waves to measure the amount of urine in a patient's bladder (Fig. 17-16). A bladder scan is often done after a patient urinates to check for any remaining urine. This urine is called *post-void residual.* Depending on the amount of post-void residual, the nurse may insert a straight catheter to empty the bladder. This type of catheter has a lower infection risk.

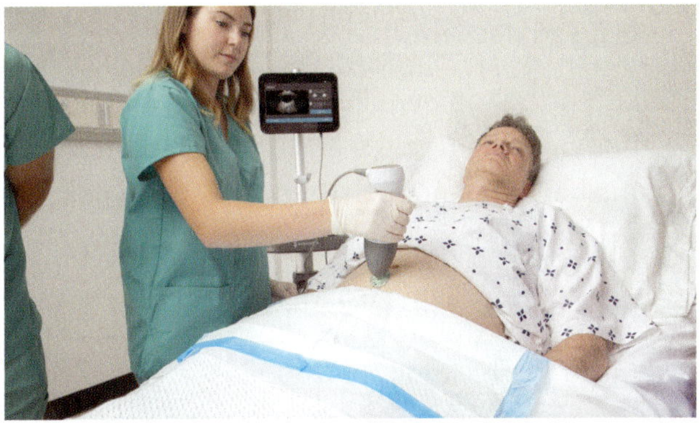

Fig. 17-16. A bladder scanner uses sound waves to measure the amount of urine in a patient's bladder.
(BLADDERSCAN I10™. USED WITH PERMISSION. ©VERATHON INC.)

A nurse decides when a bladder scanner should be used. A PCT may be assigned to do the scan. Bladder scans should not be done on patients who have wounds or nonintact skin in the suprapubic region (the area of the abdomen above the pubic bone). They should also not be done on patients who are pregnant or who have fluid buildup in the abdomen (a condition called *ascites*). PCTs should always follow instructions.

Performing a bladder scan

Equipment: bladder scanner, alcohol swabs, ultrasound gel, disposable absorbent pad, towel, gloves (if needed)

1. Identify yourself by name. Identify the patient according to facility policy.
2. Wash your hands.
3. Explain the procedure to the patient. Speak clearly, slowly, and directly. Maintain face-to-face contact whenever possible.
4. Provide for the patient's privacy with a curtain, screen, or door.
5. Adjust the bed to a safe level, usually waist high. Lock the bed wheels.
6. With the patient in supine position, ask him to raise his gown above his abdomen, roughly up to the bottom of the rib cage. Help as needed.
7. Lower the top bedding so that the abdomen is exposed. Place the absorbent pad on top of the bedding and tuck it under the top edge of the bedding.
8. Put on gloves (if needed).
9. Clean the head of the bladder scanner with an alcohol swab. Turn it on and select the correct setting for the patient. Each scanner is different, but there are separate settings for women who have not had hysterectomies and all other adults. Some scanners have settings for children.
10. Tell the patient that you will be putting ultrasound gel on his abdomen and that it may feel cold (Fig. 17-17). Put a generous amount of gel above the pubic bone. Try to squeeze the gel out smoothly so there are as few air bubbles as possible.

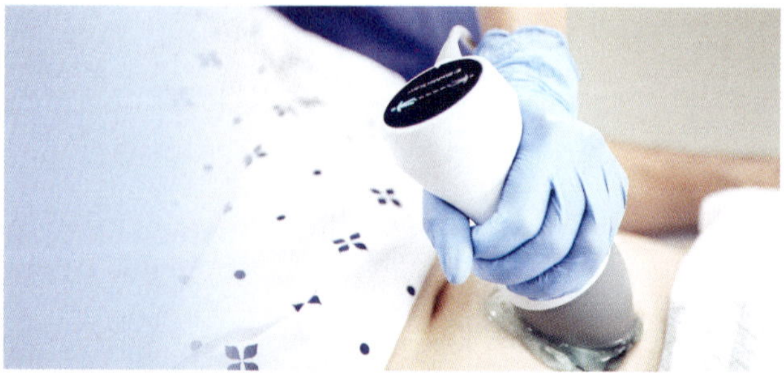

Fig. 17-17. *Let the patient know that the gel may feel cold.* (BLADDERSCAN I10™. USED WITH PERMISSION. ©VERATHON INC.)

11. Palpate (find by touch) the patient's pubic bone. Holding the scanner as shown in the manufacturer's instructions, place the scanner head on the patient's abdomen, approximately 3 centimeters (about 1 inch) above the pubic bone. Be sure there are no air bubbles between the scanner and the skin. The scanner handle usually needs to be tilted slightly toward the patient's head. This directs the sound waves toward the bladder.
12. When the scanner is positioned correctly, press the start or scan button. Some scanners have a display that shows which way to move the device to get the best result.
13. Bladder scanners give results in milliliters (mL). This is the volume of urine in the bladder. Document the result according to facility policy. You may be asked to print the scan or upload the result to a patient's medical record.
14. Use a towel to wipe the gel off the patient's abdomen (or allow him to do this if he prefers). Remove and discard the absorbent pad. Wipe the gel off the bladder scanner and then clean the head with an alcohol swab. Place the towel in the proper container. Store the device according to facility policy.
15. Return the bed to its lowest position. Remove privacy measures.
16. Place the call light within the patient's reach.
17. Remove and discard your gloves (if worn). Wash your hands.

18. Report any changes in the patient to the nurse.

5. Identify types of urine specimens that are collected

PCTs may need to collect a urine specimen from a patient. Different types of specimens are used for different tests. Some electronic records systems allow a PCT to print completed labels.

There are several factors to consider when collecting urine specimens. Body wastes and elimination needs are very private matters for most people. Having another person handle body wastes may make patients embarrassed and uncomfortable. PCTs should be sensitive to this, and be empathetic. They should think about how difficult this may be for the patient. When collecting specimens, it is important that the PCT behave professionally. If they feel that this is an unpleasant task, they should not make it known. They should not make faces, frown, or use words that let the patient know they are uncomfortable. Remaining professional when collecting specimens can help put patients at ease.

Urine specimens may be categorized as routine, clean-catch (midstream), first void, or 24-hour. A **routine urine specimen** is collected any time the patient voids, or urinates. Some patients will be able to collect their own urine specimens, while others will need help. Those patients who can collect their own specimens are directed to urinate into a specimen cup until it is at least half full. Patients who cannot collect their own specimens will void into a bedpan, urinal, commode, or hat. A **hat** is a plastic collection container sometimes put into a toilet bowl to collect and measure urine or stool (Fig. 17-18). The PCT should explain exactly how the specimen must be collected, and must label the specimen correctly (Fig. 17-19). The procedure that follows describes collecting a specimen using a bedpan, urinal, or hat.

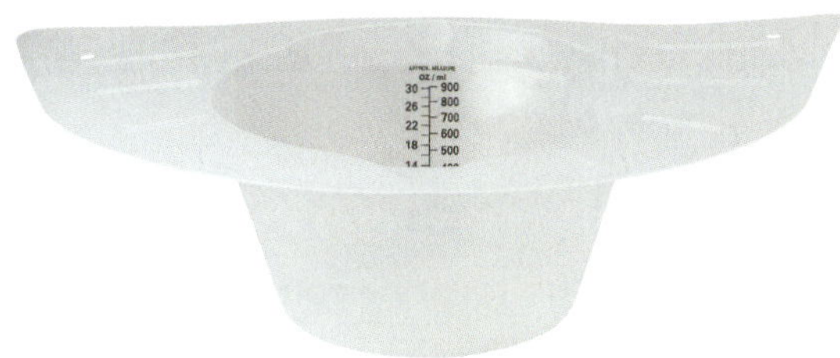

Fig. 17-18. *A hat is a container that is sometimes placed under the toilet seat to collect a specimen. Hats should be labeled and must be cleaned after each use.*

(IMAGE COURTESY OF MEDLINE INDUSTRIES, LP. USED WITH PERMISSION.)

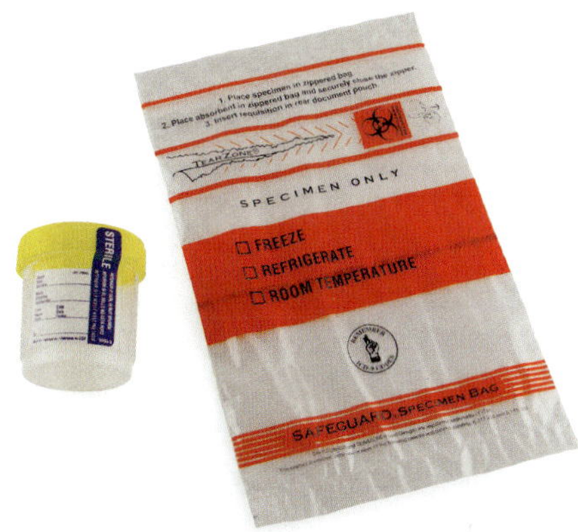

Fig. 17-19. *Specimens must always be labeled with the patient's name, date of birth, room number, and the date and time before being taken to the lab. A specimen may need to be placed in a clean specimen bag before it is transported.*

Collecting a routine urine specimen

Equipment: urine specimen container and lid; completed label (labeled with the patient's name, date of birth, room number, date, and time); specimen bag; 2 pairs of gloves; bedpan or urinal (if patient cannot use a portable commode or toilet); hat for toilet (if patient uses portable commode or toilet); plastic bag; toilet paper; disposable wipes; paper towels; supplies for perineal care; requisition

1. Identify yourself by name. Identify the patient according to facility policy.
2. Wash your hands.

3. Explain the procedure to the patient. Speak clearly, slowly, and directly. Maintain face-to-face contact whenever possible.
4. Provide for the patient's privacy with a curtain, screen, or door.
5. Put on gloves.
6. Fit the hat to the toilet or commode, or provide the patient with the bedpan or urinal.
7. Ask the patient to void into the hat, urinal, or bedpan. Ask the patient not to put toilet paper in with the sample. Provide a plastic bag to discard the toilet paper separately.
8. Make sure the bed is in its lowest position. Place the toilet paper and disposable wipes within the patient's reach. Ask the patient to clean his hands with a wipe when finished if he is able.
9. Remove and discard your gloves. Wash your hands.
10. Place the call light within the patient's reach. Ask the patient to signal when done. Leave the room and close the door.
11. When called by the patient, return and wash your hands. Put on clean gloves. Provide perineal care if help is needed.
12. Take the bedpan, urinal, or hat to the bathroom.
13. Pour the urine into the specimen container until the container is at least half full.
14. Cover the urine container with its lid. Do not touch the inside of the container. Wipe off the outside with a paper towel and discard the paper towel.
15. Apply the label, place the container in a clean specimen bag, and seal the bag.
16. Discard extra urine in the toilet and flush the toilet. Rinse the bedpan or urinal if part of facility policy. Place it in the proper area for cleaning or clean and disinfect it according to facility policy.
17. Remove and discard your gloves. Wash your hands.
18. Make the patient comfortable.
19. Return the bed to its lowest position if it was adjusted. Remove privacy measures.
20. Place the call light within the patient's reach.
21. Report any changes in the patient to the nurse.
22. Follow facility policy for getting the specimen and requisition to the laboratory. Document the procedure using facility guidelines. Note the amount and characteristics of the urine.

Connected Care

Specimens

When collecting specimens, the PCT should first explain how she will collect the specimen. This should be done in a private area, and the PCT should keep her voice low. She should also close the door to the bathroom or bedroom and pull the privacy curtain. In addition, the PCT should be discreet when removing the specimen from the room.

The **clean-catch specimen**, or midstream specimen (CCMS), does not include the first and last urine voided in the sample, reducing contamination of the specimen. The perineal area is cleaned and then the patient urinates a small amount into the toilet to clear the urethra. The patient then begins urinating again into a clean or sterile container, stopping before urination is complete. The container is removed, and the patient finishes urinating into the toilet. This specimen is collected to detect bacteria in the urine.

Collecting a clean-catch (midstream) urine specimen

Equipment: specimen kit with container and lid; completed label (labeled with patient's name, date of birth, room number, date, and time); specimen bag; cleansing wipes; gloves; bedpan or urinal (if patient cannot use a portable commode or toilet); plastic bag; toilet paper; disposable wipes; paper towels; supplies for perineal care; requisition

1. Identify yourself by name. Identify the patient according to facility policy.
2. Wash your hands.
3. Explain the procedure to the patient. Speak clearly, slowly, and directly. Maintain face-to-face contact whenever possible.
4. Provide for the patient's privacy with a curtain, screen, or door.
5. Put on gloves.
6. Open the specimen kit. Do not touch the inside of the container or the inside of the lid.
7. If the patient cannot clean his perineal area, you will do it. Use the cleansing wipes to do this. Be sure to use a clean area of the wipe or a clean wipe for each stroke. See the bed bath procedure in Chapter 9 for a reminder on how to give perineal care.
8. Ask the patient to urinate a small amount into the bedpan, urinal, or toilet, and to stop before urination is complete.
9. Place the container under the urine stream and have the patient start urinating again until the container is at least half full. Ask the patient to stop urinating and remove the container. Have the patient finish urinating in the bedpan, urinal, or toilet.
10. After urination, provide a plastic bag so the patient can discard the toilet paper. Give perineal care if help is needed. Ask the patient to clean his hands with a wipe if he is able.
11. Cover the urine container with its lid. Do not touch the inside of the container. Wipe off the outside with a paper towel and discard the paper towel.
12. Apply the label, place the container in a clean specimen bag, and seal the bag.
13. Discard extra urine in the toilet and flush the toilet. Rinse the bedpan or urinal if part of facility policy. Place it in the proper area for cleaning or clean it according to facility policy.
14. Remove and discard your gloves. Wash your hands.
15. Make the patient comfortable.
16. Return the bed to its lowest position if it was adjusted. Remove privacy measures.
17. Place the call light within the patient's reach.
18. Report any changes in the patient to the nurse.
19. Follow facility policy for getting the specimen and requisition to the laboratory. Document the procedure using facility guidelines. Note the amount and characteristics of the urine.

The *first void* specimen is collected when the patient first urinates (voids) in the morning. These specimens are more concentrated than specimens collected later in the day. First void specimens may be collected using routine or clean-catch procedures. PCTs should follow instructions for collecting these specimens.

A **24-hour urine specimen** collects all the urine voided by a patient in a 24-hour period.

It is used to test for certain chemicals and hormones. Usually the collection begins at 7 a.m. and continues until 7 a.m. the next day. When beginning a 24-hour urine specimen collection, the patient must void and discard the first urine so that the collection begins with an empty bladder. All urine must be collected and stored properly. Specimens may be stored in a cooler filled with icy water (an ice slurry) or in a refrigerator. If any urine is accidentally thrown away or improperly stored, the collection will need to be started over.

Collecting a 24-hour urine specimen

Equipment: 24-hour specimen container with lid; completed label (labeled with patient's name, date of birth, room number, date, and time); bedpan or urinal (for patients confined to bed); hat for toilet (if patient can use portable commode or toilet); gloves; toilet paper; disposable wipes; supplies for perineal care; sign to alert other team members that a 24-hour urine specimen is being collected; form for recording output (unless documentation is done electronically); requisition

1. Identify yourself by name. Identify the patient according to facility policy.
2. Wash your hands.
3. Explain the procedure to the patient. Speak clearly, slowly, and directly. Maintain face-to-face contact whenever possible. Emphasize that all urine must be saved. Ask the patient not to include toilet paper or stool (feces) with the sample.
4. Provide for the patient's privacy with a curtain, screen, or door.
5. Place a sign near the patient's bed to let all care team members know that a 24-hour specimen is being collected. The sign may read "Save all urine for 24-hour specimen."
6. When starting the collection, have the patient completely empty their bladder. Discard the urine. Note the exact time of this voiding. The collection will run until the same time the next day.
7. Label the container with the patient's name, date of birth, room number, and dates and times the collection period began and ended.
8. Wash your hands and put on clean gloves each time the patient voids.
9. Pour urine from the bedpan, urinal, or hat into the container. The container may be stored at room temperature, in a refrigerator, or on ice. Follow the nurse's instructions.
10. After each voiding, help as necessary with perineal care. Ask the patient to clean their hands with a wipe after each voiding.
11. After each voiding, place equipment in the proper area for cleaning or clean it according to facility policy.
12. Remove and discard your gloves. Wash your hands.
13. After the last void of the 24-hour period, remove the sign. Remove privacy measures. Follow facility policy for getting the specimen and requisition to the laboratory. Document the procedure using facility guidelines. Make sure to include the time of the last void before the 24-hour collection period began and the last void of the 24-hour collection period.

6. Explain types of tests performed on urine

Different types of tests can be used to detect different substances or properties in urine. Some tests can be conducted easily using chemically treated strips dipped into the urine. These strips, called *reagent strips*, or *dip strips*, have different sections that change color when they react with urine (Fig. 17-20). Reagent strips can be used to test for such things as pH level, a pregnancy hormone, glucose, ketones, blood, nitrites, and specific gravity.

Testing pH levels: The pH scale ranges from 0 to 14. The lower the number, the more acidic the fluid. The higher the number, the more alkaline the fluid. The normal pH range for urine is 4.6–8.0. A pH imbalance may be due to medication, food, or illness.

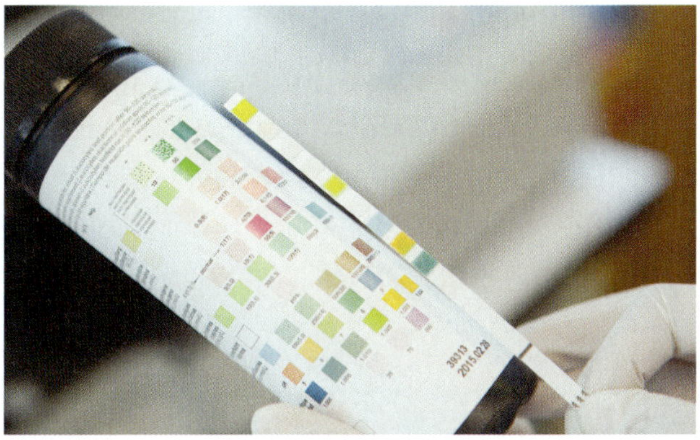

Fig. 17-20. Reagent strips change color when they react with urine. The color is then compared to a color chart to determine levels of each chemical factor.

Testing for pregnancy: Human chorionic gonadotropin (hCG) is a hormone related to pregnancy. Blood tests for hCG may be more accurate very early in pregnancy, but hCG is also in urine. Reagent strips may be used to test urine for hCG from about 10 days after conception.

Testing for glucose and ketones: These substances are associated with diabetes testing. In diabetes, the pancreas produces no insulin, too little insulin, or does not properly use insulin. Insulin is the hormone that works to move glucose, or natural sugar, from the blood and into the cells for energy for the body. Without enough insulin to process glucose, these sugars collect in the blood. Glucose is blood sugar and it can appear in urine in some cases.

Ketones are chemical substances produced when the body burns fat for energy or fuel. They are produced when there is not enough insulin to help the body use sugar for energy. Without enough insulin, glucose builds up in the blood. Since the body cannot use glucose for energy, it breaks down fat instead. When this occurs, ketones build up in the blood and spill into the urine.

In addition to strip testing, a double-voided (also called *fresh-fractional*) urine specimen may be used to test for glucose. A double-voided specimen is a urine specimen that is collected after first emptying the bladder and then waiting until another specimen can be collected. This may be ordered because testing urine that has been in the bladder for some time may not accurately reflect the amount of glucose present. With a double-voided specimen, after the person has voided, he is encouraged to drink fluids. Then approximately 30 minutes later, a second (double-voided) specimen is collected and tested.

Testing for blood: Normal urine does not contain blood. Illness and disease can cause blood to appear in urine. Blood in urine may not be visible (it is hidden, or occult) but can be detected by testing.

Testing for nitrites: This test may be performed to determine if the person has a urinary tract infection. Nitrites are substances produced by the bacteria that cause urinary tract infections.

Testing specific gravity: A specific gravity (also called *urine density*) test is performed to measure the concentration of chemical particles in the urine. The test evaluates the body's water balance and urine concentration by showing how the density of urine compares to water. Normal values range from 1.002 to 1.028. Certain disorders increase or decrease specific gravity. For example, kidney failure can decrease it. This test usually requires a clean-catch urine specimen.

PCTs may not be allowed to perform urine testing. They should follow their facility's policies.

Testing urine with reagent strips

Equipment: urine specimen as ordered, reagent strip, gloves, paper towel

1. Wash your hands.
2. Put on gloves.

3. Take a strip from the bottle and recap the bottle. Close it tightly.
4. Dip the strip into the specimen.
5. Follow the manufacturer's instructions for when to remove the strip from the specimen. Remove the strip at the correct time.
6. Follow the manufacturer's instructions for how long to wait after removing the strip. After the proper time has passed, compare the strip with the color chart on the bottle. Do not touch the bottle with the strip.
7. Read the results.
8. Store the strips. Discard used items. Discard the specimen in the toilet and flush the toilet.
9. Remove and discard your gloves. Wash your hands.
10. Document the procedure using facility guidelines.

7. Explain guidelines for assisting with bladder retraining

Injury, illness, or inactivity may cause a loss of normal bladder function. Patients may need help in reestablishing a regular routine and normal function. An occupational therapist may set a bladder training schedule and teach the patient exercises to strengthen muscles around the bladder. Problems with elimination can be embarrassing or difficult to discuss. PCTs should be sensitive to this and always remain professional when handling incontinence or working to reestablish routines.

Guidelines: Bladder Retraining

G Follow Standard Precautions. Wear gloves when handling body wastes.

G Explain the bladder training schedule to the patient. Follow the schedule carefully.

G Keep a record of the patient's bladder habits. When you see a pattern of elimination, you can predict when the patient will need a bedpan or a trip to the bathroom.

G Offer a bedpan or a trip to the bathroom before beginning long procedures (Fig. 17-21).

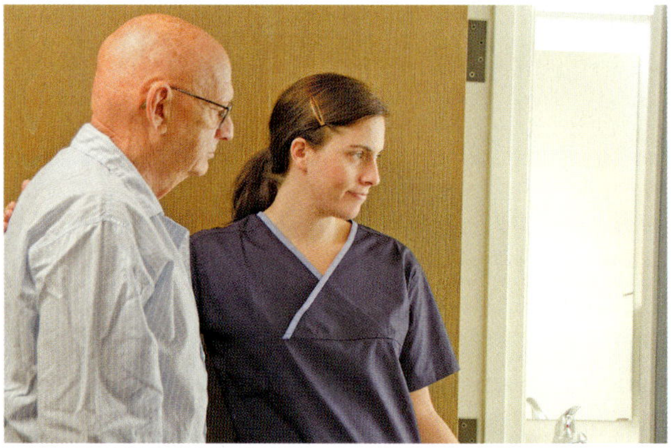

Fig. 17-21. *Offer regular trips to the bathroom.*

G Encourage the patient to drink plenty of fluids. Do this even if urinary incontinence is a problem. About 30 minutes after fluids are taken, offer a trip to the bathroom or a bedpan or urinal.

G Answer call lights promptly. Patients cannot wait long when the urge to go to the bathroom occurs. Leave call lights within reach of the patient's stronger hand.

G Provide privacy for elimination—both in the bed and in the bathroom.

G If a patient has trouble urinating, try running water in the sink. Have her lean forward slightly to put pressure on the bladder.

G Do not rush the patient during urination.

G Help patients with careful perineal care. This helps prevent skin breakdown and promotes proper hygiene. Carefully observe for skin changes.

G Discard wastes according to your facility's policies.

G Discard clothing protectors and incontinence briefs properly. Double-bag these items if ordered. This stops odors from collecting.

G Some facilities use washable bed pads or briefs. Follow Standard Precautions when rinsing before placing these items in the laundry.

G Keep an accurate record of urination. This includes any episodes of incontinence.

G Offer positive words for successes or even attempts to control the bladder. However, do not talk to adult patients as if they were children. Keep your voice low and do not draw attention to any aspect of retraining.

G Never show frustration or anger toward patients who have incontinence. The problem is out of their control. It is hard enough for patients to handle incontinence without having to worry about healthcare workers' reactions. Negative reactions will only make things worse. Be kind, supportive, and professional.

G When the patient has incontinence or cannot urinate when asked, be positive. Never make the patient feel like a failure. Praise and encouragement are essential for a successful program. Remember that each patient has different needs and may respond to different types of encouragement. Finding out each patient's needs and preferences is part of providing person-centered care.

G Some patients will always have incontinence. Be patient and kind. Offer these patients extra care and attention. Skin breakdown may lead to pressure injuries without proper care. Always report changes in skin.

Chapter Review

1. What are 2 functions of the urinary system?
2. Is urinary incontinence a normal part of aging?
3. Why should a PCT never refer to an incontinence brief as a diaper?
4. What are 4 ways that PCTs can help prevent urinary tract infections?
5. Why must PCTs always wear gloves (and additional PPE as assigned) when handling bedpans, urinals, or basins that contain wastes?
6. When performing perineal care, in what direction should the PCT wipe the patient?
7. How should a standard bedpan be positioned? How should a fracture pan be positioned?
8. Why should the catheter drainage bag always be kept lower than the hips or the bladder?
9. Why should catheter tubing be kept as straight as possible?
10. What is a syringe used for during the procedure for removing an indwelling urinary catheter?
11. How is bladder scanning used to reduce the risk of urinary tract infections?
12. What is a clean-catch urine specimen?
13. How can PCTs help reduce discomfort when assisting with specimen collection?
14. List 4 things reagent strips can detect in urine.
15. About how long after fluids are taken should the PCT offer to take a patient to the bathroom?
16. List 2 guidelines for bladder retraining that help promote dignity.

18 The Gastrointestinal System and Related Care

1. Describe the structure and function of the gastrointestinal system

The gastrointestinal (GI) system, also called the digestive system, is made up of the gastrointestinal tract and the accessory digestive organs (Fig. 18-1). The gastrointestinal tract is a long passageway extending from the mouth to the anus, the opening of the rectum. Food passes from the mouth through the pharynx, esophagus, stomach, small intestine, large intestine, and out of the body as solid waste (*feces* or *stool*). The teeth, tongue, salivary glands, liver, gallbladder, and pancreas assist in digestion. They help prepare the food so that it can be absorbed.

Food is first placed in the mouth. The teeth chew it by cutting it, then chopping and grinding it into smaller pieces that can be swallowed. Saliva moistens the food and begins chemical digestion. The tongue helps with chewing and swallowing by pushing the food around between the teeth and then into the pharynx.

The pharynx is a muscular structure located at the back of the mouth. It extends into the throat. It contracts with swallowing and pushes food into the esophagus. The muscles of the esophagus then move food into the stomach through involuntary contractions called **peristalsis**.

The stomach is a muscular pouch located in the upper left part of the abdominal cavity. It provides physical digestion by stirring and churning the food to break it down into smaller particles. The glands in the stomach lining aid in digestion. They secrete gastric juices that chemically break down food. This process turns food into a semiliquid substance called chyme. Peristalsis continues in the stomach, pushing the chyme into the small intestine.

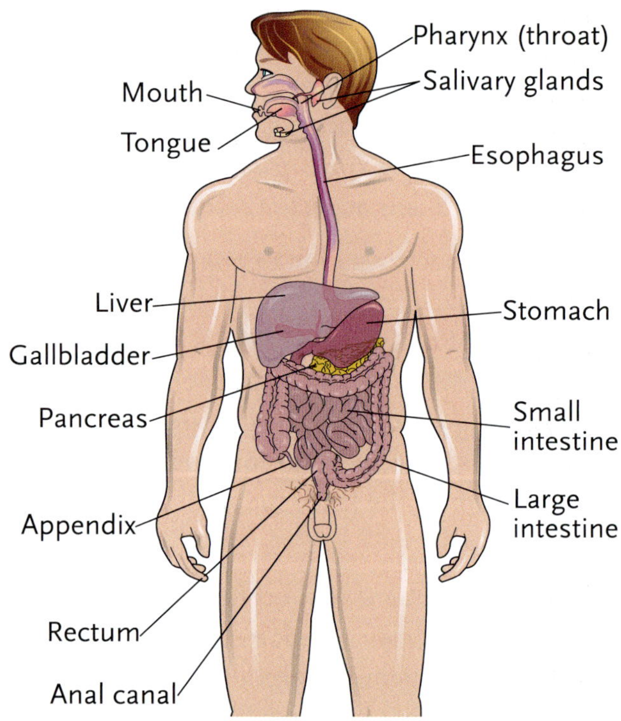

Fig. 18-1. The GI system consists of all the organs needed to digest food and process waste.

The small intestine is about 20 feet long. Here enzymes secreted by the liver and the pancreas finish digesting the chyme. Bile, a green liquid produced by the liver, is stored in the gallbladder and released into the small intestine. Bile helps break down dietary fat. The liver converts fats and sugars into **glucose**, a natural sugar that can be carried to cells by the blood. The liver also stores glucose. The pancreas produces insulin, a hormone that works to move glucose from the blood into the cells for energy for the body.

The chyme is moved by peristalsis through the small intestine. There villi, tiny projections lining the small intestine, absorb the digested food into the capillaries.

Peristalsis moves the chyme that has not already been digested through the large intestine. In the large intestine, most of the water in the chyme is absorbed. What remains is feces, a semisolid material of water, solid waste material, bacteria, and mucus. Feces passes by peristalsis through the rectum, the lower end of the colon. It moves out of the body through the anus, the rectal opening.

The gastrointestinal system has the following functions: digestion, absorption, and elimination. **Digestion** is the process of preparing food physically and chemically so that it can be absorbed into the cells. **Absorption** is the transfer of nutrients from the intestines to the cells. **Elimination** is the process of expelling wastes (made up of the waste products of food and fluids) that are not absorbed into the cells.

Observing and Reporting: Gastrointestinal System

Observe and report these signs and symptoms:

- O/R Difficulty swallowing or chewing (including denture problems, tooth pain, or mouth sores)
- O/R **Fecal incontinence** (inability to control the bowels, leading to involuntary passage of stool)
- O/R Weight gain or weight loss
- O/R Loss of appetite
- O/R Abdominal pain and cramping
- O/R Diarrhea
- O/R Nausea and vomiting (especially vomitus that looks like coffee grounds)
- O/R Constipation
- O/R Flatulence
- O/R Hiccups or belching
- O/R Bloody, black, or hard stools
- O/R Heartburn
- O/R Poor nutritional intake

2. List common conditions of the gastrointestinal system and discuss related care

Constipation

Constipation is the inability to eliminate stool (have a bowel movement), or the infrequent, difficult, and often painful elimination of hard, dry stool. Constipation occurs when the feces move too slowly through the intestine. This can result from decreased fluid intake, poor diet/lack of fiber, inactivity, medications, aging, certain diseases, or ignoring the urge to eliminate. Changes to routine and diet, such as the changes that result from hospitalization, can also cause constipation. Signs of constipation include abdominal swelling, gas, irritability, and no recent bowel movement.

Treatment includes increasing the amount of fiber eaten and fluids consumed, increasing activity level, and possibly medication. Accurate documentation of bowel movements is important. An enema or rectal suppository may be ordered to help with constipation. An **enema** is a specific amount of water, with or without an additive, that is introduced into the colon to stimulate the elimination of stool. A rectal suppository is a medication given rectally to cause a bowel movement.

Fecal Impaction

A **fecal impaction** is a hard stool that is stuck in the rectum and cannot be expelled. It results from unrelieved constipation. Symptoms include no stool for several days, oozing of liquid stool, cramping, abdominal swelling, and rectal pain. When an impaction occurs, a nurse or provider will insert 1 or 2 gloved fingers into the rectum and break the mass into fragments so that it can be passed. Prevention of fecal impactions often includes the same measures as those used for preventing constipation, i.e., high-fiber diet, plenty of fluids, an increase in activity level, and possibly medication. Early assessment of constipation may also help prevent impactions.

Hemorrhoids

Hemorrhoids are enlarged veins in the rectum, which may also be visible outside the anus. Chronic constipation, obesity, pregnancy, chronic diarrhea, overuse of laxatives and enemas, and straining during bowel movements are common causes of hemorrhoids. Rectal itching, burning, pain, and bleeding during bowel elimination are signs and symptoms of hemorrhoids. Treatment includes adding more fiber into the diet and increasing fluid intake. Medications, compresses, and sitz baths are also used to treat hemorrhoids. Surgery may be necessary. When cleaning the anal area, the PCT should be very careful to avoid causing pain and bleeding.

Diarrhea

Diarrhea is the frequent elimination of liquid or semiliquid feces. Abdominal cramps, urgency, nausea, and vomiting can accompany diarrhea, depending on the cause. Bacterial and viral infections, microorganisms in food and water, irritating foods, and medications can cause diarrhea. Treatment of diarrhea usually involves medication, an increase in hydrating fluids, and a temporary change of diet. The patient's ordered diet may focus on soft, low-fiber foods with few seasonings.

Fecal Incontinence

Fecal incontinence is the inability to control the bowels, leading to an involuntary passage of stool. Common causes are constipation, muscle and nerve damage, loss of storage capacity in the rectum, and diarrhea. Treatment includes a change in diet, medication, bowel training, or surgery.

Gastroesophageal Reflux Disease

Gastroesophageal reflux disease (**GERD**) is a chronic condition in which the liquid contents of the stomach back up into the esophagus. Stomach acid causes a burning sensation, often called *heartburn,* in the esophagus. It can inflame and damage the lining of the esophagus. It can also cause bleeding or ulcers (sores). Over time, scars from tissue damage can narrow the esophagus and make swallowing difficult.

The most common symptom of GERD is **heartburn**, which is the result of a weakening of the sphincter muscle that joins the esophagus and the stomach. When healthy, this muscle prevents the leaking of stomach acid and other contents back into the esophagus. If heartburn occurs frequently and remains untreated, it can cause **ulceration**.

Heartburn must be reported to the nurse. Heartburn and GERD are usually treated with medications. Serving the evening meal 3 to 4 hours before bedtime may help. The patient should not lie down flat until at least 2 to 3 hours after eating (Fig. 18-2). Extra pillows can be used to keep the body more upright during sleep.

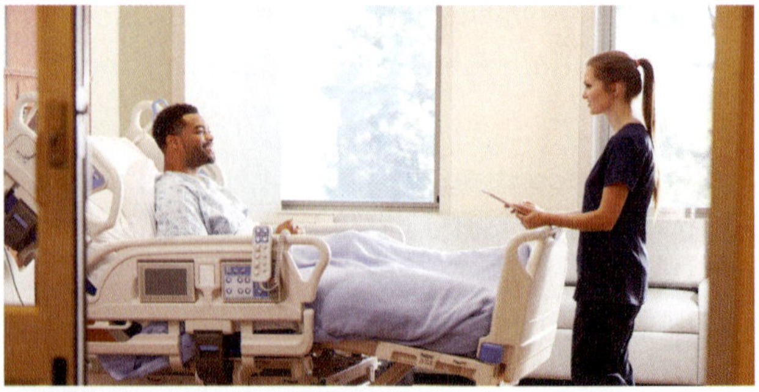

Fig. 18-2. *Sitting up in bed for at least 2 hours after eating can help prevent heartburn.*

Peptic Ulcers

Peptic ulcers or *gastric ulcers* are raw sores in the stomach. Ulcers are caused by excessive acid secretion. A digestive tract bacterium called *Helicobacter pylori*, or *H. pylori*, can also cause ulcers. Peptic ulcers cause dull or burning pain 1 to 3 hours after eating, accompanied by belching or vomiting. They can also cause bleeding, and stool may appear black (tarry). Treatment includes antacids, antibiotics and other medications, as well as a change in diet. A bland diet, which eliminates foods that produce or increase levels of gastric acid in the stomach, may be ordered.

Irritable Bowel Syndrome (IBS)

Irritable bowel syndrome (**IBS**) is a condition that causes diarrhea, constipation, or both on a regular basis. These symptoms may be accompanied by bloating, abdominal pain, and gas. Some forms of IBS cause only constipation or only diarrhea. Others cause both. Stress may worsen symptoms. Certain foods and beverages may also cause flare-ups. Fried foods, fatty foods, caffeine, and alcohol are common triggers.

Although it is not fully understood, irritable bowel syndrome relates to the function of the bowel. In other words, it is not caused by physical damage or disease. It is a result of problems in communication between the nervous system and the digestive tract. This causes the bowel to function less effectively.

There is no single treatment for IBS. Medication and diet changes are important for managing IBS.

Inflammatory Bowel Disease

Inflammatory bowel disease (**IBD**) is a term for conditions in which the bowel is chronically inflamed. It is not the same as IBS. IBD is thought to be caused by improper immune system response. Two different illnesses are considered to be forms of IBD: ulcerative colitis and Crohn's disease.

Ulcerative colitis is a chronic inflammatory disease of the large intestine. Symptoms include cramping, diarrhea, pain occurring on one side of the lower abdomen, rectal bleeding, loss of appetite, and weight loss. Ulcerative colitis is a serious illness that can cause intestinal bleeding and death if left untreated.

Crohn's disease can affect any part of the digestive tract, but most commonly affects the small intestine. The inflammation caused by Crohn's disease may occur in patches. Damaged tissue may be among healthy tissue. Ulcerative colitis causes a continuous area of damage that may spread. Crohn's disease causes symptoms similar to those of ulcerative colitis.

Medications can relieve symptoms, but they cannot cure inflammatory bowel disease. Surgical treatment may include a colostomy or an ileostomy, which is the diversion of waste to an artificial opening (**stoma**) through the abdomen. Stool is diverted through the stoma instead of the anus. There is more information on colostomy care later in the chapter.

Diverticulitis

Diverticulosis is a condition that happens when small pouches called *diverticula* form in the colon. The chance of developing these pouches increases with age. If the diverticula become inflamed, they cause **diverticulitis**. The condition causes fever and abdominal pain and tenderness. It may also cause nausea, vomiting, and diarrhea.

A mild case of diverticulitis may be treated with oral antibiotics. More severe cases may be treated at a hospital with IV antibiotics; surgery and a colostomy may be necessary.

Complications of diverticulitis can be dangerous. If an infected pouch breaks open, or ruptures, the contents of the intestines can leak into the abdominal cavity. This is a medical emergency called *peritonitis*. Scarring from diverticulitis can cause a bowel obstruction, or a blockage in the intestine.

Cancer

Colorectal cancer, also known as *colon cancer*, is cancer of the gastrointestinal tract. Signs and symptoms include changes in normal bowel patterns, cramps, abdominal pain, and rectal bleeding. Colorectal cancer must be treated with surgery. Chapter 21 contains more information about cancer.

3. Discuss how enemas are given

Putting fluid into the rectum in order to eliminate stool or feces is called an *enema*. Enemas may be given prior to surgery or a medical test, or when a person cannot eliminate stool on their own. PCTs may be trained to give enemas, depending upon the state and facility in which they work. PCTs may also assist a nurse who is giving an enema. If PCTs are allowed to give enemas, they must make sure to follow policies and procedures. Any questions a PCT may have should be discussed with the nurse before giving an enema.

Providers will write an enema order. There are 4 different types of enemas:

- Tap water enema (TWE): 500–1000 milliliters (mL) of water from a faucet
- Soapsuds enema (SSE): 500–1000 mL water with 5 mL of mild castile soap added
- Saline enema: 500–1000 mL water with 2 teaspoons of salt added
- Commercially prepared enema (also called *commercial enema* or *prepackaged enema*): 120 mL solution; may have oil or other additive

Tap water, soapsuds, and saline enemas are all considered cleansing enemas. They all require more fluid than commercially prepared enemas do. Equipment used for giving cleansing enemas includes an IV pole, the enema solution, tubing, and a clamp.

Guidelines: Assisting with Enemas

G Provide plenty of privacy for this procedure.

G Keep the bedpan nearby or make sure that the bathroom is vacant before assisting with an enema.

G Help the patient into the Sims' (left side-lying) position (Fig. 18-3). If the person is positioned on the left side, water does not have to flow against gravity.

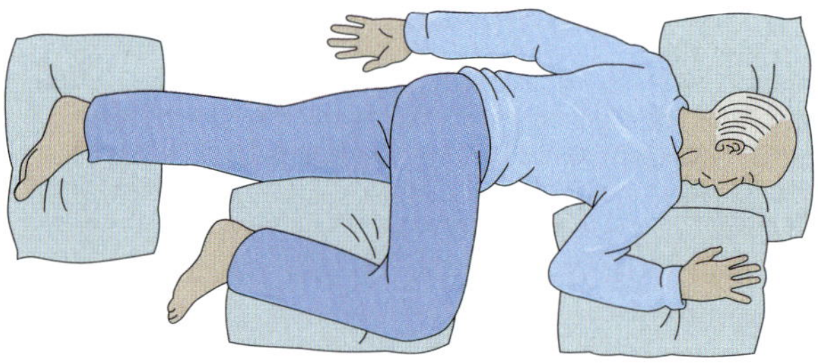

Fig. 18-3. The Sims' position (left side-lying position) is the proper position for an enema.

G While the enema is being given, encourage the patient to take slow, deep breaths to help hold the solution longer.

Connected Care

Enemas

Protecting a patient's rights during an enema includes providing plenty of privacy. The patient must be covered with a bath blanket or sheet and the anal area only exposed as needed to complete the procedure. The privacy curtain should be pulled around the bed and the door closed. Any questions that the patient has about the procedure should be answered. Questions that are not within the PCT's scope of practice should be answered by the nurse.

A commercially prepared enema usually has 120 mL of solution and may have an additive (Fig. 18-4). An oil retention enema has a type of oil in it that softens the stool to allow it to pass more easily. It is often used when a person has been constipated for a long time, resulting in a stool that is very hard, or when a person has a fecal impaction. Commercially prepared enemas do not require an IV pole, tubing, or clamp, because they are prepackaged and premixed.

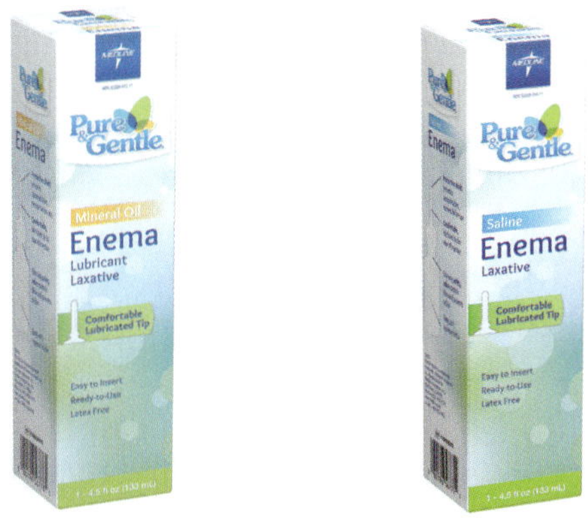

Fig. 18-4. *Commercially prepared enemas may come with additives, such as saline and mineral oil.* (IMAGES COURTESY OF MEDLINE INDUSTRIES, LP. USED WITH PERMISSION.)

4. Demonstrate how to collect a stool specimen

Stool (feces) specimens are sometimes collected so that the stool can be tested for blood, pathogens, fat (an indication that nutrients are not being absorbed properly), and for other things, such as worms or amoebas. Worms and amoebas can be detected with an ova and parasites test. If the specimen is to be examined for ova and parasites, it must be taken to the lab immediately. This examination must be made while the stool is still warm.

If the patient uses a bedpan or portable commode for elimination, that is where the PCT will collect the stool specimen. If the patient uses the toilet, a hat (collection container) will be used.

The PCT should ask the patient to let her know when he needs to have a bowel movement, and she should be ready to collect the specimen. The PCT should explain that urine or toilet paper should not be included in the sample because they can ruin the sample and create the need for a new specimen.

Collecting a stool specimen

Equipment: specimen container and lid; completed label (labeled with patient's name, date of birth, room number, date, and time); specimen bag; 2 pairs of gloves; 2 tongue blades; bedpan (if patient cannot use portable commode or toilet); hat for toilet (if patient uses portable commode or toilet); plastic bag; toilet paper; disposable wipes; paper towels; supplies for perineal care; requisition

1. Identify yourself by name. Identify the patient according to facility policy.
2. Wash your hands.
3. Explain the procedure to the patient. Speak clearly, slowly, and directly. Maintain face-to-face contact whenever possible.
4. Provide for the patient's privacy with a curtain, screen, or door.
5. Put on gloves.
6. When the patient is ready to move his bowels, ask him not to urinate at the same time and not to put toilet paper in with the sample. Provide a plastic bag to discard toilet paper and wipes separately.
7. Fit the hat to the toilet or commode, or provide the patient with a bedpan.
8. Make sure the bed is in its lowest position. Place toilet paper and disposable wipes within the patient's reach. Ask the patient to clean his hands with a wipe when finished if he is able.
9. Remove and discard your gloves. Wash your hands.
10. Place the call light within the patient's reach. Ask the patient to signal when done. Leave the room and close the door.
11. When called by the patient, return and wash your hands. Put on clean gloves. Give perineal care if help is needed.
12. Using the 2 tongue blades, take about 2 tablespoons of stool and put it in the

container. Without touching the inside of the container, cover it tightly. Apply the label and place the container in a clean specimen bag. Seal the bag.

13. Wrap the tongue blades in toilet paper and put them in the plastic bag with the used toilet paper and wipes. Discard the bag in the proper container.
14. Empty the contents of the bedpan or container carefully into the toilet. Flush the toilet.
15. Rinse the bedpan if part of facility policy. Place it in the proper area for cleaning or clean and disinfect it according to facility policy.
16. Remove and discard your gloves. Wash your hands.
17. Remove privacy measures.
18. Place the call light within the patient's reach.
19. Report any changes in the patient to the nurse.
20. Follow facility policy for getting the specimen and requisition to the laboratory. Document the procedure using facility guidelines. Note the amount and characteristics of stool.

5. Define *ostomy* and list care guidelines

An **ostomy** is the surgical creation of an opening from an area inside the body to the outside. The terms *colostomy* and *ileostomy* refer to the surgical removal of a portion of the intestines. In a patient with one of these ostomies, the end of the intestine is brought out of the body through an artificial opening in the abdomen. This opening is called a *stoma*. Stool, or feces, is eliminated through the ostomy rather than through the anus. (When a ureter is opened to the abdomen for urine to be eliminated, it is called a **ureterostomy**.) An ostomy may be necessary due to bowel disease, cancer, or trauma. It may be temporary or permanent.

The terms *colostomy* and *ileostomy* indicate what section of the intestine was removed and the type of stool that will be eliminated. A **colostomy** is a surgically created opening into the large intestine to allow stool to be expelled. With a colostomy, stool will generally be semisolid. An **ileostomy** is a surgically created opening into the end of the small intestine to allow stool to be expelled. Stool will be liquid and may be irritating to the patient's skin.

Patients who have had an ostomy wear a disposable pouching system that fits over the stoma to collect the feces (Fig. 18-5). The pouching system is attached to the skin by adhesive, and a belt may also be used to secure it.

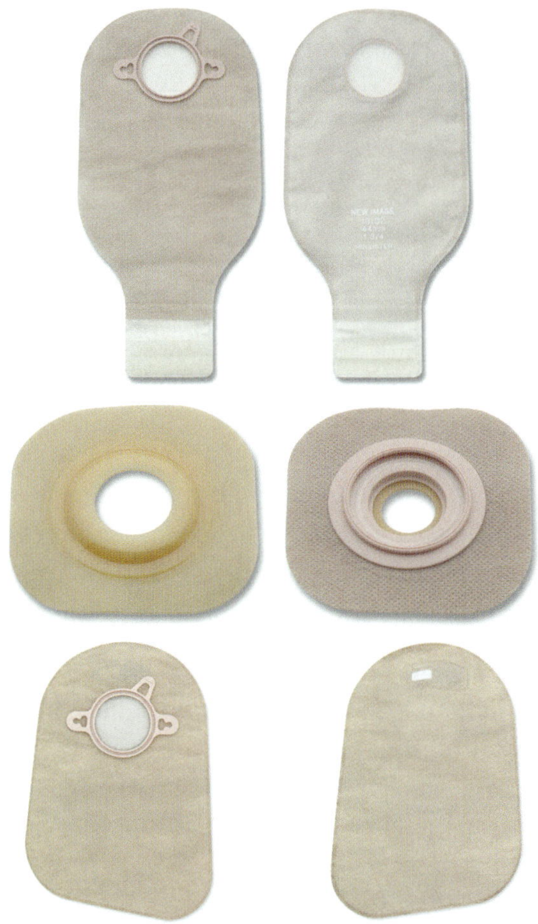

Fig. 18-5. *The top and middle photos show an ostomy drainage pouch and a skin barrier for a drainable (reusable) system. The bottom photo shows a closed (disposable) system that is only used once before being discarded.* (PHOTOS COURTESY OF HOLLISTER INCORPORATED, LIBERTYVILLE, ILLINOIS, WWW.HOLLISTER.COM)

Many people manage the ostomy appliance by themselves. Employers should provide training before PCTs provide this care and let PCTs know what specific care is allowed. Because state and local guidelines vary, PCTs should follow facility policy regarding ostomy care. If the PCT is to provide care, it is important to find out the patient's preferences and routines. The patient may have been doing this care for themselves most of their lives.

Guidelines: Ostomies

- **G** Always wash hands carefully and wear gloves when providing ostomy care. Follow Standard Precautions.
- **G** Help patients with ostomies to wash their hands properly.
- **G** It may be necessary for hair near the stoma to be shaved or clipped to prevent skin irritation. If so, shave in one direction, away from the stoma, after the skin is cleaned. Follow policy regarding ostomy care.
- **G** Make certain that the patient receives regular, careful skin care. Observe and report any changes in the skin to help prevent skin breakdown.
- **G** Empty and clean or replace the ostomy pouch whenever stool is eliminated.
- **G** Skin barriers protect the skin around the stoma from irritation from the waste products and/or the adhesive material that is used to secure the pouch to the body. Barriers may come in the form of a powder, gel, cream, ring, paste, wafer, or square.
- **G** Patients who have an ileostomy may experience food blockage. A food blockage is a large amount of undigested food, usually high-fiber food, that collects in the small intestine and blocks the passage of stool. Food blockages can occur if the patient eats large amounts of foods that are high in fiber and/or if the patient does not chew the food well. Follow the nurse's instructions when assisting with feeding.
- **G** Encourage fluids and proper diets. Patients with ileostomies need to drink plenty of fluids because they lose extra liquid in their stools. They may also be on high-potassium diets due to rapid elimination.
- **G** Many patients with ostomies feel they have lost control of a basic bodily function. They may be embarrassed or angry about the ostomy. Be sensitive and supportive when working with these patients. Always provide privacy for ostomy care. Behave professionally and do not act uncomfortable with any aspect of ostomy care.
- **G** Ostomy pouches are made to be odor resistant. If odors are present, they may be due to a leak or improper cleaning. Report odors to the nurse.
- **G** Observe how the patient is reacting to the ostomy and observe their general attitude. Report any emotional or physical problems with adjusting to the ostomy to the nurse.

Observing and Reporting: Ostomies

Report any of the following to the nurse:

- O/R Changes in color, amount, frequency, or odor of stool
- O/R Any skin changes at the stoma site, such as sores, excessive redness, or swelling
- O/R Leaking stool
- O/R Absence of stool
- O/R Watery stool with green, stringy material
- O/R Abdominal cramps
- O/R Vomiting

Caring for an ostomy

Equipment: disposable bed protector, bath blanket, clean ostomy pouching system, belt (if needed), disposable wipes (made for ostomy care), basin of warm water, washcloth, 2 towels, plastic bag, gloves

1. Identify yourself by name. Identify the patient according to facility policy.
2. Wash your hands.
3. Explain the procedure to the patient. Speak clearly, slowly, and directly. Maintain face-to-face contact whenever possible.
4. Provide for the patient's privacy with a curtain, screen, or door.
5. Adjust the bed to a safe level, usually waist high. Lock the bed wheels.
6. Put on gloves.
7. Place the bed protector under the patient. Cover the patient with the bath blanket. Pull down the top sheet and blankets. Expose only the ostomy site. Offer the patient a towel to keep clothing dry.
8. Undo the ostomy belt if used. Remove the ostomy pouch carefully. Place it in the plastic bag. Note the color, odor, consistency, and amount of stool in the pouch.
9. Wipe the area around the stoma with disposable wipes for ostomy care. Discard the wipes in the plastic bag.
10. Using a washcloth and warm water, wash the area in one direction, away from the stoma (Fig. 18-6). Rinse. Pat dry with another towel.
11. Place the clean ostomy drainage pouch on the patient. Hold in place and seal securely. Make sure the bottom of the pouch is clamped.
12. Remove and discard the bed protector. Place soiled linens in the proper container. Discard the plastic bag properly.

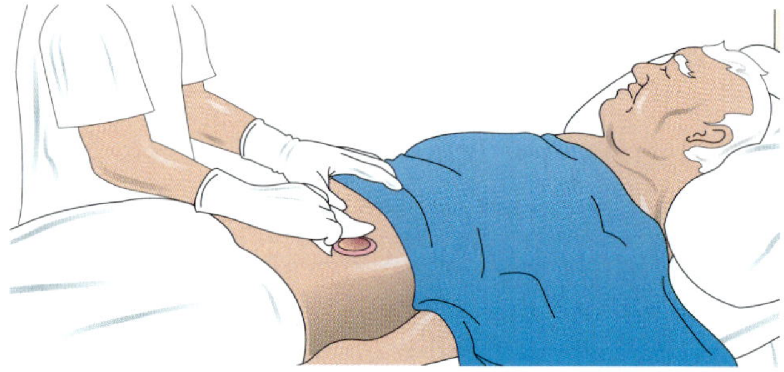

Fig. 18-6. *Wash the area gently, moving away from the stoma.*

13. Remove and discard your gloves. Wash your hands.
14. Make the patient comfortable.
15. Return the bed to its lowest position. Remove privacy measures.
16. Place the call light within the patient's reach.
17. Report any changes in the patient to the nurse. Note any changes to the stoma and surrounding area. A normal stoma is red and moist, and looks like the lining of the mouth. Call the nurse if the stoma appears irritated or discolored or if swelling or bleeding is present. Report any signs of skin breakdown around the stoma.
18. Document the procedure using facility guidelines.

6. Explain guidelines for assisting with bowel retraining

Patients who have had a disruption in their bowel routines from illness, injury, or inactivity may need help in reestablishing a regular routine and normal function. To assist with bowel retraining, the provider may order suppositories, laxatives, stool softeners, or enemas. Bowel elimination issues may be difficult for patients to discuss. PCTs should be sensitive to this and should remain professional when assisting patients with bowel retraining.

Connected Care

Bowel Retraining

Patients who have problems controlling their bowels need to be treated with dignity. The PCT should think about how he might feel in the same situation. For example, if a patient has a bowel movement in her bed, she probably feels embarrassed about this and about the fact that a PCT has to clean her and change the sheets. The PCT can help the patient maintain her dignity by being kind and supportive. He should promote the patient's right to privacy by keeping his voice low and not discussing the situation in a public area.

Guidelines: Bowel Retraining

G Follow Standard Precautions. Wear gloves when handling body wastes.

G Explain the bowel training schedule to the patient. Follow the schedule carefully.

G Keep a record of the patient's bowel habits. When you see a pattern of elimination, you can predict when the patient will need a bedpan or a trip to the bathroom.

G Encourage the patient to drink plenty of fluids.

G Encourage patients to follow special diets as ordered.

G Answer call lights promptly. Leave the call light within reach of the patient's stronger hand.

G Provide privacy for elimination—both in the bed and in the bathroom.

G Do not rush the patient during elimination.

G Help patients with careful perineal care. This prevents skin breakdown and promotes proper hygiene. Carefully observe for skin changes.

G Discard wastes according to your facility's policies.

G Discard clothing protectors and incontinence briefs properly. Double-bag these items if ordered.

G Some facilities use washable bed pads or briefs. Follow Standard Precautions when placing these items in the laundry.

G Keep an accurate record of elimination.

G Praise successes or attempts to control bowels. However, do not talk to patients as if they were children. Keep your voice low and do not draw attention to any aspect of bowel retraining.

G Never show frustration or anger toward patients who have incontinence. Remember that the problem is out of their control. Be positive and professional.

Chapter Review

1. What is chyme?
2. What do these terms mean: digestion, absorption, and elimination?
3. What may need to be increased in a patient's diet if she has constipation?
4. List 3 signs of a fecal impaction.
5. List 3 causes of diarrhea.
6. What is gastroesophageal reflux disease (GERD)?
7. What diet may be ordered for a patient with peptic ulcers?
8. What are 3 symptoms of colorectal cancer?
9. In what position must the patient be placed for an enema?
10. What 2 things should not be included in a stool specimen?
11. If a stool specimen needs to be tested for ova and parasites, what should be done immediately and why?
12. What are 3 reasons that a patient may need a colostomy or ileostomy?

13. How often should an ostomy pouch be emptied?
14. Why should a PCT keep a record of the bowel habits of a patient going through bowel retraining?

19 The Endocrine System and Related Care

1. Describe the structure and function of the endocrine system

The endocrine system is made up of glands in different areas of the body (Fig. 19-1). **Glands** are organs that produce and secrete chemicals called hormones. **Hormones** are chemical substances created by the body that control numerous body functions. Hormones are carried in the blood to various organs.

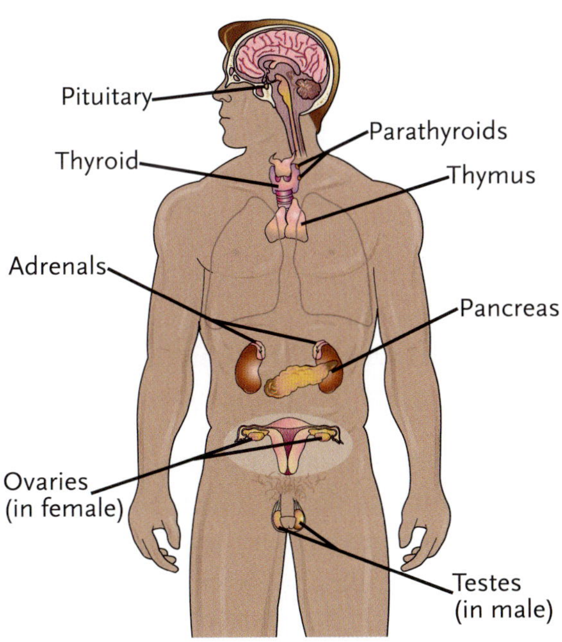

Fig. 19-1. *The endocrine system includes organs that produce hormones that regulate essential body processes.*

The pituitary gland, called the *master gland,* is located behind the eyes at the base of the brain. It secretes key hormones that cause other glands to produce other hormones. The following are some hormones secreted by the pituitary gland:

- Growth hormone, which regulates growth and development
- Antidiuretic hormone (ADH), which controls the balance of fluids in the body
- Oxytocin, which causes the uterus to contract during and after childbirth

The pituitary gland also produces hormones that regulate the thyroid gland and the adrenal glands. The thyroid gland is located in the neck in front of the larynx. It produces thyroid hormone, which regulates metabolism, the burning of food for heat and energy.

The parathyroid glands secrete a hormone that regulates the body's use of calcium. Nerves and muscles require calcium to function smoothly. A deficiency of this hormone can cause severe muscle contractions and spasms. It can be fatal if untreated.

The pancreas, a gland located in the upper midsection of the abdomen, secretes insulin. Insulin is a hormone that works to move glucose (natural sugar) from the blood and into the cells for energy for the body.

There are 2 adrenal glands and they are located at the tops of the kidneys. They produce hormones that are essential to life. These hormones are important because they help the body regulate carbohydrate metabolism. They also control the body's reaction to stress and regulate salt and water absorption in the kidneys. Adrenal glands also produce the hormone adrenaline, which regulates muscle power, heart rate, blood pressure, and energy levels during stressful situations or emergencies.

Gonads, or sex glands, produce hormones that regulate the body's ability to reproduce. The testes in the male secrete testosterone. The ovaries in the female secrete estrogen and progesterone.

The functions of the endocrine system are to maintain homeostasis through hormone secretion, influence growth and development, maintain blood sugar levels, and regulate levels of calcium and phosphate in the body. The endocrine system also regulates the body's ability to reproduce and determines how fast cells burn food for energy.

Observing and Reporting: Endocrine System

Observe and report these signs and symptoms:

- O/R Headache
- O/R Weakness
- O/R Blurred vision
- O/R Dizziness
- O/R Irritability
- O/R Sweating/excessive perspiration
- O/R Change in "normal" behavior
- O/R Confusion
- O/R Change in mobility
- O/R Change in sensation
- O/R Numbness or tingling in arms or legs
- O/R Weight gain or weight loss
- O/R Loss of appetite or increased appetite
- O/R Increased thirst
- O/R Frequent urination or any change in urine output
- O/R Hunger
- O/R Dry skin
- O/R Skin breakdown
- O/R Sweet or fruity breath
- O/R Sluggishness or fatigue
- O/R Hyperactivity

2. List common conditions of the endocrine system and discuss related care

Diabetes

Diabetes mellitus, commonly called **diabetes**, occurs when the pancreas produces no insulin, too little insulin, or does not properly use insulin. **Insulin** is a hormone that works to move glucose, or natural sugar, from the blood and into the cells for energy for the body. Without insulin to process glucose, these sugars collect in the blood and cannot get to the cells. This causes problems with circulation and can damage vital organs.

Diabetes is common in people with a family history of the illness, in the elderly, and in people who are obese. Diabetes is a chronic disease that has 2 major types: type 1 and type 2.

Type 1 diabetes is usually diagnosed in children and young adults. In type 1 diabetes, the pancreas either produces no insulin or too little insulin. The condition will continue throughout a person's life. Type 1 diabetes is managed with daily injections of insulin or an insulin pump and a special diet. Regular blood glucose testing must be done.

Type 2 diabetes is the most common form of diabetes. In type 2 diabetes, either the body does not produce enough insulin, or the body fails to properly use insulin. This is known as *insulin resistance*. Type 2 diabetes usually develops slowly and is the milder form of diabetes. It typically develops after age 35; the risk of getting this type increases with age. However, the number of younger people with type 2 diabetes is growing rapidly.

Type 2 diabetes often occurs in people who are obese or those with a family history of the disease. Type 2 diabetes can usually be controlled with diet and/or oral medications. Blood glucose levels are tested regularly.

Other types of diabetes are prediabetes and gestational diabetes. **Prediabetes** occurs when a person's blood glucose levels are above normal but not high enough for a diagnosis of type 2 diabetes. Research indicates that some damage to the body, especially to the heart and circulatory system, may already be occurring during prediabetes. Prediabetes can be delayed or prevented with certain lifestyle changes, such as a change in diet, weight loss, and regular exercise.

Pregnant women who have never had diabetes before but who have high glucose levels during pregnancy are said to have **gestational diabetes**.

People with diabetes may have these signs and symptoms:

- Excessive thirst (**polydipsia**)
- Extreme hunger (**polyphagia**)
- Frequent urination (**polyuria**)
- Unexplained weight loss
- Elevated blood sugar levels
- Glucose in the urine
- Sudden vision changes
- Tingling or numbness in hands or feet
- Feeling very tired much of the time
- Very dry skin
- Sores that are slow to heal
- More infections than usual

Diabetes can lead to further complications:

- Changes in the circulatory system can cause heart attack and stroke, reduced circulation, poor wound healing, and kidney and nerve damage.
- Damage to the eyes can cause vision loss and blindness.
- Poor circulation and impaired wound healing may cause leg and foot ulcers, infected wounds, and gangrene. Gangrene can lead to amputation.
- Hypoglycemia and diabetic ketoacidosis can be serious complications of diabetes. Chapter 6 lists signs and symptoms of each.

Diabetes must be carefully controlled to prevent complications and severe illness. The care plan must be followed closely.

Guidelines: Diabetes

G Encourage the patient to follow diet instructions exactly. The intake of carbohydrates, including breads, potatoes, grains, pastas, and sugars, must be regulated. Meals must be eaten at the same time each day. The patient must eat all that is served. If a patient does not eat what is served, or if you do not think he is following the diet, tell the nurse.

G Encourage the patient to do any ordered exercise. Exercise affects how quickly the body uses food, and it also helps improve circulation. Exercise may include walking or other active exercise (Fig. 19-2). It may also include passive range of motion exercises. Help with exercises as assigned. Be positive and try to make it fun.

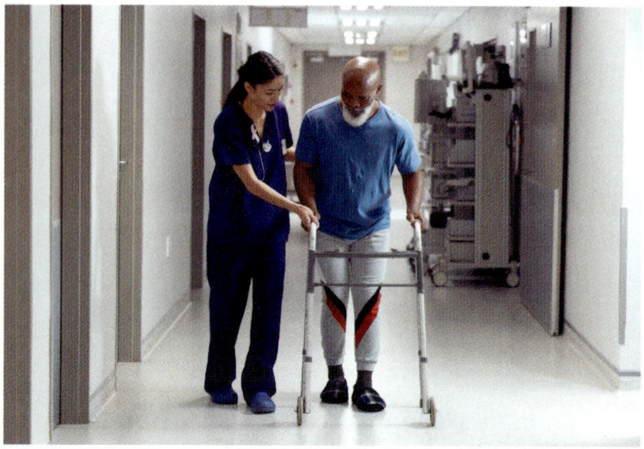

Fig. 19-2. *Exercise is very important for patients who have diabetes. Exercise helps to increase circulation.*

- **G** Observe the patient's use of insulin. Doses are calculated exactly. They are administered by the nurse at the same time each day. PCTs are not permitted to inject insulin, but it is important to know when patients take insulin and when their meals should be served. There must be a balance between the insulin level and food intake.
- **G** Perform blood tests as directed. A fingerstick blood glucose test is one type of blood test that may be used to check blood sugar. This is a simple test that is performed by quickly piercing the fingertip, then placing the blood on a chemically active disposable strip. The strip is inserted into a blood glucose meter, a special glucose monitoring machine (Fig. 19-3). The strip will indicate the result.

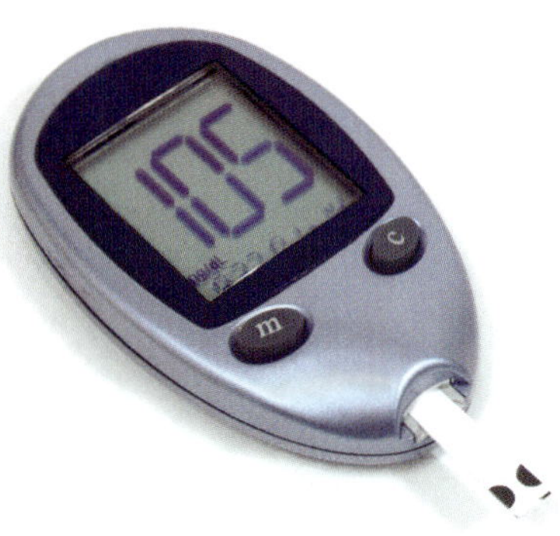

Fig. 19-3. *There are different types of equipment to measure glucose levels in the blood.*

Some patients may have a continuous glucose monitoring (CGM) system in place. CGM systems track a person's blood glucose level frequently and report how glucose levels change. The system consists of a small wearable sensor that is inserted under the skin, usually in the arm or on the stomach. The sensor sends data wirelessly to a monitoring unit or a smartphone. Sometimes readings from these systems need to be confirmed by fingerstick testing. More information about blood glucose testing is located in Chapter 22.

- **G** Proper foot care is vitally important for people with diabetes. Because diabetes causes poor circulation, even a small sore on the leg or foot can grow into a large wound that may not heal. This can result in amputation. Careful foot care, including regular inspection, is very important (Fig. 19-4). Nurses usually perform foot care for patients with diabetes. PCTs should report any observations of sores on the feet or legs right away.

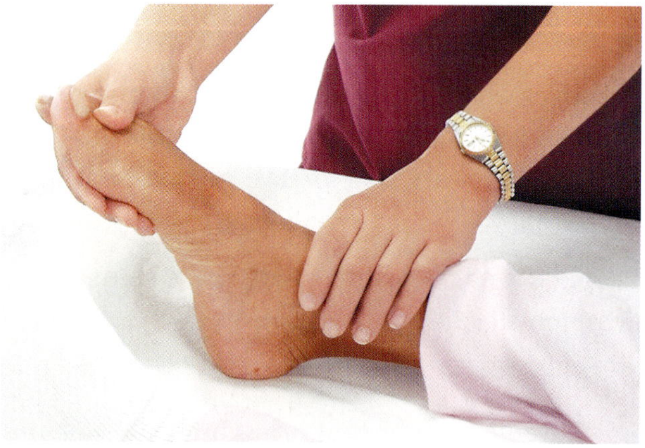

Fig. 19-4. *Observe the legs and feet carefully. Poor circulation can increase the risk of infection and the loss of toes, feet, or legs to gangrene.*

- **G** To avoid injuries to the feet, patients with diabetes should not go barefoot. In a hospital, patients with diabetes usually wear the same nonskid socks given to all patients. Socks should not be too tight. PCTs should never trim or clip a patient's toenails. Only a nurse or provider should do this.

Observing and Reporting: Diabetes

Report any of these to the nurse:

- O/R Any sign of skin breakdown, especially on the feet and toes
- O/R Change in appetite (patient overeating or not eating enough)
- O/R Weight changes
- O/R Change in mental status
- O/R Increased thirst
- O/R Change in urine output, any signs of urinary tract infection, fruity or sweet-smelling urine
- O/R Nausea or vomiting
- O/R Irritability or confusion
- O/R Nervousness or anxiety
- O/R Feeling faint or dizzy
- O/R Visual changes, especially blurred vision
- O/R Change in mobility
- O/R Change in sensation
- O/R Sweet or fruity breath
- O/R Numbness or tingling in arms or legs

Hyperthyroidism (Overactive Thyroid Gland)

Hyperthyroidism is a condition in which the thyroid produces too much thyroid hormone. Metabolism increases and body processes speed up, causing weight loss, a rapid heartbeat, sweating, and nervousness. Hyperthyroidism is usually treated with medication. Occasionally, part of the thyroid is surgically removed.

Graves' disease, an autoimmune disorder, often causes hyperthyroidism. Signs and symptoms include rapid heart rate, palpitations (abnormal heartbeats), dizziness, tremors, weight loss, and exophthalmia, or bulging eyes. It is treated with medications that reduce the effect of the thyroid hormones. Radioactive medications to destroy the thyroid gland or surgical removal may be necessary. In this case, the patient will need to take medication to replace thyroid hormones.

Thyrotoxic crisis, also known as *thyroid storm*, is a life-threatening condition caused by a rapid rise in thyroid hormone levels. It can be caused when hyperthyroidism is not treated or is seriously undertreated. It may also happen if antithyroid medications are suddenly stopped. Signs and symptoms include rapid or irregular heartbeat, confusion, and difficulty breathing. It is treated by removing the thyroid gland surgically or by medication that prevents it from producing hormones.

Hypothyroidism (Underactive Thyroid Gland)

Hypothyroidism is a condition in which the body lacks thyroid hormone. This causes body processes to slow down. Hypothyroidism is often caused by **Hashimoto's thyroiditis**, a type of autoimmune disorder. The body produces antibodies that attack the thyroid, interfering with the production of thyroid hormone. Metabolism slows, causing fatigue, weight gain, constipation, and intolerance to cold (Fig. 19-5). Dry skin, hair loss, slow heart rate, and low blood pressure are other symptoms. Hypothyroidism is treated with medications that replace the thyroid hormone.

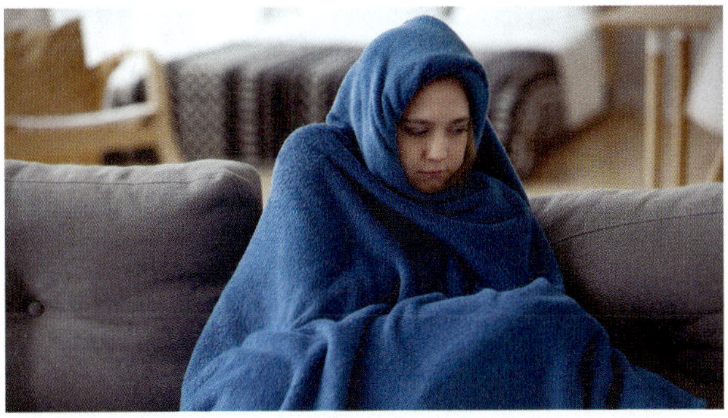

Fig. 19-5. *Slower metabolism, fatigue, and cold intolerance are some signs and symptoms of hypothyroidism.*

Congenital hypothyroidism (formerly called *cretinism*) is a form of hypothyroidism that affects infants and children. The most common cause is iodine deficiency during pregnancy. The deficiency stunts the development of the thyroid gland. This disorder can stunt growth and development and cause intellectual deficits. It is treated with hormone replacement.

Myxedema is a complication of untreated hypothyroidism that can affect teenagers and adults. It causes dry skin, hair loss, intolerance to cold, fatigue, and, in females, heavy bleeding during menstruation. It can be life-threatening if untreated. It is treated with thyroid hormone replacement.

Chapter Review

1. What are glands?
2. What are the functions of the endocrine system?
3. Where is the pituitary gland located and what does it control?
4. What is the most common form of diabetes?
5. Why is proper foot care especially important for a patient with diabetes?
6. Why is it important for a PCT to encourage a patient with diabetes to follow diet directions exactly?
7. What kinds of symptoms occur in people with hyperthyroidism?
8. Which autoimmune disorder can cause hyperthyroidism? Which autoimmune disorder can cause hypothyroidism?
9. What type of dietary deficiency during pregnancy can cause congenital hypothyroidism in infants?

20
The Reproductive System and Related Care

1. Describe the structure and function of the reproductive system

The reproductive system is made up of the reproductive organs, which are different in men and women. The reproductive system allows human beings to **reproduce**, or create new human life. Reproduction begins when a male's and female's sex cells (sperm and ovum) join. These sex cells are formed in the male and female sex glands. These sex glands are called the *gonads.*

The Male Reproductive System

In the male, the sex glands or gonads are the testes or testicles. The 2 oval glands are located outside the body in the scrotum. The scrotum is a sac made of skin and muscle that is suspended between the thighs. The testes produce the male sex cells, called sperm, and testosterone (Fig. 20-1). Testosterone is the male hormone needed for the reproductive organs to function properly. Testosterone also promotes development of male secondary sex characteristics, which include the following:

- Facial hair
- Pubic and underarm hair
- Hair on the chest, legs, and arms
- Deepening of the voice
- Development of muscle mass

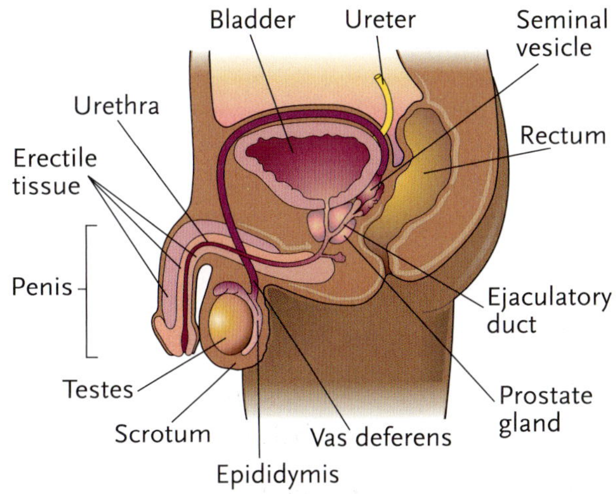

Fig. 20-1. *The male reproductive system.*

Sperm travel from the testes through a coiled tube, the epididymis, and another tube called the vas deferens. Sperm then pass into the seminal vesicle where semen is produced. Semen carries sperm out of the body.

The ducts coming from each seminal vesicle unite to form the ejaculatory ducts. They pass through the prostate gland, where more fluid is added to the semen. In the prostate, the ejaculatory ducts join the urethra, the tube through which both urine and semen pass. The urethra continues through the penis, the sex organ located outside the body, in front of the scrotum. The penis is composed of erectile tissue that becomes filled with blood during sexual excitement. As the penis fills with blood, it becomes enlarged and erect. It then can enter the vagina, the female reproductive tract, where it releases semen containing sperm.

The Female Reproductive System

In the human female, the gonads are 2 oval glands called the ovaries. There is 1 ovary on each side of the uterus (Fig. 20-2). The ovaries make the female sex cells or eggs (ova). They release the female hormones, estrogen and progesterone. Each month, from puberty to menopause, an egg is released from an ovary. This cycle is maintained by estrogen and progesterone. These hormones control development of female secondary sex characteristics, which include the following:

- Increased breast size
- Wider and rounder hips
- Pubic and underarm hair
- A slightly deeper voice

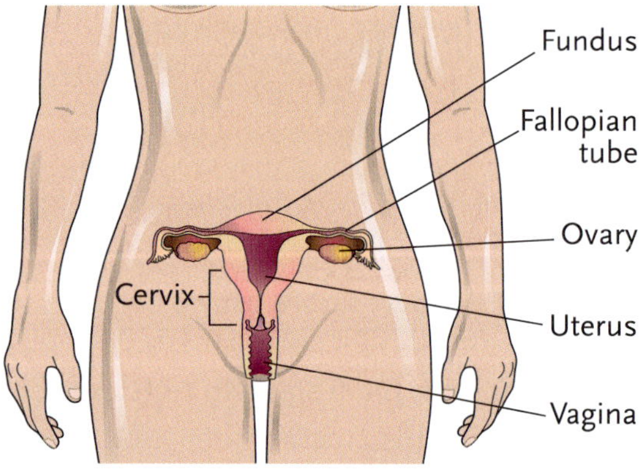

Fig. 20-2. *The female reproductive system.*

Once an egg is released from an ovary, it travels through the fallopian tube to the uterus. The uterus is a hollow, pear-shaped, muscular organ that is located within the pelvis. It lies behind the bladder and in front of the rectum. If sexual intercourse takes place while the egg is in the fallopian tube, the egg may be fertilized by sperm in the fallopian tube. The fertilized egg then travels down into the uterus. It implants in the endometrium, the lining of the uterus. Stimulated by hormones, the endometrium builds up during the menstrual cycle. It has many blood vessels supplying it for the growth and feeding of an embryo. If the egg is not fertilized, the hormones decrease. The blood supply to the endometrium decreases. The endometrium then breaks up in a process called menstruation.

The main section of the uterus is the fundus. This is where the fetus develops after the fertilized egg is implanted. The narrow neck of the uterus extending into the vagina is the cervix. The cervix has an opening through which menstrual fluid can pass and semen can enter the vagina.

The vagina is the muscular canal that opens to the outside of the body. The external vaginal opening is partially closed by the hymen membrane. The vagina is kept moist by secretions from glands in the vaginal walls. The vagina receives the penis during sexual intercourse. It also serves as the birth canal. The baby passes through the cervix, which is made thin by pressure from the baby's head during contractions. Once the cervix opens, the baby can move out through the vagina. There is more information about pregnancy and childbirth in Learning Objective 3.

For males, the function of the reproductive system is to manufacture sperm and the male hormone testosterone. For females, the reproductive system manufactures ova (eggs) and the female hormones estrogen and progesterone. It also provides an environment for the development of a fetus and produces milk for the nourishment of a baby after birth.

With age, sperm production decreases in males but does not stop. Testosterone levels may go down gradually. In females, the levels of estrogen and progesterone drop and menstruation ends. Menopause is the end of menstruation; it occurs when a woman has not had a menstrual period for 12 months. The decrease in estrogen may lead to a loss of calcium. This can cause brittle bones and, potentially, osteoporosis.

Observing and Reporting: Reproductive System

Observe and report these signs and symptoms:

- O/R Discomfort or difficulty with urination
- O/R Discharge from the penis or vagina
- O/R Swelling of the genitals
- O/R Blood in urine or stool
- O/R Breast changes, including size, shape, lumps, or discharge from the nipple
- O/R Sores on the genitals
- O/R Redness or rash on the genitals
- O/R Genital itching
- O/R Patient reports erectile dysfunction (ED; trouble getting or maintaining an erection)
- O/R Patient reports painful intercourse

Connected Care

Gender Identity and Health Care

For people who are transgender, or *trans*, gender identity does not correspond to sex assigned at birth. Trans patients require attentive, person-centered health care. *Transition* is a term used to describe the measures a transgender person takes to align their gender expression with their gender identity. For some transgender patients this may include using names, pronouns, and clothing associated with their experienced gender. Patients may also be prescribed hormonal treatments to reduce traits associated with their sex assigned at birth and develop traits associated with the gender with which they identify. Reconstructive surgery (known as *gender-affirming surgery*) may or may not be a part of a transgender patient's transition. Medical aspects of transition are managed by a variety of experienced providers. Standards of care for transgender patients are based on medical research.

Transgender people, including transgender youth, experience higher levels of depression, anxiety, and suicide than other groups. Puberty can be a difficult time for transgender youth. The development of secondary sex characteristics associated with their sex assigned at birth can cause intense distress. *Gender-affirming care* is the accepted medical standard of care. It involves treating transgender children and youth so that their gender identity is respected. For children who have not reached puberty, this means using chosen names and pronouns and allowing clothing and grooming choices that match gender identification. Medications to delay puberty may be prescribed. This reversible treatment gives the patient, family, and care team time to determine the best approach to transition if that is what the patient chooses. Most surgical procedures are not performed until a patient is at least 18, although breast reduction may be performed in some cases. Gender-affirming care is provided by a team that may include specialists in endocrinology and behavioral health, among others. It is patient-led.

LGBTQ patients, as a group, have poorer health outcomes than other groups. One reason is that LGBTQ patients experience discrimination and judgment that leads them to avoid medical care. PCTs can provide professional, person-centered care by treating all patients without judgment or bias.

2. List common conditions of the reproductive system and discuss related care

Sexually Transmitted Infections

Sexually transmitted infections (STIs), or sexually transmitted diseases (STDs), are caused by sexual contact with an infected person. Sexually transmitted infections do not always have apparent signs and symptoms.

These infections are mostly transmitted through sexual contact, which includes sexual intercourse (vaginal and anal), contact of the mouth with the genitals or anus, and contact of the hands with the genital area. Some STIs can also be transmitted during pregnancy or childbirth. The human immunodeficiency virus (HIV) and some kinds of hepatitis can be transmitted via needles, as well as through sexual contact. (HIV and AIDS are discussed in detail in Chapter 21.)

Sexually transmitted infections cause a variety of signs and symptoms and health problems, which are detailed below. The transmission of some STIs can be reduced or stopped by using latex or polyurethane condoms (Fig. 20-3).

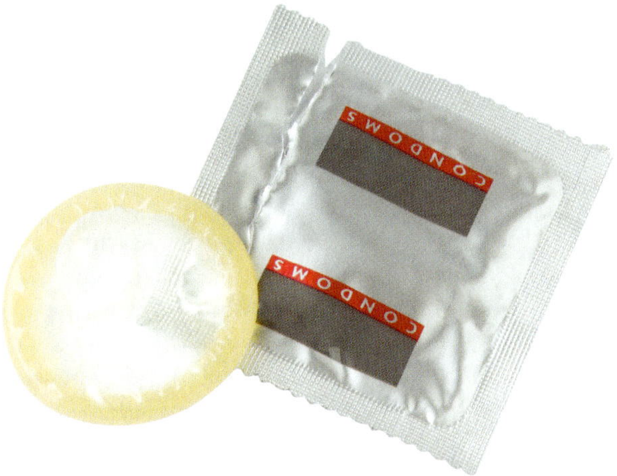

Fig. 20-3. Latex or polyurethane condoms can reduce or stop the transmission of some sexually transmitted infections.

Patients may be unaware of or embarrassed by symptoms of this type of infection. The PCT should remain professional when discussing STIs and should report signs and symptoms to the nurse.

Chlamydia is a bacterial infection caused by organisms introduced into the mucous membranes of the reproductive tract. Chlamydia can cause serious infection, including pelvic inflammatory disease (PID) in women. PID can lead to sterility. Signs and symptoms of chlamydia include yellow or white discharge from the penis or vagina, burning during urination, swelling of the testes, painful intercourse, and abdominal and low back pain. Chlamydia is treated with antibiotics.

Syphilis is a bacterial infection. It can be treated effectively in the early stages, but if left untreated, it can cause brain damage, mental illness, and even death. Babies born to mothers infected with syphilis may be born blind or with other serious birth defects. Syphilis is easier to detect in men than in women. This is due to open sores called **chancres** that develop on the penis soon after infection. In women, these sores may form inside the vagina. The chancres are painless and can go unnoticed. If untreated, the infection progresses to rashes, headache, fever, weight loss, and muscle aches. Then, over time, if the infection is still not treated with penicillin or other antibiotics, it spreads to the heart, brain, and other vital organs. Untreated syphilis will eventually be fatal. The sooner the disease is treated, the better the person's chances of preventing long-term damage and avoiding infection of others.

Gonorrhea is a bacterial infection. Like syphilis, it is easier to detect in men than in women because many women with gonorrhea show no early symptoms. Men infected with gonorrhea will typically have a white, yellow, or green discharge from the penis. Painful or swollen testes and burning during urination are other common symptoms in men. Symptoms in women include cloudy vaginal discharge, along with vaginal bleeding between periods. Rectal itching, soreness, bleeding, or painful elimination of stool can occur in both men and women. If untreated, gonorrhea can cause blindness, joint infection, sterility, and pelvic inflammatory disease. Gonorrhea is treated with antibiotics.

Genital herpes, unlike the STIs discussed previously, is caused by a virus—herpes simplex type 1 (HSV-1) or type 2 (HSV-2). HSV-2 is generally the cause of genital herpes. Genital herpes cannot be treated with antibiotics, nor can it be cured. Once infected with genital herpes, a person may suffer repeated outbreaks of the disease for the rest of their life. A herpes outbreak includes burning, painful, red sores on the genitals that may take weeks to heal. The sores are infectious, but a person with genital herpes can spread the infection even when sores are not present.

Some people infected with genital herpes never experience repeated outbreaks, and the later episodes may not be as painful as the initial outbreak. Treatment with antiviral medication can help people stay symptom-free for longer periods of time. The medication can also help lessen the duration and intensity of the episodes. Babies born to women infected with genital herpes can be infected during birth. Pregnant women experiencing an outbreak usually give birth by Cesarean section, or C-section.

Genital HPV infection is a sexually transmitted infection caused by human papillomavirus (HPV). HPV is a different virus than HIV and HSV (herpes). Genital HPV infection is spread primarily through genital contact and can infect the genital area of both men and women. This includes the penis, vulva, lining of the vagina, cervix, rectum, or anus. Many people have no signs or symptoms of HPV. Some HPV infections cause women to have an abnormal Pap test (a test that checks cells from the cervix for abnormal changes). Genital warts may appear. They may also lead to the development of cervical cancer. Treatment to remove warts is done in a provider's office or through the use of medication. There is no cure for HPV. However, HPV vaccines are available (Fig. 20-4). They may help prevent genital warts and cervical, anal, vaginal, and vulvar cancers in women, and genital warts and anal cancer in men.

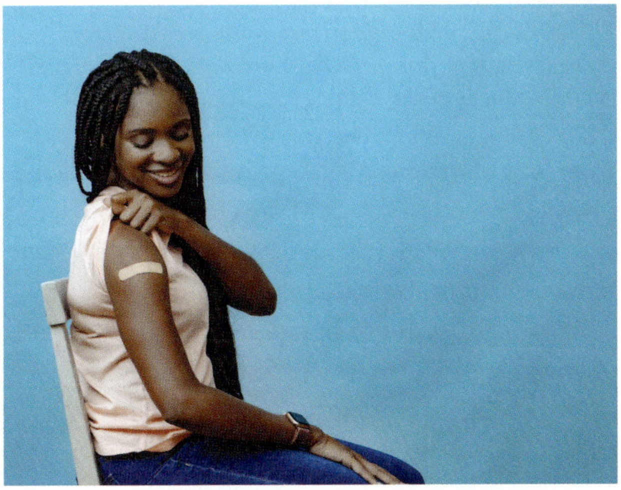

Fig. 20-4. *In women the HPV vaccine can help prevent genital warts and cervical cancer, along with other less common cancers.*

The human immunodeficiency virus (HIV) can be transmitted sexually as well and is discussed in the next chapter.

Conditions of the Male Reproductive System

Hydrocele is a condition in which fluid accumulates in the membrane around the testes. This causes swelling in the scrotum. It is painless. About 10% of male infants are born with a hydrocele. In older males hydrocele can develop due to injury or inflammation. Hydrocele usually resolves on its own. In rare cases, surgery may be required.

Benign prostatic hyperplasia (**BPH**) is a disorder common in men over the age of 60. The prostate becomes enlarged and causes pressure on the urethra. This pressure leads to frequent urination, dribbling of urine, and difficulty in starting the flow of urine. Urinary retention (urine remaining in the bladder) may also occur, causing urinary tract infection. Urine can also back up into the ureters and kidneys, causing damage to these organs. The cause of benign prostatic hyperplasia is unknown. Medications and/or surgery are used to treat this disorder.

Prostate cancer is one of the most common types of cancer in men. As men age, they are at increased risk for prostate cancer. Prostate cancer is usually slow-growing and responsive to treatment if detected early. Signs and symptoms include difficulty urinating, pain during urination or with bowel movements, and blood in the urine. Treatment includes hormone therapy to slow the cancer's growth, surgical removal of cancerous tissue, chemotherapy, and radiation.

While prostate cancer is most common in older men, **testicular cancer** can occur in adolescents and young adults. It is usually aggressive and fast-growing. There are few signs and symptoms in the early stages. As the disease progresses, symptoms may include pain in the groin or scrotum. Cancer treatment is discussed in Chapter 21.

Conditions of the Female Reproductive System

Vaginitis is an inflammation of the vagina. It may be caused by bacteria, protozoa (one-celled organisms), or a fungus (yeast). Bacterial vaginosis occurs when there is an overgrowth of normal bacteria inside the vagina. Yeast infections are caused by an overproduction of a fungus called *Candida albicans*. Vaginitis may also be the result of hormonal changes after menopause. Women who have vaginitis have a white vaginal discharge. Itching and burning are common symptoms. Treatment of vaginitis may include oral medications as well as vaginal creams or suppositories.

Uterine fibroids are growths that occur in or on the uterus. They are almost always benign (non-cancerous). There may be a single fibroid or multiple fibroids and they can vary in size, ranging from very small to the size of a grapefruit. They may grow slowly or quickly. Risk factors include family history, race (Black people are at a higher risk), hormones, diet, and obesity. Uterine fibroids are common but often do not cause symptoms. Symptoms that do occur include the following: heavy periods, painful periods, bleeding between periods, frequent urination, back pain, pain during sex, pregnancy complications, and a feeling of fullness in the pelvic area. Uterine fibroids are treated with medications for mild pain and iron supplements to prevent anemia from heavy periods. Birth control pills or progesterone injections may be given to control bleeding as well. Imaging tests such as ultrasounds may be done periodically to check the fibroid's growth. Surgery may be performed for moderate or severe symptoms.

Endometriosis is a condition that causes tissue that normally lines the inside of the uterus (endometrial tissue) to grow on the outside of the uterus. This can create scar tissue that attaches to structures surrounding the uterus. Signs and symptoms include abnormal periods, painful periods, pelvic pain, and difficulty getting pregnant. It is treated with oral contraceptives and other medications to relieve symptoms. Surgery may be performed to remove some of the abnormal growths. In severe cases, a hysterectomy (removal of the uterus) may be performed.

Breast cancer is one of the most common types of cancer in women. Its cause is unknown. However, the female hormones estrogen and progesterone are linked to the growth of some tumors. Signs and symptoms include a lump in the breast, nipple discharge, and changes to the skin of the breast, such as dimpling of skin in the breast or nipple. **Mammograms**, a special form of X-ray, are the best tool for detecting breast cancer (Fig. 20-5).

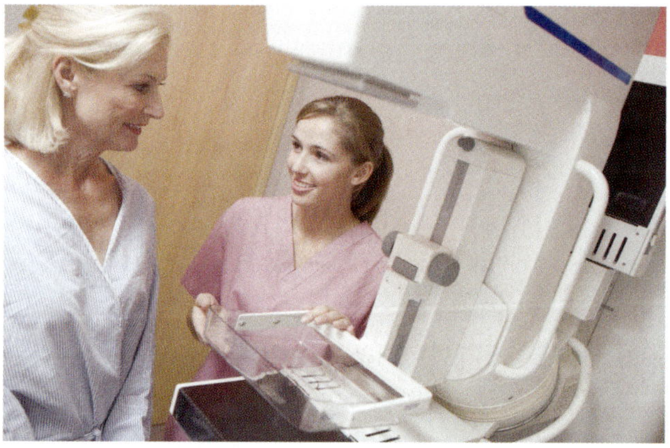

Fig. 20-5. *During a mammogram the breast is compressed between flat surfaces to produce horizontal and vertical images of the breast structures.*

Cervical cancer is a slow-growing cancer of the uterine cervix. The risk of developing cervical cancer is higher for women with multiple sex partners and those who have unprotected sex. This is because these practices increase the risk of exposure to human papillomavirus (HPV). Cervical cancer is usually painless in the early stages. Symptoms include vaginal discharge or bleeding and pain with intercourse.

Cancer can also affect one or both ovaries or the uterus. The risk of these forms of cancer increases with age. Cancer treatment is discussed in the next chapter.

3. Discuss pregnancy, childbirth, and postpartum care

Pregnancy

Prenatal care refers to the care of women during pregnancy. This care is usually provided by an obstetrician/gynecologist, but may also be provided by a family practice physician or a **certified nurse-midwife** (**CNM**). CNMs have graduate-level training to provide gynecological, prenatal, and postpartum care. CNMs usually care for women with low-risk pregnancies. Prenatal care is sometimes provided at clinics associated with a hospital's labor and delivery unit.

Pregnancy is divided into 3 trimesters. Each one lasts approximately 12 weeks. During the first trimester the menstrual period stops. A woman's breasts may be tender and she may have nausea, fatigue, and mood changes.

During the second trimester the woman usually begins to gain weight. She feels the baby move for the first time. The fatigue and nausea of the first trimester are likely to improve.

Weight gain continues in the last trimester. The woman may have indigestion, heartburn, and urinary frequency as the growing fetus fills the abdominal space. Fatigue may return. Swelling is common, but sudden swelling in a pregnant patient should be reported immediately.

Abortion

Termination of pregnancy is also known as **abortion**. Most abortions take place during the first trimester. Prior to 10 weeks of pregnancy either a medication or surgical abortion may be performed. Medication abortions use drugs that first stop the growth of the embryo or fetus and then cause the body to expel the contents of the uterus. Surgical procedures such as dilation and curettage (D&C) are used after 10 weeks. D&C involves dilating the cervix and surgically removing tissue from the uterus. All but approximately 1% of abortions occur before 21 weeks. Later abortions are generally performed for medical reasons: severe abnormalities in the fetus or danger to the mother's life. States set laws related to abortion. Some states may not allow abortion at all. Others may allow it only in certain circumstances or at certain stages of pregnancy.

PCTs who work in states where abortion is legal must understand that the choice to have an abortion belongs entirely to the patient if that patient is an adult. (Most states have laws requiring that parents either consent or be notified when a minor has an abortion.) Professional and ethical conduct requires that PCTs not share any personal opinions about abortion with a patient.

Pregnancy is a normal process, but complications may cause problems for the mother or the fetus.

Gestational diabetes is the development of high blood sugar in pregnancy. Patients are tested during pregnancy to screen for this condition. Treatment includes medications and changes in diet to control blood sugar levels.

Hyperemesis gravidarum is the medical term for excessive nausea and vomiting during pregnancy. It usually occurs in the first trimester. Medications can reduce symptoms. In extreme cases, patients may need to be hospitalized to replace lost fluids.

The **placenta** is an organ that forms inside the uterus. The fetus is connected to the placenta by the umbilical cord. The placenta supplies the fetus with oxygen and nutrients and removes wastes. Problems with the placenta can create complications during pregnancy. In **placenta previa**, the placenta implants too low in the uterus. The provider may prescribe bedrest or hospitalization to monitor the patient and the fetus. Depending on the location of the placenta, a C-section may be necessary. (There is more information about C-sections later in this learning objective.) **Placental abruption** is the sudden complete or partial separation of the placenta from the uterine wall. In severe cases, the fetus may need to be delivered early.

Preeclampsia is the sudden development of hypertension in pregnancy. Symptoms can be severe and include blurred vision, headaches, and seizures. Treatment includes managing symptoms. Early delivery may be required.

Miscarriage, sometimes called *spontaneous abortion*, is the death of an embryo or fetus before 20 weeks of pregnancy. It may be caused by problems with the fetus, illness in the mother, infection, or injury. Signs and symptoms include vaginal bleeding, passing of amniotic fluid or tissue, and cramping.

All of the fetal tissue is often expelled in miscarriages that occur in the first weeks of pregnancy. If needed, a surgical procedure may be performed to remove the remaining tissue. **Stillbirth** occurs when a baby dies before or during delivery. This term is generally used to describe the death of a fetus from 20 weeks of pregnancy and beyond.

Childbirth

Fetuses move and change positions often during pregnancy. Terms to describe fetal position include *cephalic, breech,* and *transverse.* In cephalic position, the head is facing downward. The *vertex position* is the most common type of cephalic position. In vertex position the fetus's head is tucked so that it can move more easily through the delivery process. By the final months of pregnancy most babies will be turned head down in preparation for delivery. Babies in the breech position remain upright in the uterus. Breech deliveries pose a higher risk for mother and infant. The transverse, or side-lying, position is the most difficult. Babies in this position cannot be delivered vaginally. Cesarean delivery, or C-section, is required. In a C-section the baby is delivered through a surgical incision in the abdomen.

Delivery, or childbirth, normally occurs between 37 and 42 weeks of pregnancy. Delivery before 37 weeks is considered a **preterm birth**. Most infants are delivered vaginally. A C-section may be necessary due to the position of the fetus, complications during childbirth, or a health condition in the mother.

Contractions of the uterus that happen regularly for more than 2 hours mean **labor** has started. This is the beginning of the childbirth process. The length of time from the beginning of labor to childbirth varies widely. If the patient is giving birth for the first time, labor often lasts 12–24 hours. Second births and beyond usually involve a shorter labor. During the course of labor, the cervix dilates, or widens, to allow the infant's head to pass through to the vagina. Labor can be painful. Many women choose to receive medication that blocks pain during labor. In a procedure called an *epidural,* anesthesia is injected into the back in the area around the spinal nerves. Women may also use breathing techniques, position changes, or other nonmedical methods to manage pain.

Once the cervix is fully dilated, contractions become very strong and the woman may feel an urge to push, or bear down. As the woman pushes, the baby moves out of the uterus, through the vagina, and is born. After the infant is born, the umbilical cord is clamped and cut. The provider then delivers the afterbirth, which includes the placenta and fetal membranes. The placenta is inspected carefully to ensure that it is intact (complete). Incomplete delivery of the placenta can lead to hemorrhage and can become life-threatening.

Part of the cord remains attached to the newborn's umbilical cord. It will dry and detach around 1–3 weeks after birth (Fig. 20-6). The infant's caregivers should be educated on the importance of keeping the umbilical area clean and dry. The cord should be kept dry. Sponge baths should be performed until the cord detaches. Discoloration, swelling, or discharge around the cord should be reported to the nurse.

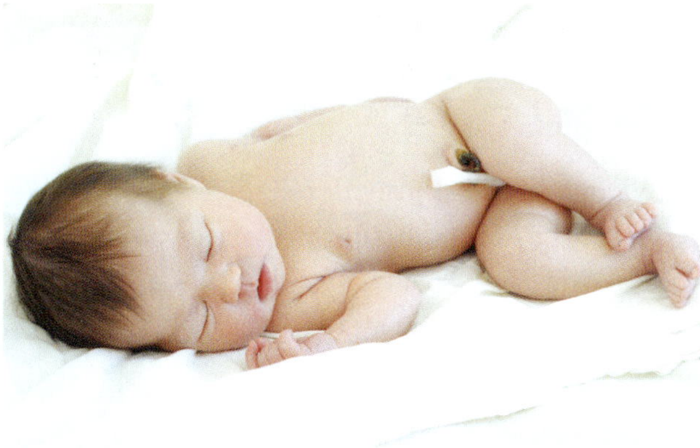

Fig. 20-6. *The umbilical cord does not require cleaning. It should be kept dry and the area around it clean until it falls off.*

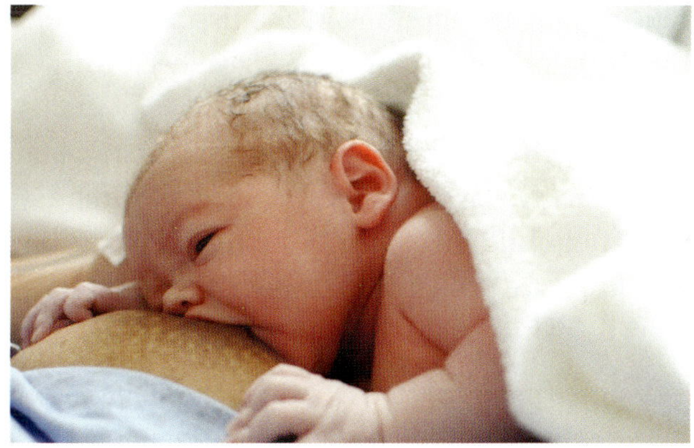

Fig. 20-7. *Even if a mother does not plan to breastfeed her infant she may choose to nurse the child in the first moments after birth.*

Neonate is the term for an infant from birth through the first 4 weeks of life. Neonatal care is usually given by a pediatrician. The neonate is first evaluated at birth in the hospital. The infant's color, cry, and reflexes are assessed and the infant is given an *Apgar score*. This score relates to how well the infant managed the birth process and the change to life outside the womb.

The Apgar score is measured 1 minute after birth and again at 5 minutes. A score ranging from 0 to 2 points is assigned to 5 different elements: appearance, pulse rate, reflexes, activity, and respiration. These are combined to form an Apgar score of 0 to 10 points. Neonates with a low score may be assessed again, usually at 10 minutes. If Apgar scores are still low, the baby may require NICU care.

The neonate's length, weight, and head circumference are also measured immediately after birth. Body temperature is measured often. Infants lose heat easily. Neonates may be placed under warming lights or wrapped in blankets to retain heat. A cap is normally placed on the head. The neonate's oxygen saturation may be measured. Neonates are often placed on the mother's chest as soon as possible after birth. This preserves body heat and promotes bonding. The infant may nurse for the first time at this point (Fig. 20-7).

Postpartum Care

Postpartum care refers to the care of the mother after childbirth. The mother's care is still managed by the obstetrician/gynecologist or CNM. Contractions called *afterpains* are normal. Vital signs should be monitored closely. Blood pressure sometimes rises after childbirth. Postpartum hypertension can increase risk of a heart attack or stroke. Vaginal discharge known as *lochia* usually lasts for several weeks after delivery. Lochia comes from the uterine wall where the placenta was attached. Similar to monthly menses, the discharge is at first bright red in color. In the days after childbirth, the flow changes color from bright red to duller red and then to pink. It then changes from pink to a yellowish white. These changes usually happen over 7–10 days. During this time the flow also decreases and then finally disappears. The PCT may be asked to report the number of sanitary pads a new mother uses. Any changes in flow or color must be reported to the nurse. Increased flow or brightening of the color should be reported immediately. Postpartum hemorrhage (heavy bleeding after giving birth) can be very dangerous and can even cause death.

PCTs may be assigned to help patients who have given birth with sitz baths. A sitz bath can relieve pain and swelling of the tissues around the vagina. These tissues may have been torn or a surgical incision called an *episiotomy* made during delivery. Patients who give birth at a hospital usually stay in the hospital for the first day or 2 after childbirth. One or more postpartum checkups are scheduled between 3 and 6 weeks after delivery.

The postpartum period is a time of enormous physical and emotional changes. A form of depression can occur during this time called *postpartum depression*. This is associated with the hormonal changes that occur after birth. Stress and exhaustion can also play a role. Signs and symptoms include tearfulness, fatigue, feelings of hopelessness, lack of energy, sleep and eating disorders, and anxiety. Signs of depression must be reported to the nurse. This condition can be life-threatening.

During the first 6 months of life, an infant receives all nourishment from breast milk or formula. Breastfeeding has many health benefits. This provides the infant with nutrition and transfers immune defenses that help to prevent infection. It is easy to digest. Infant formula provides a safe, nutritional option for parents who are unable to breastfeed or choose not to. Neonates normally consume 1–2 ounces of formula every 2–3 hours.

Chapter Review

1. What is the function of the reproductive system?
2. What are the secondary sex characteristics of a human male? What is the name of the hormone that promotes these developmental changes?
3. Where is the uterus located in the body? What is its function?
4. How can PCTs provide professional, patient-centered care for transgender patients?
5. What is a sexually transmitted infection?
6. What causes endometriosis? What are the symptoms of endometriosis?
7. Which medical providers typically provide care to patients during pregnancy and childbirth?
8. In which trimester of pregnancy will the mother begin to feel the fetus move for the first time?
9. A birth is considered *preterm* if the baby is delivered prior to how many weeks?
10. What 5 areas are assessed for a newborn infant's Apgar score?
11. What might the PCT be asked to report about a patient who has just given birth?
12. What are the benefits of a sitz bath for patients who have just given birth?

21

The Immune and Lymphatic Systems and Related Care

1. Describe the structure and function of the immune and lymphatic systems

The immune system protects the body from disease-causing bacteria, viruses, and microorganisms in 2 ways. **Nonspecific immunity** protects the body from disease in general. **Specific immunity** protects against a particular disease that is invading the body at a given time.

Nonspecific Immunity

To protect itself against disease in general, the body has several defenses:

- Anatomic barriers include the skin and the mucous membranes. They provide a physical barrier to keep foreign materials—bacteria, viruses, or microorganisms—from invading the body. Saliva, tears, and mucous secretions also help protect the body by washing away substances.
- Physiologic barriers include body temperature and acidity of certain organs. Most organisms that cause disease cannot survive high temperatures or high acidity. When the body senses foreign organisms, it can raise its temperature (by running a fever) to kill off the invaders. The acidity of organs like the stomach keeps harmful bacteria from growing there.
- Inflammatory response refers to the body's ability to fight infection through inflammation or swelling of an infected area. When inflammation occurs, it indicates that the body has sent extra disease-fighting cells and extra blood to the infected area to fight the infection.

Specific Immunity

To protect itself against specific diseases, the body makes different types of cells to fight different invaders. Lymphocytes are specialized white blood cells. There are 2 kinds of lymphocytes: B cells (or *B lymphocytes*) and T cells (or *T lymphocytes*). B cells produce antibodies to fight against disease. T cells destroy toxins and foreign substances that invade the body.

Foreign substances in the body that create an immune system response are called *antigens*. After a person is exposed to an antigen, their B cells create antibodies that "fit" the antigen like a lock and key. Once the antibody binds to the antigen it can destroy it. Antibodies are carried in the blood plasma (the liquid part of the blood). They can prevent a disease from threatening the body a second time. Another name for specific immunity is *acquired immunity*. This is because the body acquires, or gains, this immunity. Immunity may be acquired actively by fighting an infection or by getting a vaccination. For example, a person can gain active immunity to a disease such as the measles in 2 ways:

1. The person gets measles. His body forms antibodies to the disease to make sure he will not get it again.

2. The person gets a vaccine for the measles. This causes his body to produce the same antibodies to protect him from the disease.

Immunity may also be acquired passively. This means the person's own body does not produce the antibodies. *Passive immunity* is usually not as long-lasting as active immunity. Passive immunity occurs in 2 ways:

1. A mother's antibodies are transferred to her baby through the placenta and in breast milk. This is a natural form of passive immunity.
2. A person who has been exposed to an infectious disease can be treated with antibodies from someone who was infected before. This is an artificial way of gaining passive immunity.

The lymphatic system removes excess fluids and waste products from the body's tissues. It also helps the immune system fight infection. It is closely related to both the immune and the circulatory systems. The lymphatic system consists of lymph vessels and lymph capillaries in which a fluid called lymph circulates (Fig. 21-1). **Lymph** is a clear yellowish fluid that carries disease-fighting cells called lymphocytes.

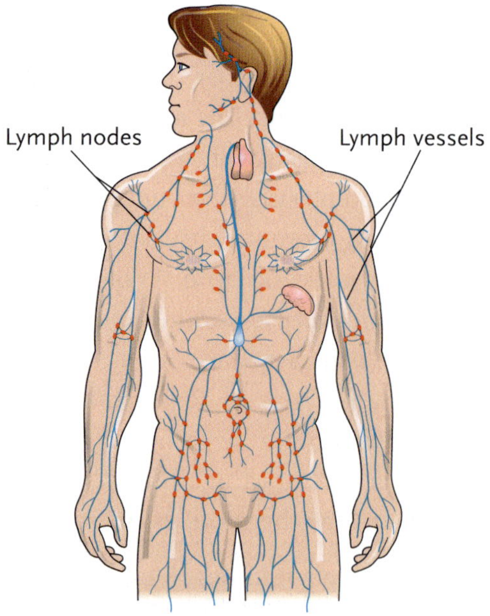

Fig. 21-1. *Lymph nodes work to fight infection and are located throughout the body.*

When the body is fighting an infection, swelling may occur in the lymph nodes. These are oval-shaped bodies that can be as small as a pinhead or as large as an almond. Located in the neck, groin, and armpits, the lymph nodes filter out germs and waste products carried from the tissues by the lymph fluid. After lymph fluid has been purified in the lymph nodes, it flows into the bloodstream.

Unlike the circulatory system, in which the heart functions as a pump to move the blood, the lymph system has no pump. Lymph fluid is circulated by muscle activity, massage, and breathing. A sore muscle may feel better if it is rubbed. The rubbing action helps the lymph fluid circulate, carrying waste products away from the tired muscle.

The functions of the immune and lymphatic systems are to protect the body against disease-causing bacteria, viruses, and microorganisms and to remove excess fluids and waste products from the body's tissues.

Observing and Reporting: Immune and Lymphatic Systems

Observe and report these signs and symptoms:

- O/R Recurring infections (such as pneumonia, fevers, and diarrhea)
- O/R Swelling of the lymph nodes
- O/R Increased fatigue

2. List common conditions of the immune and lymphatic systems and discuss related care

Allergies

Allergic reactions happen when a generally harmless substance triggers an immune response. Allergies can cause local or systemic signs and symptoms. An *allergen* is something that causes an allergic reaction. Common allergens include pollen, bee stings, milk, eggs, peanuts, and medications. Allergies can be mild, causing a sniffly nose or a small area of hives and itching, or they can be life-threatening. Anaphylaxis is a life-threatening reaction to an allergen and must be treated immediately (Fig. 21-2). It can cause sudden and severe swelling of the lips, tongue, and throat. This may block the airway and stop breathing.

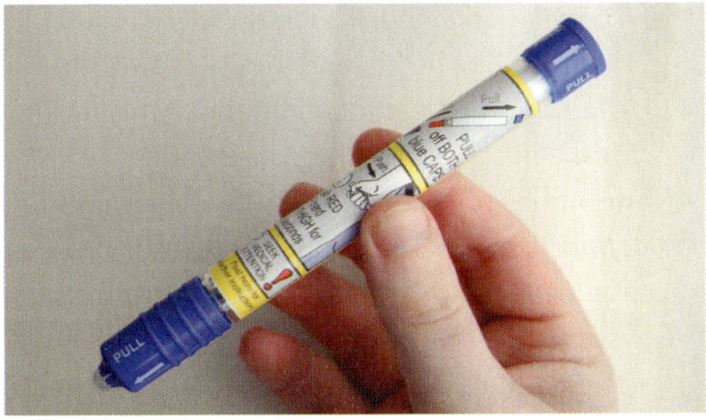

Fig. 21-2. Patients with known serious allergies may be trained to use injector pens. The pens contain a drug called epinephrine, *which can reverse an anaphylactic reaction.*

Bacterial and Viral Infections

The appendix is an organ located on the right side of the lower abdomen. It has roles in the digestive and lymphatic systems. Appendicitis is the inflammation of the appendix. It is caused by a bacterial infection. Signs and symptoms include abdominal pain and tenderness, nausea and vomiting, and fever. Appendicitis is treated with antibiotics, medications to reduce fever, and an *appendectomy*, or surgery to remove the appendix. The appendix may rupture and spread the infection throughout the abdomen if appendicitis is not treated.

The Epstein-Barr virus (EBV) can cause a number of different illnesses. One of the most common is **mononucleosis** (often called *mono*). It causes flu-like symptoms including extreme fatigue, sore throat, and fever. EBV can also cause other illnesses. It can affect the immune system. It also may cause the bone marrow to create too many white blood cells. It can have serious effects on the nervous system. People with weakened immune systems are at higher risk from EBV infection.

Lymphedema

Lymphedema is the abnormal buildup of lymph fluid in the body's tissues. It happens when there is a blockage in the lymphatic vessels. It is most common in the extremities, but it can also affect other areas of the body. Lymphedema often occurs after cancer surgery. Lymphatic vessels and nodes may be removed or damaged during cancer treatment. This disrupts lymph drainage in that area of the body. Lymphedema can also be an inherited condition. Signs and symptoms include swelling of the extremity, pain, and limited mobility (Fig. 21-3). It can also lead to cellulitis, which must be treated with antibiotics.

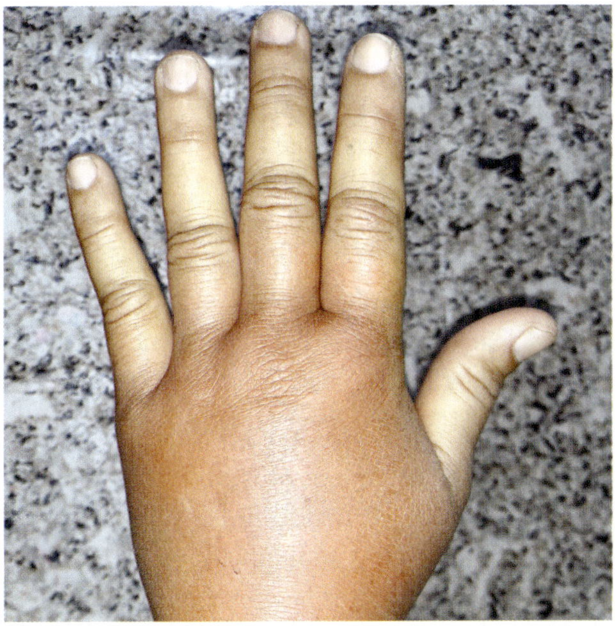

Fig. 21-3. Lymphedema is abnormal swelling caused by a blockage of the lymphatic vessels.

Treatment for lymphedema includes draining the excess lymph fluid from the extremities. This is done through exercise, special massage therapy called *manual lymph drainage*, and compression devices that help move lymph fluid. Patients who have lymphedema should try to prevent injury and infections. Blood pressure measurement and venipuncture should not be done in the affected limb.

Autoimmune Illnesses

Autoimmune illnesses can affect many different body systems. Rheumatoid arthritis, which is an autoimmune condition, is covered in Chapter 13. Multiple sclerosis is covered in Chapter 14.

Lupus is also an autoimmune disease. It is a chronic disease in which the body attacks its own healthy tissues. This causes inflammation that can be painful and damaging. There are different types of lupus. The most common form is systemic lupus erythematosus (SLE). SLE can cause symptoms in many parts of the body, but the skin, kidneys, and joints are most often affected.

Treatment involves several different drugs, including *immunosuppressants*, or drugs that suppress the immune system. These drugs slow the damaging immune response caused by lupus. Patients with lupus may be more prone to infection, however, because of these medications.

Acquired Immunodeficiency Syndrome (AIDS)

The human immunodeficiency virus (HIV) is a virus that attacks the body's immune system and gradually weakens and disables it. There are 3 stages of HIV infection:

1. **Acute HIV infection**: This early stage lasts from initial infection until HIV can be detected by an HIV antibody test (about 2 to 4 weeks). During this stage, the virus is multiplying quickly and the person is very infectious. The person may experience flu-like symptoms.

2. **Chronic HIV infection**: During this stage, HIV levels gradually increase and the number of CD4 cells decreases. CD4 cells are a type of T cell, and their decrease indicates that the immune system is being damaged. The person may not be experiencing HIV symptoms. A treatment called *antiretroviral therapy* (*ART*) can prevent HIV from destroying the immune system and advancing to AIDS.

3. AIDS: **Acquired immunodeficiency syndrome** (**AIDS**) is the final stage of HIV infection, in which infections, tumors, and central nervous system symptoms appear due to a weakened immune system that is unable to fight infection. The diagnosis of AIDS is made when a person's CD4 count falls to 200 or below or if the person has certain opportunistic infections. An *opportunistic infection* (*OI*) is an infection that occurs more often or is much more serious in people who have weakened immune systems rather than in people with healthy immune systems. Examples of opportunistic infections include lymphoma, *Pneumocystis* pneumonia (PCP), pneumonia, tuberculosis (TB), and Kaposi's sarcoma (KS), a form of skin cancer that appears as purple, red, or brown skin lesions.

Signs and symptoms of HIV infection include the following:

- Flu-like symptoms, including fever, chills, muscle aches, cough, weakness, and severe or constant fatigue
- Rash
- Night sweats
- Sore throat
- Swollen lymph nodes
- Mouth ulcers

Signs and symptoms of AIDS include the following:

- Rapid weight loss
- Recurring fever or extreme night sweats
- Extreme fatigue
- Prolonged swelling of the lymph glands in the armpits, groin, or neck

- Diarrhea lasting longer than one week
- Sores of the mouth, anus, or genitals
- Pneumonia
- Discolored blotches on or under the skin or inside the mouth, nose, or eyelids
- Memory loss
- Depression

In the late stages of AIDS, a form of dementia called *AIDS dementia complex* (*ADC*) can develop due to a damaged central nervous system. Symptoms of ADC include memory loss, poor coordination, slowed movements, and behavioral changes.

There is no vaccine to prevent the disease. Although recently new treatments have cured a small number of people with HIV, they are still experimental. They are not widely available. Patients who are at a higher risk for exposure to HIV may take a drug regimen called *pre-exposure prophylaxis* (*PrEP*). PrEP involves giving antiretroviral medications to patients who do not have HIV. It can prevent HIV infection.

Many people are living longer with HIV by taking combinations of medications every day. Antiretroviral therapy (ART) has been shown to control the HIV virus. Three or more medications are used for this therapy. Medicines must be taken at precise times. They have many unpleasant side effects: gastrointestinal symptoms like nausea, vomiting, and diarrhea, as well as fever and skin rashes. The medications are less effective for some people than for others. Other aspects of HIV treatment include relief of symptoms and prevention and treatment of infection.

In the United States, HIV is most commonly transmitted by the following:

- Having unprotected or poorly protected anal sex with an infected person
- Having unprotected or poorly protected vaginal sex with an infected person
- Sharing drug needles, syringes, and other injection equipment with an infected person

In healthcare settings, HIV transmission is rare. When transmission does occur, it is usually caused by contact with contaminated needles or other sharp objects. The best way for a healthcare worker to protect herself is to follow Standard Precautions and to handle and discard needles and other sharps properly.

Connected Care

The Facts about HIV and AIDS

A handshake or a hug cannot spread the HIV virus. The disease cannot be transmitted by telephones, doorknobs, tables, chairs, toilets, mosquitoes, or by breathing the same air as an infected person. PCTs should spend time with patients who have HIV or AIDS. These patients need the same thoughtful, personal attention that PCTs give to all patients.

Guidelines: HIV and AIDS

G Follow Standard Precautions. Follow Transmission-Based Precautions in addition to Standard Precautions if ordered.

G People with poor immune system function are more sensitive to infections. Wash your hands often and keep everything clean.

G Involuntary weight loss occurs in almost all people who develop AIDS. High-protein, high-calorie, and high-nutrient meals can help maintain a healthy weight.

G Some people with HIV/AIDS lose their appetites and have difficulty eating. These patients should be encouraged to relax as much as possible before meals and to eat in a pleasant setting. Report appetite loss or difficulty eating to the nurse. If appetite loss continues to be a problem, the provider may prescribe an appetite stimulant.

G Patients who have infections of the mouth and esophagus may need food that is low in acid and neither cold nor hot. Soft or pureed foods may be ordered. Drinking liquid meals and fortified drinks, such as milkshakes, may ease the pain of chewing. Warm rinses may help painful sores of the mouth. Careful mouth care is vital.

- **G** A person who has nausea or vomiting should eat slowly. A bland diet may be ordered. Cool foods that have little odor are usually easier to eat than hot foods. When nausea and vomiting persist, liquids and salty foods may help. Patients should drink fluids in between meals. Care must be taken to maintain proper intake of fluids to balance lost fluids.
- **G** Patients who have mild diarrhea may have a diet ordered that is low in fat, fiber, and dairy products.
- **G** Diarrhea rapidly depletes the body of fluids. Fluid replacement is necessary. IV fluids may be ordered. Good rehydration fluids include water, juice, caffeine-free soda, and broth. Caffeinated drinks should be avoided.
- **G** **Neuropathy**, or numbness, tingling, and pain in the feet and legs, is usually treated with pain medications. Wearing loose, soft slippers may be helpful. If blankets and sheets cause pain, a bed cradle can keep sheets and blankets from resting on legs and feet.
- **G** Give emotional support as well as physical care. Patients with HIV/AIDS may suffer from anxiety and depression. In addition, they may be judged by other people. Some people avoid a person with AIDS due to **homophobia**, or prejudiced speech or actions toward LGBTQ people. Some people blame them for their illness. People with HIV/AIDS may have tremendous stress. They may feel uncertainty about their illness, health care, and finances. They may also have lost friends who have died from AIDS. Listen closely to patients to understand their individual needs and concerns. This is part of providing person-centered care. Treat them with respect, and help provide needed emotional support.

  Patients with this disease need support from others. This support may come from family, friends, religious and community groups, and support groups, as well as the care team. Report to the nurse if you feel that patients need more resources and services.
- **G** Withdrawal, apathy, avoidance of tasks, and mental slowness are some symptoms of HIV infection. Medications may also cause side effects of this type. AIDS dementia complex may develop, causing further mental problems. There may also be muscle weakness and loss of muscle control, making falls a risk. Patients in this stage of the disease will need a safe environment and close supervision in their activities of daily living.

The right to confidentiality may be especially important to a person who has HIV or AIDS. Others may pass judgment on people with this disease. HIV testing requires consent; a person cannot be tested for HIV unless he agrees. HIV test results are confidential and cannot be shared with a person's family, friends, or employer without his consent. A person with HIV or AIDS cannot be fired from a job because of the disease. However, a healthcare worker with HIV or AIDS may be reassigned to duties that have a lower risk of transmitting the disease.

Cancer

Lymphoma is cancer of the lymphatic system. There are 2 types of lymphoma: Hodgkin's lymphoma and non-Hodgkin's lymphoma. In both types, cancer spreads through the body via the lymph nodes. The cause is unknown. Signs and symptoms include swollen lymph nodes, fatigue, loss of appetite, weight loss, and fever.

Multiple myeloma is cancer of the plasma cells (a type of white blood cells). Cancerous plasma cells do not produce normal antibodies. The number of these cells can also cause an imbalance in the normal blood components. This reduces the space available for red and other white blood cells. The cause is unknown. Patients with multiple myeloma have anemia, fatigue, weakness, weight loss, and frequent infections. There is more information about cancer in the next learning objective.

3. Discuss cancer and related care

Cancer is a general term used to describe a disease in which abnormal cells grow in an uncontrolled way. Cancer usually occurs in the form of a tumor or tumors growing on or within the body. A **tumor** is a cluster of abnormally growing cells. **Benign tumors** are considered noncancerous. They usually grow slowly in local areas. **Malignant tumors** are cancerous. They grow rapidly and invade surrounding tissues.

Diagnostic imaging may be ordered when cancer is suspected. A biopsy may also be done. A *biopsy* is the removal of tissue to test for malignancy (cancer). Some biopsies may be done in a medical office. More complex biopsies are done in outpatient surgery facilities.

Cancer invades local tissue and can spread to other parts of the body. When cancer spreads from the site where it first appeared (metastasizes), it can affect other body systems. In general, treatment is more difficult, and cancer is more deadly after this has occurred. Cancer often appears first in the breast, colon, rectum, uterus, prostate, lungs, or skin. There is no known cure for cancer. However, some treatments are effective. They are discussed later in the chapter.

Known causes of cancer include the following:

- Genetic factors
- Tobacco use
- Alcohol use
- Poor diet
- Obesity
- Lack of physical activity
- Certain infections
- Environmental exposure, such as radiation
- Sun exposure

When diagnosed and treated early, cancer can often be controlled. The American Cancer Society (cancer.org) has identified some warning signs of cancer:

- Unexplained weight loss
- Fever
- Fatigue
- Pain
- Skin changes, such as a change in skin color
- Change in bowel or bladder function
- Sores that do not heal
- Unusual bleeding or discharge
- Thickening or lump in the breast, testicle, or other parts of the body
- Indigestion or difficulty swallowing
- New mole or recent change in appearance of an existing mole, wart, or spot
- Nagging cough or hoarseness

People with cancer can live longer and sometimes recover when treated using the following methods. These treatments are most effective when tumors are discovered early. Often these treatments are combined.

Surgery is the front line of defense for most forms of cancer. It is the key treatment for malignant tumors of the skin, breast, bladder, colon, rectum, stomach, and muscle. Surgeons attempt to remove as much of the tumor as possible to prevent cancer from spreading.

Chemotherapy refers to medications given, usually intravenously, to fight cancer (Fig. 21-4). Certain drugs destroy cancer cells and limit the rate of cell growth. However, many of these drugs are toxic to the body. They destroy healthy cells as well as cancer cells. Chemotherapy can have severe side effects, including nausea, vomiting, mouth sores, diarrhea, temporary hair loss, fatigue, weakness, anxiety, depression, and decreased resistance to infection.

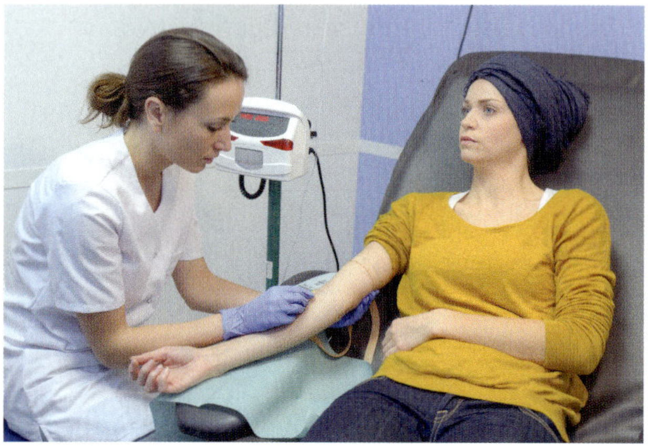

Fig. 21-4. *Surgery is often followed by chemotherapy.*

Radiation therapy (radiotherapy) directs radiation to a limited area to kill cancer cells. However, normal or healthy cells in the radiation's path are also destroyed. By controlling cell growth, radiation can reduce pain. Radiation can cause the same side effects as chemotherapy, including an increased risk of infection. The skin on the area exposed to radiation may become sore, irritated, and sometimes burned.

Targeted therapy is a specific type of chemotherapy. Traditional chemotherapy typically destroys healthy cells as well as cancer cells. Scientists have developed targeted chemotherapy drugs using the differences between cancer cells and normal cells. These drugs can attack cancer cells and the cells that help cancer grow. Side effects of these drugs can be similar to those associated with other chemotherapy drugs, and can also include high blood pressure, rashes or other skin changes, bleeding and clotting problems, and more.

Immunotherapy is a general term for treatment that uses a person's own immune system to fight disease. Immunotherapy can be helpful in treating some forms of cancer. It can work by making the immune system work harder to fight the cancer or by adding something to the immune system, like man-made proteins, to change how it works. Immunotherapy for cancer includes cancer vaccines, which make the immune system attack specific types of cancer cells. These may be used to help treat cancer or to stop cancer from coming back after other treatments. Different immunotherapy drugs have different side effects, but in general they have fewer side effects than chemotherapy drugs.

Hormone therapy is used to treat cancers that use hormones to grow, like breast and prostate cancers. Hormone therapy blocks the body's ability to produce certain hormones or changes how hormones behave. This type of therapy is usually used along with other types of treatment for cancer. Side effects include hot flashes, nausea, diarrhea, and fatigue.

Guidelines: Cancer

- G Each case is different. Cancer is a general term and refers to many individual situations. Patients may live many years or only several months. Treatment affects each person differently. Do not make assumptions about a patient's condition.
- G Patients may want to talk or may avoid talking. Respect each patient's needs. Listen if a patient wants to share feelings or experiences with you. However, never push a patient to talk. Be honest. Never tell a patient, "Everything will be okay." Be sensitive. Remember that cancer is a disease, and its cause is unknown. Maintain a positive attitude and focus on concrete details. For example, comment if a patient seems stronger, or mention that the sun is shining outside.
- G Proper nutrition is important for patients with cancer. Follow the care plan carefully. Patients frequently have poor appetites.

Encourage a variety of food and small portions. Liquid nutrition supplements may be used in addition to, not in place of, meals. If nausea or swallowing is a problem, foods such as soups, gelatins, or starches may appeal to the patient. Plastic utensils may be requested for a patient receiving chemotherapy. It makes food taste better. Metal utensils cause a bitter taste.

- G Cancer can cause great pain, especially in the late stages. It can affect the ability to sleep, eat, and move. Be alert for signs of pain. Report them to the nurse. Help with comfort measures, such as repositioning, and providing distractions, such as conversation, music, or reading materials (Fig. 21-5). Report to the nurse if pain seems to be uncontrolled.

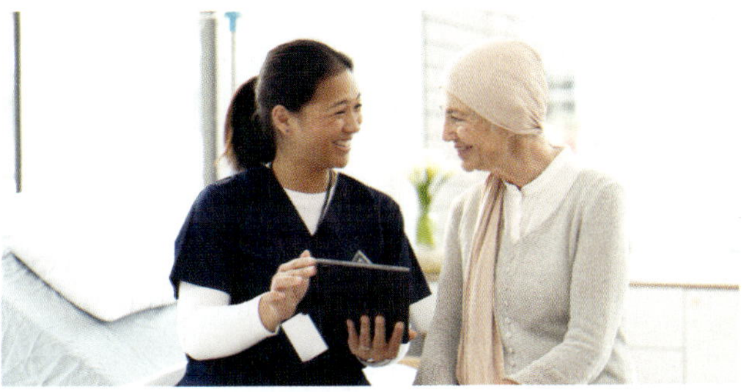

Fig. 21-5. *Give patients with cancer as much emotional support as possible. Distractions such as conversation can help a person deal with pain.*

- G Offer a back rub/massage to provide comfort and increase circulation. (See later in the chapter for a procedure on how to give a back rub.) For patients who spend many hours in bed, special pads or other positioning devices may make them more comfortable. Moving to a chair for some period of time may improve comfort as well. Reposition patients who are very weak or immobile at least every 2 hours.

- G Check the skin often to help prevent pressure injuries. Keep the skin clean and dry. Use lotion regularly on dry or delicate skin. Do not apply lotion to areas receiving radiation therapy. Do not remove markings that are used in radiation therapy. Follow any skin care orders (for example, no hot or cold packs, no soap, lotion, or cosmetics, or no tight stockings).

- G Help patients brush teeth regularly. Chemotherapy medications, nausea, vomiting, or mouth infections may cause pain and a bad taste in the mouth. You can help ease discomfort by using a soft-bristled toothbrush, rinsing with baking soda and water, or using a prescribed rinse. Do not use a commercial mouthwash. The alcohol in mouthwash can further irritate a patient's mouth. For patients with mouth sores, using oral swabs rather than toothbrushes may be preferable. The swabs can be dipped in a rinse and gently wiped across the gums. Mouth sores can make oral care very painful; be very gentle when giving patients care.

- G Chemotherapy and radiation can cause a condition called *neutropenia*. This is a reduced number of white blood cells called neutrophils. It makes it harder for the body to fight infections. *Neutropenic precautions* may be ordered for patients with cancer. Neutropenic precautions may include limiting visitors, requiring masks for visitors, not allowing flowers or plants, and using dedicated equipment for vital signs and other care. Follow all ordered precautions.

- G People with cancer may suffer from poor self-image because they are weak and their appearance has changed. For example, hair loss is a common side effect of chemotherapy. Assist with grooming if desired. Your concern and interest can help improve self-image.

- G If visitors help cheer your patient, encourage them and do not intrude. If some times of day are better than others, suggest this to visitors. Support groups exist for people with cancer and their families. The nurse may have a social worker visit the patient and family to share resources. It may help a person with cancer to think of something besides cancer and treatment for a while. Pursue other topics and get to know your patients' interests. As always, report any signs of depression immediately.

G Having a family member with cancer can be very difficult. Be alert to needs that are not being met or stresses created by the illness. Report observations.

Observing and Reporting: Cancer

Report any of these to the nurse:

- O/R Increased weakness or fatigue
- O/R Weight loss
- O/R Nausea, vomiting, or diarrhea
- O/R Changes in appetite
- O/R Fainting
- O/R Shortness of breath
- O/R Signs of depression or anxiety (see Chapter 4)
- O/R Confusion
- O/R Blood in stool or urine
- O/R Change in mental status
- O/R Changes in skin
- O/R New lumps, sores, or rashes
- O/R Increase in pain or unrelieved pain
- O/R Blood in the mouth

Care after a Mastectomy

A **mastectomy** is the surgical removal of all or part of the breast and sometimes other surrounding tissue. This operation is usually performed because of a tumor. After a mastectomy, the care plan may include arm exercises for the side of the body on which the surgery was performed. The goal of arm exercises is to strengthen the arm and chest muscles and reduce swelling in the arm and underarm. Exercises may include raising the arm, opening and closing the hand, and bending and straightening the elbow. The patient should wear loose, comfortable clothing while doing arm exercises.

The care plan's instructions may include using a compression sleeve to reduce the risk of lymphedema and keeping the arm on the affected side raised on pillows (Fig. 21-6). The patient may use a sling to keep the arm elevated. In addition, deep breathing exercises may be ordered. Blood pressure measurements and blood draws should not be done on the affected side.

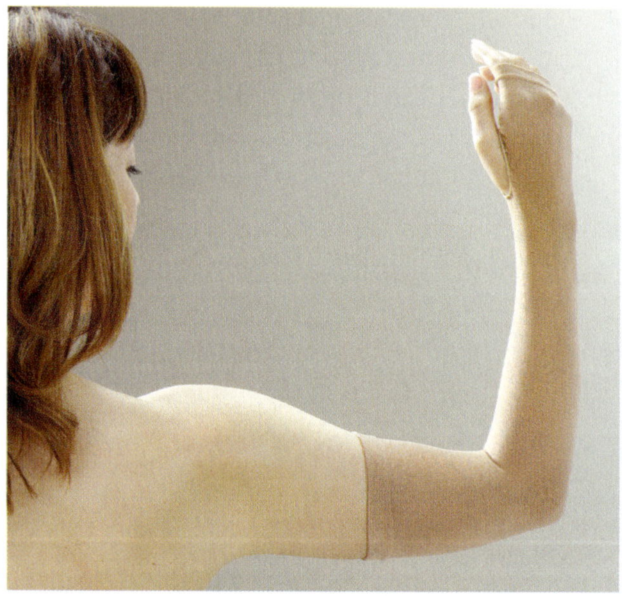

Fig. 21-6. *A compression sleeve can reduce the risk of lymphedema after a mastectomy.* (IMAGE COURTESY OF ENCOMPASS GROUP, LLC)

Back rubs help relax tired muscles, relieve pain, and increase circulation. After giving a back rub, any changes in a patient's skin should be noted.

Giving a back rub

Equipment: cotton blanket or towel, lotion

1. Identify yourself by name. Identify the patient according to facility policy.
2. Wash your hands.
3. Explain the procedure to the patient. Speak clearly, slowly, and directly. Maintain face-to-face contact whenever possible.
4. Provide for the patient's privacy with a curtain, screen, or door.

5. Adjust the bed to a safe working level, usually waist high. Lower the head of the bed. Lock the bed wheels.
6. Position the patient so he is lying on his side (lateral position) or his stomach (prone position). Cover the patient with a cotton blanket, then fold back the bed covers. Expose the patient's back to the top of the buttocks. Back rubs can also be given with the patient sitting up.
7. Warm the lotion bottle in warm water for 5 minutes. Run your hands under warm water to warm them. Pour the lotion on your hands and rub them together to spread it. Always put the lotion on your hands first, rather than directly on the patient's skin. Warn the patient that the lotion may still feel cool.
8. Place your hands on each side of the upper part of the buttocks. Use the full palms of your hands. Make long, smooth upward strokes with both hands. Move along each side of the spine, up to the shoulders (Figs. 21-7 and 21-8). Circle your hands outward. Then move back along the outer edges of the back. At the buttocks, make another circle. Move your hands back up to the shoulders. Without taking your hands off the patient's skin, repeat this motion for 3 to 5 minutes.

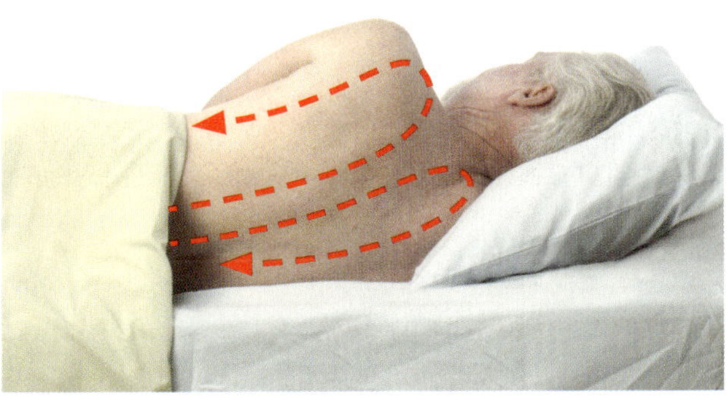

Fig. 21-7. *Move along each side of the spine, up to the shoulders.*

9. Knead with the first 2 fingers and thumb of each hand. Place them at the base of the spine. Move upward together along each side of the spine. Apply gentle downward pressure with the fingers and thumbs. Follow the same direction as with the long strokes, circling at the shoulders and buttocks.

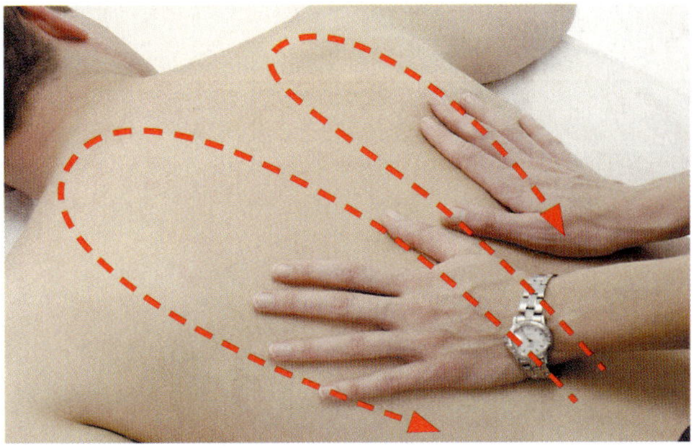

Fig. 21-8. *Long, upward strokes help release muscle tension.*

10. Gently massage bony areas (spine, shoulder blades, hip bones) with circular motions of your fingertips, using little or no pressure. Gentle massage stimulates circulation and helps prevent skin damage. However, if any of these areas are discolored, do not massage the area or put any pressure on it. The discoloration indicates that the skin is already irritated and fragile. Include this information in your report to the nurse.
11. Let the patient know when you are almost through. Finish with some long, smooth strokes, like the ones you used at the beginning of the massage.
12. Dry the back if extra lotion remains on it.
13. Remove the blanket and towel.
14. Help the patient put on a clean gown. Help the patient into a comfortable position.
15. Return the bed to its lowest position. Remove privacy measures.
16. Store supplies. Place the blanket or towel in the proper container.
17. Place the call light within the patient's reach.
18. Wash your hands.

19. Report any changes in the patient to the nurse.
20. Document the procedure using facility guidelines.

Chapter Review

1. What is nonspecific immunity? What is specific immunity?
2. What is the function of the lymphatic system?
3. How is lymph fluid moved through the body?
4. What type of allergic reaction causes life-threatening conditions such as swelling of the throat? What might reverse this reaction?
5. What is lymphedema? What is one common cause?
6. What are the 3 stages of HIV infection?
7. Which stage of HIV infection is classified as acquired immunodeficiency syndrome (AIDS)?
8. What is antiretroviral therapy and why is it used for patients who have HIV?
9. Because people who have HIV/AIDS are sensitive to infections, what steps should the PCT follow?
10. What are the types of cancer that directly affect the lymphatic and immune systems?
11. What types of testing are used to diagnose cancer?
12. What are 6 types of treatment for cancer? When is cancer treatment most effective?
13. What are the side effects of chemotherapy and radiation?
14. What are neutropenic precautions and what might they include?
15. What care instructions might the PCT receive for a patient who has had a mastectomy?

22 Phlebotomy

1. Discuss venipuncture and capillary puncture and identify common blood tests

Most blood specimens are collected by venipuncture, or the puncture of a vein. Specimens can also be collected by capillary puncture (also called *dermal puncture*). This involves puncturing the skin on a finger (adults and children) or heel (infants) (Fig. 22-1).

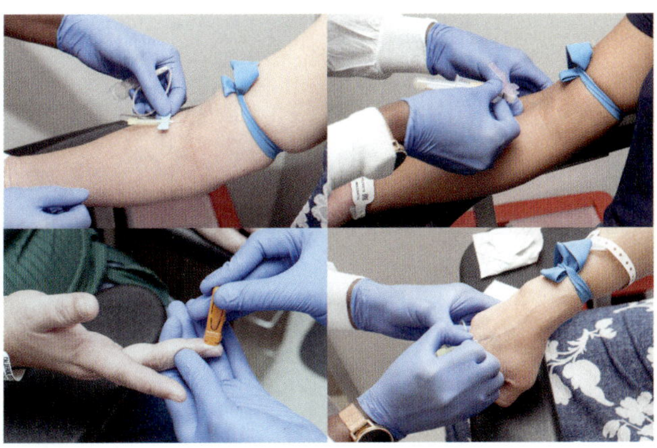

Fig. 22-1. *Blood specimens are collected by puncturing a vein or by puncturing the skin to access the capillaries below.*

Venous and capillary blood specimens are usually collected in tubes of different sizes and shapes. Some tubes contain chemicals that prepare the blood for testing. Tubes for venipuncture specimens are larger than tubes for capillary specimens. Pediatric tubes are smaller than tubes for adults. Some tests do not require blood to be collected in a tube at all. One example is point-of-care blood tests. These tests are often done by placing blood from a capillary puncture directly onto a test strip. The strip is inserted into a machine for analysis. One test done on newborns involves dripping capillary blood from a heel puncture onto filter paper.

Blood tests are ordered as part of routine medical care, to help with diagnosis, or to monitor a medication or condition. Sometimes the number or behavior of specific blood cells is observed. Sometimes specimens are tested for specific substances. **Blood cultures** test for bacterial or fungal infections. Electrolyte, enzyme, antibody, vitamin, and mineral levels can all be tested. The levels of a medication in the blood can be measured. Blood can also be tested to make sure a medication is working and is not causing damage. Blood may also be checked for illegal drugs or alcohol. The substance measured in a test is called an *analyte*.

Venipuncture is the most common way to collect blood in adults and children over 1 year old. A single specimen tube may be used for several different tests. Test **panels** are groups of tests. They either have related analytes (e.g., electrolyte panel, lipid panel) or they relate to a specific condition or organ (e.g., renal panel, hepatic panel). Table 22-1 lists common blood tests.

Capillary puncture is necessary for some tests. Point-of-care tests are done with capillary blood. Monitoring glucose for patients with diabetes and blood clotting times for patients taking the blood thinner warfarin are some of the most

TEST NAME	NOTES
Basic metabolic panel (BMP): • Glucose (blood sugar) • Calcium • Sodium (electrolyte) • Potassium (electrolyte) • Carbon dioxide (electrolyte) • Chloride (electrolyte) • Blood urea nitrogen (BUN; waste product related to kidney function) • Creatinine (waste product of muscles, related to kidney function)	• Serum separator tube (usually mottled red/gray or gold) • Heparin tube (green) may be used when results are needed right away (*stat* testing) • Fasting sometimes requested
Comprehensive metabolic panel (CMP): • All tests involved in basic metabolic panel • Albumin (protein produced in liver) • Total protein • Alkaline phosphatase (ALP; enzyme related to liver/bone health) • Alanine aminotransferase (ALT; enzyme related to the liver and kidneys) • Aspartate aminotransferase (AST; enzyme related to the liver and heart) • Total bilirubin (waste product generated in the liver)	• Serum separator tube • Heparin tube may be used for stat testing • Fasting sometimes requested
Lipid panel: • Total cholesterol • High-density lipoprotein (HDL) cholesterol • Low-density lipoprotein (LDL) cholesterol • Triglycerides	• Serum separator tube • Heparin tube may be used for stat testing • Usually requires fasting
Complete blood count (CBC): • White blood cell count (with or without differential) • Red blood cell count and measurements • Hemoglobin (Hgb; oxygen-carrying protein in the blood) • Hematocrit (Hct; ratio of RBCs to other components) • Platelet count	• EDTA tube (usually lavender) • Especially important to avoid rough handling

Table 22-1. *These test panels are often ordered as part of a routine physical.*

common point-of-care tests. The number of tests that can be performed in this way is growing.

Capillary blood may also be used to create a peripheral blood smear, often called a *blood smear.* This may be ordered if a complete blood count shows abnormal results. The blood smear allows blood cells to be viewed under a microscope.

Capillary puncture may be used to collect blood from certain patients, including the following:

- Patients who are obese
- Patients whose arms are burned, heavily scarred, or cannot be reached (e.g., due to a body cast)
- Patients with a history of blood clots in the veins
- Patients whose veins must be used only for treatments such as chemotherapy
- Patients whose veins are very fragile or damaged
- Patients whose veins are hard to puncture
- Patients who are infants

Blood specimens for children under 1 year old are usually collected by heel puncture. Babies over 6 months old who weigh 10 kilograms (22 pounds) or more may have blood collected by finger stick. **Iatrogenic anemia** is anemia caused by removing too much blood. It is an important concern when drawing blood from small children. The small amount of blood needed for a capillary puncture specimen is safer to remove than a larger venipuncture specimen.

Newborns often develop **jaundice**, a condition caused by too much of a substance called bilirubin in the blood. Specimens for testing bilirubin levels in infants are collected by capillary puncture. Newborns also have a series of tests for dangerous conditions that can be treated if they are found early. The blood for these tests is collected by capillary puncture. Blood is allowed to drip from the heel onto a special type of filter paper. (There is more information about these tests later in the chapter.)

Not all blood tests can be performed on a capillary specimen. Erythrocyte sedimentation rate is a test that measures the time it takes for red blood cells to settle to the bottom of a container. This test requires more blood than a capillary specimen has. So do some tests of blood clotting, or **coagulation**.

Capillary blood is a mixture of venous and arterial blood and tissue fluids. Because of this, some analytes are different in capillary blood. The type of specimen collected should always be documented clearly.

2. Describe the importance of avoiding errors before and during specimen collection

If a blood specimen is not collected properly, the results may not be accurate. Errors in handling, processing, or transportation can also affect results. The provider may make decisions based on the wrong information. If a patient or specimen is not identified correctly, the errors can be deadly.

Errors that happen before a specimen is tested are called *preanalytical errors*. Most of these errors can be avoided. Incorrect identification of a patient or specimen is one of the most common errors. Before a specimen is drawn, the PCT must identify the patient by 2 unique identifiers (following facility policy). Usually this means asking the patient to state and spell her first and last names and state her date of birth. The patient's wristband (if used), the requisition, and all specimen labels must match what the patient says (Fig. 22-2). Some facilities may have barcode patient identification systems. With these systems, scanning a barcode on the patient's wristband confirms identity. It may also allow the PCT to print specimen labels for the tests ordered for that patient.

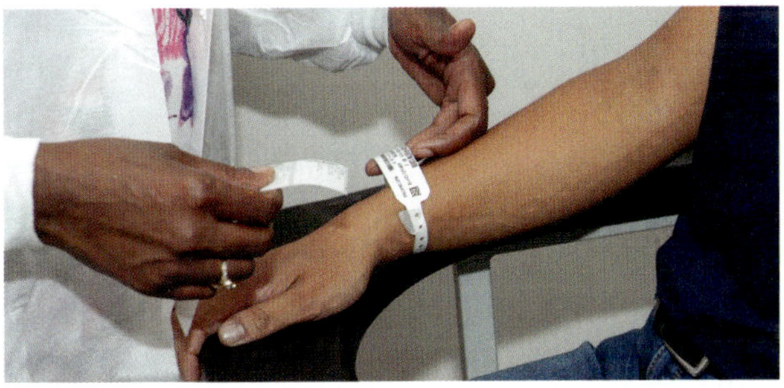

Fig. 22-2. *A patient's stated name and date of birth must be checked against the wristband, requisition, and specimen labels.*

Errors can also happen when a requisition is not checked carefully or if it contains an error. Requisitions for ordered tests are usually found in the patient's EHR. PCTs may also be given a paper requisition form, which should match orders in the EHR. If anything is unclear, the PCT should check with the nurse before drawing blood.

A requisition may list special requirements for timing or patient preparation. The PCT must make sure that the patient meets any special requirements before the blood draw. **Fasting** is a common requirement. This means not eating or drinking anything except water for 8–12 hours before the draw. Sometimes a *basal state* is required. A basal state is a rested state in which the patient has not had food or drink (except water) in the last 12 hours and has done no strenuous exercise. When testing medication levels or effects, the nurse may need to give the medication to the patient a certain amount of time before the test.

Preanalytical errors can happen at every stage of blood collection. These are errors a PCT must avoid, followed by the learning objective (LO) where more detailed information is found:

- Use of the wrong needles or collection equipment (LO 3)
- Use of wrong tubes (wrong additive) for the tests ordered (LO 4)
- Not properly mixing the specimen with the tube's chemical additive (LO 4)
- Not following the correct order for filling tubes, called *order of draw* (LO 4)
- Not filling tubes to the right level (LO 4)
- Not using careful technique during the blood draw (LO 8)
- Not handling or transporting specimens properly (LO 10)

3. Identify equipment used to collect blood specimens

In venipuncture a hollow needle is used to access (get into) the patient's vein. In most cases, a double-sided needle called a *multisample needle* is used. Multisample needles allow the PCT to fill all of the tubes needed for testing with a single puncture. One side of the needle goes into the patient's vein. The other side has a hub that screws into a rigid plastic holder. It punctures the stoppers of collection tubes. Air is removed from the tubes when they are manufactured, creating a vacuum. This lets them draw in the exact amount of blood needed for the specimen. The multisample needle, holder, and tube together are called an *evacuated tube system* (Fig. 22-3).

There are many different needle and holder styles. All systems include safety devices to reduce chances of accidental needle sticks. Most needles have shields that slide or swing into place after use. All of these collection systems work the same way (Fig. 22-4). The multisample needle is either preattached or screwed into a tube holder. After use, the safety device is activated. The needle and holder are immediately placed in a sharps container.

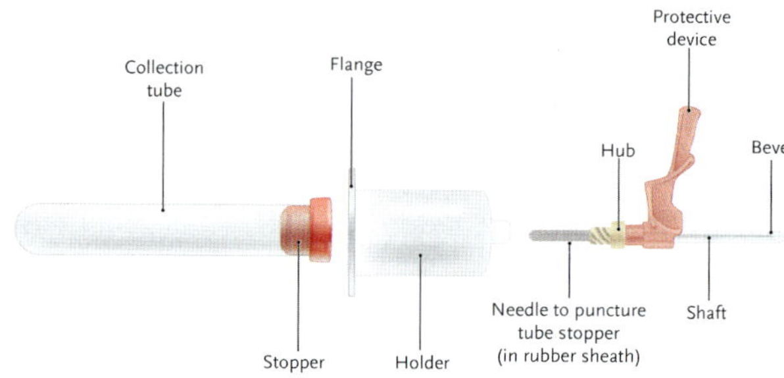

Fig. 22-3. *In an evacuated tube system, a double-sided needle is attached to a holder. Multiple tubes can be inserted and filled with a single venipuncture.*

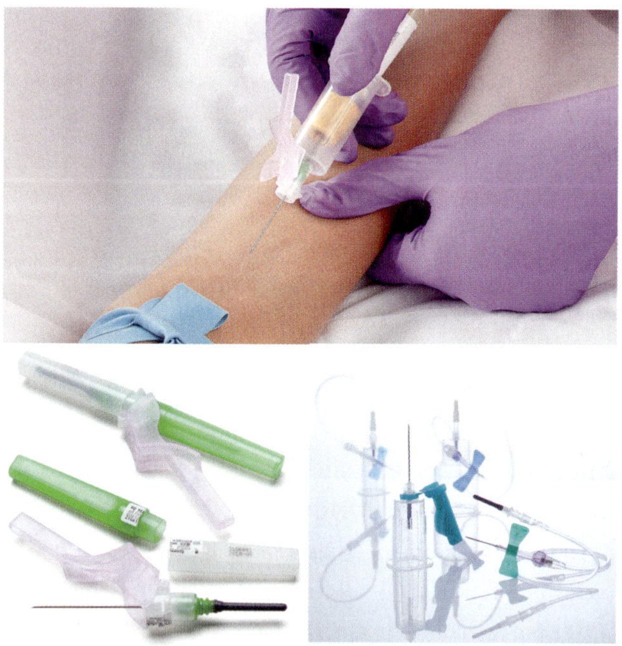

Fig. 22-4. *Multisample needles and holders come in a variety of styles and with different safety mechanisms.* (TOP AND LEFT PHOTOS COURTESY AND © BECTON, DICKINSON AND COMPANY; BOTTOM RIGHT COURTESY OF GREINER BIO-ONE, WWW.GBO.COM)

The opening of a venipuncture needle is slanted. This makes a sharp point for piercing the skin. This angled opening is called a *bevel* (Fig. 22-5). Multisample needles are usually 1"–1.5" long. They come in a range of needle widths. The hollow space inside the needle is called the *lumen*. The needle's **gauge** is based on the width of the lumen. The lower the gauge number, the wider the needle's lumen. The higher the gauge number, the thinner the lumen. Blood is usually drawn from adults using a 21-gauge needle. For adult patients with small or fragile veins or for pediatric patients, 22- or 23-gauge needles may be used. Pediatric draws may require an even smaller needle. The hubs of needles are color-coded based on gauge. Most manufacturers use green for 21-gauge needles. PCTs should know the color codes used at their facilities.

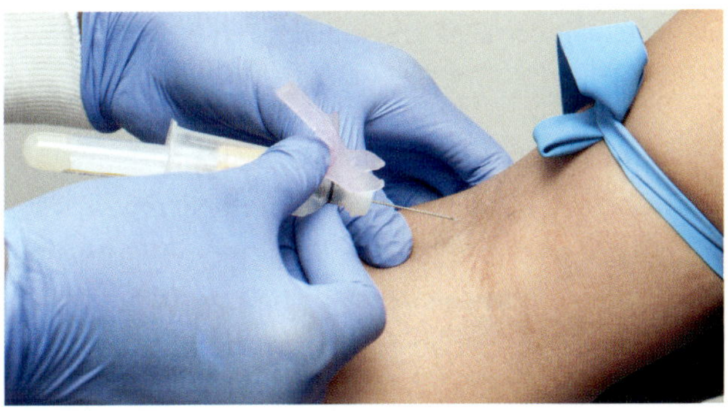

Fig. 22-5. *The needle's bevel is the angled opening that allows it to puncture the skin.*

PCTs may also use a winged collection set. This is usually called a *butterfly needle* (Fig. 22-6). It is shorter than a straight needle (3/4"–1"). At the base of the needle there is a pair of flaps ("wings"). Holding these wings, the PCT can guide the needle as it is inserted in the patient's skin and vein. This style of needle does not connect directly to a tube holder. Instead, it has thin, flexible tubing that connects to the tube holder. The PCT can change tubes without moving the needle or putting pressure on the patient's vein.

Butterfly needles come in many gauges. The most common are 21- and 23-gauge, but 25-gauge winged needles are also available. This type of needle is often used when drawing blood from patients with small or fragile veins. It is also used when blood is drawn from the back of the hand. Some collections, such as blood cultures, are almost always done with a butterfly needle. Butterfly needles are often used when drawing a specimen with a syringe. There is more information about these types of blood draws later in the chapter.

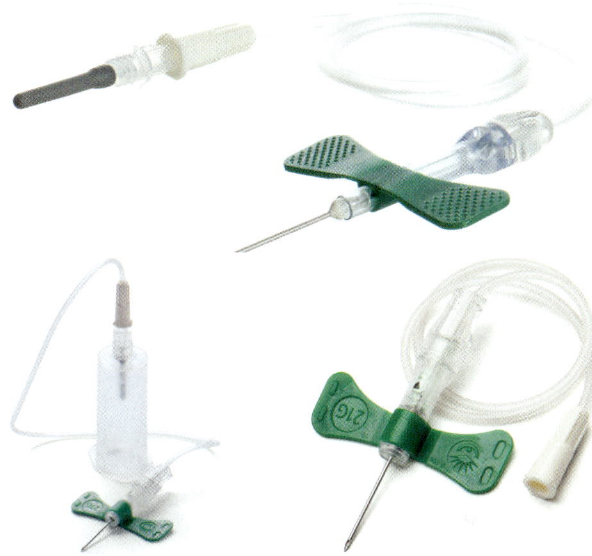

Fig. 22-6. *Winged collection, or butterfly, systems are often used for patients who are elderly, very young, or medically fragile (seriously ill patients who may have complicated or difficult treatments).* (TOP PHOTO COURTESY OF GREINER BIO-ONE, WWW.GBO.COM; BOTTOM PHOTOS COURTESY AND © BECTON, DICKINSON AND COMPANY)

Collection tubes come in many different sizes (Fig. 22-7). Larger tubes put more pressure on a patient's vein. Children's veins are smaller than adults'. They are more likely to collapse from the pressure created by a large tube. It is also important to draw as little blood as possible from children to avoid iatrogenic anemia. For these reasons, pediatric collection tubes are smaller (1–2 mL) than tubes used for adults (3–5 mL). Smaller tubes may also be used for patients who are elderly or ill (such as cancer patients), or for patients whose blood is drawn often.

Because of the pressure created by evacuated tubes, they are not the best choice for all patients. Thin or fragile veins may collapse. This can cause the blood flow to stop. It may harm the specimen. In these situations, the PCT needs to use a syringe and a syringe transfer device. A **syringe** is a barrel-shaped device with a plunger that is pulled to draw in blood.

The needle (usually a winged collection set) is attached to the syringe. The PCT collects the blood by gently pulling back on the plunger. Blood is then transferred to evacuated tubes using the syringe transfer device. This procedure is described later in the chapter.

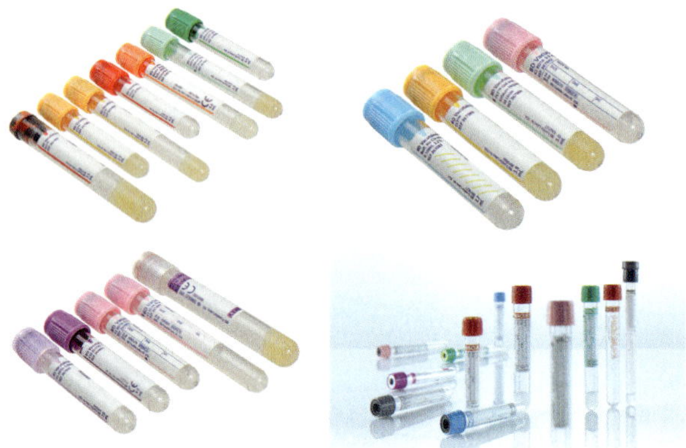

Fig. 22-7. *Venipuncture collection tubes range widely in size.* (TOP AND BOTTOM LEFT PHOTOS COURTESY AND © BECTON, DICKINSON AND COMPANY; BOTTOM RIGHT PHOTO COURTESY OF GREINER BIO-ONE, WWW.GBO.COM)

In addition to the devices used for puncturing the vein and collecting blood, PCTs also need the following supplies:

- **Gloves**. New gloves must be used for each patient. Gloves should always be checked for holes and discarded if defective.
- **Antiseptic solution**. The venipuncture site must be cleaned before blood is drawn. In most cases a 70% isopropyl alcohol prep pad is used to do this. Chlorhexidine gluconate (ChloraPrep is a common brand name) is often used for blood culture preparation.
- **Tourniquet**. A tourniquet is a band that slows the return of venous blood below the area where it is applied (Fig. 22-8). This makes it easier to find and access the patient's veins. It can be left on the patient's arm for up to 1 minute before it must be removed. Most facilities use disposable, nonlatex tourniquets. Reusing tourniquets is a contamination risk.
- **Gauze**. Gauze is applied to the puncture site right after the needle is removed. Applying pressure on the gauze helps stop the flow of blood.

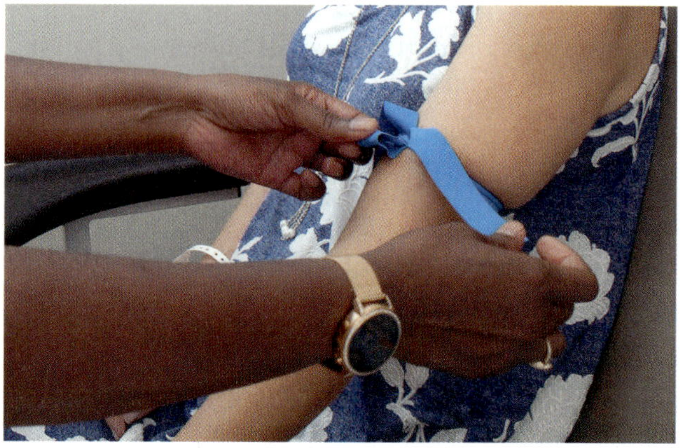

Fig. 22-8. *Tourniquets are applied above the venipuncture site. The veins below fill and expand. This makes it easier to find and puncture a vein.*

- **Bandage**. After bleeding has stopped, an adhesive bandage or a self-adhesive wrap is placed over the gauze. This prevents the clot at the puncture site from being disturbed (Fig. 22-9). Coban is a common brand name for wrap bandages. In patients with very fragile skin, gauze may be wrapped around the arm before a wrap bandage is applied.

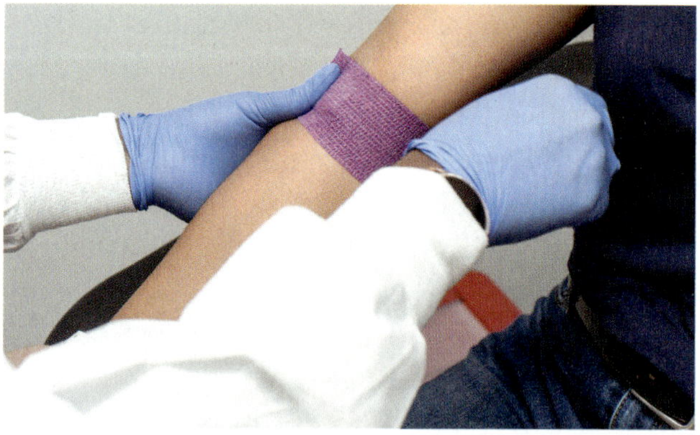

Fig. 22-9. *Self-adhesive wrap bandages are often used after blood draws. They are gentle on the patient's skin and easy to remove.*

In some situations, warming packs may be needed to make a patient's veins easier to find. Some facilities have electronic devices to locate veins. PCTs will be trained to use these devices if they are available. They may be helpful in caring for patients who are obese. Veins may be harder to locate in these patients.

Much of the equipment used for venipuncture is also used for capillary puncture. Gloves, alcohol prep pads, gauze, and bandages are all needed. Collection tubes may be used as well, but capillary collection tubes are different. They are not evacuated (vacuum) tubes and they hold much less blood. Most collection tubes for capillary puncture have a volume of 125–600 microliters. One microliter is one thousandth (1/1000) of a milliliter. They may be called *microcollection tubes.*

Some microcollection tubes have a straw-like attachment. This allows blood to flow from the puncture site into the tube. Others have spout-like openings under their caps. Sometimes capillary blood is not collected in tubes with lids but in very thin, straw-like tubes that hold a very small amount of blood (Fig. 22-10). These tubes are sealed with clay or another substance. Some are *heparinized,* or treated with the anticoagulant drug heparin. Heparinized capillary tubes are usually marked with a red or green line. Tubes without heparin are marked with a blue line.

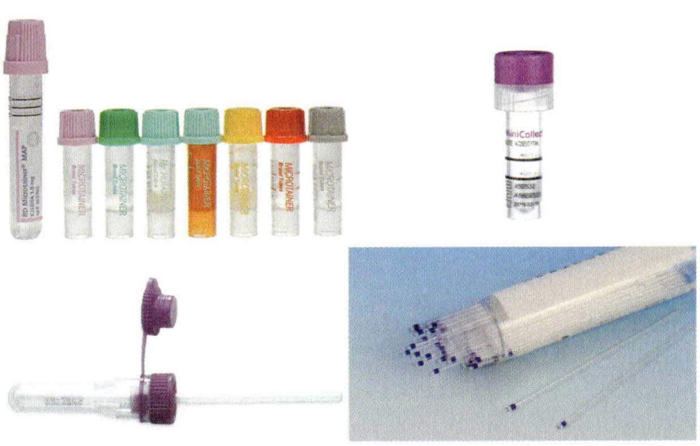

Fig. 22-10. *Capillary collection tubes are much smaller than venipuncture tubes. They might have straw-like lids to make collection easier. Capillary blood may also be collected in tiny straw-like tubes.* *(TOP LEFT PHOTO COURTESY AND © BECTON, DICKINSON AND COMPANY; TOP RIGHT PHOTO COURTESY OF GREINER BIO-ONE, WWW.GBO.COM; BOTTOM LEFT PHOTO COURTESY OF MARKETLAB, INC., WWW.MARKETLAB.COM; BOTTOM RIGHT PHOTO COURTESY OF GLOBE SCIENTIFIC, INC., WWW.GLOBESCIENTIFIC.COM)*

A lancet is used to start blood flow for capillary specimens. There are several types of lancets. Some are activated by a button. Others are activated when they are pressed against the patient's skin. When the lancet is activated, a blade or needle punctures the skin and then retracts (pulls back). All lancets are disposable, single-use items. They are discarded in a sharps container after use. Lancets come in many sizes. Each punctures the skin at a specific depth. Depths range from 0.85 millimeters (mm) for premature infants to 2.4 mm (Fig. 22-11). The range of 1.8 mm–2.2 mm is recommended for adults. The maximum puncture depth for small children is 2 mm.

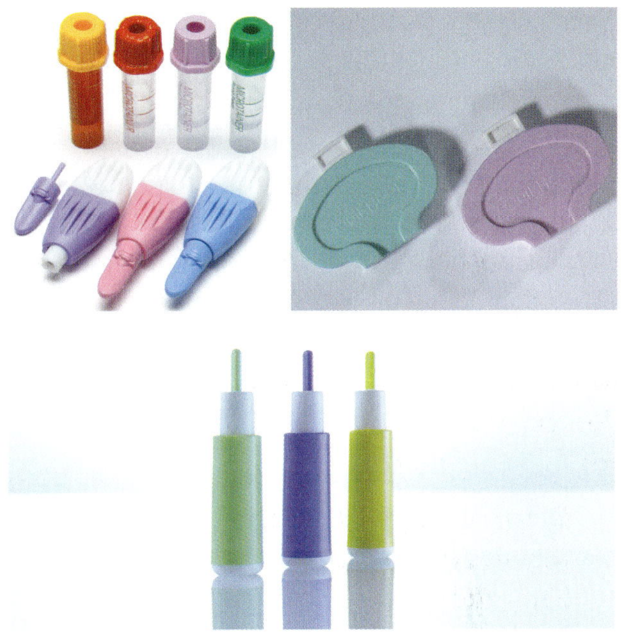

Fig. 22-11. *Lancets for finger sticks and infant heel sticks come in a variety of styles.* *(TOP PHOTOS COURTESY AND © BECTON, DICKINSON AND COMPANY; BOTTOM PHOTO COURTESY OF GREINER BIO-ONE, WWW.GBO.COM)*

To improve blood flow, warming packs may be used before capillary puncture. Other equipment may include filter paper for certain blood tests (e.g., newborn screening) or test strips for glucose monitoring and blood clotting time (a test called *PT/INR*). Adhesive bandages are used after capillary puncture for most patients, but never on small children. Bandages are choking hazards for infants and toddlers.

4. Identify additives to blood specimens and discuss order of draw

As blood is collected, additives in the collection tubes start preparing it for testing. Using a tube with the right additive makes sure the analytes for each test are preserved properly. Complete blood counts, for instance, must be done on whole blood. Blood will clot in a collection tube without an additive. Specimens for complete blood counts are collected in tubes with an anticoagulant additive. Requisitions often list the type of tube needed for each test. Most EHR systems print specimen labels that show the type of tube required.

Tube stoppers are color coded based on the type of additive inside. Colors may vary between manufacturers, but are usually similar. The tubes are also labeled with the name of any additives, as well as an expiration date (Fig. 22-12). They may have a line or arrow to show how far to fill the tube. PCTs should check all of this information before using a collection tube.

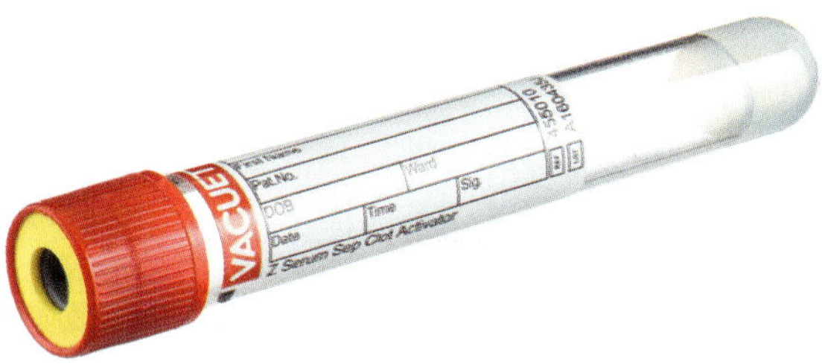

Fig. 22-12. *It is important to check the tube label as well as the stopper. Not all manufacturers use the same shades or colors for each additive. Some stopper colors are used for more than one type of additive.* (PHOTO COURTESY OF GREINER BIO-ONE, WWW.GBO.COM)

There are 2 categories of tubes: tubes with anticoagulants and tubes without. Many tests are done on blood serum. **Serum** is the liquid that is left after blood has clotted in the collection tube. Specimens used for serum testing must clot completely before tests can be done. Some tubes have clot activators to make specimens clot faster.

Different anticoagulants act in different ways. Some make calcium in the blood unavailable. Calcium is important to blood clotting, so this stops clots from forming. Other anticoagulants stop the action of thrombin. Thrombin is an enzyme involved in clotting. These different ways of stopping coagulation make each additive suited to particular blood tests.

After collection, blood specimens are sometimes prepared for testing by spinning in a machine called a centrifuge. When a specimen with anticoagulants is spun in a centrifuge, it divides into plasma and solid components (blood cells and platelets). Because of this, anticoagulant tubes are sometimes called *plasma tubes*. *Serum tubes* allow the blood to clot, leaving serum and clotted cells. In addition to additives that act on the blood, tubes may contain a separator gel. When the specimen is centrifuged, this gel separates the liquids and solids.

It is important to mix blood specimens with tube additives correctly. Right after a blood draw, a specimen with an additive must be gently turned upside down and then brought upright several times. This motion is called an *inversion*. Tubes should never be shaken. More information about inversions is in Learning Objective 8.

Color codes for plasma and serum tubes are listed in Tables 22-2 and 22-3. Other tubes may be used in addition to the common tubes listed in these tables. Tan-topped tubes contain the same additive as lavender tubes, but are lead-free. They are used to test lead levels. PCTs should always use the collection tubes shown on the requisition and/or specimen label. They should ask the nurse if there is any doubt.

Chemical additives can carry over from one tube to the next when the tubes are changed. Because of this, a specific tube order is needed when more than one tube is used. This **order of draw** is very important. It prevents clot activators, for example, from getting into a tube with an anticoagulant. Following the order of draw also reduces the risk of contamination of a blood culture specimen. Contamination is a serious problem. It can produce errors in the results and harm patient care.

SERUM TUBES	
Red. Tubes with red stoppers either contain a clot activator (plastic tubes) or no additive (glass tubes). They are used for chemistry, serology, and immunology tests. *Serology* is the study of blood serum.	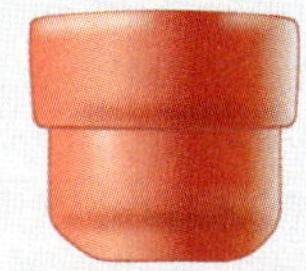
Gold or mottled red and gray (tiger top). Tubes with either gold or mixed red and gray stoppers contain both a clot activator and a separator gel. They are commonly called serum separator tubes (SSTs). They are used for chemistry, serology, and immunology tests. They should not be used to test therapeutic drug levels.	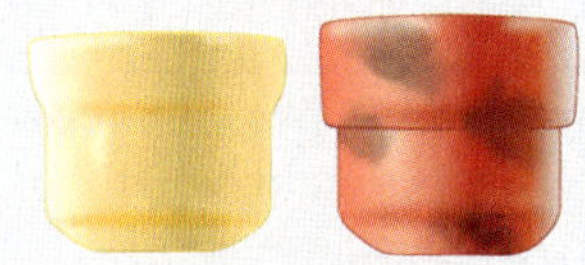
Orange. Tubes with an orange stopper are stat serum tubes. They contain a fast-acting clot activator and are available with or without separator gel. They may be used when test results are needed quickly.	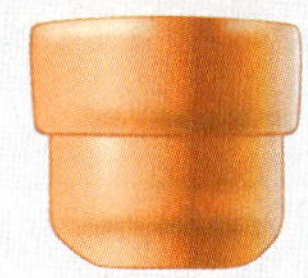

Table 22-2. *Serum tubes may or may not contain clot activators and/or separator gel.*

ANTICOAGULANT (PLASMA) TUBES	
Light blue. Tubes with light blue stoppers contain sodium citrate. They are often called *citrate tubes* and are used for coagulation studies. Sodium citrate acts by binding calcium. Its action is reversible. These tubes must always be filled completely.	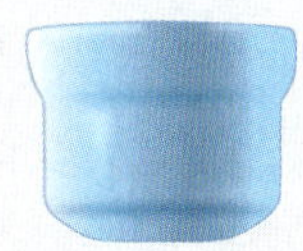
Green. Tubes with green stoppers of any shade contain heparin. Sodium heparin and lithium heparin are 2 different additives, both with the same anticoagulant action (deactivating thrombin). Tubes with separator gel usually have light green stoppers. These tubes may be called *plasma separator tubes* (*PSTs*). Green-topped tubes are used for routine or stat chemistry tests and certain types of genetic testing.	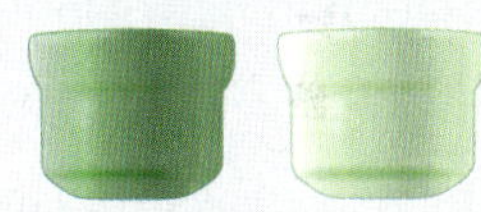
Lavender, pink, or white. Tubes with lavender (light purple), pink, or pearly white stoppers contain EDTA. EDTA acts by stopping the action of calcium in a patient's blood. These tubes are used for hematology studies (e.g., complete blood count). Pink-topped tubes are used for blood bank specimens (blood type and matching for transfusion, called *type and crossmatch*).	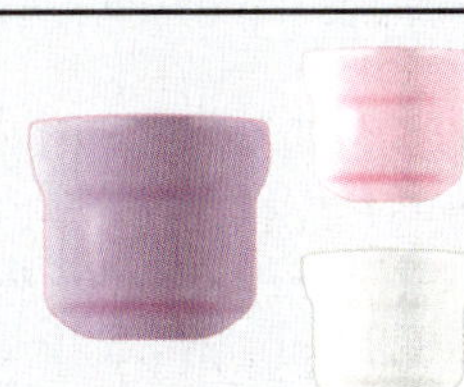
Gray. Tubes with gray stoppers usually contain 2 types of additives: sodium or potassium oxalate (anticoagulants) and sodium fluoride, which prevents the breakdown of glucose. This breakdown, called *glycolysis*, can affect some test results if it is not prevented. Gray-topped tubes (called *oxalate tubes*) are used for glucose testing. **Note:** Oxalate/sodium fluoride is the most common additive combination in gray-topped tubes, but some may contain EDTA as an anticoagulant. All gray-topped tubes contain sodium fluoride to prevent glycolysis.	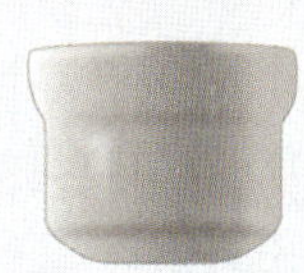

ANTICOAGULANT (PLASMA) TUBES (cont'd)	
Yellow. Tubes with yellow stoppers contain either acid citrate dextrose (ACD) or sodium polyanethole sulfonate (SPS). They are not as commonly used as the other anticoagulant tubes. ACD tubes are used for DNA analysis (e.g., paternity testing) or testing before organ transplant. SPS tubes are used for microbiology studies such as blood culture. *It is very important to check the label to verify the additive in a yellow tube.*	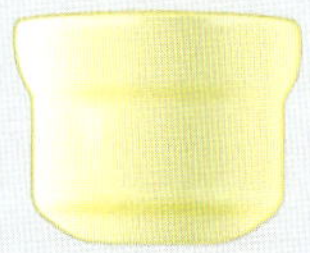
Royal blue. Tubes with royal blue stoppers usually contain EDTA, although they may also contain heparin or no additive. A colored stripe on the label shows the additive: lavender for EDTA, green for heparin, or red for no additive. Royal blue-topped tubes are free of *trace elements*, or chemicals present in tiny amounts. They are used for trace element, toxicology, and nutrition testing. *It is very important to check the label to verify the additive in a royal blue tube.*	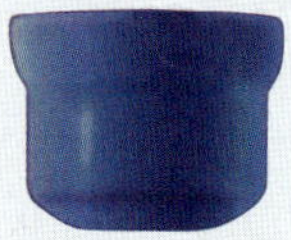

Table 22-3. *Different anticoagulant additives are used for specific diagnostic tests.*

The Clinical & Laboratory Standards Institute (CLSI) sets standards for blood draws that are used by medical facilities around the world. This is CLSI's venipuncture order of draw:

- Blood culture (may be yellow-topped SPS tubes or special blood culture bottles)
- Sodium citrate tubes (light blue tops)
- Serum tubes, with or without separator gel or clot activator (mottled red/gray, gold, red, or orange tops)
- Heparin tubes (green tops, all shades)
- EDTA tubes (lavender, pink, or pearly white tops)
- Oxalate tubes (gray tops)

Not all tubes are listed in the CLSI order of draw. PCTs should follow facility policy for collecting other tubes and for collecting gel and non-gel tubes of the same type (e.g., heparin tubes with and without separator gel).

Order of draw for capillary puncture specimens is different. In venipuncture draws, additives can be carried over when tubes are changed. This is not a problem in capillary collections. Instead, the order of draw is based on the qualities of capillary blood. As time passes after capillary puncture, the blood changes. The first blood collected is similar to arterial blood. As the collection continues, the blood becomes more like venous blood. As time passes, platelets collect at the puncture site. This causes the blood to be less similar to the rest of the patient's blood.

This is the CLSI order for capillary collection:

- Specimens to measure blood gases (this test is most often done on arterial blood, but the first capillary blood can be similar to arterial blood)
- EDTA tubes (often used for complete blood count, and should be filled before too many platelets collect)
- Tubes with other additives
- Serum tubes

For both types of blood collection, it is important to fill each tube to the proper level.

5. Understand the importance of safety during the collection of blood specimens

Before collecting a blood specimen, the PCT must have the correct equipment to safely perform the draw. This includes the equipment listed in Learning Objective 3. It also includes the proper safety equipment. If Transmission-Based Precautions are ordered, the PCT must use the correct PPE, such as a mask/respirator, gown, and goggles.

Gloves must be worn for all patients. Gloves should be easy to reach in case a pair needs to be replaced (Fig. 22-13). A sharps container should be in arm's reach during a blood draw. It should be less than 2/3 full. If it is over 2/3 full, a new container is needed before another blood draw is done. All phlebotomy needles and lancets have safety devices. Before starting a draw, the PCT should make sure he understands how the safety devices work.

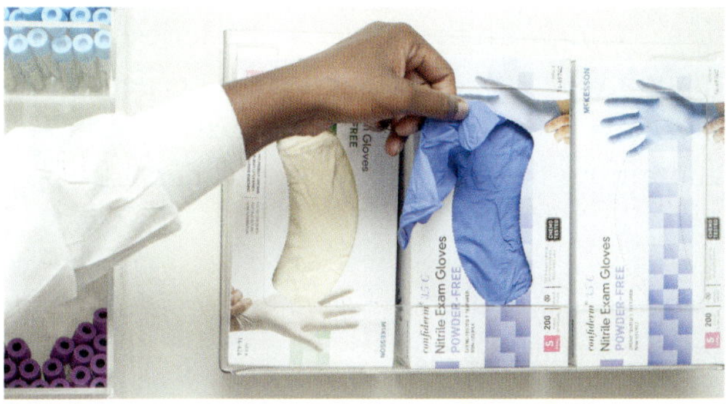

Fig. 22-13. A good supply of gloves makes sure the PCT is prepared to work safely.

In a hospital, blood is often drawn at a patient's bedside. Equipment is carried in a caddy or tray. This should be placed on a flat, clean surface. It should not be placed on the patient's bed. Needles should never be placed on the bed, before or after use.

A pillow may be used to support the patient's arm. Facilities may also have foam wedges or other devices to help with positioning. Any device or equipment (e.g., a caddy) that is used for more than one patient must be disinfected after each use, according to facility policy.

Drawing blood is a task delegated to PCTs by licensed healthcare providers. PCTs do not decide which tests are done or how much blood is drawn. However, PCTs should know the danger of drawing too much blood. Iatrogenic anemia is a serious risk for infants and for ICU patients. Sometimes multiple providers order tests for the same patient. If a PCT has any concern about the amount of blood they are asked to draw from a patient, they should check with the nurse. This is a safety issue that may be improved by careful observation and communication.

Another part of safe blood collection is being mentally prepared for each procedure. If a PCT is mentally prepared, when something unexpected happens, such as a patient fainting or having a seizure, she is ready. Safety is about using the proper equipment and procedures. It is also about state of mind.

6. Identify appropriate sites for venipuncture and capillary puncture

Blood is usually drawn in the area inside the elbow, called the *antecubital fossa*. Several veins are often easy to find here. The first choice for the PCT should always be the **median cubital vein**. There are many advantages to using this vein. The median cubital vein is usually well anchored. This means it is not likely to move back and forth. Using this vein also has the lowest risk of accidentally hitting an artery or a nerve.

Hitting a nerve can cause serious, sometimes permanent, damage. Nerve damage causes pain and/or loss of feeling. Puncturing an artery can be dangerous. Blood flows through the arteries at a higher pressure. Bleeding from an arterial puncture can be harder to stop than bleeding from a vein. Analytes are often present in different amounts in arterial blood. Most test result ranges are for blood from veins. Testing arterial blood can give incorrect results.

Figure 22-14 shows the common patterns of veins in the antecubital area. In some people the veins form a slanted "H" shape. In some they form an "M" shape. The "H" formation is more common. In this pattern the median cubital vein crosses between the cephalic vein and the basilic vein. In the "M" formation, the median cubital vein and the median cephalic vein form the inside, slanting parts of the letter "M."

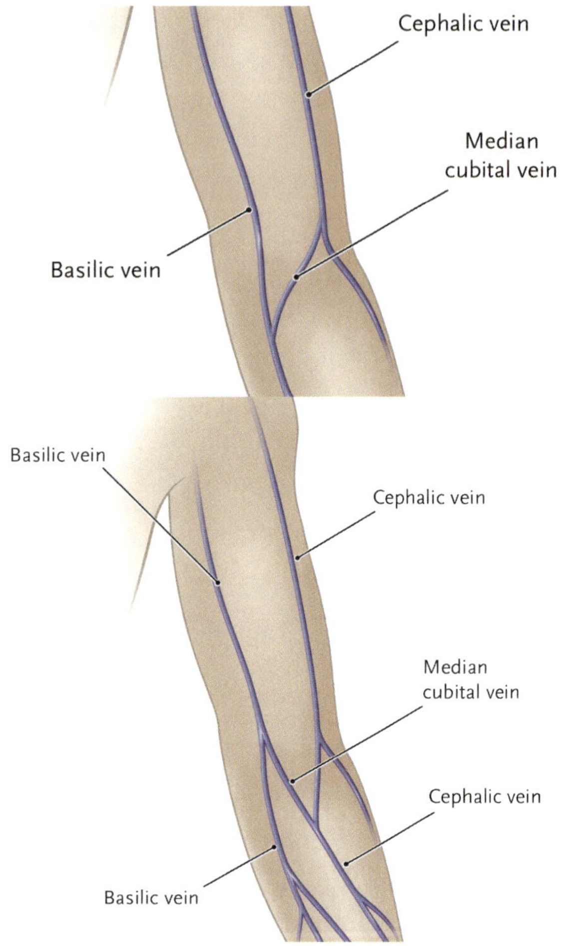

Fig. 22-14. *An illustration of the "H" formation is on top and an illustration of the "M" formation is on the bottom.*

Preventing Blood Draw Injury

Accidental artery puncture or nerve contact is less likely when a PCT follows proper procedures. It is still important to know how to manage these situations if they happen. Arterial blood is easy to recognize. It is bright red and pulses as it enters the tube. If an artery is accidentally punctured, the PCT should make sure that bleeding has stopped after removing the needle. Pressure must be applied to the site for a longer period of time. It may help to hold the arm up above the level of the heart. Patients taking anticoagulants may bleed more from an arterial puncture than other patients. The patient should not be bandaged or left alone until bleeding has stopped completely. The specimen should be clearly labeled as arterial blood. Shooting pain, tingling, numbness, or an "electric" feeling in the arm can be caused by nerve contact. The needle must be removed right away if a patient reports these feelings. Nerve damage can cause permanent disability.

Patient safety is the most important factor when choosing a venipuncture site. PCTs should never draw blood from an arm on the side of the body where a mastectomy was performed. This may increase the chance of infection or lymphedema. They should never use an arm that has an IV or a fistula, which is a connection made between an artery and a vein for dialysis. Locations close to arteries and nerves and sites where the vein is hard to see or palpate (find by touch) should also be avoided. These sites are more likely to be hard to draw from; they may cause pain or injury. Figure 22-15 shows the veins of the antecubital fossa, along with the nerves and arteries. Although the nerves and arteries are deeper than the veins, there is still a risk of missing a vein and hitting the brachial artery or a nerve.

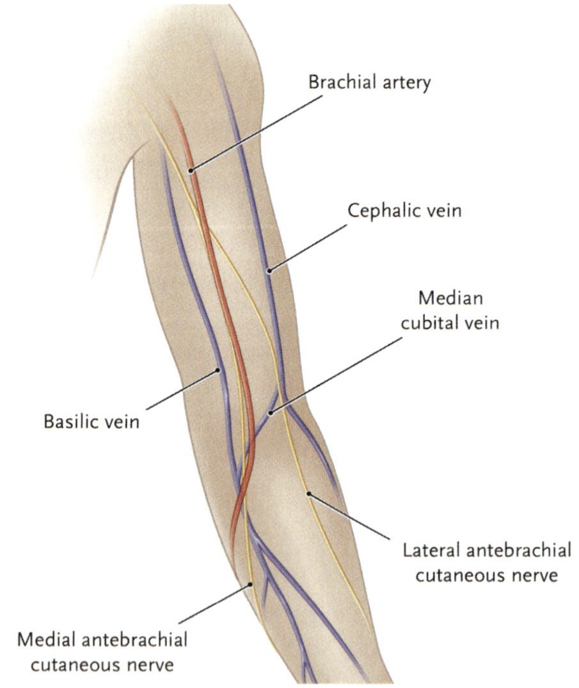

Fig. 22-15. *Nerves and arteries are located in the antecubital fossa, along with the veins used for venipuncture.*

In order of preference, the veins that a PCT should consider for venipuncture are as follows:

- Median cubital vein
- Cephalic vein
- Basilic vein

The basilic vein is the last choice because it is close to an artery and nerves. It is also the site most likely to cause pain. Before choosing this vein the PCT should first check both arms for a better choice. Veins should be examined by palpation as well as sight. People with different skin colors, physical builds, and ages may have veins that look different (Fig. 22-16). Palpation is the best way to locate a good vein for venipuncture.

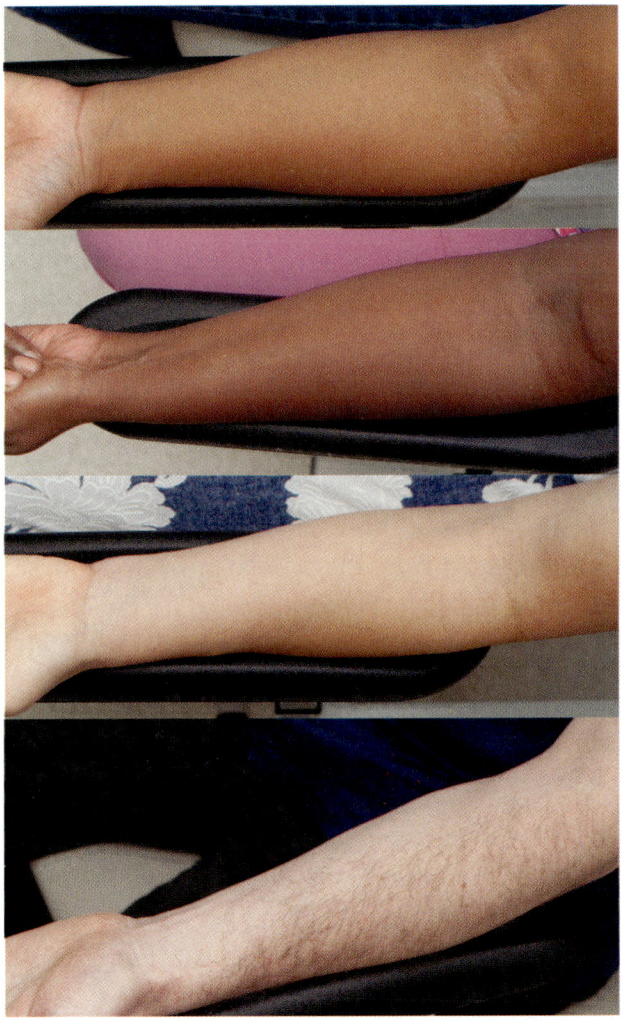

Fig. 22-16. *The antecubital area looks different in different people.*

When palpating a vein, the PCT should line a finger up with the vein and gently press and release to feel the vein. This motion is repeated until the PCT has found a good vein to use. If the PCT is wearing gloves during palpation, she should not tear the finger off of the glove. PCTs should follow facility policy about wearing gloves during palpation. Gloves must always be worn if the patient has broken skin or a rash or has Contact Precautions ordered. Palpation can give information about these factors:

Vein health. A healthy vein feels springy and uniform. It should not be hard or bumpy.

Vein depth. Veins are located at different depths in different patients. The age and weight of a patient can affect vein depth. The veins of patients who are obese may be hard to see. Palpation is especially important with these patients. If a patient's veins are deep under the skin, a longer needle must be used.

Anchoring of the vein. Veins in the median antecubital area are usually well anchored. They do not often move or roll away. Some patients have veins that tend to roll no matter where they are located. Palpation can show whether vein rolling is likely during venipuncture.

Diameter (width) of the vein. Knowing how wide the patient's vein is helps the PCT to choose the right needle gauge. It also helps the PCT to insert the needle in the center of the vein.

When a patient's veins are hard to find, the PCT can try these techniques:

- The patient can be asked to hang her arm straight down for a few minutes. This causes blood to pool in the arm. It can make finding a vein easier.
- A warm washcloth or a commercial heating pack can be applied to the area. The heat causes veins to dilate, or expand.
- The patient can make a fist, which causes blood to surge. The patient should not pump her fist. This can cause blood cells to build up. This buildup is called *hemoconcentration*. Fist pumping can also cause *hemolysis*, or destruction of red blood cells. Hemoconcentration and hemolysis can both cause errors in test results.

The PCT can ask the patient where venipuncture has worked well in the past. Patients often know which sites are best. However, if the PCT thinks the vein a patient suggests is unsuitable, the PCT should not use it.

PCTs should *never* slap or flick the patient's skin to cause the veins to show more clearly. This was once considered a good way to make veins easier to find. Now it is seen as unprofessional. Patients may consider it abusive.

Petechiae

Some patients may develop a rash-like condition called *petechiae* after a tourniquet is applied. These small, flat red, brown, or purple dots are caused by blood leaking from capillaries. Petechiae may relate to several different health conditions. Their appearance is not a cause for removing the tourniquet or stopping the blood draw. However, the PCT should watch carefully after the draw is finished to make sure bleeding has stopped completely. Patients who get petechiae may bleed longer than other patients.

If a good vein in the antecubital area is not found after checking *both arms* by sight and palpation, the PCT should check the veins on the back of the hand. This part of the hand is called the *dorsal aspect* (Fig. 22-17). The PCT should know that drawing blood from the back of the hand is usually more painful for the patient. The veins in the wrist are *never* an acceptable site for venipuncture. Nerves, tendons, and arteries are all close to the surface of the skin in the wrist. The risk of injury is high.

Connected Care

Site Selection

The first priority when selecting a site for venipuncture should be the safety and health of the patient. Drawing blood from sites close to nerves or arteries, or from sites that are unsafe for other reasons, can harm or even permanently disable patients. A patient's comfort is also important. Venipuncture may cause some amount of pain no matter how carefully it is done. Even so, a PCT should try to choose the site that will cause the least discomfort.

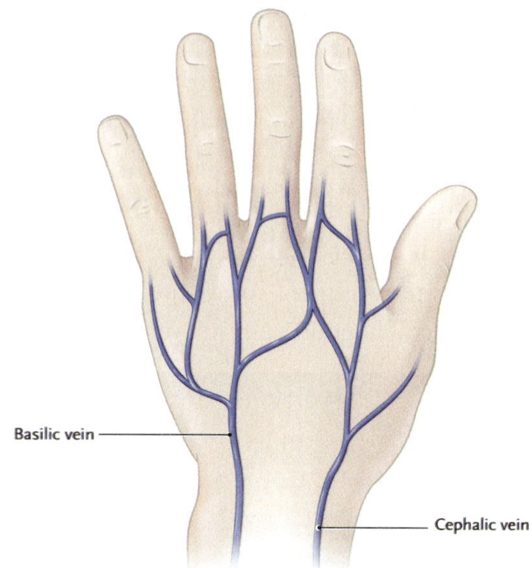

Fig. 22-17. *Veins on the back of the hand may be the best choice if the veins in the antecubital fossa cannot be located or cannot be used.*

In most cases capillary specimens are collected from the middle or ring finger of an adult's or child's nondominant hand. The *nondominant* hand is the hand the person uses less. In infants, the side of the heel is used. Capillary blood used to be collected from the earlobe or from the first toe (the "big toe"). The earlobe should not be used. The big toe is not a preferred site but is allowed if other sites cannot be used.

These points are important to consider when choosing a fingerstick site:

- The fingers on a person's dominant hand are more likely to be calloused. The *dominant* hand is the hand the person uses more. This makes puncturing the skin more difficult. It may also be more painful.
- The index finger (also called the second finger) of either hand may be calloused, or have thicker skin. This finger also has more nerve endings. It is more sensitive to pain.
- The bones of the smallest finger (the pinky finger or fifth finger) are closer to the skin than the bones of the other fingers. It is not a good choice for capillary collection.

- There is a pulse point in the thumb (considered the first finger). This increases bleeding risk. Because of this, the thumb should not be used.
- If a patient has capillary puncture done often, the selected finger/site should be rotated. The same site should not be used twice in a row.
- A finger stick may only be performed on an infant over 6 months old weighing 10 kilograms (22 pounds) or more. Heel stick must be used for younger infants and infants who weigh less. There is more about heel stick later in this learning objective.

Once a finger is chosen, the best area for making the puncture is the fleshy part near the tip. The puncture should be toward either side of the finger, but not completely on the side (Fig. 22-18). The medical term for this site is the palmar surface of the distal segment of the finger. The very tip should not be used. The bone is closer to the surface here. The chance of injury is higher. A fingertip puncture may also be more painful and more likely to reopen and bleed after the procedure is done.

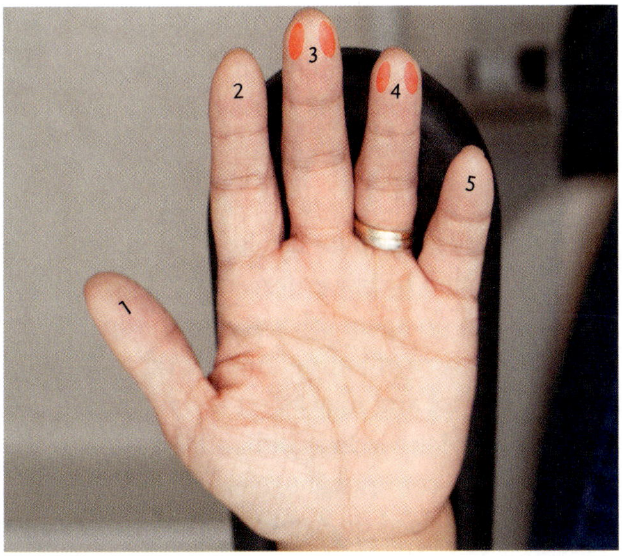

Fig. 22-18. *The third and fourth fingers of the nondominant hand are best for capillary puncture. The best sites are near the fingertip on the palm side of the hand, toward one side or the other.*

These situations may cause problems with a capillary puncture site:

- Cyanotic fingernail beds are a sign of poor circulation. Poor circulation makes it hard to collect blood from a finger stick.
- Patients with edema, or swelling, of the hands are not good candidates for capillary puncture. Their capillary blood is likely to contain a lot of fluid.
- Patients whose fingers are burned, injured, scarred, bruised, or covered with a rash are not good candidates for capillary puncture.
- Blood draws of any kind should not be performed on the same side as a mastectomy. If a patient has had a bilateral (double) mastectomy, the provider must give permission before blood is taken from either side. This is true no matter how long ago the surgery happened.
- Dehydration makes any type of blood collection more difficult. It may not be possible to collect enough capillary blood from a dehydrated patient.

If capillary collection is ordered for patients in these situations, the PCT should check with the nurse before continuing.

When doing a heel stick on an infant, it is important to avoid locations where the bone is very close to the surface of the skin. Hitting the heel bone, or calcaneus, with the lancet can cause a bone infection called *osteomyelitis*. The arch of the foot, the bottom surface of the heel, and the very back of the heel should not be used. The sole of the foot is called the *plantar surface*. The medial (inside) and lateral (outside) plantar surfaces of the heel are good sites for infant heel stick (Fig. 22-19). The lateral plantar surface is the part of the heel roughly in line with the smallest toe. The medial plantar surface lines up with the outer half of the big toe.

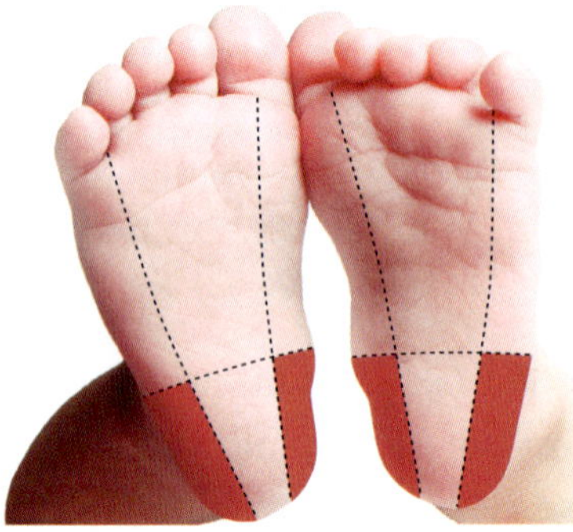

Fig. 22-19. The sides of the bottom surface of the heel (shaded in this picture) are the sites where infants' heel bones are located deep enough beneath the skin to allow capillary puncture.

7. Describe site preparation and proper needle/lancet placement

Once a site has been selected, it must be cleaned. This reduces the risk of harmful microorganisms entering the puncture wound or the specimen. An alcohol prep pad is generally used (Fig. 22-20). If commercial pads are not available, a gauze square can be wet with 70% isopropyl alcohol and used to clean the site. CLSI standards emphasize using friction and a back-and-forth motion when cleaning a venipuncture site.

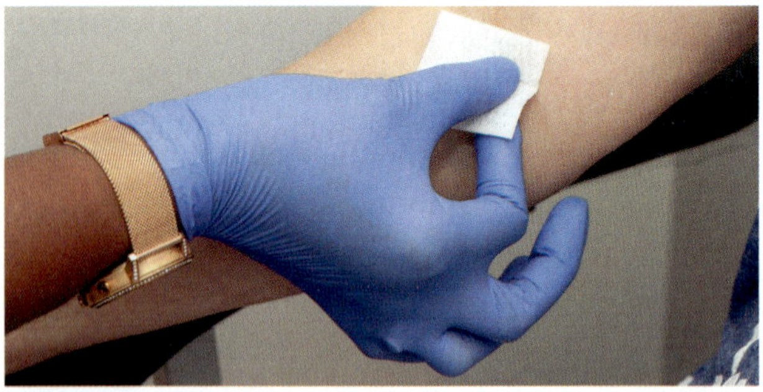

Fig. 22-20. A commercially prepared alcohol prep pad or a gauze square soaked in alcohol is used to clean the site of a blood draw.

Care must be taken not to damage the patient's skin. PCTs should be especially careful when cleaning the skin of pediatric and elderly patients. After cleaning, the skin must be allowed to air-dry before the blood draw is performed. The alcohol must dry completely. This gives it time to destroy microorganisms. It may also prevent stinging at the puncture site. Let the alcohol dry naturally. This takes about 15 seconds. A dry site should not look shiny. Do not blow on the site to dry it. Do not fan the site. This can spread pathogens. After the site has been cleaned, it must not be touched again. If the vein is palpated again before venipuncture, the site must be cleaned again.

When a blood culture is ordered, as many microorganisms as possible must be removed from the patient's skin. Microorganisms on the skin can contaminate the culture. Isopropyl alcohol may be used for blood culture, but the alcohol prep pad must be in contact with the skin for a longer time. If alcohol is used, the site is usually cleaned with 2 or 3 different pads for a total of 30–60 seconds.

Blood culture sites are more often prepared using a chlorhexidine gluconate product. ChloraPrep is one brand. A 2% tincture of iodine may also be used. When iodine is used, it is later removed from the skin with an alcohol prep pad. If it is not removed, it can pass through the skin and into the patient's bloodstream. Some patients are allergic to iodine, and patients with a shellfish allergy may also react to iodine-based antiseptics. A PCT should follow her facility's policies. It is important to follow the time requirements for cleaning and drying. Contamination of blood cultures is a common problem. It causes inaccurate results and can harm patients.

When blood is tested for alcohol content (as in a test requested by law enforcement), the site is cleaned with an agent other than isopropyl alcohol or tincture of iodine. Both of these agents contain alcohol and may affect test results. Instead, povidone-iodine and antiseptic soap and water are commonly used. Povidone-iodine should not be used on patients with iodine or shellfish allergies.

After equipment is chosen and the best site located and cleaned, the PCT is ready to puncture the vein or skin. For venipuncture, the thumb of the PCT's nondominant hand is used to anchor the vein. To do this, the PCT pulls down on the skin below the puncture site. The needle is placed at the site, bevel up, and inserted into the skin at an angle of 30 degrees or lower (Fig. 22-21). It is then moved forward (advanced) gently until blood starts to flow. It is very important to insert the needle at the lowest angle possible. A deeper angle creates a higher risk of hitting an artery or nerve (Fig. 22-22). It raises the risk of putting the needle straight through, rather than into, the patient's vein. This is often called a *blown vein*. This is why, for patients who are obese or whose veins seem to be deep under the skin, a longer needle is used. The needle is still inserted at 30 degrees or lower.

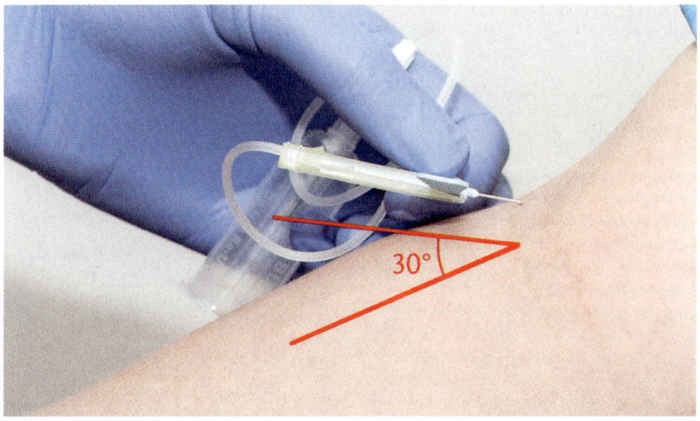

Fig. 22-21. *Inserting the needle at an angle of 30 degrees or lower reduces risk to the patient. It improves the chance of a successful draw.*

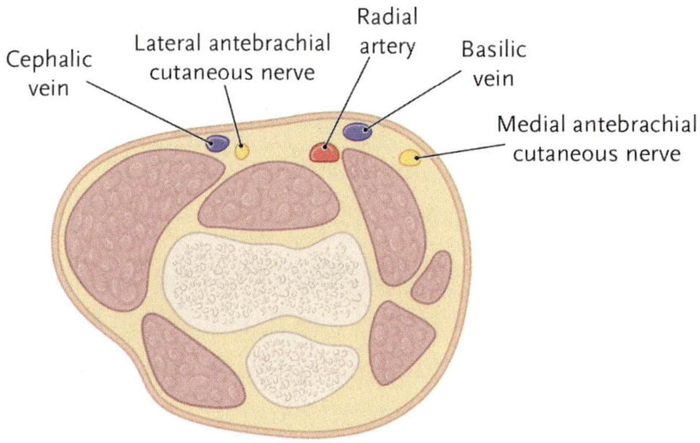

Fig. 22-22. *This cross-section of an arm at the elbow shows the depth of veins, arteries, and nerves. Puncturing the skin at a low angle is the safest way to ensure that a vein is punctured.*

Once the needle has been inserted, a number of problems can prevent blood flow. The patient's vein may have moved, or rolled. The needle may have gone through the entire vein. The bevel may not be fully inserted into the vein, or the vein may have collapsed against the bevel (Fig. 22-23).

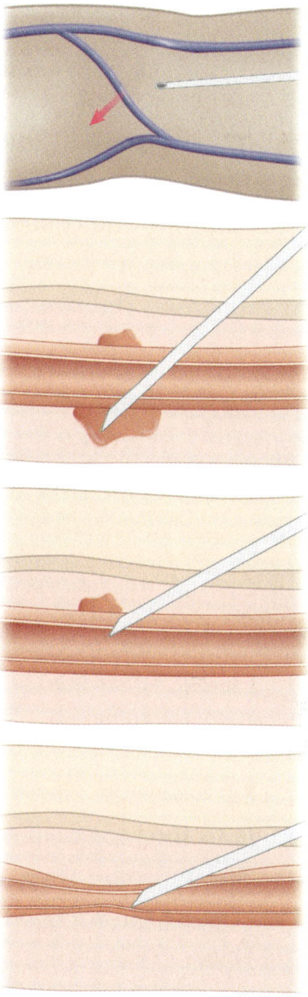

Fig. 22-23. *Veins may roll or may be punctured all the way through ("blown"). The bevel may not be completely inside the vein, or the vein may have collapsed onto it.*

If blood flow does not start right away, the PCT must not move the needle around blindly. This is called *probing for a vein*. It is painful for the patient and can also create a **hematoma**. A hematoma is an area of leaked blood under the patient's skin. Hematomas can develop even after a blood draw is complete. They can put pressure on nerves and may cause damage. Blood drawn from a site inside a hematoma may create errors in test results.

After puncturing the patient's skin, the PCT can gently adjust the needle slightly forward or slightly back (never side to side). If blood does not start to flow, the tourniquet should be released and the needle removed. Another site should be chosen. **A PCT should not make more than 2 venipuncture attempts on a patient.** If, after 2 attempts, blood flow has not started, the PCT should tell the nurse.

When doing a capillary puncture, the angle of a blade-style lancet is important. Blood can run into fingerprint lines. This makes it harder to get the blood to drip into the collection device. It is less likely to happen if the lancet is placed perpendicular to (across) the fingerprint lines (Fig. 22-24).

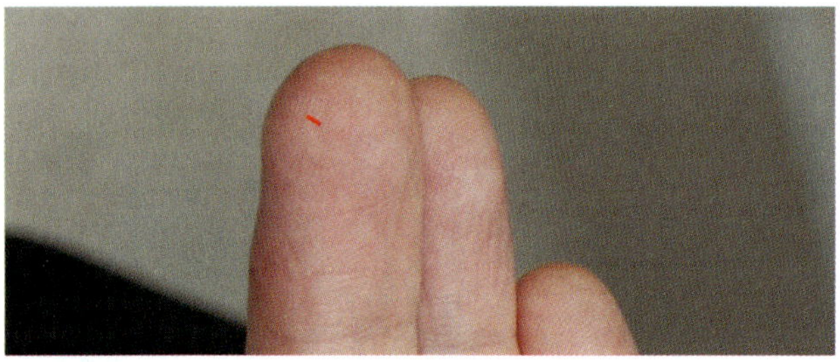

Fig. 22-24. *Cutting across, rather than along, fingerprint lines makes capillary collection easier.*

In the same way, it is best to place the lancet at a 90-degree angle to the length of a baby's foot for a heel stick. The PCT can then squeeze the heel gently. This opens the incision slightly and increases blood flow.

Some lancets activate automatically when pressed to the skin. Others are button-activated. When using a button-activated lancet, a PCT should not press the lancet into the patient's skin. This can make an incision that is too deep.

Before a capillary puncture, the PCT should have all equipment ready and within easy reach. Capillary collections must be made quickly and efficiently. The longer the procedure takes, the more likely the specimen will begin to clump. The blood flow may stop completely. Squeezing the puncture site too hard to keep blood flowing can harm the specimen. It can also cause the patient pain. The best solution is to use the right lancet and to be prepared to collect the blood right away.

8. Describe procedures for routine venipuncture and capillary puncture

Venipuncture is usually done in the antecubital area of the arm with a straight, 21-gauge needle and evacuated tubes. Changes are usually based on the patient's age or condition. If a butterfly needle is not necessary due to the patient's age or condition or the test ordered, the PCT should use a straight multisample needle. These needles are easier to handle. They have less risk of accidental needle stick.

Connected Care

Phobias Are Real

A large number of people, children and adults, have phobias about needles and/or blood. Phobias are often described as *illogical* or *irrational*, but the fears are real for the people who have them. Telling a patient that there is nothing to be afraid of is not helpful. It does not show respect for a patient's rights. PCTs can support patients with phobias by treating them with dignity. When a patient is afraid of needles or blood, a PCT should not dismiss the fear. The PCT can suggest that the patient look away while equipment is prepared and during the draw. He should still tell the patient before inserting the needle. The PCT should never try to "trick" a patient, inserting the needle when it is not expected. This can increase anxiety and fear.

Before venipuncture the PCT should ask the patient if she has ever had trouble with blood draws in the past. This helps the PCT prepare. The PCT should also confirm that the patient meets any requirements (such as fasting) for the blood draw. She should make sure there is no gum or food in the patient's mouth. All equipment should be checked carefully for defects. Expiration dates must be checked as well. Expired or damaged equipment must be properly discarded.

Limiting Tourniquet Time

A tourniquet cannot stay on a patient's arm for more than 1 minute. Longer use causes hemoconcentration and damages the specimen. It may also be uncomfortable for the patient. When a patient has veins that are easy to see, palpate, and puncture, a PCT may be able to finish a blood draw within a 1-minute period. This is a very tight timeline, though. It creates pressure to finish the draw quickly. It is better to release the tourniquet as soon as a site is selected. The released tourniquet can stay on the arm, not tightened, while the PCT cleans the site and prepares the needle and holder. It can then be reapplied right before the vein is punctured. The loose ends of the tourniquet must not touch the selected site. This is considered contamination. The site would need to be cleaned again. After the vein is punctured, the tourniquet is released as soon as blood flow begins.

For all types of blood draws, if the patient is a young child and a parent or guardian is present, the PCT should request that the parent or guardian hold the child during the procedure. This comforts the child and also helps to keep the child still.

Performing routine venipuncture with multisample needle and evacuated tube(s)

Equipment: gloves (additional PPE if required based on patient condition); tourniquet; alcohol prep pad (or other antiseptic agent); multisample needle of the correct gauge; needle holder; collection tubes for ordered tests; specimen labels; 2"x2" gauze; adhesive or self-adhesive bandage; pillow or wedge to support patient's arm; requisition; pen

1. Identify yourself by name. Identify the patient according to facility policy. For some tests (e.g., testing blood type for transfusion) a nurse may need to verify identification.
2. Explain the procedure to the patient. Speak clearly, slowly, and directly. Maintain face-to-face contact whenever possible.
3. Provide for the patient's privacy with a curtain, screen, or door.
4. If drawing blood from a patient in bed, adjust the bed to a safe level, usually waist high. Lock the bed wheels.
5. Put your equipment on a clean, flat surface (not the patient's bed).
6. Wash your hands. Put on gloves and other PPE as required. (In the case of some Transmission-Based Precautions this will have been done outside the patient's room.)
7. Ask the patient to extend her arms for a visual inspection. Ask the patient if one arm is better than the other for venipuncture. Choose an arm based on the appearance of the veins and the patient's input.
8. Apply the tourniquet to the selected arm, 3–4 inches above the bend in the elbow. Ask the patient to make (but not pump) a fist.
9. With a gloved index finger, palpate the arm to find an acceptable vein (Fig. 22-25). If a good site is not found, remove the tourniquet. Apply it to the other arm.

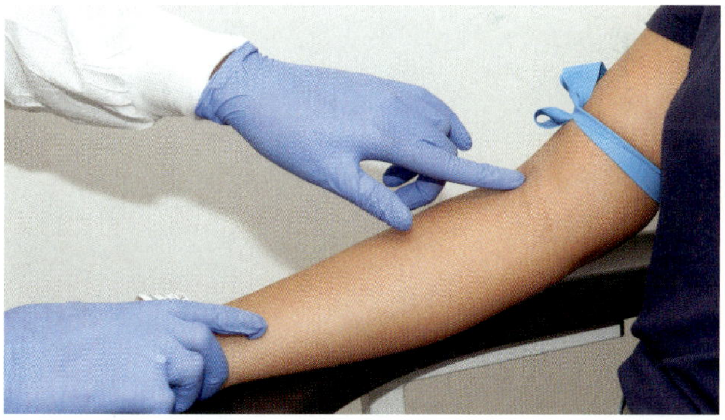

Fig. 22-25. *Palpate the arm with your index finger to find an acceptable vein.*

10. When a good site is located, release the tourniquet. Put the wedge or pillow under the patient's arm so it is supported. Clean the site thoroughly. Apply friction with the alcohol prep pad (or other antiseptic agent). It may help to make a mental note of a physical marker of the site, such as a freckle or a crease in the skin.

11. Allow the alcohol to dry fully. Do not blow on, fan, or wipe the skin to speed drying. This can recontaminate the site. While the alcohol dries, assemble the needle and holder (Fig. 22-26). The first tube may be placed in the holder, but should not be inserted fully until the patient's vein is punctured.

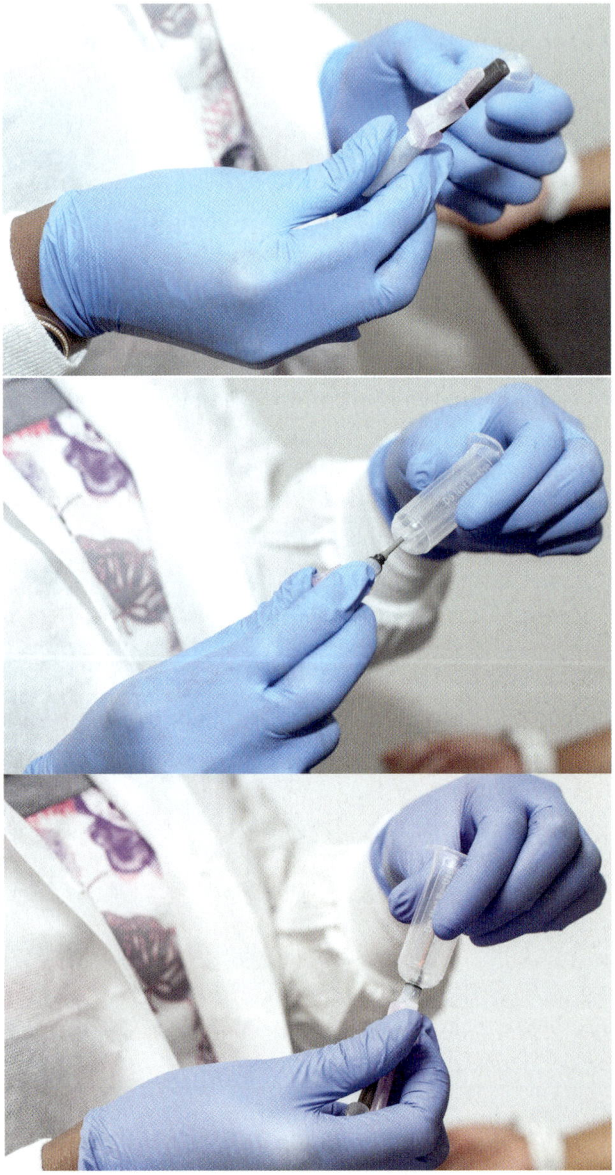

Fig. 22-26. *Assemble equipment while the patient's arm dries.*

12. Reapply the tourniquet.
13. Anchor the vein by holding the patient's forearm with your nondominant hand. Use your thumb to apply pressure and pull the skin toward the wrist 1 or 2 inches below the venipuncture site. Do not anchor from above the site. This is a needlestick risk.
14. Tell the patient that she may feel brief pain as the needle enters the skin. In a single, fluid motion, insert the needle into the skin to puncture the selected vein. The angle of the needle to the skin should be 30 degrees or lower (Fig. 22-27).

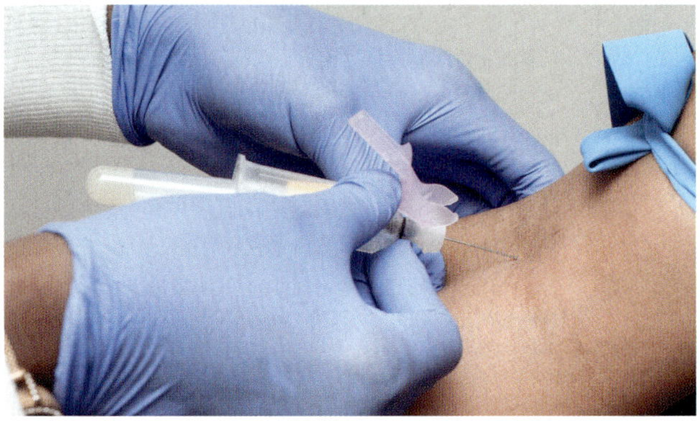

Fig. 22-27. *Be gentle but decisive when puncturing the patient's skin to access the vein.*

15. Insert the first collection tube, pressing it in to the point marked on the tube. As soon as blood flow begins, release the tourniquet. Let it hang loose. Allow the tube to fill completely. The vacuum should draw in exactly the right amount of blood.
16. If more than 1 tube is needed, replace the first filled tube with the next tube. Use the proper order of draw. Continue until all needed tubes are filled. Remove the last tube from the holder.
17. Place a piece of gauze, folded into quarters, over the needle.
18. Remove the needle from the patient's arm. Engage the safety device. Discard the needle and holder in a sharps container. Keep pressure on the gauze. The patient can help if she is able (Fig. 22-28). Do not allow the patient to bend her arm up. This can create a hematoma.

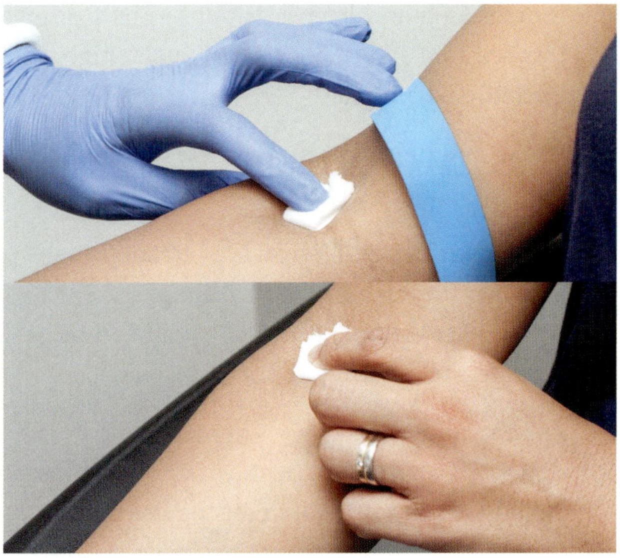

Fig. 22-28. Apply pressure to the gauze right after the needle is removed. The patient can hold pressure if she is able.

19. Mix tubes based on manufacturer directions. Most citrate and serum tubes require 3–5 inversions; most other tubes require 8–10. This is done by gently turning the tube upside down and then right side up again (Fig. 22-29). This counts as one inversion. Mix tubes right away. If more than one tube is needed, the tube collected first can be mixed while the next tube fills.

20. Label the tubes in front of the patient if the labels are not preprinted with the patient's information. Initial each tube. Document the time and date of collection according to facility policy. Ask the patient to check that the identifying information on the label is correct. Follow facility policy for preparing the specimens for transport. Properly discard any waste.

21. Check to make sure that the patient has stopped bleeding. This can take as long as 5 minutes for patients on anticoagulant medication.

22. Place a bandage over the gauze at the puncture site. Self-adhesive bandages are less likely to damage skin. They may be better for patients with fragile skin. Tell the patient to leave the bandage in place for the next 15 minutes.

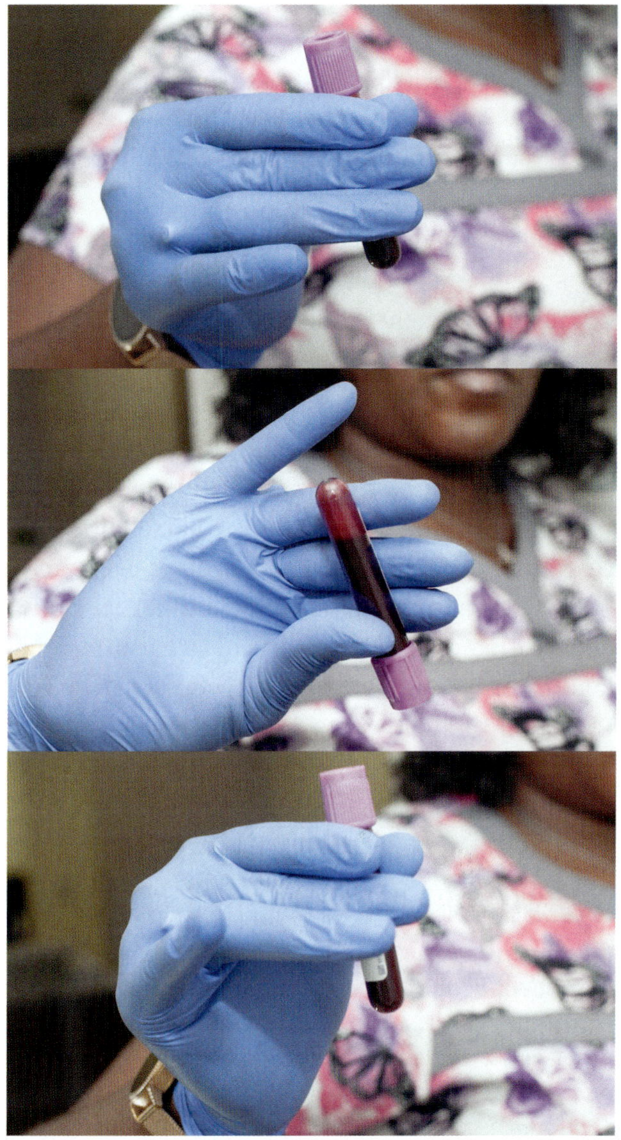

Fig. 22-29. Never shake tubes to mix them. Smooth, gentle inversions mix the specimen and prevent hemolysis (destruction of red blood cells).

23. Observe the patient for any signs of dizziness or discomfort. Do not leave the patient if she seems unsteady or says that she feels faint.

24. Remove and discard your gloves. Wash your hands.

25. Remove the pillow/wedge. If a wedge was used, place it in the proper area for

disinfecting or clean and disinfect it according to facility policy.

26. Return the bed to its lowest position. Remove privacy measures.
27. Place the call light within the patient's reach.
28. Report any changes in the patient to the nurse.
29. Follow facility policy for getting the specimen(s) and requisition to the laboratory. Document the procedure using facility guidelines.

Patients with small or fragile veins may have blood drawn using a syringe. A transfer device is used to move the blood from the barrel of the syringe to evacuated tubes. This type of draw may be done using a straight needle, but it is usually done with a butterfly set. A vein in the antecubital area or on the back of the hand may be used. Photos in the following procedure show a draw from the back of the hand.

Collecting a blood specimen using a syringe and transfer device

Equipment: gloves (additional PPE if required based on patient condition); tourniquet; warming pack (as needed for vein location); alcohol prep pad (or other antiseptic agent); winged needle set of the correct gauge; syringe; medical tape for securing needle (optional); specimen labels; 2"x2" gauze; adhesive or self-adhesive bandage; collection tubes for ordered tests; syringe transfer device; requisition; pen

1. Identify yourself by name. Identify the patient according to facility policy.
2. Explain the procedure to the patient. Speak clearly, slowly, and directly. Maintain face-to-face contact whenever possible.
3. Provide for the patient's privacy with a curtain, screen, or door.
4. If drawing blood from a patient in bed, adjust the bed to a safe level, usually waist high. Lock the bed wheels.
5. Put your equipment on a clean, flat surface (not the patient's bed).
6. Wash your hands. Put on gloves and other PPE. (In the case of some Transmission-Based Precautions, this will have been done outside the patient's room.)
7. Ask the patient to extend her hands, palms down, for a visual inspection. Choose a hand based on the appearance of the veins. (If drawing from the antecubital fossa, select a site as described in steps 7–9 of the previous procedure.) A warming pack can make the veins easier to find.
8. Apply the tourniquet 3–4 inches above the selected area. Ask the patient to make (but not pump) a fist.
9. With a gloved index finger, palpate the vein and choose the best site for puncture. If a good site is not found, remove the tourniquet. Apply it to the other side.
10. When a good site is found, release the tourniquet. Clean and dry the site as described in steps 10 and 11 of the previous procedure.
11. Assemble the needle and syringe (Fig. 22-30).

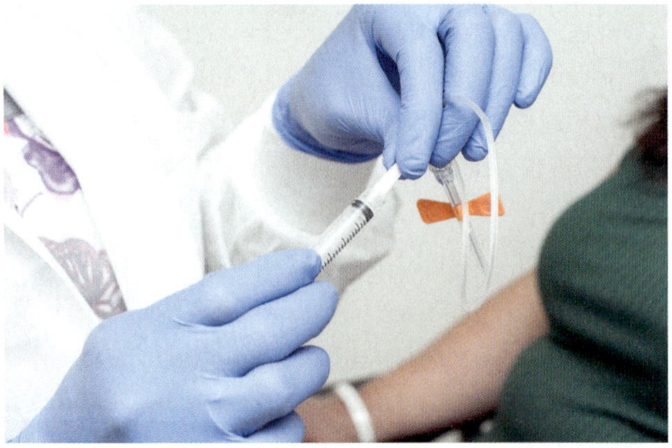

Fig. 22-30. *The tubing of a winged needle set is screwed onto the syringe.*

12. Prepare the syringe for use. Draw the plunger back to break the seal. Press it back in to push air out of the barrel (Fig. 22-31).

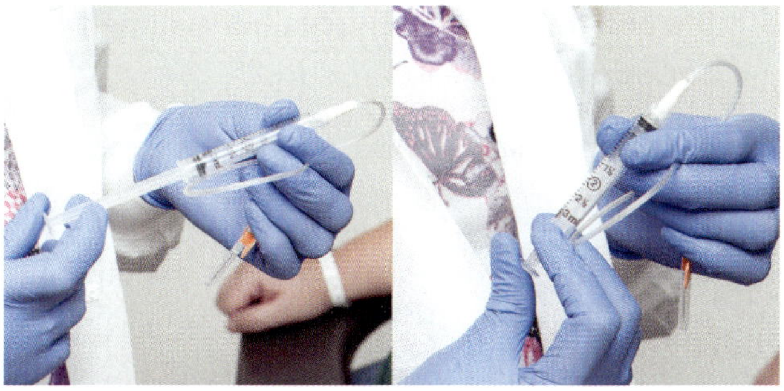

Fig. 22-31. *The plunger of the syringe is pulled out and pushed back in before it is used to draw blood.*

13. Reapply the tourniquet.
14. Anchor the vein. Grasp the patient's hand (or arm) with your nondominant hand. Use your thumb to apply pressure and pull the skin toward you, below the venipuncture site. Do not anchor from above the site. This is a needlestick risk.
15. Tell the patient that she may feel brief pain as the needle enters the skin. In a single, fluid motion, insert the needle into the skin to puncture the selected vein. The angle between the needle and skin should be as low as possible (Fig. 22-32).

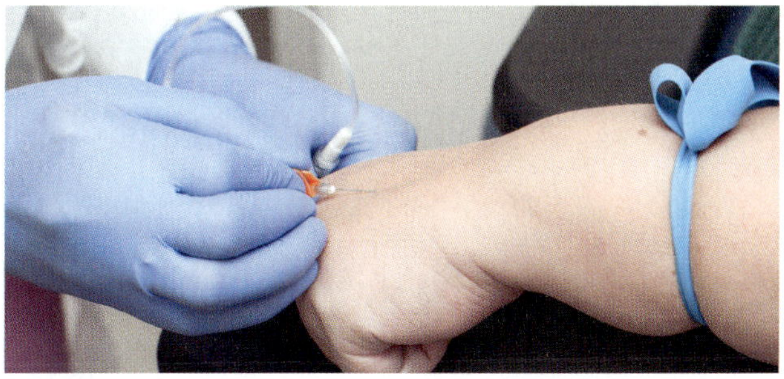

Fig. 22-32. *A low angle of insertion is safest and least painful.*

16. Secure the needle of a winged collection set throughout the draw. This is required by CLSI standards. Either hold the needle with one hand or tape the needle in place.
17. Pull back gently and steadily on the syringe plunger until the needed amount of blood is drawn (Fig. 22-33). Do not pull the plunger back forcefully. This can collapse the vein. It can also damage the specimen.

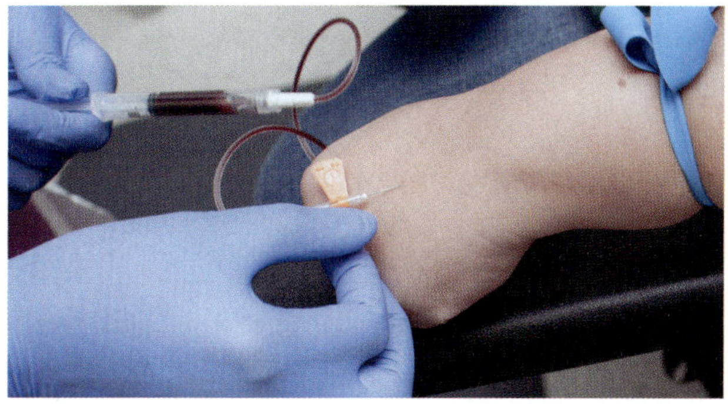

Fig. 22-33. *The needle can be secured with one hand and the plunger gently pulled back with the other.*

18. Place a piece of gauze, folded into quarters, over the needle.
19. Remove the needle from the patient's vein. Engage the safety device. Keep pressure on the gauze. The patient can help if she is able.
20. Remove the flexible tubing from the syringe. Discard the needle and tubing in a sharps container.
21. Immediately screw the syringe onto the syringe transfer device (Fig. 22-34).

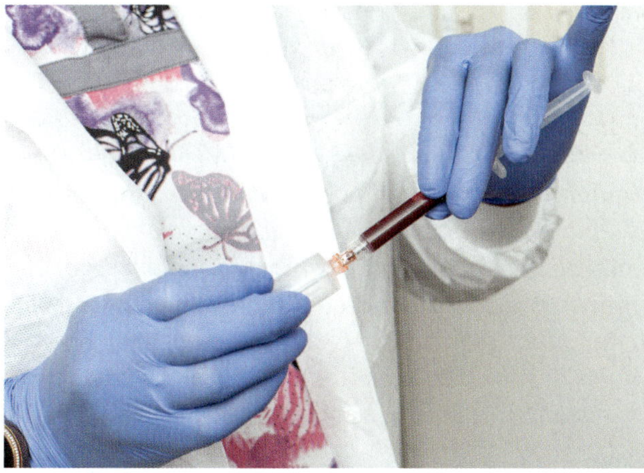

Fig. 22-34. *A syringe transfer device looks similar to an evacuated tube holder. It is designed to attach securely to a syringe.*

22. Insert the needed collection tube(s), following order of draw. Do not press on the syringe plunger as the blood transfers. The vacuum in the tube will draw blood in (Fig. 22-35).

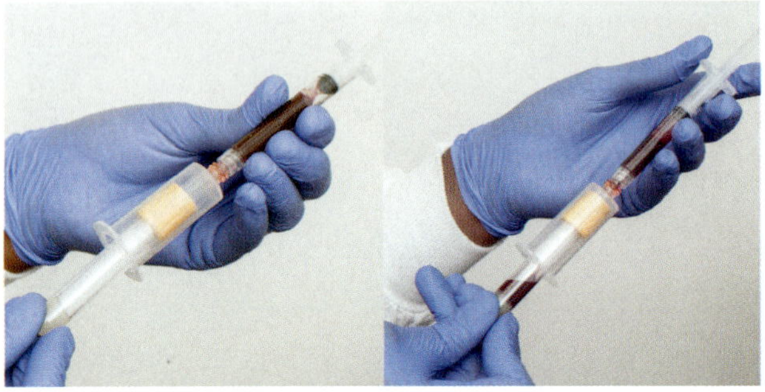

Fig. 22-35. *Tubes are inserted into syringe transfer devices just as in evacuated tube holders.*

23. Discard the syringe and transfer device in a sharps container.
24. Finish with steps 19–29 from the previous procedure.

When performing capillary puncture, after cleaning the puncture site and preparing the lancet, the PCT should have these items close by:

- Gauze
- Collection device
- Point-of-care testing machine if needed
- Bandage (for patients over 2 years old)

Performing routine capillary puncture

Equipment: gloves (additional PPE if required based on patient condition); warming pack; alcohol prep pad (or other antiseptic agent); proper lancet for the patient and specimen needed; collection device(s) required for ordered test(s); specimen labels; 2 pieces of 2"x2" gauze; adhesive bandage (for older children and adults); requisition; pen

1. Identify yourself by name. Identify the patient according to facility policy.
2. Explain the procedure to the patient. Speak clearly, slowly, and directly. Maintain face-to-face contact whenever possible.
3. Provide for the patient's privacy with a curtain, screen, or door.
4. If drawing blood from a patient in bed, adjust the bed to a safe level, usually waist high. Lock the bed wheels.
5. Put your equipment on a clean, flat surface (not the patient's bed).
6. Wash your hands. Put on gloves and other PPE as required. (In the case of some Transmission-Based Precautions this will have been done outside the patient's room.)
7. Ask the patient to extend her hands, palms up, for a visual inspection. (For infants under 6 months old and who weigh less than 10 kg [22 lbs.], the puncture site is the medial or lateral plantar surface of either heel.) Choose a site free of bruising, rashes, broken skin, swelling, and cyanosis.
8. Warm the site for up to 5 minutes using a commercial warming pack to improve blood flow, following facility policy. Asking the patient to wash her hands in warm water can also warm the finger.
9. Clean the selected puncture site thoroughly with the alcohol prep pad or other antiseptic (as ordered), creating gentle friction (Fig. 22-36). Allow the site to dry fully.

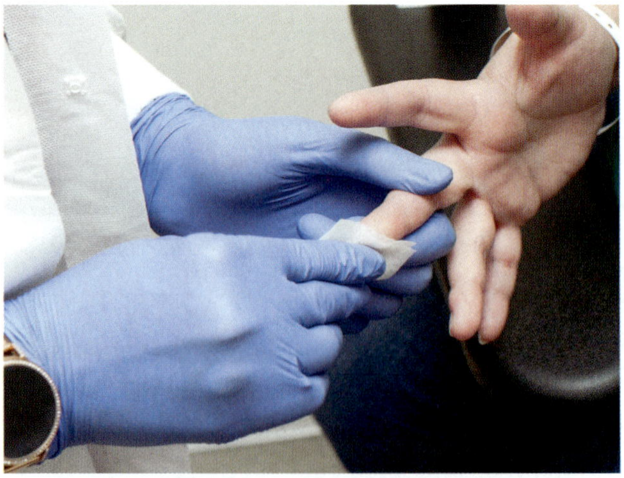

Fig. 22-36. *The puncture site should be cleaned carefully and allowed to dry completely.*

10. Prepare the lancet and collection devices for use. Remove the packaging or cap from the lancet (Fig. 22-37). Once the lancet is prepared, use it immediately or discard it. If the lancet is put down, it is contaminated.

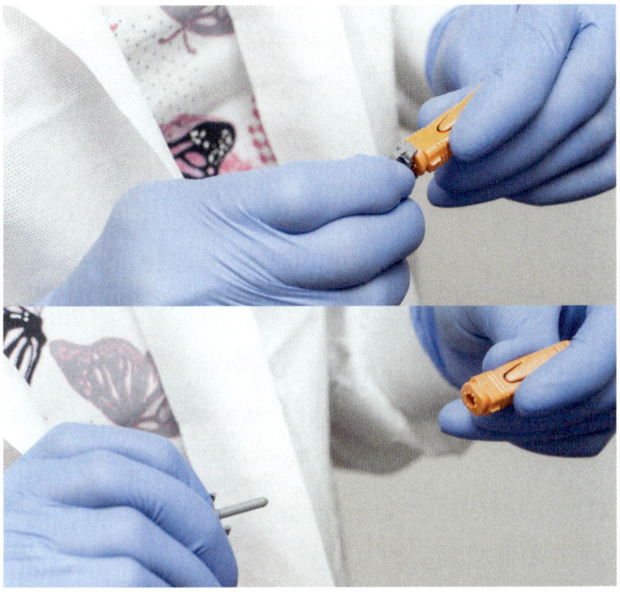

Fig. 22-37. *Different styles of lancets are operated differently. This lancet has a cap that is removed before use.*

11. Tell the patient that she may experience brief pain when the lancet is activated. Place the lancet on the patient's skin at the selected site and activate it to puncture the skin (Fig. 22-38).

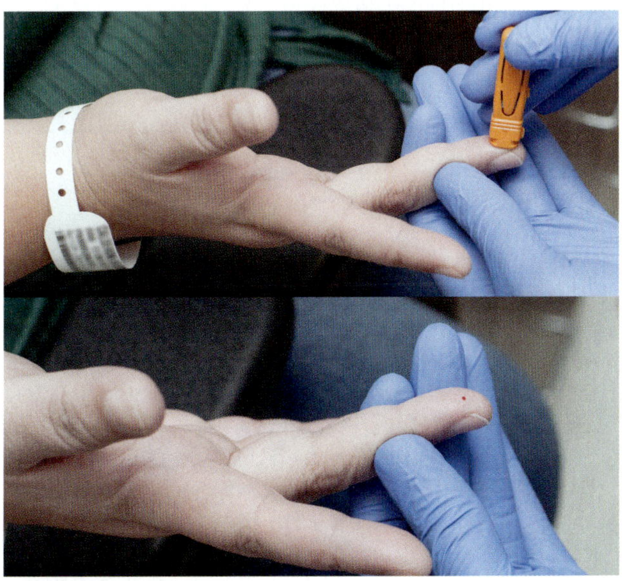

Fig. 22-38. *A lancet creates blood flow quickly and with the least possible pain.*

12. Discard the used lancet in a sharps container.

13. Use a gauze square to wipe away the first drop of blood (Fig. 22-39). (This step may not be needed for some tests.)

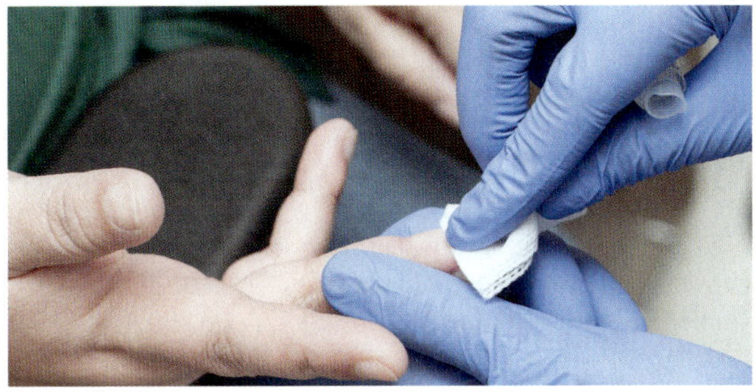

Fig. 22-39. *The first drop of capillary blood is usually wiped away before a specimen is collected.*

14. Collect the patient's blood in the required container(s). Apply gentle pressure. Do not squeeze hard or "milk" the finger or heel. Gently apply and then release pressure. Do not touch the spout or any part of the collection device to the patient's skin. Instead, allow the blood to drip into the tube and create a channel down the side of the tube (Fig. 22-40). Scraping the skin can cause hemolysis. It can also start platelet activation. This slows down the collection. It can damage the specimen. Gently tapping the collection tube as the blood enters helps mix the specimen.

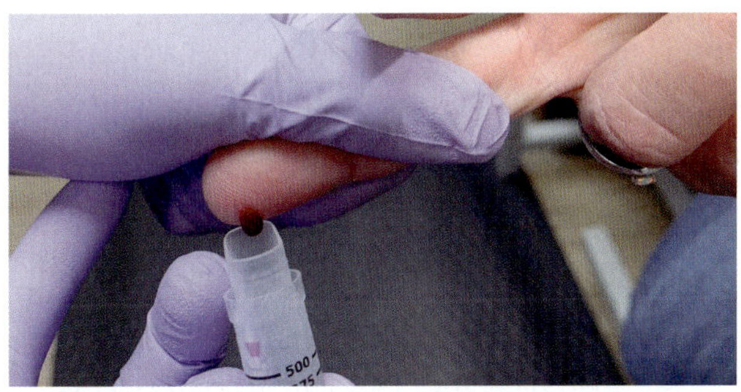

Fig. 22-40. *Allow blood to enter the collection container without scraping, scooping, or excessive squeezing.*

15. Continue to hold the patient's finger or heel and the collection device in place until the container is filled to the proper level (Fig. 22-41). After filling, cap/seal the specimens as instructed. Mix them promptly (as needed).

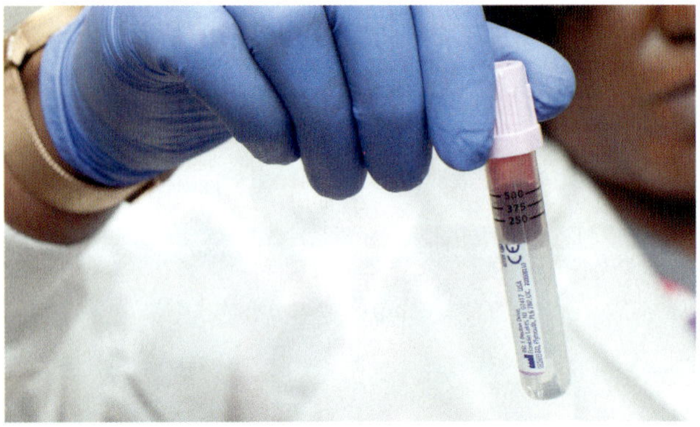

Fig. 22-41. *Fill containers to the proper level to make sure there is enough blood for testing. This also makes sure the balance of blood to additive is correct.*

16. After all needed containers are filled, place gauze over the puncture site. Apply pressure. The patient can hold pressure if she is able.
17. Label the tubes in front of the patient (Fig. 22-42). Initial each one. Document the time and date of collection according to facility policy. Ask the patient to check that the identifying information on the label is correct. Follow facility policy to prepare the specimens for transport. Properly discard any waste.

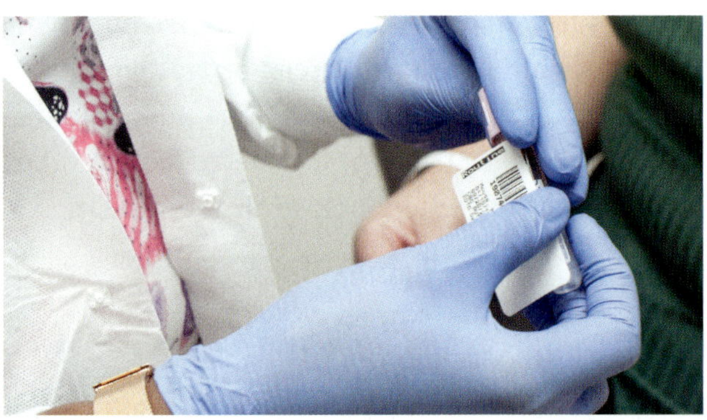

Fig. 22-42. *Always label specimens in front of the patient. Check that the identification details are correct.*

18. Check to make sure that the patient has stopped bleeding. This can take as long as 5 minutes for patients on anticoagulant medication.
19. Place a bandage over the puncture site if the patient is over 2 years old (Fig. 22-43). Advise the patient to leave the bandage in place for the next 15 minutes.

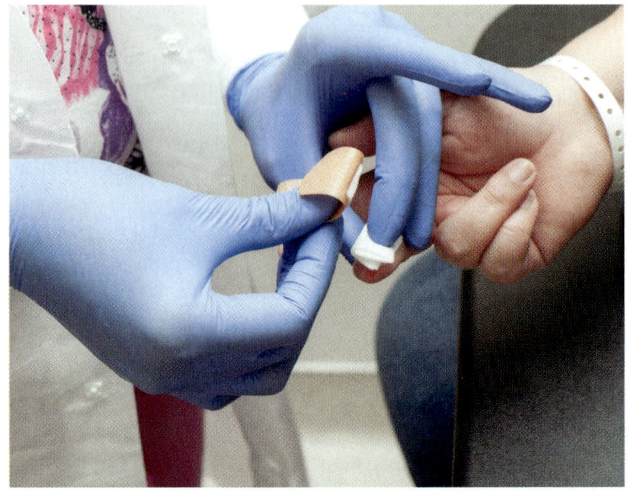

Fig. 22-43. *Apply a bandage after bleeding has stopped.*

20. Observe the patient for any signs of dizziness or discomfort. Do not leave the patient if she seems unsteady or says that she feels faint.
21. Remove and discard your gloves. Wash your hands.
22. Return the bed to its lowest position. Remove privacy measures.
23. Place the call light within the patient's reach.
24. Report any changes in the patient to the nurse.
25. Follow facility policy for getting the specimen(s) and requisition to the laboratory. Document the procedure using facility guidelines.

Responding to Fainting (Syncope)

It is not unusual for a patient to faint or feel faint during a blood draw. Patients who have fainted before may know that it is a risk. They can tell the PCT. This is why it is important to ask if a patient has had trouble with blood draws in the past. Fainting may also happen with little or no warning. If a patient says she is feeling faint before a blood draw, a cool washcloth can be placed on the forehead or neck. The patient can rest. Juice or a snack can be offered if the patient is not fasting. After the patient has rested, the blood draw should be done with the patient in a reclined or supine position. This position should also be used for patients who have a history of fainting.

The risk of an accidental needle stick goes up when a patient faints. If a patient faints, the PCT should first release the tourniquet and then remove the needle. The needle's safety mechanism must be activated and the needle discarded in a sharps container. If a patient faints when she is already reclined or lying down, there is less risk of harm. If the patient faints while sitting upright, the PCT's priority after removing and discarding the needle is to keep the patient safe from falling. Head injury can occur if the patient falls.

9. Describe special collections and procedures

Infant Metabolic Screening

Before leaving the hospital, newborn babies are tested for certain illnesses. If detected early, these illnesses can be treated. Tests vary by state. All states test for **phenylketonuria**, or **PKU**, a rare condition that can cause brain damage. Many other tests are performed at the same time. These conditions relate to the body's ability to make or process hormones and enzymes. Because of this the screening is called *metabolic screening*. It is often simply referred to as *PKU*. Capillary puncture is performed as a heel stick, but the test differs from other capillary collections in these ways:

- Blood is not collected in a capillary tube or microcollection device. Instead, it is dripped onto special filter paper. The paper is marked with circles for each blood drop required (Fig. 22-44).
- When collecting this specimen, the paper is not touched to the baby's foot. The blood is allowed to drip onto each circle.
- Each circle should be fully covered and soaked through. Blood should be visible on both the front and back of the paper.
- The blood should only be dripped onto the front side of the filter paper.

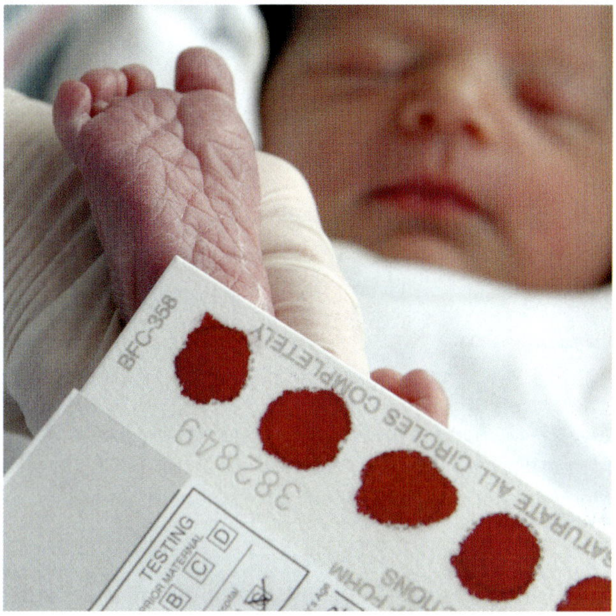

Fig. 22-44. *Newborn metabolic screening is conducted using blood collected on filter paper sheets.* (PHOTO COURTESY OF MARCH OF DIMES, MARCHOFDIMES.ORG, 571-257-2307)

- Only 1 drop should be placed in each circle.
- Filter paper collection forms vary. All information must be either preprinted or completed by the PCT before the form is sent for testing.

Blood Culture

A blood culture is ordered when a patient may have a bacterial or fungal infection in her blood. This can happen when a smaller, localized infection spreads to the blood. It is especially dangerous for people whose immune systems are compromised. When a blood culture is ordered, blood is introduced, or *inoculated*, into 2 bottles prepared with a liquid called a *broth*. The broth encourages the growth of any bacteria or fungi in the blood. One blood culture bottle is called the *aerobic bottle*. The other is the *anaerobic bottle* (Fig. 22-45). Each bottle encourages the growth of a different type of microorganism. Aerobic microorganisms require oxygen. Anaerobic microorganisms do not. The bottles are left to develop for a set time. They are then studied to see if infectious microorganisms have grown.

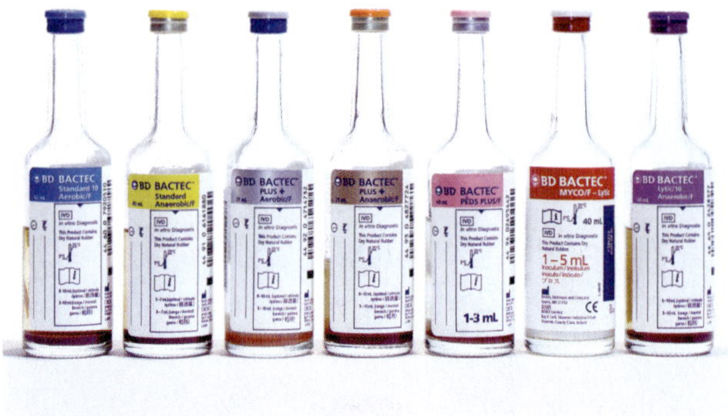

Fig. 22-45. Aerobic and anaerobic bottles are inoculated with a patient's blood. This photo shows several types of blood culture bottles from one manufacturer. (COURTESY AND ©BECTON, DICKINSON AND COMPANY)

The following changes are made when collecting venipuncture specimens for a blood culture:

- A winged collection set is used in most cases. The flexible tubing allows the blood culture bottle to be kept upright as it fills. This prevents the broth from entering the patient's blood. It also allows the PCT to see clearly when the bottle is completely filled.
- The site is cleaned more thoroughly. Cleaning with a 70% isopropyl alcohol prep pad is often followed (after drying) by cleaning with a chlorhexidine gluconate swab. The second cleaning is timed and usually lasts at least 30 seconds. This depends on the manufacturer's instructions. The second antiseptic must also be allowed to dry fully.
- Some blood culture bottles work with evacuated tube systems and can be inserted in a holder just like any tube. Other systems require that blood be collected using a syringe and transfer device. Blood cultures may also be collected in tubes containing the anticoagulant additive sodium polyethanol sulfonate (SPS), and later transferred to culture bottles. PCTs should collect blood for culturing according to facility policy. Each transfer increases the risk of specimen contamination.
- The rubber stoppers on blood culture bottles must be cleaned. A new alcohol prep pad is used for each bottle. The alcohol must be allowed to dry before collection. If blood is collected in an SPS tube, the tube stopper must be cleaned and dried before collection.
- In most cases, the aerobic bottle should be filled first. This avoids getting air from the winged set's tubing into the anaerobic bottle. Tubes or bottles must always be filled to the correct volume. Too much or too little blood can cause incorrect results.
- Sometimes blood cultures are ordered to be collected at 2 different venipuncture sites. If so, both aerobic and anaerobic bottles are filled from each site. This increases the chance of a correct diagnosis.
- If additional tests are ordered, blood culture specimens are always drawn first.

Blood Alcohol Testing

Ethanol, sometimes abbreviated *EtOH*, is the intoxicating ingredient in alcoholic beverages. When a person is suspected of driving drunk, or if for any other reason a provider needs to know how much alcohol is in a person's body, a blood test may be ordered.

In a hospital, blood alcohol testing is most likely to be done in the ED. In most ways blood collection for alcohol testing is like any routine collection. Possible exceptions include the following:

- In some states, having a driver's license is considered to be implied consent for blood alcohol testing. PCTs should follow facility policy and the direction of law enforcement in these situations.
- When drawing blood for alcohol testing, many facilities use an antiseptic agent other than isopropyl alcohol. This avoids any possible risk that the alcohol used for cleaning will cause inaccurate results.

- This test may be done as part of a legal action. Because of this, the specimen may require **chain of custody** documentation. This documentation notes the exact path a specimen takes from collection to analysis. It provides legal proof that the specimen has not been changed or tampered with.

Point-of-Care Testing

A point-of-care test (POCT) is one that is done where care is given rather than at a lab. In a hospital, this is usually the patient's bedside. Most POCTs are *CLIA waived*. This means the tests have little risk of error. CLIA rules allow them to be done by any trained healthcare worker. Point-of-care devices are used in doctor's offices, hospitals, long-term care facilities, and other healthcare settings (Fig. 22-46). Glucose and PT/INR testing are common types of POCTs. They usually require only a single drop of blood. They are very fast, with results usually available right away.

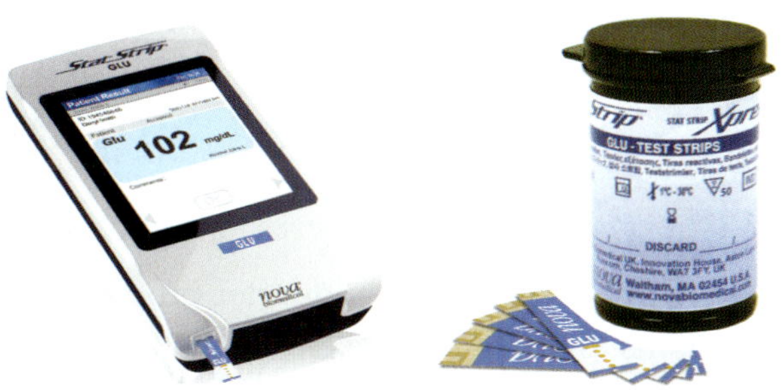

Fig. 22-46. *Point-of-care tests make routine testing quicker and simpler for patients and healthcare workers.* *(PHOTOS COURTESY OF NOVA BIOMEDICAL, NOVABIOMEDICAL.COM, 781-894-0800)*

The capillary puncture procedure in Learning Objective 8 is used during point-of-care testing. However, the process of collecting the specimen may be different. In most cases, a test strip is placed into a testing machine. A single drop of blood is allowed to drip directly from the puncture site onto the strip. Manufacturer instructions should say whether the first drop of blood can be used. In most capillary collections it is wiped away. For some point-of-care tests blood is collected in a small container and then inserted into the machine.

Guidelines: Point-of-Care Blood Tests

- **G** Follow all facility procedures for patient identification and infection prevention.
- **G** Do not use a testing device you are not trained to use. If you are asked to use a new machine, ask for training.
- **G** Follow manufacturer instructions. You may need to do a quality control procedure before testing. Quality control procedures check that the machine is working correctly. They are usually done daily. Follow facility policy to document results.
- **G** Check expiration dates on test strips and any other supplies. Make sure that the strips have been stored properly. Out-of-date or damaged test strips can cause errors in results.
- **G** Only touch test strips with clean gloves. Change gloves if a test is repeated or if a second strip is needed. Do not touch fresh strips with dirty gloves.
- **G** Make sure that requirements about diet or medication have been met.
- **G** Document any changes in medication or diet (e.g., if a patient being tested for PT/INR has missed a dose of warfarin).
- **G** Follow facility procedures for communicating and documenting test results.
- **G** Do not discuss results with patients. Point-of-care testing gives results right away, but the nurse or provider must discuss the results with the patient.
- **G** Many point-of-care tests have critical values. These are results that require immediate attention. Point-of-care tests are usually repeated if results are in critical ranges. This confirms that the first result was not an

error. Know critical values for any tests you perform. Report critical value results to the nurse, even if a second test is within normal range. Report both test results.

G Discard test strips or containers properly. These items are considered biohazardous waste.

G Follow facility procedures for cleaning testing devices. The machines must be cleaned thoroughly after every use.

Discontinuing a Peripheral IV

In some states PCTs are allowed to discontinue (remove) a peripheral IV. A small number of states allow PCTs to insert a peripheral IV line. Peripheral IVs are often inserted in the same veins used for venipuncture. They are started using a catheter device that is inserted with the use of a needle (Fig. 22-47). The needle is used to access the patient's vein. The catheter, which is like a sheath around the needle, is pushed down and threaded into the patient's vein. The needle is then removed. This is beyond scope of practice for most PCTs. (For states where this is allowed, there is a handout provided in the instructor's guide for this textbook.)

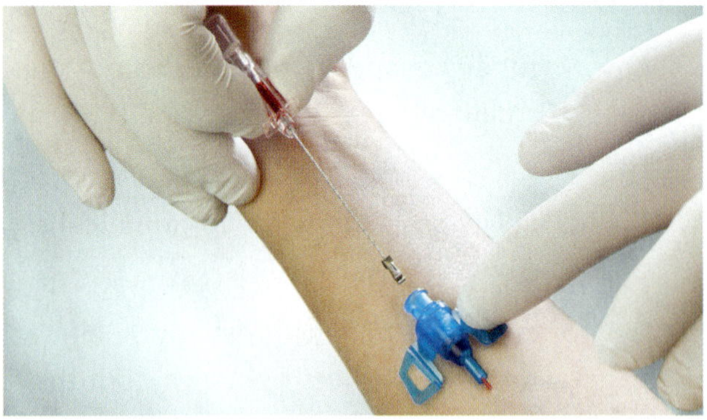

Fig. 22-47. *A peripheral IV is started using an over-the-needle IV catheter.* (PHOTO COURTESY OF B. BRAUN MEDICAL INC.)

If assigned and allowed to remove a peripheral IV, a PCT should confirm the order with the nurse. The procedure must be explained to the patient and the nurse must stop the IV pump. After washing hands and donning gloves, the PCT should gently remove and discard dressings while holding the catheter still. This will reduce discomfort for the patient. It can also prevent a hematoma from forming.

Holding a piece of gauze over the catheter, the PCT should slowly and steadily remove it by pulling it straight back and out of the patient's vein. As soon as the catheter is removed, pressure should be held on the site for 2–3 minutes. Longer hold times may be needed if a patient is taking an anticoagulant. When bleeding has stopped, a bandage is placed on the site (unless the patient is a toddler or infant).

Before discarding an IV catheter in a biohazard container, it is very important for the PCT to check that it is intact. This means it should be checked to be sure no part of the catheter is missing. If part of a catheter breaks off inside a patient's vein, it can cause serious problems such as an embolism. If the catheter is not intact, this should be reported immediately to the nurse. Removal of a peripheral IV must always be documented, following facility policy.

10. Identify guidelines for transporting specimens

Either right after collection or after processing, specimens are taken to the lab for testing. Specimens must be transported in biohazard containers that are clearly marked. Here are some common forms of specimen transport:

- The PCT personally delivers specimens (processed or not) to the lab where testing is done. This may happen in a large outpatient office that has its own lab.
- Specimens are placed in a box or other container. They are collected by a courier or by a lab employee. Even facilities with a lab may send some specimens out for special testing.
- Specimens are sent through an automated system from the area where they are drawn to

the testing area. One example is a pneumatic tube system similar to those used in drive-through banking. This is most common in hospitals. PCTs must follow facility policy on pneumatic tube systems carefully. If they are not used correctly, these systems can damage specimens and/or create an infection risk.

Some analytes are sensitive to temperature and/or light. They must be handled with special care. Bilirubin is an example of a light-sensitive analyte. Amber collection tubes may be used when an analyte is light-sensitive. Tubes may also be wrapped in aluminum foil. Special containers may be used to transport these specimens, but any container that blocks light may be used.

Most analytes are stable at room temperature. Some specimens, however, must be kept cold or warm. Equipment for keeping specimens cold or warm includes

- Heating blocks, which hold tubes upright and at a set temperature
- Cooling or warming packs to wrap around specimens
- Refrigerators/freezers

The following guidelines are important to managing specimen temperature:

Guidelines: Temperature-Sensitive Specimens

G For specimens that must be kept at body temperature (98.6°F/37°C), collect the specimen in a prewarmed tube. Then place it in a heating block (Fig. 22-48).

G Make sure specimens stay at the correct temperature until they are delivered for testing. Follow facility procedures. Some facilities use color-coded transport bags showing the required temperature.

G When a specimen must be kept cold, do not pack it with cubed ice. This causes uneven cooling. Store and transport it in an ice slurry. An ice slurry is a mixture of crushed ice and water. Cold packs may also be used.

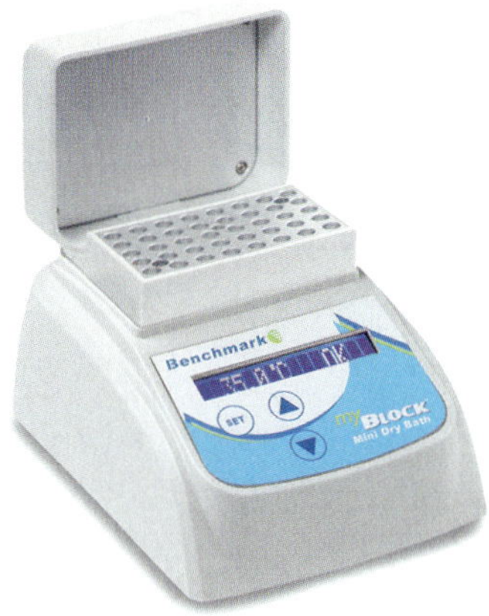

Fig. 22-48. *Heating blocks can be set to keep specimens at an exact temperature.* (PHOTO COURTESY OF BENCHMARK SCIENTIFIC, WWW.BENCHMARKSCIENTIFIC.COM)

After preparing specimens for transport, the PCT can remove and discard PPE and wash his hands. Surfaces where specimens were handled must also be disinfected. PCTs should follow facility policy for cleaning equipment such as heating blocks.

Temperature- and Light-Sensitive Specimens

PCTs should remember these common analytes that must be protected from light or kept at a specific temperature. This list is not complete. PCTs should always check requisitions for any special instructions.

Protect from light

- Bilirubin
- Many vitamins
- Carotene
- Folate

Keep cold (ice slurry)

- Ammonia
- Gastrin
- Lactate/lactic acid
- pH

Keep at body temperature (98.6°F/37°C)

- Cold agglutinins
- Cryoglobulin
- Cryofibrinogen

Chapter Review

1. What is the most common way to collect blood in adults and children over the age of 1?
2. What are 2 common types of point-of-care tests requiring capillary puncture?
3. What is it called when an error is made before a specimen is tested? Give 2 examples of this type of error.
4. What are 2 styles of needles used for venipuncture collection?
5. What is the most common needle gauge for venipuncture collection on an adult patient?
6. Describe how blood specimens are mixed with additives after filling a tube. What is this action called?
7. What organization sets standards for blood draws in medical facilities throughout the world?
8. Why is it important to follow the order of draw when collecting specimens by venipuncture and for capillary collection?
9. Which vein is considered the best choice for a blood draw by venipuncture? Where is it located?
10. How should a healthy vein feel when it is palpated?
11. What serious complication can happen if a lancet hits an infant's heel bone during a heel stick? How can this be avoided?
12. What is the most common antiseptic used to clean the skin before a routine blood draw?
13. In what direction can a PCT move the needle if blood flow does not start after the patient's skin is punctured?
14. How many unsuccessful venipuncture attempts is a PCT allowed to make on a patient before he must alert the nurse?
15. Where should the lancet be placed in relation to fingerprint lines when performing capillary puncture? Why?
16. What is the maximum amount of time the tourniquet should be left on a patient's arm? Why should it be released after this amount of time has passed?
17. Describe how to anchor the vein before inserting the needle for a blood draw.
18. How long should the PCT (or patient) hold pressure on the gauze over the puncture site after a blood draw?
19. What is a syringe transfer device? When might blood be collected using a syringe and a syringe transfer device?
20. What is the best position for blood specimen collection for a patient who has a history of fainting during blood draws?
21. What special collection procedure requires cleaning the skin more thoroughly, sometimes with more than one cleaning agent?
22. What should the PCT do if he receives a critical value result on a point-of-care test?
23. What important step must a PCT perform before discarding an IV catheter that he has removed from a patient's vein?
24. What may be used to protect light-sensitive specimens?
25. When a specimen must be kept cold, why is an ice slurry better than cubed ice?

23 Electrocardiograms (EKGs) and Related Tests

1. Describe the electrical activity of the heart and how it is recorded by EKG machines

An EKG shows the electrical activity of the heart. The heart's electrical activity causes the muscle contractions that pump blood. This activity occurs in patterns. These patterns are shown on the EKG. *Cardiac conduction* is the movement of electrical signals in the heart. It was first described in Chapter 15. Normal cardiac conduction starts in the upper part of the heart. It moves on a set path through the heart. Conduction is continuous. Changes in its pattern may be a sign of a heart problem.

Cardiac cells can change their electrical charge. The charge changes from negative to positive and back to negative again. These changes are what is shown on an EKG. *Depolarization* is a change in electrical charge from negative to positive. Each heartbeat begins with one small area of the heart muscle depolarizing. The depolarization then quickly spreads to the next cell and throughout the heart. This causes the heart muscle to contract and pump blood.

Repolarization is a change in electrical charge from positive back to negative. This causes the heart muscle to relax. Each cardiac cycle has a depolarization phase and a repolarization phase. This cycle causes the atria and the ventricles to contract and relax at opposite times. As this happens, the chambers fill and then pump blood.

The **sinoatrial node**, also called the *SA node* or *sinus node*, is in the upper part of the right atrium. It is the main, or primary, pacemaker of the heart. This means it sets the timing of the heart's contractions.

From the SA node, the electrical impulse moves to the atrioventricular node, also called the *AV node*. The AV node is at the bottom of the right atrium. As the impulse enters the AV node it is slowed down by a fraction of a second. Without this delay the atria and ventricles would contract at the same time. Instead, the atria can empty and the ventricles can fill before they contract.

The electrical impulse then moves through an area called the *atrioventricular (AV) junction* to the *bundle of His*, or *AV bundle*. The bundle of His is located in the upper part of the wall between the left and right ventricles.

The bundle of His divides into the right and left bundle branches. These branches carry the electrical impulse to the walls of the ventricles. The bundle branches divide into smaller and smaller branches and then form the Purkinje fibers (Fig. 23-1).

EKG machines are connected to patients using **electrodes**. These are pads that conduct electricity. Electrodes are attached to lead wires (also sometimes called *EKG cables* or *electrode cables*). The lead wires transmit the heart's electrical signals to the EKG machine. The EKG machine can measure the electrical activity of the heart in several ways. It takes information from different electrodes to create different "views" of the heart. These different views are called **leads**. Each lead gives different information about the heart.

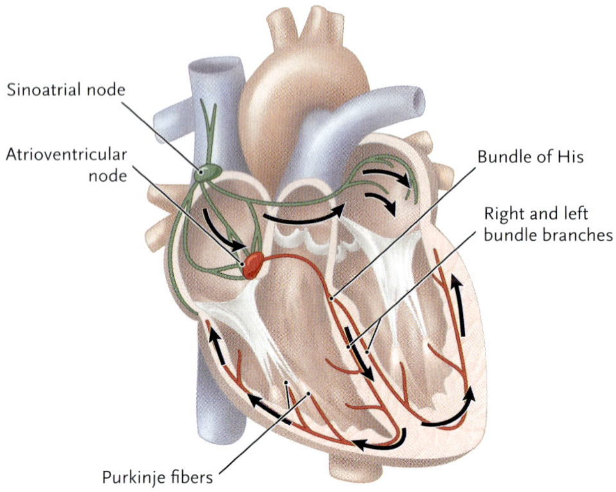

Fig. 23-1. *When the heart is healthy, electrical impulses move in this way. This causes the heart muscles to contract in a regular rhythm and pump blood.*

Electrodes Are Not Leads

Many people, even healthcare workers, use the word *leads* to refer to the electrodes used in EKG tests. This can be confusing because in cardiology, the word *leads* has a specific meaning. Leads are measurements of the heart's electrical activity. Each EKG lead provides information about a different part of the heart. More than 1 electrode is used to create each measurement. In this book, the word *lead* is only used to describe these views of the heart. The word *electrode* is always used to describe the pads applied to the patient's skin.

The muscle contractions of the heart are the heart's *mechanical activity*. EKGs do not give direct information about the heart's mechanical activity. They only record the heart's electrical activity. They give information about the location, rate, and rhythm of that activity. The heart's electrical activity prompts, or causes, the heart's contractions. Because of this relationship, EKGs provide important information about heart health. In most cases, if the heart's electrical activity is normal, its mechanical activity is also normal. When EKGs are not normal, more testing may be needed. If the provider needs direct information about the mechanical activity of the heart, other types of diagnostic tests may be ordered. Echocardiograms, CT (computerized tomography) scans, and MRIs (magnetic resonance imaging) are tests that show the mechanical activity of the heart.

2. Understand EKG waves and identify normal features in an EKG

An EKG machine records the changes in electrical charge created by depolarization and repolarization. Graph paper moves through the machine at a controlled speed, creating the EKG tracing (Fig. 23-2). Trained healthcare professionals read, or interpret, these tracings (sometimes called *EKG strips*).

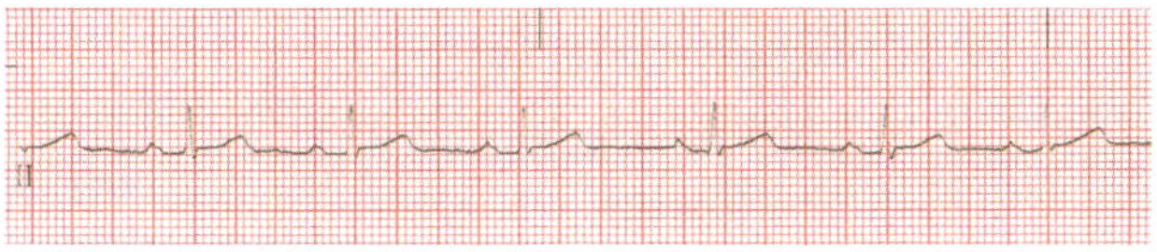

Fig. 23-2. *This is an example of a clear, accurate, EKG tracing.*

Reading an EKG tracing is beyond the scope of practice for a PCT. The PCT's job is to get a good tracing. To do this, PCTs need to know what a tracing should look like and what each part of the tracing shows.

Basic EKG features are shown in Figure 23-3. The *isoelectric line,* also called the *baseline,* is the straight line between the upward and downward movements. Those upward and downward movements are called *waves.* A deflection, or movement, upward from the baseline is a positive wave. A deflection downward is a negative wave. The area between 2 waves, where the EKG goes back to the baseline, is called a *segment.* A wave and a segment taken together form an *interval.* Several waves together are called a *complex.*

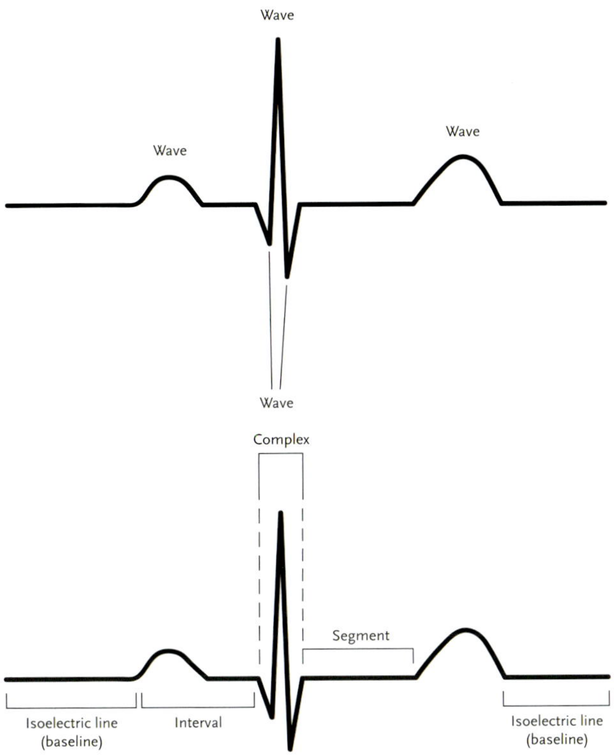

Fig. 23-3. *The isoelectric line, waves, segments, intervals, and complexes are the key features of the EKG.*

When the heart is functioning normally, the EKG shows a pattern called **normal sinus rhythm** (**NSR**). Normal sinus rhythm on an EKG can look different from person to person. It also looks different in different leads on the same person. However, it will show some version of the features described in this learning objective.

The basic features of a normal EKG complex in lead II—the view used for routine monitoring—are shown in Figure 23-4. Each part of the tracing is given a letter name that is used to label and describe waves, intervals, and complexes in EKG analysis. These letters do not stand for words or have meaning. They are just labels to refer to the features of the EKG.

When the heart is working properly, there is a correlation between the electrical and mechanical actions of the heart. In other words, each electrical change matches up with a mechanical action (as shown in the following orange box).

The P wave is the first positive deflection, or upward movement, in the complex. It represents atrial depolarization. The mechanical activity related to the P wave is the contraction of the atria.

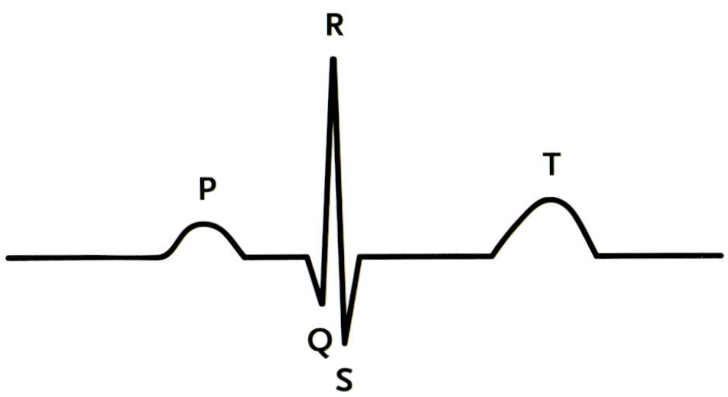

Fig. 23-4. *This image shows a normal sinus rhythm EKG. Each wave is named by a letter. P, Q, R, S, and T waves are the waves seen most often.*

The QRS complex is made up of 3 waves:

- The Q wave is the first negative deflection, or downward movement, after the P wave (though it is not always seen in all leads).
- The R wave is the next positive deflection.
- The S wave is the next negative deflection.

The QRS complex represents ventricular depolarization. The related mechanical action is the contraction of the ventricles. The T wave comes after the QRS complex. It shows ventricular repolarization. When this happens, the ventricles relax.

EKG Features

EKG feature	Electrical activity	Mechanical activity
P wave	Atrial depolarization	Contraction of the atria
QRS complex	Ventricular depolarization	Contraction of the ventricles
T wave	Ventricular repolarization	Relaxation of the ventricles

The way different waves and complexes look on an EKG can give providers important information. For example, the P wave has to do with the contraction of the atria. Changes in the P wave may be caused by a problem like atrial enlargement. Abnormal QRS complexes may show a problem with the ventricles.

When PCTs know the normal appearance of these features, they can see when something is not right. The provider should be notified.

3. Describe the types of EKG-based tests and how each is used

PCTs may perform several types of EKG tests. Different tests use different numbers and types of electrodes and leads. A provider orders a specific type of EKG based on the information she needs. If the patient's EKG must be monitored for an extended time, either 3 or 5 leads will be used. This type of monitoring is often done in emergency departments. It allows the provider to continuously check the patient's rate and rhythm (Fig. 23-5).

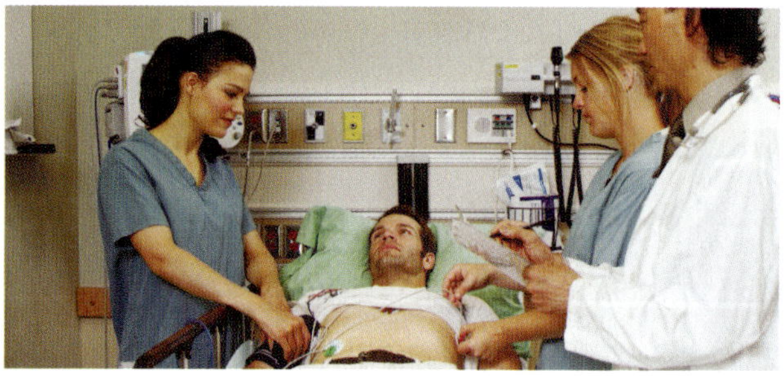

Fig. 23-5. *EKG technology allows for constant monitoring of a patient's heart.*

Telemetry monitoring is used in large facilities. It monitors a patient's EKG on an ongoing basis (Fig. 23-6). The patient wears a small device with 5 lead wires. The device transmits information to a central monitoring station. Trained healthcare workers view the patient's cardiac activity. They alert a nurse or provider if the patient's heart rate or rhythm changes.

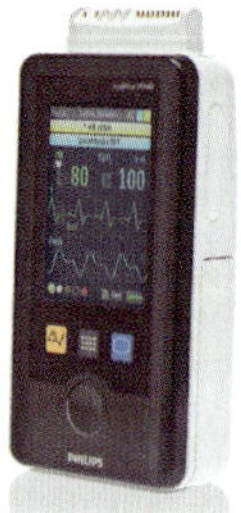

Fig. 23-6. *This telemetry pack stays with the patient. It allows the patient to be monitored remotely.* (COURTESY OF ROYAL PHILIPS.)

Ambulatory monitoring is used when a patient is not hospitalized and a provider needs information about the heart over a longer period of time. An ambulatory monitor stays with the patient. Holter monitors are a common type of ambulatory monitor. These monitors are usually placed on the patient in a medical office and removed after 24–48 hours (Fig. 23-7). The information stored in the machine is then evaluated by the provider.

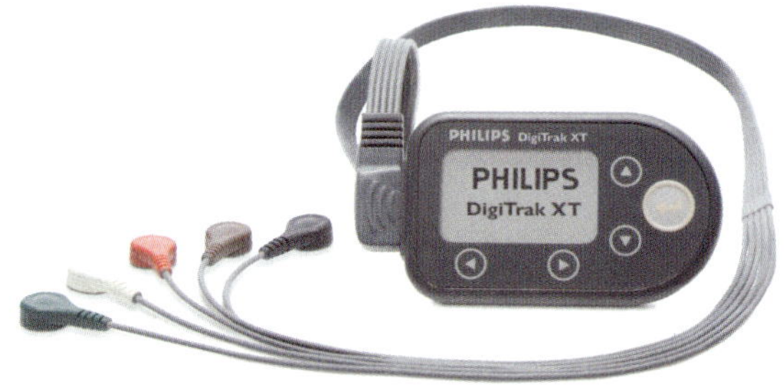

Fig. 23-7. *A Holter monitor allows the patient to continue everyday life while being monitored.* (COURTESY OF ROYAL PHILIPS.)

Event monitors are another type of ambulatory monitor. They only record the heart's electrical activity when the patient presses a button. Pressing the button indicates that he is having symptoms. Sometimes these monitors are returned to the provider's office for evaluation. Sometimes the information is sent in by telephone or through an internet connection. Mobile cardiac telemetry is another type of ambulatory monitoring. It automatically alerts a healthcare professional if an irregular heart rate or rhythm is detected.

The most common EKG test is the **12-lead EKG**. It is often the first test done when a patient has chest pain or other symptoms of heart problems. It only takes a few minutes to complete a 12-lead EKG. The 12-lead EKG is also used during stress tests. These tests check how the heart responds to physical activity on a treadmill or stationary bicycle (Fig. 23-8). If the patient cannot exercise for a stress test, the stress can be created by giving the patient medications that speed up the heart.

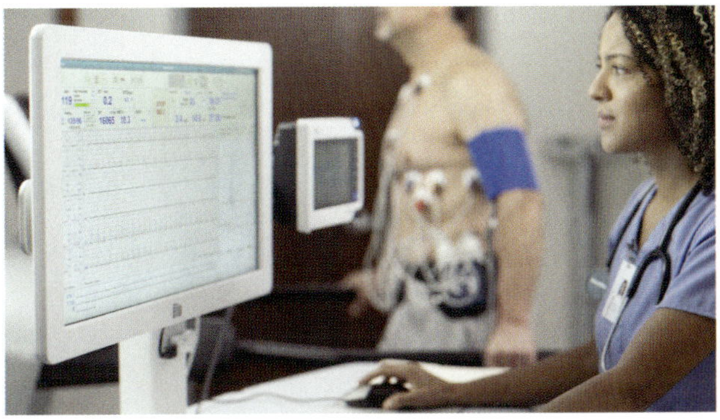

Fig. 23-8. An exercise stress test uses a treadmill or a stationary bicycle to increase a patient's heart rate. Blood pressure and a 12-lead EKG are monitored during the test.

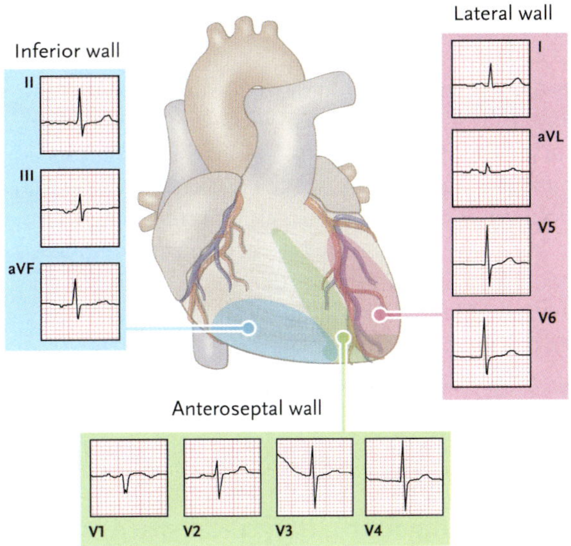

Fig. 23-9. Different leads provide information about the electrical activity in different areas of the heart.

4. Describe EKG leads and electrode placement

All of the leads used in EKG tests have names and are arranged into groups. The groups also have names. Leads I, II, and III are called the **limb leads**. They are created by measuring electrical activity between electrodes placed on or near a patient's limbs. The first, most basic EKG recordings were from the limb leads. These leads are also called *bipolar leads*. This refers to the way the electrical activity is measured for these leads.

Leads aVR, aVL, and aVF are called the **augmented limb leads**. They use the same electrodes as leads I, II, and III but are *unipolar leads*. They measure electrical activity differently than the bipolar leads.

Leads V1, V2, V3, V4, V5, and V6 are known together as the **precordial leads**, or *chest leads*. The electrodes that measure these leads are placed in a line across the chest. These leads are also unipolar.

Each lead on the EKG gives information about a specific area of the heart (Fig. 23-9). Each one has a specific appearance on the tracing. By looking at different leads, a provider can get information about the health of all areas of the heart. Lead II is the lead most commonly used for general monitoring.

To record EKG leads the PCT needs to know where to place electrodes on the patient. Incorrect electrode placement creates errors in EKG tracings. Most EKG tests use either 3, 5, or 12 leads with 3, 5, or 10 electrodes. Some leads in a 12-lead EKG share the same electrodes, so only 10 electrodes are needed.

The electrodes used for 3-lead testing are called the *right arm*, *left arm*, and *left leg* electrodes, but these electrodes are placed on the torso (Fig. 23-10). This allows the patient to move more freely. It can give a more accurate reading. The right arm electrode (RA) is placed on the right upper torso, the left arm electrode (LA) on the left upper torso, and the left leg electrode (LL) on the left lower torso.

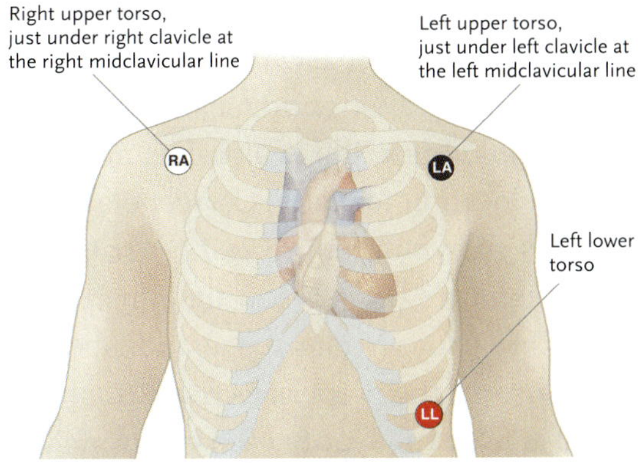

Fig. 23-10. In 3-lead applications there are right arm, left arm, and left leg electrodes.

Limb Lead Reversal

One of the most common mistakes in electrocardiography is the reversal of limb leads. This error causes the EKG tracing to be incorrect. It could make the tracing look like the patient has a heart problem and could lead to an incorrect diagnosis. PCTs should *always* double-check electrode placement. The right arm electrode must be on the patient's right side. The left arm electrode must be on the patient's left side.

In 5-lead testing, the right arm, left arm, and left leg electrodes are placed as in 3-lead testing. The V1 electrode is placed to the right of the sternum at the fourth intercostal space. An *intercostal space* is a space between ribs. The fourth intercostal space is just below the fourth rib. The right leg electrode (RL) is placed on the right lower torso (Fig. 23-11). This electrode is also sometimes known as the *ground electrode.*

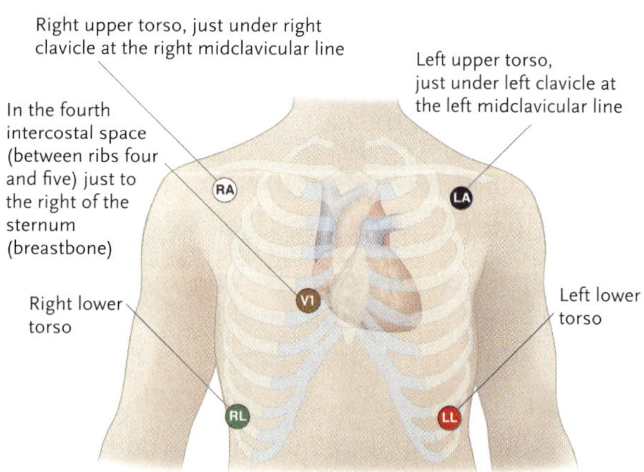

***Fig. 23-11.** In 5-lead applications, the same electrodes are used as in 3-lead applications, plus the right leg (ground) electrode and V1 electrode.*

The 12-lead EKG uses 10 electrodes. They are placed in 4 limb locations and 6 chest locations. The PCT should know the anatomical name and the physical location for each. Correct electrode placement is shown in Figure 23-12. Anatomical descriptions are listed below the illustration. Lead wires are usually color-coded and labeled with the name of the proper electrode. A standard color is used to identify each electrode location, as shown in the illustration.

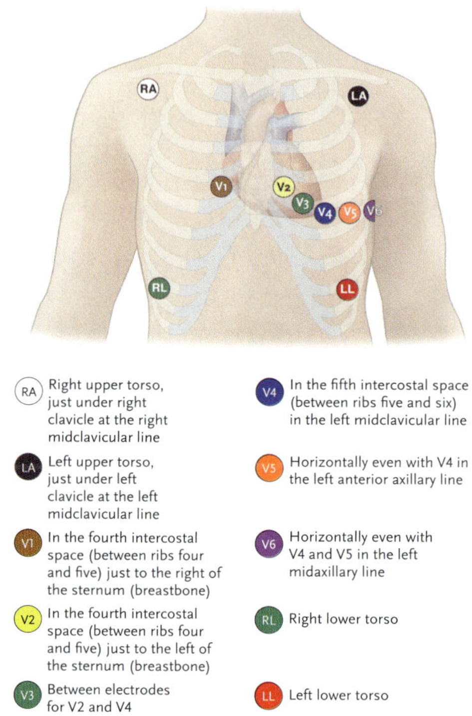

***Fig. 23-12.** A 12-lead EKG uses 10 electrodes. Some leads share the same electrodes.*

In 3-lead and 5-lead EKG applications the limb electrodes are placed on the torso. This leaves the patient free to move more normally. This is important because 3- and 5-lead applications are often used over several hours or even days. A resting 12-lead EKG only takes a few minutes to complete. During this test the limb electrodes may be placed on the limbs or on the torso. These variations are shown in Figure 23-13. For stress testing these electrodes are placed on the torso to allow free limb movement.

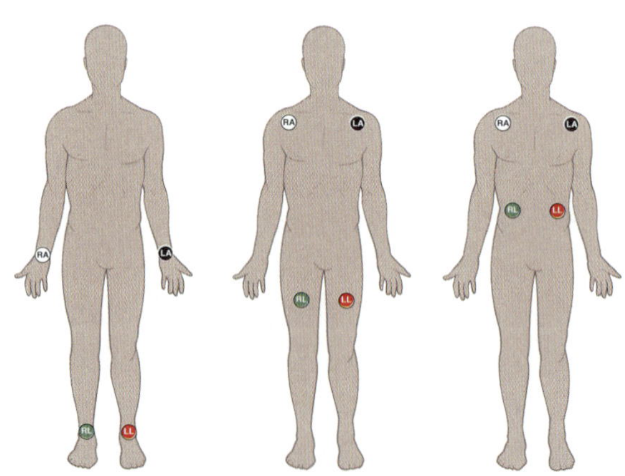

***Fig. 23-13.** The arm and leg electrodes can be placed either on the torso or on the limbs themselves.*

Adaptations, or adjustments to the EKG procedure, may be needed for some patients. For most resting EKGs, the patient is in the supine position with standard electrode placement. Electrode placement may be different for some pediatric patients. Positioning and electrode placement are changed for certain conditions as well. Any time electrodes are placed in alternate locations, the PCT must document the changes. Changes should also be written directly on the EKG tracing. The provider needs to know about adaptations because they can change how the EKG looks.

PCTs may need to change electrode placement in these situations:

Dextrocardia: *Dextrocardia* is a rare heart condition. It causes the heart to point to the right side of the chest rather than the left side. The chest electrodes must be placed over the heart on the right side of the chest (Fig. 23-14). Otherwise the EKG will not be accurate. The patient usually knows about this condition or it is noted in the patient's record.

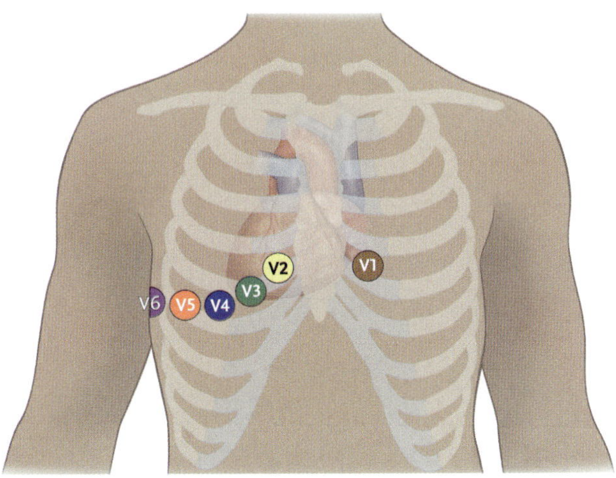

***Fig. 23-14.** Right-sided placement of the chest electrodes is a mirror image of left-sided placement.*

Limb amputation/injury: Limb electrode placement must be changed for patients with limb amputations. The electrodes may be placed on the torso, as close as possible to the amputated limb. They may also be placed on the limb itself but closer to the torso (Fig. 23-15). The electrodes should not be placed over scar tissue. The electrode for the unaffected limb should be placed in a mirror image position. The PCT should also use this adaptation for a patient who has a limb with open wounds, a cast, or a thick bandage. All other electrodes are placed in the standard locations.

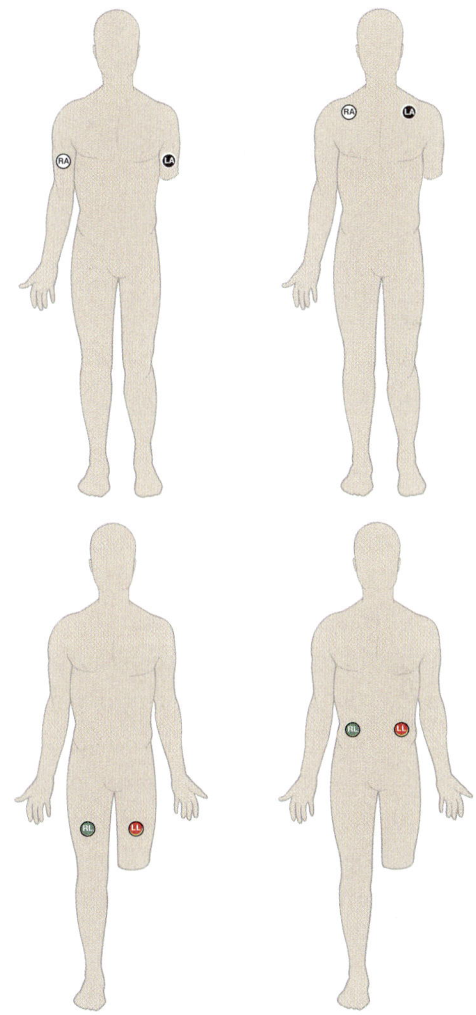

***Fig. 23-15.** For a patient with an amputation, the electrodes may be moved closer to the torso or may be placed on the torso rather than on the limbs. The unaffected side should mirror the affected side.*

Scar tissue or injury on the chest wall: The PCT should not place electrodes on scar tissue from a mastectomy or other chest wall surgery. Scar tissue can be fragile and may be injured when the electrode is removed. Instead, electrodes should be placed as close as possible to the standard locations (Fig. 23-16).

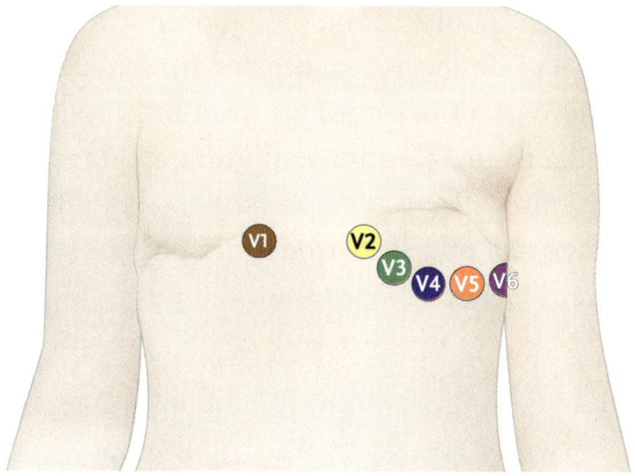

Fig. 23-16. Electrodes can be placed around mastectomy scars and other scar tissue from chest surgery.

Medical implants: Electrodes should not be placed over implanted medical equipment like a pacemaker, or over breast implants. Instead, the PCT should place the electrodes to the side of the implant. They should be as close as possible to the standard positions.

Large breasts: If a patient has large breasts the breast tissue should be moved away from the electrode site as much as possible. This allows placement of the electrodes on the chest wall. The PCT should explain the process to the patient. The patient can lift her own breast tissue or the PCT can move the breast using the back of her hand. The PCT should get the patient's consent before doing this. Electrodes should be placed as close to standard positions as possible. They should not be placed on top of breast tissue.

Pediatric patients: The heart takes up more room in the chest of an infant or small child than in an adult. The right ventricle extends past the right side of the sternum. Because of this, electrodes may be placed differently. In most cases, these changes are made in children 5 years old and younger. The most common change is to place the V4 electrode on the right side of the chest. This placement is called V4R. It is a mirror image of V4: at the fifth intercostal space on the right midclavicular line (Fig. 23-17). The PCT should label the EKG tracing to note this change.

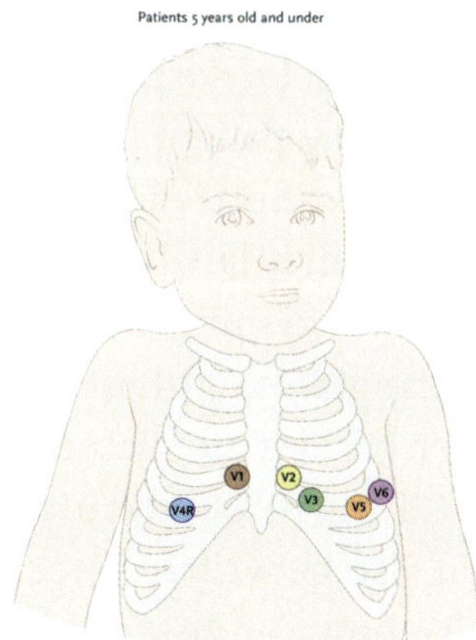

Fig. 23-17. Pediatric patients may have electrodes applied differently than adult patients.

Some facilities may make other adjustments for pediatric EKGs. Extra electrodes may be placed on the chest and/or on the back. The PCT should follow facility policy. She should check with a nurse if she has questions about electrode placement.

Posterior EKG: Sometimes a provider will order an EKG that uses posterior leads. This can help diagnose a type of heart attack called an inferior wall myocardial infarction. The PCT will use the V4, V5, and V6 lead wires and place the electrodes on the patient's back. These locations are called V7, V8, and V9 (Fig. 23-18). The patient is seated upright while the electrodes are placed on her back. She is then put in the supine position, as usual, for the EKG.

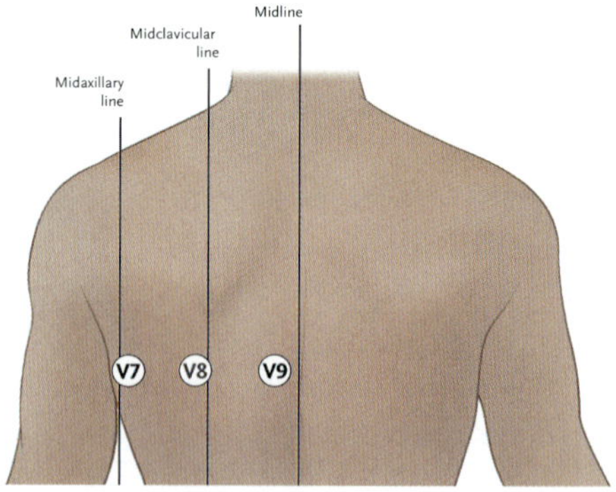

Fig. 23-18. In a posterior EKG, V7 takes the place of V4, V8 takes the place of V5, and V9 takes the place of V6.

V7 is used in place of V4. It is located on the left side of the back in the same horizontal line normally used for V4–V6, along the posterior axillary line. V8 is used in place of V5 and is placed just below the tip of the left shoulder blade (scapula) in the same horizontal line as V7. V9 is used in place of V6. It is placed to the left of the spine in the same horizontal line as V7 and V8. It is very important for the PCT to label the EKG as a posterior EKG (Fig. 23-19).

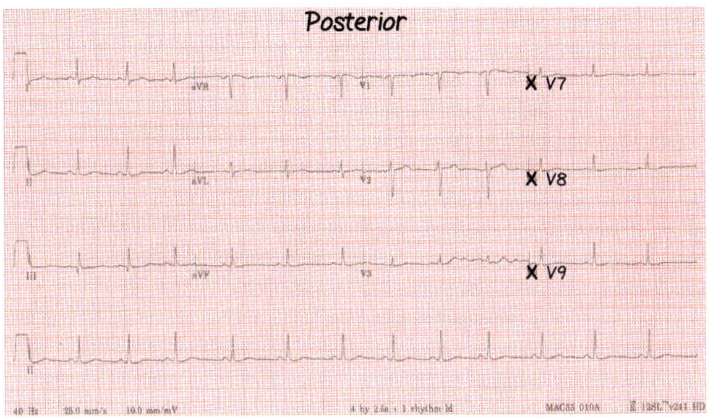

Fig. 23-19. *The tracing from a posterior EKG must be clearly marked. Leads V4, V5, and V6 should be crossed out and replaced with V7, V8, and V9 and POSTERIOR written at the top.*

Alternate patient positions are also sometimes needed. A patient who is over 6 months pregnant should not be placed in the supine position for an EKG. Lying down in the supine position could cause the fetus to compress the patient's vena cava. This reduces blood return to the heart. The patient could become weak and possibly faint. A pregnant patient should lie down and be tilted slightly to the left. A rolled-up blanket or a pillow can help make the patient more comfortable.

A patient with respiratory or heart problems may not be comfortable in a supine position for the EKG. If a patient has orthopnea (difficulty breathing while lying down), they should be placed in a semi-Fowler's position (45-degree angle). This will help them breathe during the test.

5. Demonstrate the performance of a 12-lead EKG

The EKG machine must be set up properly before testing. This makes it more likely that the tracing will be accurate and will not show interference or distortion, known as **artifact**. (Causes of artifact and ways to correct it are described in Learning Objective 9.) Most EKG machines run an automatic self-test when they are turned on. If the machine fails the self-test, it will display an error message. The PCT should follow manufacturer directions to correct any errors shown.

The EKG machine should be placed close to the patient during testing. This reduces tension on lead wires and electrodes. Some machines are on rolling carts. Others have handles so they can be carried. Smaller machines can be placed on a bedside or overbed table. If possible, the machine should be placed to the left of the patient. Electrodes for the precordial leads are placed on the left side of the chest.

The lead wires must be plugged into the machine if they are not already attached. The wires can be laid over the machine or beside the patient. The electrodes can be attached to the lead wires before or after they are placed on the patient. Attaching the lead wires to the electrodes before applying them to the patient reduces pressure on the patient's skin.

Before starting an EKG, the PCT should be sure enough paper is loaded. The paper comes in rolls and only a small amount is needed for each test. EKG paper has preprinted grids made up of 1-millimeter blocks. The PCT can adjust the speed of the paper going through the machine. The default (standard) paper speed is 25 millimeters per second (mm/s). The EKG machine prints the paper speed on each electrocardiogram (Fig. 23-20).

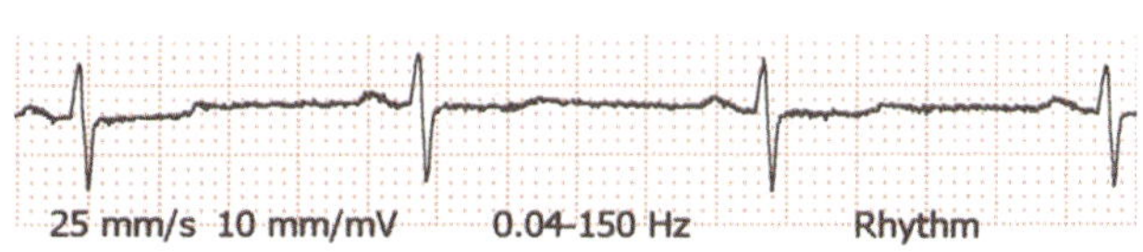

Fig. 23-20. *An EKG tracing at the default paper speed of 25 mm/s.*

Paper speed can be increased to 50 mm/s if the provider requests it. The faster speed spreads out the tracing. It makes waves easier to see. This can be especially helpful for fast heart rhythms

(Fig. 23-21). Instructions for loading and changing paper speed may vary. They can be found in the manufacturer's manual.

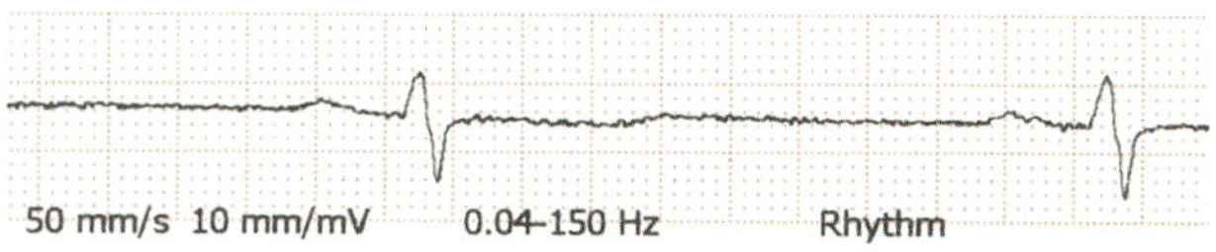

***Fig. 23-21.** An EKG tracing at the paper speed of 50 mm/s. The tracing is spread out over a wider space, which is especially helpful in viewing fast rhythms.*

The gain control on an EKG machine can be used to change the sensitivity of the machine. *Gain* is a measurement of how high or low the stylus (the part of the machine that makes the marks on the paper) moves. Gain is measured in millimeters per millivolt (mm/mV). Millivolts are a measurement of electricity. The gain setting controls how many millimeters the stylus will move to record each millivolt of electricity. Standard gain (the default gain setting) is 10 mm/mV. This means that a 1-millivolt signal makes a mark on the EKG tracing that measures 10 mm.

The EKG tracing includes a calibration marker that looks like a rectangle with the bottom line missing (Fig. 23-22). When the machine is used at standard speed and gain settings, the mark should be 5 mm wide by 10 mm tall.

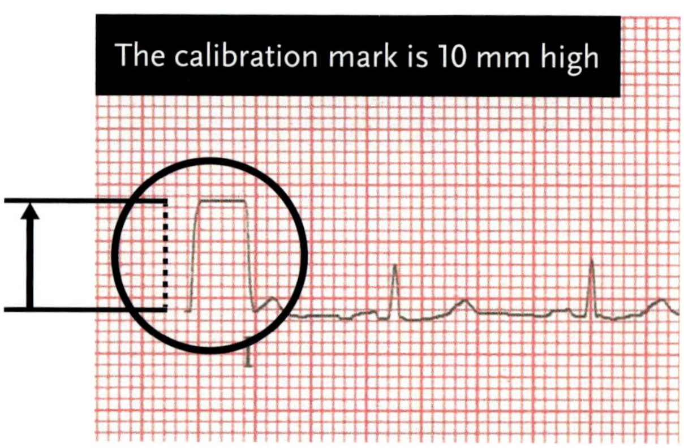

***Fig. 23-22.** The rectangular calibration mark on an EKG tracing shows the gain and speed settings.*

Adjusting the gain control changes how the EKG tracing looks (Fig. 23-23). Increasing gain can make features on the EKG easier to see.

There may be specific machine settings shown in mm/mV: 5 mm/mV (one half of standard), 10 mm/mV (equal to standard), 20 mm/mV (2 times standard), and so on. PCTs should use standard gain unless the provider asks for a different setting.

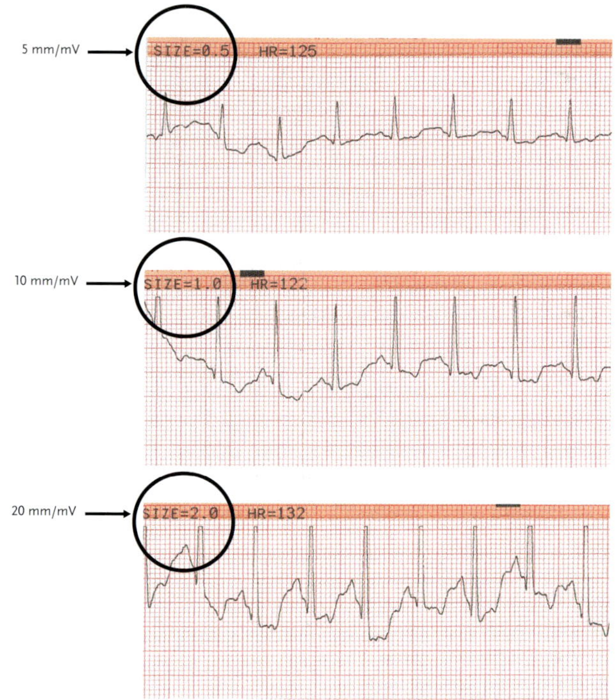

***Fig. 23-23.** Higher gain makes a taller tracing. Lower gain makes a shorter tracing. These tracings show gain at 5 mm/mV, 10 mm/mV, and 20 mm/mV.*

A 12-lead EKG test is used in many settings. It may be done to screen for heart problems. It is also useful as a diagnostic tool when a patient has cardiac symptoms.

Connected Care

Pediatric Patients

Children may be scared of medical procedures. It is important to tell pediatric patients that EKG tests do not hurt and only take a few minutes. Children may not understand medical terms. The PCT should describe the tests in words they are sure to understand. Electrodes can be called *stickers*. The thorax can be *chest and tummy* or *chest and stomach*, depending on the child's age. Children should also be given a chance to ask any questions they may have before the test is given. Follow facility policy about positioning pediatric patients. Small children may be able to be held by a parent or guardian. This is reassuring and may also help the child stay still for testing.

Obtaining a 12-lead EKG

Equipment: EKG machine loaded with paper, lead wires, electrodes, gloves (if needed), towel, clippers

1. Identify yourself by name. Identify the patient according to facility policy.
2. Wash your hands.
3. Explain the procedure to the patient. Speak clearly, slowly, and directly. Maintain face-to-face contact whenever possible. For a male patient, explain that chest hair may need to be clipped for proper electrode contact. Reassure the patient that the test is painless and takes only a few minutes.
4. Provide for the patient's privacy with a curtain, screen, or door.
5. Adjust the bed to a safe level, usually waist high. Lock the bed wheels.
6. Put on gloves (if needed).
7. Assist the patient into a supine position (lying flat on his back).
8. Place the EKG machine beside the bed and plug it into an electrical outlet.
9. Turn the machine on and wait until it completes self-tests.
10. Enter the patient's information into the machine. Be sure the machine is showing the right patient information.
11. Prepare the patient's skin, if needed, by drying or removing lotion or by clipping hair that would stop electrodes from sticking. Throughout the procedure, expose only the areas necessary to prepare the skin and run the test.
12. Open the package of electrodes and attach 1 electrode to each lead wire by snapping or clipping.
13. Attach the electrodes in the correct positions, keeping the patient covered as much as possible. Avoid bony areas, broken skin, scar tissue, and skin over implanted devices.
14. Ask the patient to relax and be as still as possible.
15. When the tracing is clear on the monitor or when the machine shows a green light, print the EKG according to the manufacturer's instructions.
16. Check the EKG for evidence of lethal dysrhythmias or ST segment abnormalities (more information in Learning Objectives 10 and 11). If any are seen, tell the nurse or provider immediately.
17. Disconnect lead wires, taking care not to pull or tug on the patient's skin (Fig. 23-24). Remove the electrodes gently and discard them. The patient may remove the electrodes herself if she prefers.

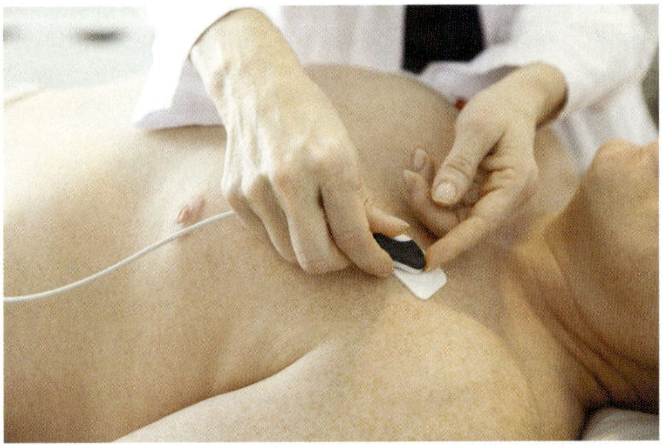

***Fig. 23-24.** Be careful to avoid patient discomfort when removing lead wires from electrodes.*

18. Remove and discard your gloves (if used). Wash your hands.
19. Upload or file the EKG into the patient's medical record.
20. Return the bed to its lowest position. Remove privacy measures.
21. Place the call light within the patient's reach.
22. Clean and store the EKG machine and equipment. This may include cleaning the

electrode clips and wiping the lead wires with a cleaning agent.

23. Wash your hands.

24. Report any changes in the patient to the nurse.

25. Document the procedure using facility guidelines.

NOTE: Follow facility policy regarding reuse of electrodes if more than one EKG is conducted on the same patient. Some electrodes are not as effective after they have conducted electrical activity.

Electrode and Wire Placement

Electrodes can be attached first to the patient or to the lead wires. If attaching electrodes first to the patient, take special care when snapping or clipping the lead wires in place. Avoid pulling the patient's skin when attaching clip-style electrodes. Do not apply unnecessary pressure when attaching snap-style electrodes.

6. Explain patient preparation for continuous monitoring and telemetry

Continuous cardiac monitoring may be ordered when a patient is in a hospital. It may be used when a patient in the ED is considered to be at risk for dangerous heart problems for any reason. It may also be used for a period of time after a heart attack or other heart problem. This type of monitoring is usually done with either 3 or 5 electrodes. The locations for placing electrodes are shown in Figures 23-10 and 23-11 in Learning Objective 4.

Another form of cardiac monitoring is telemetry. A telemetry pack (also called a *telemetry unit*) is used to monitor a patient's heart rate and rhythm. Telemetry technicians monitor signals from multiple patients' telemetry packs at a remote location. They notify a nurse or provider of changes (Fig. 23-25).

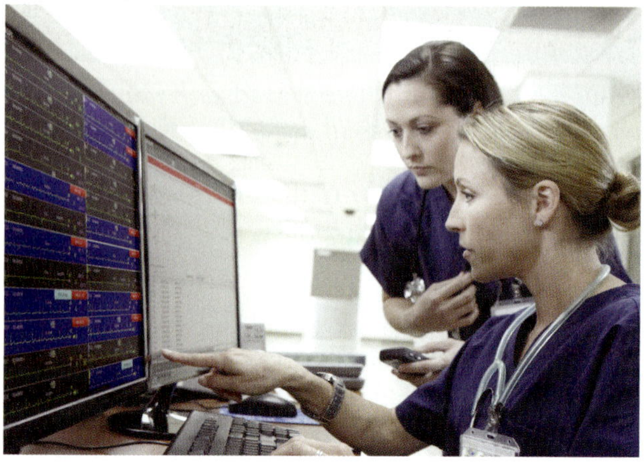

Fig. 23-25. *Specially trained workers monitor several patients at once in telemetry monitoring rooms or stations.* (COURTESY OF ROYAL PHILIPS.)

Most telemetry units come in a small pouch. The pouch has straps that allow the patient to tie the unit around her neck (Fig. 23-26). Some facilities have patient gowns with a small pocket in the front for a telemetry unit. The patient should be told not to remove the electrodes or wires. The patient must notify the PCT or the nurse if the electrodes or wires become loose or fall off. PCTs may be told to alert the telemetry department before removing electrodes (e.g., to assist a patient with showering). The patient can get out of bed and move around the facility while wearing the telemetry pack.

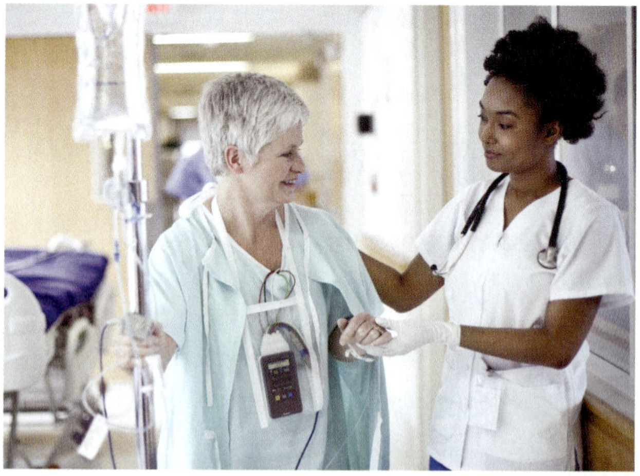

Fig. 23-26. *Telemetry packs can be worn around the neck or in the pocket of a hospital gown. Patients wearing a telemetry pack are free to move around.* (COURTESY OF ROYAL PHILIPS.)

Applying a telemetry pack

Equipment: telemetry pack with fresh batteries, lead wires, electrodes, gloves (if needed), towel, clippers

1. Identify yourself by name. Identify the patient according to facility policy.
2. Wash your hands.
3. Explain the procedure to the patient. Speak clearly, slowly, and directly. Maintain face-to-face contact whenever possible. For a male patient, explain that chest hair may need to be clipped for proper electrode contact.
4. Provide for the patient's privacy with a curtain, screen, or door.
5. Adjust the bed to a safe level, usually waist high. Lock the bed wheels.
6. Put on gloves (if needed).
7. Prepare the patient's skin, if needed, by drying or removing lotion or by clipping hair that would stop electrodes from sticking. Throughout the procedure, expose only the areas necessary to prepare the skin and apply the electrodes.
8. Open the package of electrodes and attach 1 electrode to each lead wire by snapping or clipping.
9. Attach the electrodes in the correct positions, keeping the patient covered as much as possible. Avoid bony areas, broken skin, scar tissue, and skin over implanted devices.
10. Attach the lead wires to the telemetry pack and turn the unit on.
11. Contact the telemetry monitor room to confirm the unit is working properly.
12. Tell the patient to inform you or the nurse if electrodes fall off or the unit is disconnected.
13. Help the patient to store the telemetry pack in a gown pocket or pouch.
14. Give the patient any instructions required by facility policy (how to manage bathing, what to do if an electrode falls off, etc.).
15. Remove and discard your gloves (if used). Wash your hands.
16. Return the bed to its lowest position. Remove privacy measures.
17. Place the call light within the patient's reach.
18. Wash your hands.
19. Report any changes in the patient to the nurse.
20. Document the procedure using facility guidelines.

7. Discuss stress testing

A stress test measures how the heart functions under controlled stress. Stress tests can assess heart function. They can also help predict future heart problems. They may be helpful in planning more invasive heart procedures on a patient. Patients who have had heart surgery usually have a stress test once a year.

Depending on the patient's condition, cardiac stress can be induced (created) in different ways. Exercise on a treadmill or stationary bicycle is the most common way of raising the patient's heart rate. The provider may inject medications to raise the heart rate in patients who cannot exercise. Other names for this test are *exercise stress test, exercise tolerance test,* and *treadmill test.* When medications are used, the test may be called a *pharmacologic stress test.*

A nuclear stress test is another type of cardiac stress test. During this test a harmless radioactive substance called a tracer is injected into the patient. Before the stress test is done, the patient is put in a supine position with her arms over her head. A camera records the motion of the tracer through the heart. This is repeated after the stress test is done. This type of testing gives the provider more detailed information about possible blockages in coronary arteries.

To prepare for a stress test, patients should be instructed to

- Avoid caffeine (coffee, tea, soft drinks, chocolate, certain headache medications) for 24 hours before the exam.
- Follow the provider's instructions about taking any regular medications for 24 hours before the test. Some medications may need to be stopped temporarily. If the patient is hospitalized, the nurse will hold medications as ordered.
- Not eat or drink anything except water for 3 hours before the test. Patients who have diabetes may have different instructions.
- Wear comfortable, loose clothing and rubber-soled shoes or athletic shoes.
- Bring all of their medications on the day of the test. A patient who is hospitalized should have all medications listed in the EHR.

The patient should be told that the entire procedure will last 2–4 hours and that a medical professional will be present or nearby for the entire test.

A 12-lead EKG is conducted before the patient starts exercising and then continuously during the test. The EKG is repeated at 5, 10, and 15 minutes after the exercise is completed. The patient's vital signs are also monitored every 2.5 minutes during the test.

In order for a stress test to be considered valid, the patient's heart must reach a particular heart rate. The goal is for the patient to reach 85% of a rate called the *age-predicted maximal heart rate.* This rate is calculated by subtracting the patient's age from 220, as shown below:

220 – patient's age = age-predicted maximal heart rate

Age-predicted maximal heart rate × 0.85 = target heart rate (goal) for stress test

For example, a 54-year-old's maximal heart rate would be calculated in this way:

220 – 54 = 166 beats per minute (BPM), the age-predicted maximal heart rate

The heart rate the patient should reach during the test is 85% of 166:

166 × 0.85 = 141 BPM, the target heart rate for the test

This patient must reach a heart rate of 141 beats per minute for the test to be valid.

Stress testing should only be done by people who are trained in CPR. The facility must have oxygen, an automated external defibrillator (AED), and a crash cart ready. (A crash cart has supplies needed immediately for a medical emergency). The test should be stopped immediately if the patient has any of the following:

- Dizziness
- Chest pain
- Shortness of breath
- A sudden increase or decrease in systolic or diastolic blood pressure
- Systolic blood pressure greater than 250 mm Hg
- Diastolic blood pressure greater than 115 mm Hg
- Leg cramps
- Severe fatigue
- Severe diaphoresis (excessive sweating)
- ST segment changes (described in Learning Objective 10)
- Worsening or possibly dangerous dysrhythmias (described in Learning Objective 11)

The test should also be stopped if the patient wants to stop or if the heart rate does not rise above 120 BPM.

A PCT or other healthcare worker continues to monitor the patient after the test is completed until the patient's vital signs return to baseline. The patient should be told to rest and avoid stimulants for the rest of the day.

8. Discuss Holter and other ambulatory monitoring

Holter monitors allow a provider to check cardiac activity over a 24- to 48-hour period. Patients with some types of heart conditions may have Holter or other ambulatory monitoring ordered when they are discharged from a hospital. The patient wears a small recording device with lead wires. These are attached to electrodes on the patient's chest. Other types of ambulatory monitors may be worn for longer periods of time. Placing electrodes securely is very important in ambulatory monitoring. The patient will wear the monitor for 24 hours or more and will continue regular activities.

Most ambulatory monitors use 5 electrodes. The skin may have to be cleaned with soap and water or gently abraded (rubbed) with a piece of gauze. This helps the electrodes adhere (stick) to the skin (Fig. 23-27). The PCT should ensure that the monitor batteries are fresh before attaching the electrodes to the patient. Some facilities give patients extra batteries, along with instructions for changing them if the installed batteries fail.

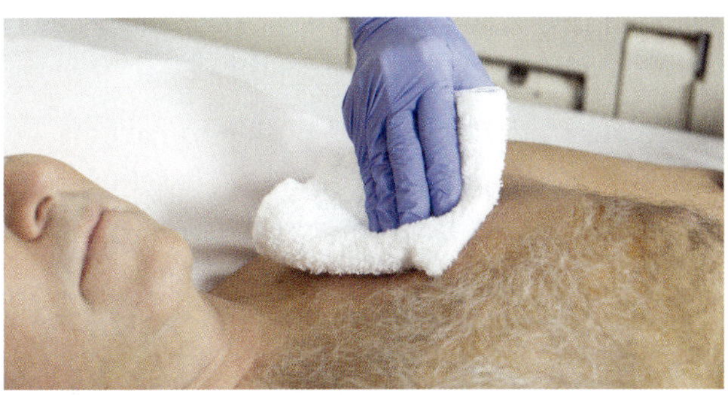

Fig. 23-27. *Gently preparing the skin ensures that electrodes adhere properly.* (SOURCE REFERENCE: CLEANING SKIN OF HAIR. COURTESY OF 3M. © 3M 2015. ALL RIGHTS RESERVED.)

Because patients using an ambulatory monitor continue their everyday activities, electrodes and lead wires may be tugged or strained. This can disrupt the EKG recording or make it harder to read. Some electrodes for ambulatory monitoring have a built-in clip or slot. This allows the PCT to create a loop with the lead wire. This is called a *stress loop*. It can reduce tension placed on the electrodes by the patient's movements (Fig. 23-28). A stress loop can also be created by looping the lead wire and then placing tape over the loop.

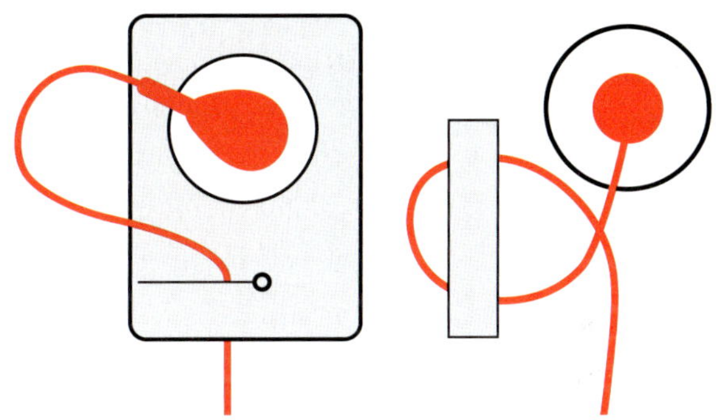

Fig. 23-28. *Stress loops can reduce tugging on the electrodes. This gives a better reading in ambulatory monitoring.*

The PCT should provide information to the patient about ambulatory monitoring when the monitor is applied (Fig. 23-29). Directions vary for each type of monitoring.

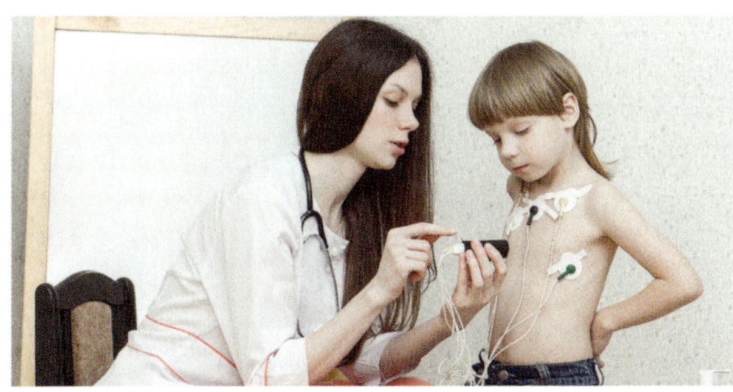

Fig. 23-29. *Patient education is an important part of setting up ambulatory monitoring.*

Patients who have Holter monitoring should be told to

- Call the provider if the electrodes become loose or fall off.
- Not remove the lead wires.
- Not get the monitor wet or shower or swim with the monitor in place.

- Continue their normal activities.
- Keep an activity and symptom diary and press the event button on the monitor for any symptom.
- Call 911 for severe chest pain, weakness, or shortness of breath.
- Return all equipment as directed when the test is complete.

Most facilities have printed instructions in brochures or booklets for the patient to take home and refer to if needed.

9. Demonstrate solutions to different types of EKG artifact

Both patient and environmental factors can interfere with EKG tracings. Newer EKG machines have artifact filters that detect and correct artifact automatically. PCTs should still know how to recognize and fix different types of artifact.

Any patient muscle movement will show up on an EKG tracing. This can create 2 types of artifact: somatic tremor and wandering baseline.

Somatic tremor artifact makes a fine, choppy distortion on the EKG tracing. This makes the EKG difficult or impossible to read. This interference is usually caused by tremors or shivering (Fig. 23-30).

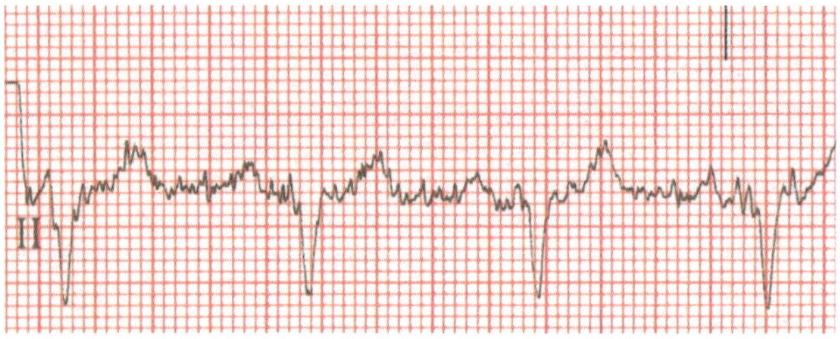

Fig. 23-30. *Somatic tremor may occur if a patient is cold or has an illness that causes tremors.*

These are ways to reduce somatic tremor artifact:

- Patients who have Parkinson's disease or other conditions that cause tremors can be positioned with their hands under their buttocks. This reduces tremors.
- Placing limb electrodes on the torso, rather than on the limbs, may also help.
- Patients who are shivering should be given a blanket. The room temperature should be adjusted if possible. Pillows can also help make a patient more comfortable and reduce patient movement.
- Anxious or nervous patients should be reassured that the test is painless.

In wandering baseline artifact, the normally flat baseline goes up and down across the tracing (Fig. 23-31).

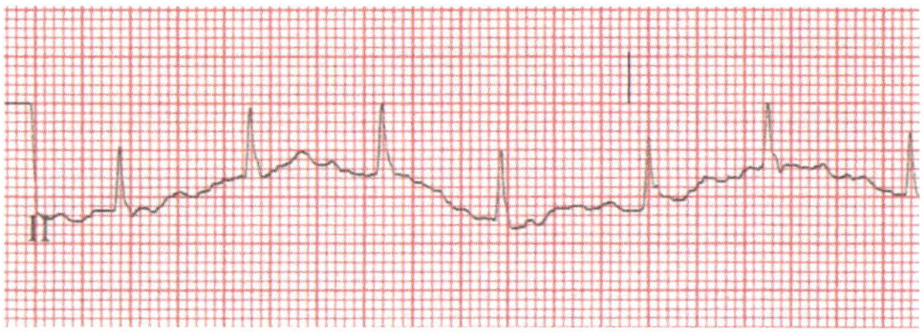

Fig. 23-31. *Wandering baseline makes it hard to see the features of the EKG tracing. Sometimes the tracing runs off the paper.*

It may be hard for the provider to read the EKG. In some cases the tracing goes off the paper. The movement of the muscles used for breathing can cause wandering baseline artifact. The PCT should remind patients to breathe as normally as possible and to stay quiet and still during the test. Placing the electrodes for the limb leads on the wrists and ankles can reduce wandering baseline caused by breathing.

Loose electrodes or poor electrode contact are also common causes of wandering baseline. Sweaty or wet skin, oily or soiled skin, dry skin, and body hair can all interfere with electrode contact. Careful skin preparation is the best way to correct this:

- Sweat or moisture can be removed with a towel, paper towel, or gauze pads. Skin oil or lotion can be removed with soap and water.
- The outer layer of dead skin cells can be removed by gently rubbing (abrading) the

skin. This lets the electrode come in contact with more conductive tissue. Dry gauze or a special skin-abrading product may be used for this purpose (Fig. 23-32).

- Body hair may need to be removed to increase contact between skin and electrode.

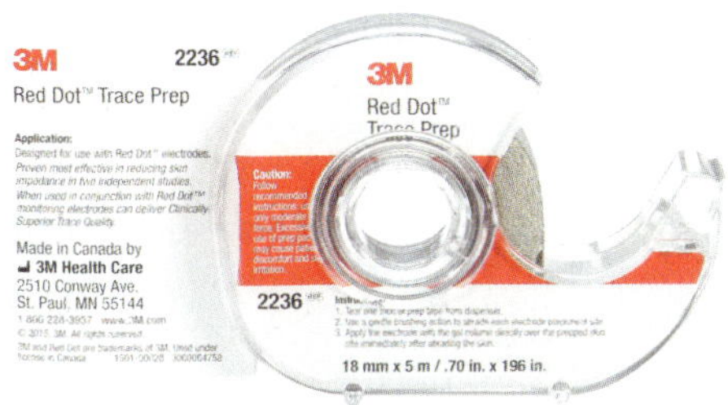

Fig. 23-32. *The use of abrading tape can improve skin-electrode contact.* (SOURCE REFERENCE: ELECTRODE TRACE PREP. 3M™ RED DOT™ TRACE PREP. COURTESY OF 3M. © 3M 2016. ALL RIGHTS RESERVED.)

Body hair that prevents electrode contact should only be removed with medical clippers (Fig. 23-33). Medical clippers are usually powered by rechargeable batteries. They have disposable cutting heads. A standard shaving razor should not be used. It can create microcuts, which increase the chance of infection. The PCT can also place paper tape over an electrode to help increase skin contact.

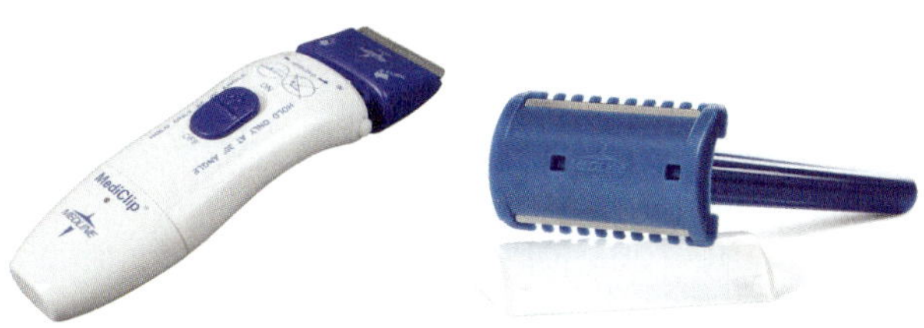

Fig. 23-33. *Medical razors or clippers should be used to remove body hair if necessary. Most facilities use electric clippers for this purpose.* (IMAGES COURTESY OF MEDLINE INDUSTRIES, LP. USED WITH PERMISSION.)

Electrodes that are expired or dried out may cause wandering baseline. They may prevent the EKG machine from picking up any signals at all. Electrodes should be stored in an airtight container. Any that are dried out or expired should be thrown away. Tension on the lead wires or wires that are not secured well can also cause wandering baseline artifact.

Artifacts called *electrical interference* and *broken recording* can be caused by factors in the care environment. Electrical interference is also called *alternating current (AC) interference* or *60-cycle interference*. It can be caused by other equipment in use near the EKG machine (Fig. 23-34).

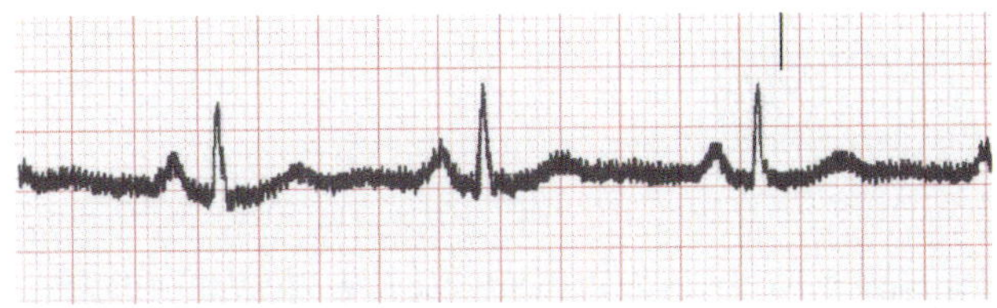

Fig. 23-34. *An EKG tracing showing electrical interference is difficult or impossible to read.*

The PCT will need to look for the source of electrical interference and try to stop it. Electrical interference may be stopped by

- Turning off other electrical equipment
- Plugging the EKG machine into a different outlet
- Not using an extension cord
- Making sure the machine is properly grounded. The machine must be plugged into a grounded 3-prong outlet.
- Turning off fluorescent lights

Broken recording, also called *interrupted baseline*, happens when the EKG machine cannot find a signal. The stylus goes from side to side as the machine searches for a signal (Fig. 23-35). The most common cause of broken recording is frayed or broken lead wires. The PCT should check the EKG machine before each use to make sure the lead wires are in good shape. If the lead wires are broken or frayed, he should not use them.

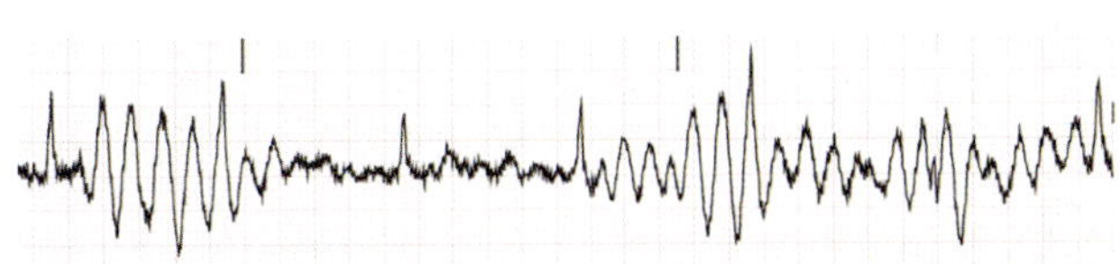

Fig. 23-35. *Broken recording is usually a result of frayed wires.*

10. Identify normal and abnormal heart rhythms

PCTs are responsible for getting a good EKG tracing for the provider to review. They should also be able to see when a heart rhythm may be dangerous. In some cases the nurse or provider must be informed right away.

As described in Learning Objective 2, EKG features give the provider information about a patient's heart rhythm. *Heart rhythm* and *heart rate* are not the same. The heart rate is the speed at which the heart is beating. The heart rhythm is the overall pattern of the heartbeat. These are some of the factors the provider considers when analyzing heart rhythm:

- **Regularity**: A normal rhythm has a clear, repeating pattern.
- **P wave**: This wave relates to the depolarization and contraction of the atria. A normal rhythm has a clear P wave that is the same from beat to beat.
- **QRS complex**: This complex relates to the depolarization and contraction of the ventricles. A wide, spread-out QRS complex may be a sign of a problem.

Normal sinus rhythm (NSR) is the standard, normal heart rhythm. It has a heart rate between 60 and 100 BPM and a regular rhythm. It has an identical, positive P wave before each QRS complex. The QRS complex is not spread out (Fig. 23-36). Rhythms that do not have these features are dysrhythmias. They may be too fast or too slow. They may start in an area of the heart other than the SA node.

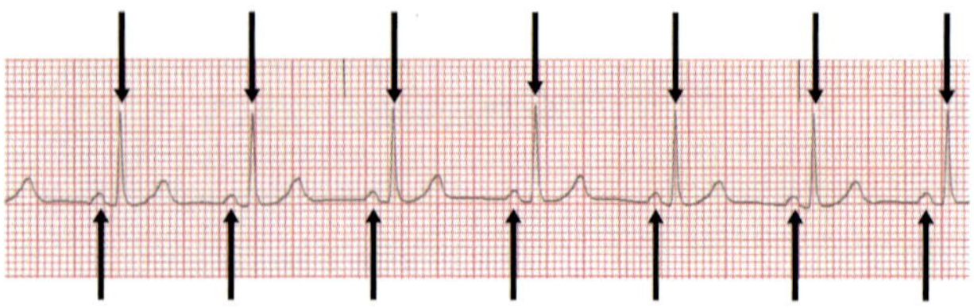

***Fig. 23-36.** EKG tracing showing NSR.*

A fast heart rhythm, with a rate over 100 beats per minute, is called *tachycardia*. A slow rhythm, with a rate below 60 beats per minute, is called *bradycardia*. In some rhythms, electrical signals are firing very quickly in the heart. The heart muscle contracts in a chaotic way and does not pump blood as it is supposed to. This type of rhythm is called *fibrillation*.

AFib Is Common and Serious

Atrial fibrillation is the most commonly treated cardiac dysrhythmia. The risk for developing AFib goes up with age, and it is more common in women than in men. It is also more common in people of European ancestry.

AFib does not always cause serious symptoms, but it can be very dangerous. People with AFib have twice the risk of death from cardiac problems and 5 times the risk of stroke. Not all patients understand these risks. Providers can help explain how patients can reduce the danger.

Patients who use smartwatches or other personal EKG devices may be alerted to AFib rhythms. If a PCT sees any irregular rhythm on a patient's EKG, she should alert the nurse or provider. Only the provider can make a diagnosis. Treatments for AFib may include blood thinners to prevent pooled blood from clotting, which increases stroke risk. Medications that control heart rate or regulate heart rhythm may also be ordered.

Heart rate can change based on activity, stress, or medical conditions. The normal range also varies by age. Many differences in heart rate are not dangerous for the patient. Athletes may have a slow heart rate, for instance. With any irregular rate or rhythm, the provider considers whether it is causing symptoms or problems for the patient.

Dysrhythmias often start in areas of the cardiac conduction system other than the SA node. These rhythms look different from NSR on an EKG:

Atrial rhythms have abnormal P waves. For example, the P wave may be wider or taller than normal, may have a notch, or may look different in each beat (Fig. 23-37a).

Junctional rhythms may have P waves that go down, rather than up, from the baseline. P waves may also be hidden (Fig. 23-37b).

Ventricular rhythms have QRS complexes that are wider than normal. Ventricular rhythms can be dangerous (Fig. 23-37c). Ventricular tachycardia and ventricular fibrillation can both be deadly.

Heart block rhythms usually have long spaces between the P wave and the R wave. This is called a long PR interval (Fig. 23-37d).

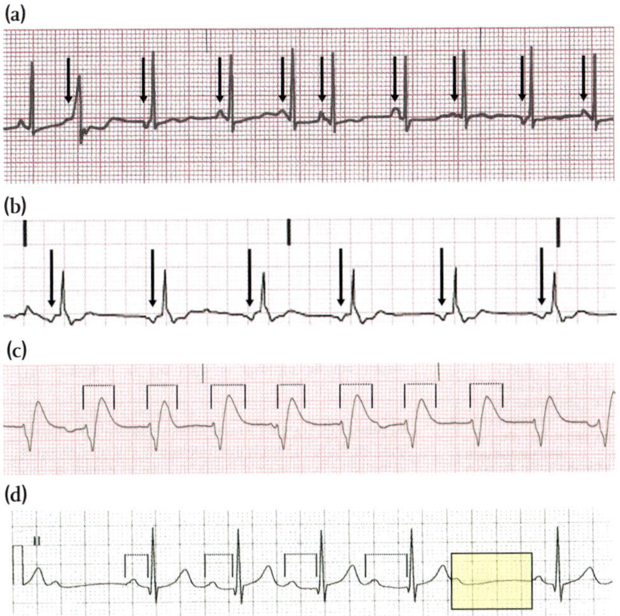

Fig. 23-37. Examples of EKG changes in (a) atrial, (b) junctional, (c) ventricular, and (d) heart block rhythms (yellow highlighting shows a completely blocked beat).

Some irregularities on EKG tracings are not from dysrhythmias or abnormal heartbeats. An artifical pacemaker is put in when a patient's natural cardiac pacemakers (e.g., the SA node) fail (Fig. 23-38). They can change how EKG tracings look. Dysrhythmias (especially very slow rhythms), heart blocks, cardiomyopathy, and heart failure are conditions that may be treated with a pacemaker.

Pacemaker impulses make a spike-like wave on EKG tracings (Fig. 23-39). PCTs may see these spikes when doing an EKG on a patient with a pacemaker.

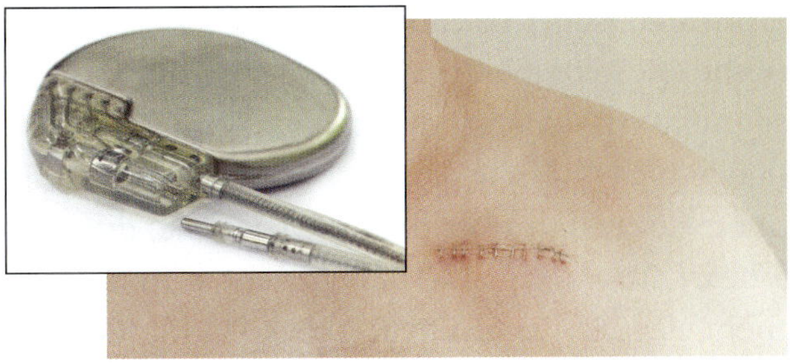

Fig. 23-38. An artificial pacemaker and a patient with a scar from pacemaker placement.

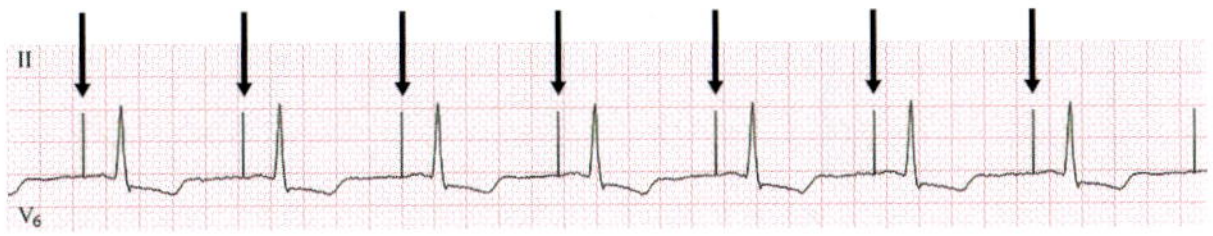

Fig. 23-39. Pacemaker spikes appear before the P wave in this EKG tracing. The pacemaker is stimulating the atria.

EKG tracings may also show changes when something is going wrong with the heart at the moment the EKG is performed. Myocardial infarction and cardiac ischemia are some of the conditions that EKGs can detect. These conditions are caused by lack of blood flow and oxygen to an area of the heart. On the EKG this can cause ST segment depression. This means that the part of the tracing between the S wave and the T wave goes below the isoelectric line (Fig. 23-40). Lack of oxygen to the heart can also cause the T wave to go down, rather than up, from the isoelectric line. If ischemia is not treated immediately, tissue death in the heart will occur.

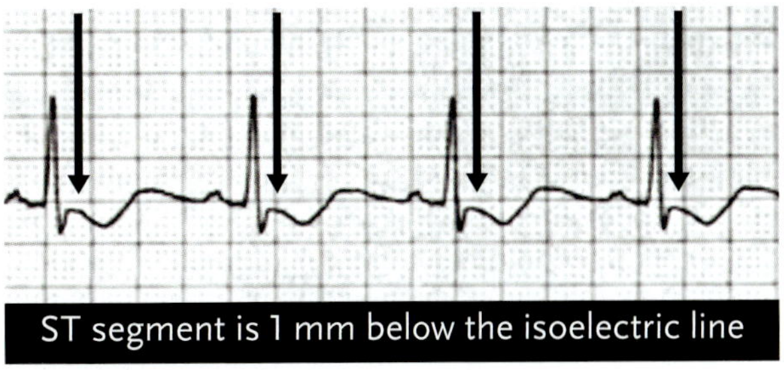

Fig. 23-40. ST segment depression can mean that part of the heart is not getting enough blood and oxygen.

Untreated ischemia can lead to MI. The shapes of the QRS complex, the T wave, and the ST segment may change during some heart attacks due to heart muscle damage. The ST segment is often elevated (higher than the baseline) during a heart attack (Fig. 23-41). A patient with ST segment elevation needs to be checked by a provider right away.

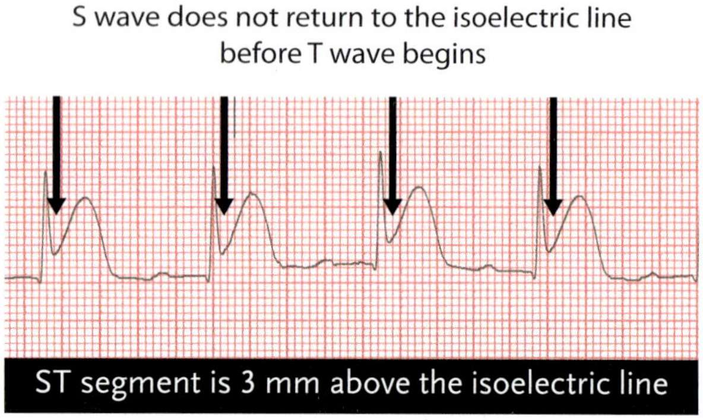

Fig. 23-41. *ST segment elevation is a sign of MI.*

Knowing Normal

PCTs may be the first healthcare workers to view EKG tracings. They need to know how to identify a normal EKG. Anything abnormal—unusual P waves, widened or strange QRS complexes, or elevated ST segments—is then easier to see and report.

11. Identify potentially lethal EKG changes and describe emergency response

PCTs should always observe patient condition carefully. During EKG testing, PCTs may be the first to see a change that means emergency care is needed. Not all heart attacks cause ST segment changes. If a patient reports any of these symptoms, or the PCT observes any of these signs, the provider should be called immediately. This is true even if the EKG tracing looks normal.

Symptoms of a cardiac emergency

- Increased shortness of breath
- Chest pain or pressure
- Arm, neck, shoulder, or back pain
- Increased weakness or fatigue
- Any other change from baseline

Signs of a cardiac emergency

- Increased respiratory rate
- Hypotension (low blood pressure)
- Hypertension (high blood pressure)
- Diaphoresis (excessive sweating)
- Cyanosis
- Bradycardia (heart rate under 60 beats per minute)
- Tachycardia (heart rate over 100 beats per minute)
- Unconsciousness
- Altered mental status
- Any other change from baseline

Table 23-1 shows potentially deadly EKG changes a PCT should recognize. The PCT must always check both the EKG tracing and the patient's condition. If EKG changes do not match the patient's condition (e.g., there is no EKG activity but the patient is conscious and seems normal), the tracing may be showing artifact or error. The PCT should still call a provider to assess the patient, even if the patient seems fine.

Chapter 6 contains detailed information on responding to emergencies, including MI. PCTs should always follow facility policy when responding to any emergency. In a hospital, a code team usually manages care in a cardiac emergency. If directed to do so, a PCT may use an automated external defibrillator (AED) when a patient has a cardiac emergency. Some dangerous heart rhythms can be corrected by a shock. The AED has pads that attach to the patient's bare chest. It analyzes the heart rhythm and delivers a shock if it is needed. AEDs come in many makes and models. All AEDs are designed

EKG CHANGES TO REPORT IMMEDIATELY

ST segment elevation: ST segment >1 mm above isoelectric line

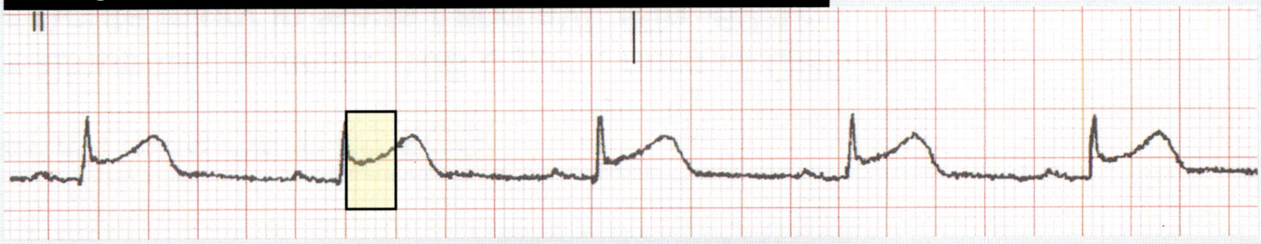

ST segment depression: ST segment >2 mm below isoelectric line

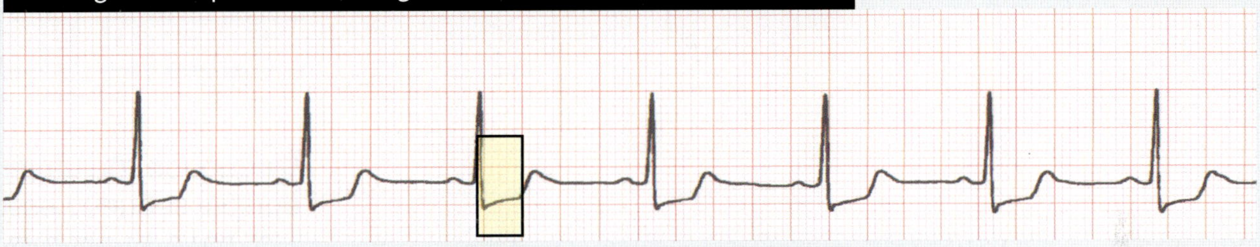

New-onset dysrhythmia: sudden changes should be reported immediately

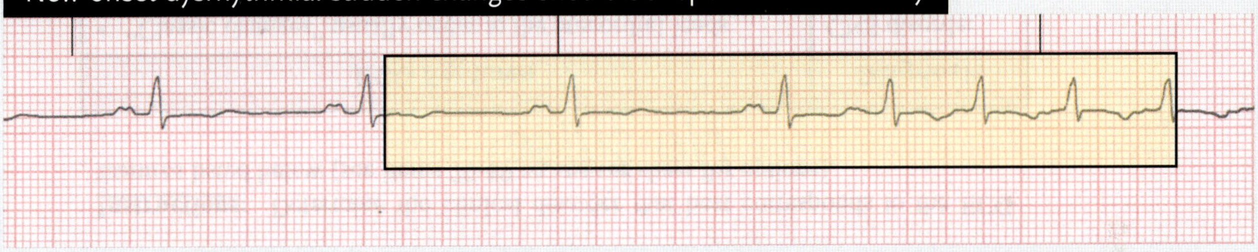

LETHAL DYSRHYTHMIAS

Ventricular tachycardia: rapid rate with no P waves and wide, bizarre QRS complexes

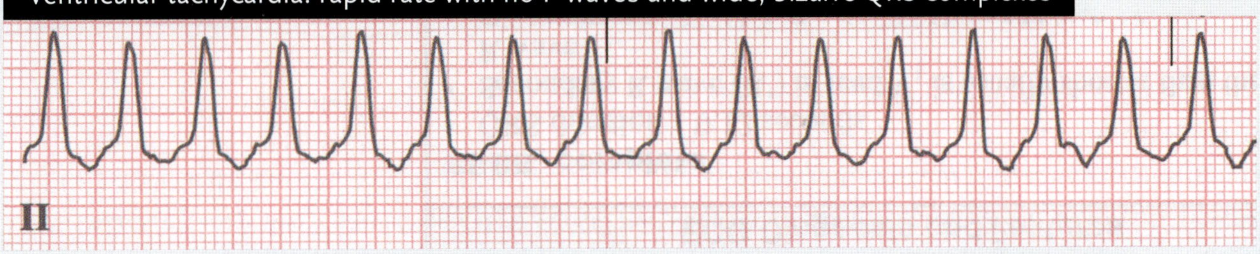

Ventricular fibrillation: chaotic and disorganized with no recognizable waves or complexes

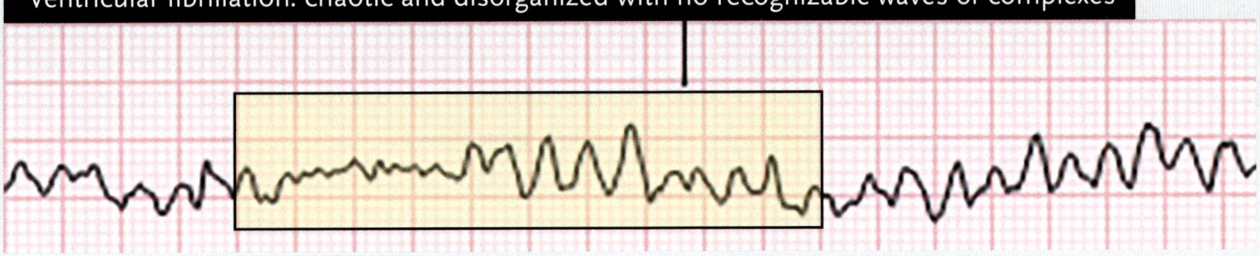

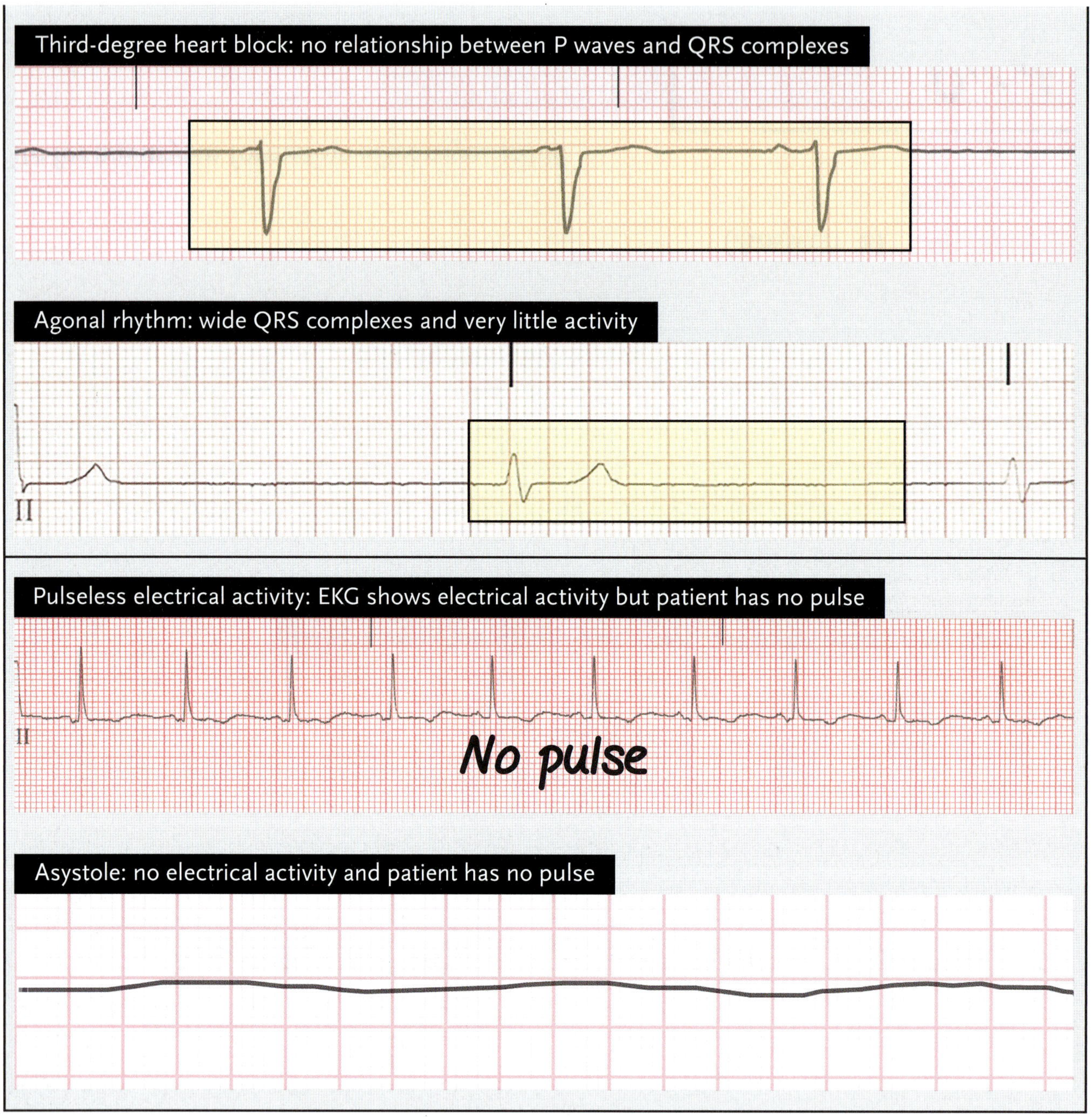

Table 23-1. *The PCT should check the patient's condition and call the nurse immediately if any of these changes are seen.*

to guide even an untrained person through using the device (Fig. 23-42). This includes cues for when to start or stop CPR. Visual and verbal prompts from the machine direct the process.

Certain medications may be administered during cardiac emergencies. Oxygen, aspirin, and nitroglycerin are drugs often used to treat cardiac symptoms.

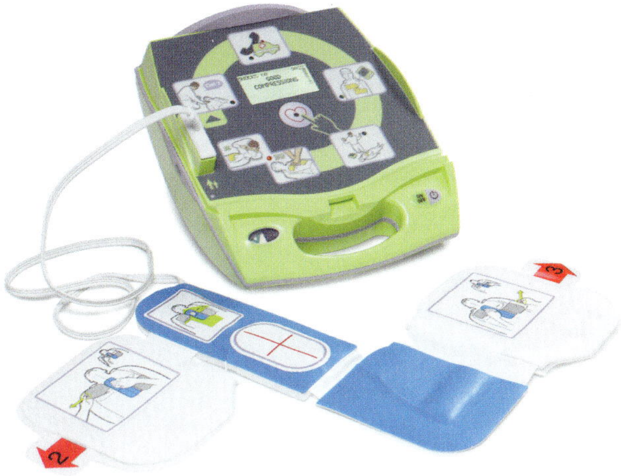

Fig. 23-42. *AEDs are made to be used easily by healthcare workers or members of the public.* (PHOTO COURTESY OF ZOLL MEDICAL CORPORATION, WWW.ZOLL.COM.)

Chapter Review

1. What physical activity in the heart is caused by depolarization? What activity is caused by repolarization?
2. What is the primary pacemaker of the heart? Where does the electrical impulse go from there?
3. Describe 4 types of tests done with EKG technology.
4. Which leads are called the limb leads? What is another name for these leads?
5. What is the difference between electrodes and leads?
6. How many electrodes are put on the patient for a 12-lead EKG?
7. Describe 3 situations when alternate electrode placement is used.
8. Why should an EKG machine be close to a patient during testing?
9. What does a higher gain control setting do to an EKG tracing?
10. When may continuous cardiac monitoring be ordered?
11. Calculate the age-predicted maximal heart rate for a 60-year-old patient who is having a stress test.
12. What should happen if a patient's heart rate does not rise above 120 BPM during a stress test?
13. How many electrodes are used for most ambulatory monitoring?
14. What is the purpose of a stress loop?
15. List 3 situations that may cause somatic tremor artifact. Describe what a PCT can do to address each situation.
16. What artifact might be caused by lotion on a patient's skin? How could the PCT prevent or correct it?
17. What part of the heart may be involved if a patient's EKG shows abnormal P waves?
18. What activity of the heart does the QRS complex relate to?
19. What may be happening to the patient when there are ST segment changes on an EKG?
20. How does a pacemaker change what an EKG tracing looks like?
21. What should a PCT do when an EKG tracing shows a potentially lethal change?
22. What drugs may be given during a cardiac emergency?

24 End-of-Life Care

1. Describe the stages of grief and the grief process

Death can occur suddenly without warning, or it can be expected. Older people or people with terminal illnesses may have time to prepare for death. A **terminal illness** is a disease or condition that will eventually cause death. Preparing for death is a process that affects the dying person's emotions and behavior.

Grief is deep distress or sorrow over a loss. It is an adaptive, or changing, process and usually involves healing. Dr. Elisabeth Kübler-Ross studied and wrote about the grief process. She theorized that dying people share a common grief process. Her book, *On Death and Dying*, describes 5 stages that dying people and their families or friends may experience before death. These 5 stages are described below. Not all people go through all the stages. Some may stay in one stage until death occurs. Others may move back and forth between stages during the process.

Denial: People in the denial stage may refuse to believe they are dying. They often believe that a mistake has been made. They may demand lab work be repeated. They may talk about the future and avoid discussion of their illnesses. They may simply act like it is not happening. This is the "No, not me" stage.

Anger: Once people start to face the possibility of their death, they may become angry. They may be angry because they think they are too young to die. They may be angry because they feel they have always lived a healthy life and have always taken care of themselves. This anger may be directed at healthcare workers, visitors, roommates, family, or friends. Anger is a normal and healthy reaction. Even though it may be upsetting, it is important to try not to take anger personally. This is the "Why me?" stage.

Bargaining: Once people have begun to believe that they really are dying, they may make promises to God or a higher power, care providers, or others. They may somehow try to bargain for their recovery. This is the "Yes me, but..." stage.

Depression: As dying people become weaker and their symptoms get worse, they may become deeply sad or depressed (Fig. 24-1). They may cry or withdraw. They may be unable to perform simple activities. They need additional support. It is important to listen and be understanding.

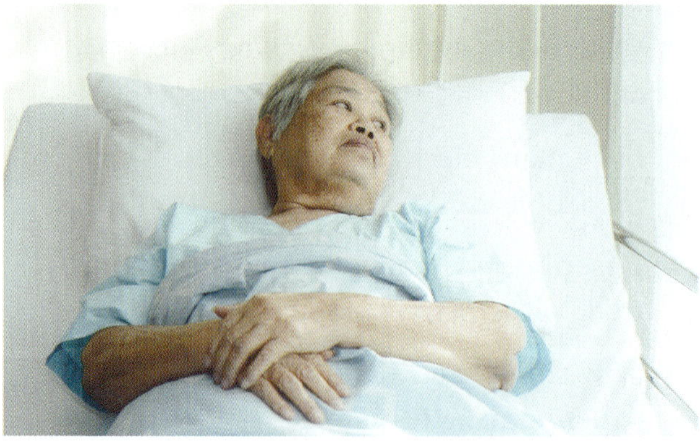

Fig. 24-1. *A person who is dying may become depressed and withdrawn. The PCT should give extra emotional support to these patients.*

Acceptance: Peace or acceptance may or may not come before death. Some people who are dying are eventually able to accept death and prepare for it. They may make arrangements with attorneys and accountants. They may arrange with loved ones for the care of important people or things. They may make plans for their last days or for the ceremonies that may follow their death. At this stage, people who are dying may seem emotionally detached.

These stages may not be possible for someone who dies suddenly, unexpectedly, or quickly. People cannot force anyone to move from stage to stage; they can only listen and be ready to offer their help.

Dealing with grief after the death of a loved one is a process as well. Grieving is an individual experience. No two people will grieve in exactly the same way. Religious leaders, counselors, or social workers can provide help for people who are grieving. These are some reactions that family members or friends may have to the death of a loved one:

Shock: Death may be expected or unexpected. Even when it is expected, family members and friends may still be shocked when it occurs. Many people do not know what to expect after the death of a loved one and may be surprised by their feelings.

Denial: It is easy to want to believe that everything will quickly return to normal after a death. Denying or refusing to believe they are grieving can help people deal with the initial hours or days after a death. But eventually it is important to face feelings. Grief can be so overwhelming that some people may take years to face their feelings. Professional help can be very valuable.

Anger: Although it is hard to admit it, many people feel angry after a death. They may be angry at themselves, at God, at the doctors, or even at the person who died. There is nothing wrong with feeling anger as a part of grief.

Guilt: It is very common for families, friends, and other caregivers to feel guilty after a death. They may wish they had done more for the dying person. They may simply feel that the person did not deserve to die. They may feel guilty that they are still living or that they feel relieved.

Regret: Often people regret what they did or did not do for the dying person. They may regret things they said or did not say to the person who has died. Many people have regrets for years.

Relief: People may feel relieved that the person who has died is no longer suffering. They may be relieved that they no longer have a responsibility (emotional, physical, or financial) regarding care.

Sadness: It is very common to feel depressed or emotionally unstable after a death. People may suffer headaches or insomnia when they cannot express their sadness.

Loneliness: Missing someone who has died is very normal. It can bring up other feelings, such as sadness or regret. Many things may remind people of the person who died. The memories may be painful at first. With time, those who survive usually feel less lonely, and memories are less painful.

Connected Care

Coping Mechanisms

People who are dying and their loved ones are managing many emotions. These feelings are natural. There are positive and negative ways to cope with these feelings. It is normal to feel angry, for example, but some people may express anger in a harmful way. Dying patients or their family members may lash out at healthcare workers or at each other. They may seem rude or ungrateful for the care they are receiving. These are negative coping mechanisms. A social worker or a spiritual leader may provide support to patients who are behaving this way. Report any inappropriate behavior to the nurse.

2. Define the goals of a hospice program

Hospice care is the term for the special care that a dying person needs. It is a compassionate way to care for people who are dying and their families. Hospice care emphasizes a holistic, person-centered approach. It treats the dying person's physical, emotional, spiritual, and social needs.

Hospice care can be given 7 days a week, 24 hours a day. It is available with a provider's order. There is always a nurse on call to answer questions, make a visit, or solve a problem. Hospice care may be given in a hospital, at a care facility, or in the home. A hospice can be any location where a person who is dying is treated with dignity by caregivers.

Any caregiver may provide hospice care, but often specially trained nurses, social workers, and volunteers provide hospice care. The hospice team may include doctors, nurses, social workers, counselors, patient care technicians, therapists, religious leaders, dietitians, and volunteers.

Hospice care helps meet all needs of the patient who is dying. The patient is directly involved in care decisions, as are family and friends. The patient is encouraged to participate in family life and decision-making as long as possible.

In other types of care, goals focus on the patient's recovery or on the patient's ability to care for herself as much as possible. In hospice care, however, the goals are the comfort and dignity of the patient. This type of care is called **palliative care**, which is care that is provided for people who are dying that emphasizes relieving pain, managing symptoms, promoting comfort, and preventing side effects and complications. However, it is important to note that palliative care is not only given to people who are dying. It is also given to people who have serious, chronic diseases, such as cancer, congestive heart failure, and AIDS.

Patients who are dying need to feel independent for as long as possible. Healthcare workers should allow patients to have as much control over their lives as possible. Eventually, healthcare workers may have to meet all of the patient's basic needs.

Guidelines: Hospice Care

G Be a good listener. It is hard to know what to say to someone who is dying or to his relatives or friends. Most often, people need someone to listen to them (Fig. 24-2). A good listener can be a great comfort. Some people, however, will not want to confide in healthcare workers, and you should never push someone to talk.

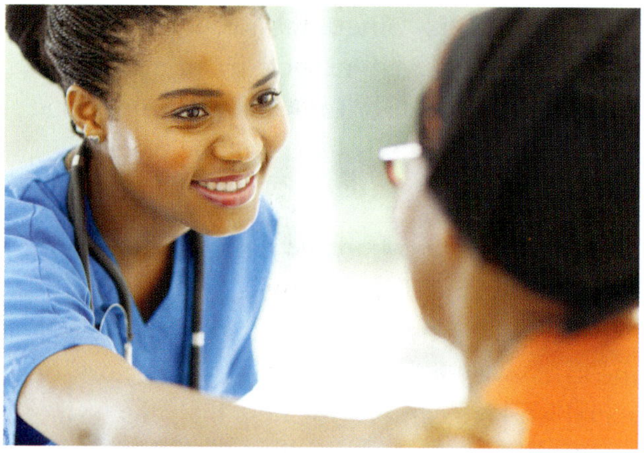

Fig. 24-2. *Being a good listener can be a great help to a patient who is dying.*

G Respect privacy and independence. Relatives, friends, religious leaders, and others may visit a patient who is dying. Make it easy for these difficult visits to take place. Stay out of the way when you can. Do not join in the conversation unless asked to do so. Understand that some people wish to be alone with their dying loved ones. Dying patients can have some independence even when they need total care. Let the patient make choices when possible, such as when to bathe and what to eat or drink.

G Be sensitive to individual needs. Different patients and families will have different needs. The more you know what is needed, the more you can help. Some patients need a quiet and calm atmosphere. Others appreciate a cheery presence and might like you to talk or stay close by. Ask family members or friends how you can help.

G Be aware of your own feelings. Caring for people who are dying can be draining. Know your limits and respect them. Discuss feelings of frustration or grief with another care team member.

G Recognize the stress. Just realizing how stressful it is to work with patients who are dying is a first step toward caring for yourself. Talking with a therapist about your experiences at work can help you understand and work through your feelings. Remember, however, that specific information must be kept confidential. A supervisor may be able to make a referral to a therapist or support group.

G Take care of yourself. Eating right, exercising, and getting enough rest are ways of taking care of yourself. Remember that caring for your emotional health is important too. Talk about and acknowledge your feelings. Take time to do things for yourself, such as reading a book, taking a bubble bath, or doing another activity that you enjoy. If you are a religious or spiritual person, these needs may be met by attending religious services, reading, praying, meditating, or just taking a quiet walk (Fig. 24-3). Meeting your needs allows you to best meet other people's needs.

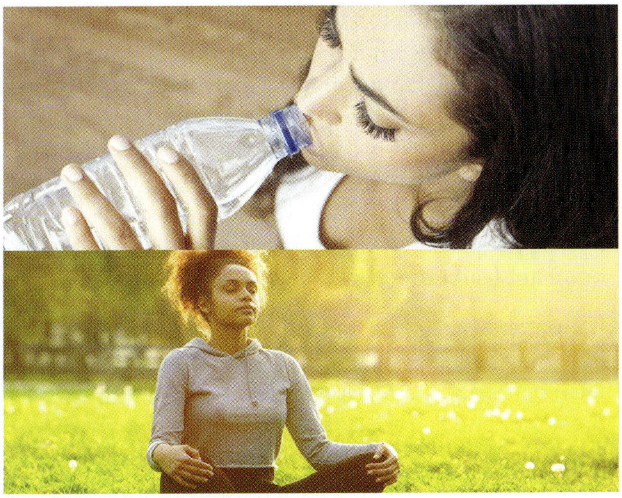

Fig. 24-3. *Taking care of yourself, including eating right, drinking plenty of water, and relaxing, is a way to help you tend to your needs while caring for people who are dying. Exercise, meditation, prayer, or reading are also ways to meet your needs.*

G Take a break when you need to. Find 10 minutes to sit down and relax or stand up and stretch. This may be enough of a break in some situations.

3. Discuss how to care for a patient who is dying

Care for a patient who is dying should focus on meeting physiological needs, as well as providing comfort and emotional support. Promoting independence and person-centered care is important.

Guidelines: Patient Who Is Dying

G **Diminished senses**: Vision may begin to fail. Reduce glare and keep room lighting low (Fig. 24-4). Hearing is usually the last sense to leave the body, so speak in a normal tone. Tell the patient about care that is being done or what is happening in the room. Do not expect an answer. Ask few questions. Encourage the family to speak to the patient, but to avoid subjects that are disturbing. Observe body language to anticipate a patient's needs.

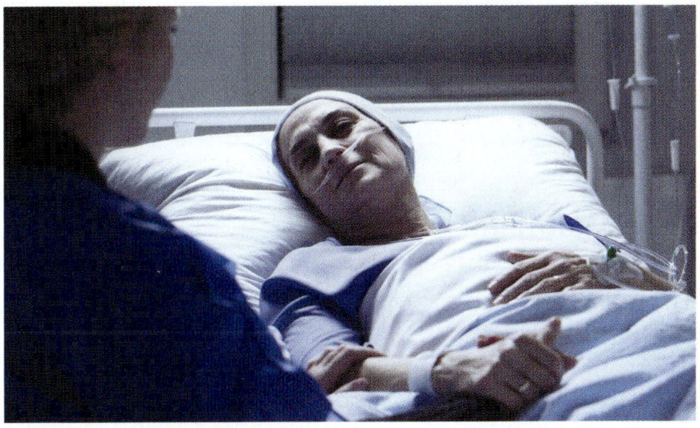

Fig. 24-4. *Keep a dying patient's room softly lit without glare.*

G **Care of the mouth and nose**: Give mouth care often. If the patient is unconscious, give mouth care every 2 hours. The lips and nostrils may be dry and cracked. Apply lubricant, such as balm, to the lips and nose.

- G **Skin care**: Give bed baths and incontinence care as needed. Bathe perspiring patients often. Skin should be kept clean and dry. Change sheets and clothes for comfort. Keep sheets wrinkle-free. Giving regular skin care and repositioning the patient often can help prevent pressure injuries.
- G **Pain control and comfort**: Patients who are dying may be in pain. Pain relief is critical. Observe and report signs of pain to the nurse immediately. Patients may be connected to a patient-controlled analgesia (PCA) device. A PCA device allows patients to administer pain medication to themselves with the press of a button. Report any complaints of pain or discomfort to the nurse immediately. Because some patients may not be able to communicate that they are in pain, observe body language and watch for other signs.

  Frequent changes of position, back massage, skin care, mouth care, and proper body alignment may help. Body temperature usually rises when a person is dying. Many patients are more comfortable with light covers. However, fever may cause chills. Use extra blankets if patients need more warmth.
- G **Environment**: Play music if the patient requests it. Make sure the room is comfortable, appropriately lit, and well ventilated. When leaving the room, place the call light within reach, even if the patient is unaware of his surroundings.
- G **Emotional and spiritual support**: Patients who are dying may be afraid of what is happening and of death. Listening may be one of the most important things you can do. Allow the patient to fully express his feelings, and do not change the subject even if it makes you uncomfortable. Pay attention to these conversations. Report any comments about fear to the nurse.

  People who are dying may also need the quiet, reassuring, and loving presence of another person. Touch can be very important. Holding the patient's hand as you sit quietly can be very comforting.

  Do not avoid the dying person or his family. Do not deny that death is approaching, and do not tell the patient that anyone knows how or when it will happen. Do give accurate information in a reassuring way. No one can take away a person's fear of death. However, your supportive and reassuring presence can help.

  Some patients who are dying may also seek spiritual comfort from a religious or spiritual leader. Tell the nurse immediately if a patient requests a religious leader, and provide privacy for visits. Respect any cultural or religious practices the patient may want to follow as death nears. Do not discuss your religious or spiritual beliefs with patients or their families or make recommendations.

  Take the time to sort out your own feelings about death. If you are not comfortable with the topic, patients will feel it. Speak to the nurse if you need resources to help you deal with your feelings.

Advance Directives and Related Medical Orders

Advance directives and medical orders were first introduced in Chapter 2. Advance directives allow people to choose what medical care they want or do not want if they cannot make those decisions themselves. A DNR order tells healthcare workers not to perform CPR. DNR orders may be issued for a person who has a terminal illness, someone who almost certainly will not be saved by CPR, a person who is not expected to live long, and/or a person who does not want to interfere with natural processes.

If a patient has an advance directive in place, the PCT may be asked to continue to monitor vital signs, such as temperature, pulse, respirations, and blood pressure, and to report the readings to the nurse. Comfort measures, such as pain medication, will continue to be used. However, depending on what the advance directive states, performing CPR or any extraordinary measures may be prohibited, no matter how the vital signs have changed or declined.

Extraordinary measures are measures used to prolong life when there is no reasonable expectation of recovery. When a person with a DNR order stops breathing or the heart stops, she will die unless the heart or breathing restarts on its own. This is not likely to happen. By law, advance directives must be honored. PCTs must respect each patient's decisions about advance directives.

4. Explain common signs of approaching death

Death can be sudden or gradual. Certain physical changes occur that can be signs and symptoms of approaching death. Vital signs and skin color are often affected. Disorientation, confusion, and reduced responsiveness may occur. Vision, taste, and touch usually diminish. However, hearing is often present until death occurs.

Common signs of approaching death include the following:

- Blurred and failing vision
- Unfocused eyes
- Impaired speech
- Diminished sense of touch
- Loss of movement, muscle tone, and feeling
- A rising or below-normal body temperature
- Decreasing blood pressure
- Weak pulse that is abnormally slow or rapid
- Alternating periods of slow, irregular respirations and rapid, shallow respirations, along with short periods of apnea, called *Cheyne-Stokes* respirations
- A rattling or gurgling sound as the person breathes
- Cold, pale skin
- Mottling (bruised appearance), spotting, or blotching of skin caused by poor circulation
- Perspiration
- Incontinence (both urine and stool)
- Disorientation or confusion

5. List changes that may occur in the human body after death

When death occurs, the body will not have a heartbeat, pulse, respiration, or blood pressure. The eyelids may remain open or partially open with the eyes in a fixed stare. The mouth may remain open. The body may be incontinent of urine and stool. Between 2 to 6 hours after death, the muscles in the body become stiff and rigid. This is a temporary condition called ***rigor mortis***, which is Latin for *stiffness of death*. Though these things are a normal part of death, they can be frightening. The PCT should inform the nurse immediately to help confirm the death. A provider will officially certify the death.

6. Describe postmortem care

Postmortem care is care of the body after death. It takes place after the patient has been declared dead. It is important for PCTs to be sensitive to the needs of the family and friends after death. Family members may wish to sit by the bed to say goodbye. They may wish to stay with the body for a while. They should be allowed to do these things. PCTs should be aware of religious and cultural practices that the family may want to observe. Not touching the body for a certain time after death and having a family member bathe the patient's body are examples. Facilities have different policies about postmortem care. PCTs should follow their facility's policies and only perform assigned tasks.

Guidelines: Postmortem Care

G After death, the muscles in the body become stiff and rigid. This may make the body difficult to move. Talk to the nurse if you need help performing postmortem care.

G Be sure to follow Standard Precautions and any ordered Transmission-Based Precautions.

G Respect any requests from the family about personal, cultural, or religious practices. If you have a question about a request, talk to the nurse. If family members have questions about how or why postmortem care is given, refer them to the nurse. Do not continue with care if the family objects.

G If instructed to do so, put dentures back in the mouth and close the mouth. You may need to place a rolled towel under the chin to support the closed mouth position. If this is not possible, place dentures in a denture cup near the patient's head.

G Follow facility policy about personal items. Check to see if you should remove jewelry. Always have a witness if personal items are removed or given to a family member. Document what was given and to whom.

G When the body is gone, strip the bed.

G Tidy the area, and open windows to air the room if part of facility policy.

Performing postmortem care

Equipment: 2 pairs of gloves, drainage pads, shroud kit or sheets, identification tag(s), clean gown, washcloths or wipes, wash basin of warm water, mild soap, towel

1. Identify the patient according to facility policy.
2. Wash your hands.
3. Explain the procedure to the patient's family and ask them to step outside. Be courteous and respectful.
4. Provide for the patient's privacy with a curtain, screen, or door.
5. Adjust the bed to a safe level, usually waist high. Lock the bed wheels.
6. Be gentle with the body throughout the process. Treat the body with respect.
7. Put on gloves.
8. Turn off equipment such as oxygen or suction if directed by the nurse. Do not remove any tubes or other equipment unless you are directed to do so. A nurse or someone at the funeral home usually performs these tasks. You may be directed to cut the tubes to a length of 1" and tape them in place.
9. Gently close the eyes.
10. Position the body in proper alignment, on the back with legs straight. Fold the arms across the abdomen.
11. Gently close the mouth. Place a rolled towel under the chin.
12. Gently bathe the body, using mild soap if directed to do so.
13. Comb or brush the patient's hair carefully.
14. Place drainage pads where needed. Most often this is under the head and/or under the perineal area and buttocks.
15. Put a clean gown on the body.
16. Place a sheet over the body, leaving the face and head uncovered.
17. Remove and discard all used supplies. Place used linen in the proper container. Tidy the area around the bed.
18. Follow facility policy for any personal items.
19. Remove and discard your gloves. Wash your hands.
20. Return the bed to its lowest position. Remove privacy measures. Turn the lights down and let the family know they can return to spend time with the patient. Leave the room so they can have privacy.

21. When the family leaves, return and put on clean gloves.
22. Place a shroud on the patient and follow instructions for completing ID tags. The shroud may be a standard sheet or may be part of a kit for postmortem care. Follow facility policy for placement over the body. Tags may be placed both under the shroud (usually on the large toe) and outside the shroud. If the patient died of a communicable illness, follow facility procedure for noting this on the tags.
23. Remove and discard your gloves. Wash your hands.
24. Document the procedure using facility guidelines.

Organ Donation

Organ donation is the removal of organs and tissues for the purpose of transplanting into someone who needs them. Organ donors can be people who have recently died or living people. If a patient has designated himself an organ donor after death, specific policies and procedures will need to be followed. Some organs must be taken from the body very soon after a person dies. PCTs should follow the nurse's instructions regarding special preparations.

Connected Care

Acknowledging Grief

It is normal for a PCT to feel grief after the death of a patient. If a PCT needs resources to help deal with their feelings, they should speak to the nurse. Care team members can also help each other. If coworkers notice that a team member may need help dealing with their grief, they should notify the nurse. There are also online and in-person support groups for healthcare workers dealing with grief.

Chapter Review

1. Describe one behavior that a PCT might see at each stage of grief.
2. Describe 5 possible feelings/responses in the grief process.
3. In what setting(s) does hospice care take place?
4. What is the focus in palliative care? Is palliative care only for patients who are close to death?
5. Give 3 examples of how a PCT can promote dignity and independence for a patient receiving hospice care.
6. How might a PCT being aware of their own feelings about death help make the PCT a better caregiver?
7. Which sense is usually present until death occurs?
8. What are some of the ways that a PCT might provide emotional and spiritual support for a patient who is dying?
9. What measures may help a patient who is dying and in pain?
10. List 10 common signs of approaching death.
11. List 5 changes that may occur in the human body after death.
12. What is postmortem care?
13. What should the PCT do with valuable personal items in the room or on the patient's body after he has died?
14. Where are drainage pads most often needed during postmortem care?

Abbreviations

ā	before
abd	abdomen
ABR	absolute bedrest
ac, a.c.	before meals
ad lib	as desired
ADLs	activities of daily living
adm.	admission
AED	automated external defibrillator
AFib	atrial fibrillation
AIDS	acquired immunodeficiency syndrome
AIIR	airborne infection isolation room
AMA	against medical advice
amb	ambulate, ambulatory
amt	amount
ant	anterior
ap	apical
AROM	active range of motion
ASAP	as soon as possible
as tol	as tolerated
A, T, D	admission, transfer, and discharge
ax.	axillary (armpit)
BID, b.i.d.	2 times a day
BM	bowel movement
BP, B/P	blood pressure
BPM	beats per minute
BR	bedrest
BRP	bathroom privileges
BSC	bedside commode
bx	biopsy
c̄	with
C	Celsius
CA	cancer
CAD	coronary artery disease
cath.	catheter
CBC	complete blood count
CBR	complete bedrest
CCU	cardiac care unit, cardiovascular care unit
CDC	Centers for Disease Control and Prevention
C. diff	*Clostridioides difficile*
CHF	congestive heart failure
ck, ✓	check
cl liq	clear liquid
CMS	Centers for Medicare & Medicaid Services
CNA	certified nursing assistant
CNP	certified nurse practitioner
CNS	central nervous system
c/o	complains of
COPD	chronic obstructive pulmonary disease
CPM	continuous passive motion
CPR	cardiopulmonary resuscitation
CS	Central Supply
CV	cardiovascular
CVA	cerebrovascular accident, stroke
CVP	central venous pressure
CXR	chest X-ray
DAT	diet as tolerated
DM	diabetes mellitus
DNR	do not resuscitate
DO	doctor of osteopathy
DOA	dead on arrival
DOB	date of birth
DON	director of nursing
Dr., DR	doctor
DRE	digital rectal exam
drsg	dressing
DVT	deep vein thrombosis
Dx, dx	diagnosis
ECG, EKG	electrocardiogram
ECHO	echocardiogram
ED	emergency department
EEG	electroencephalogram
EMS	emergency medical services
ENT	ears, nose, throat

ER	emergency room
ETOH	alcohol
exam	examination
F	Fahrenheit
FBS	fasting blood sugar
FS	finger stick
FSBS	fingerstick blood sugar
ft	foot
F/U, f/u	follow-up
FUO	fever of unknown origin
FWB	full weight-bearing
fx	fracture
FYI	for your information
g	gram
GB	gallbladder
GE	gastroenterology
GI	gastrointestinal
GP	general practitioner
GSW	gunshot wound
GYN, gyn	gynecology
H_2O	water
h, hr, hr.	hour
H/A, HA	headache
HBV	hepatitis B virus
HIPAA	Health Insurance Portability and Accountability Act
HIV	human immunodeficiency virus
HOB	head of bed
ht	height
HTN	hypertension
Hx	history
hyper	above normal, too fast, rapid
hypo	low, less than normal
ICU	intensive care unit
inc	incontinent
inf	inferior
I&O	intake and output
isol	isolation
IV, I.V.	intravenous (within a vein)
K	potassium
kg	kilogram
L	liter
L, lt	left
lab	laboratory
lb.	pound
L&D	labor and delivery
LE	lower extremity
lg	large
LOC	level of consciousness
LPN	licensed practical nurse
LTC	long-term care
LTCF	long-term care facility
LVN	licensed vocational nurse
MD, M.D.	doctor of medicine
MDRO	multidrug-resistant organism
meds	medications
med/surg	medical/surgical unit
mg	milligram
MI	myocardial infarction
min	minute
mL	milliliter
mm	millimeter
MMGM	mammogram
mm Hg	millimeters of mercury
mod	moderate
MRI	magnetic resonance imaging
MRSA	methicillin-resistant *Staphylococcus aureus*
MSW	medical social worker
MVA	motor vehicle accident
NA	nursing assistant
N/A	not applicable
N/C	no complaints, no call
neg	negative
neur.	neurology
NG, ng	nasogastric
NICU	neonatal intensive care unit
NKA	no known allergies
NKDA	no known drug allergies
NPO	nothing by mouth
NSR	normal sinus rhythm
NVD	nausea, vomiting, and diarrhea

Abbreviation	Meaning
NWB	non-weight-bearing
O_2	oxygen
OB	obstetrics
OB/GYN	obstetrics and gynecology
Obs	observation
OOB	out of bed
OPD	outpatient department
OR	operating room
ord.	ordered
ortho	orthopedics
OSHA	Occupational Safety and Health Administration
OT	occupational therapist/therapy
oz	ounce
$\bar{p}$	after
PA	physician assistant
PACU	postanesthesia care unit
PAD	peripheral artery disease
pc, p.c.	after meals
PCA	patient-controlled analgesia
PE	pulmonary embolism
ped, peds	pediatrics
PEG	percutaneous endoscopic gastrostomy
peri care	perineal care
PET	positron emission tomography
pharm	pharmacy
PHI	protected health information
P&N	psychiatry and neurology
PNS	peripheral nervous system
PO	by mouth
pos.	positive
post-op	after surgery
PPE	personal protective equipment
pre-op	before surgery
p.r.n., prn	when necessary
PROM	passive range of motion
psych.	psychiatry
pt	patient
PT	physical therapist, physical therapy
PVD	peripheral vascular disease
PWB	partial weight-bearing
$\bar{q}$	every
q2h	every 2 hours
q3h	every 3 hours
q4h	every 4 hours
qh, qhr	every hour
R	respirations, rectal
R, rt.	right
RBC	red blood cell, red blood count
RDT	registered dietitian
reg.	regular
rehab	rehabilitation
req.	requisition
resp.	respiration
RF	restrict fluids
RN	registered nurse
R/O	rule out
ROM	range of motion
RR	respiratory rate
RT	respiratory therapist, respiratory therapy
Rx	prescription, treatment
$\bar{s}$	without
SCA	sudden cardiac arrest
SCD	sequential compression device
SDS	safety data sheet
SLP	speech-language pathologist
SNF	skilled nursing facility
SOB	shortness of breath
SP	Standard Precautions
spec.	specimen
S&S, S/S	signs and symptoms
SSE	soapsuds enema
staph	*staphylococcus*
stat, STAT	immediately
std. prec.	Standard Precautions
STI	sexually transmitted infection
strep	*streptococcus*

surg.	surgery
T., temp	temperature
TB	tuberculosis
TBI	traumatic brain injury
T, C, DB	turn, cough, and deep breathe
TDWB	touch-down weight-bearing
TIA	transient ischemic attack
t.i.d., tid	3 times a day
TPN	total parenteral nutrition
TPR	temperature, pulse, and respiration
TTWB	toe-touch weight-bearing
TWE	tap water enema
U/A, u/a	urinalysis
U/C	urine culture
UE	upper extremity
UGI	upper gastrointestinal
URI	upper respiratory infection
urol.	urology
US	ultrasound
UTI	urinary tract infection
VRE	vancomycin-resistant *Enterococcus*
VS, vs	vital signs
VT	ventricular tachycardia
WBC	white blood cell, white blood count
w/c, W/C	wheelchair
WNL	within normal limits
wt.	weight
yo	years old

Symbols

©	copyright
☣	biohazard
△	change, heat
°	degree
♀	female
♂	male
%	percent
☢	radiation

Appendix

Abbreviations are useful but can be misunderstood. Misread abbreviations can cause dangerous errors in care. Because of this, in 2004 the Joint Commission created an official *Do Not Use* list. This list contains abbreviations that should never be used because they may not be clear. The Joint Commission requires that facilities have policies about the use of standardized abbreviations. These policies must reflect the Joint Commission's *Do Not Use* list. They may include additional abbreviations that staff should not use. Healthcare workers should follow their facility's policies.

Official "Do Not Use" List		
Do Not Use	**Potential Problem**	**Use Instead**
U, u (unit)	Mistaken for "0" (zero), the number "4" (four) or "cc"	Write "unit"
IU (International Unit)	Mistaken for "0" (zero), the number "4" (four) or "cc"	Write "International Unit"
Q.D., QD, q.d., qd (daily) Q.O.D., QOD, q.o.d, qod (every other day)	Mistaken for each other Period after the Q mistaken for "I" and the "O" mistaken for "I"	Write "daily" Write "every other day"
Trailing zero (X.0 mg)* Lack of leading zero (.X mg)	Decimal point is missed	Write X mg Write 0.X mg
MS MSO_4 and $MgSO_4$	Can mean morphine sulfate or magnesium sulfate Confused for one another	Write "morphine sulfate" Write "magnesium sulfate"

*Exception: A "trailing zero" may be used only where required to demonstrate the level of precision of the value being reported, such as for laboratory results, imaging studies that report size of lesions, or catheter/tube sizes. It may not be used in medication orders or other medication-related documentation. *(The Joint Commission, 2023 https://www.jointcommission.org/resources/news-and-multimedia/fact-sheets/facts-about-do-not-use-list/ accessed 10/12/23.)*

Glossary

12-lead EKG: a common type of EKG that records the electrical activity of the heart in 12 different directions (leads).

24-hour urine specimen: urine specimen consisting of all urine voided in a 24-hour period.

abdominal thrusts: a method of attempting to remove an object from the airway of someone who is choking.

abduction: moving a body part away from the midline of the body.

abortion: termination of a pregnancy.

absorption: the transfer of nutrients from the intestines to the cells.

abuse: purposeful mistreatment that causes physical, mental, or emotional pain or injury to a person.

active assisted range of motion (AAROM): exercises to put a joint through its full arc of motion that are performed by the affected person with some help from another person.

active range of motion (AROM): exercises to put a joint through its full arc of motion that are performed by the affected person alone, without help.

adduction: moving a body part toward the midline of the body.

advance directive: a legal document that allows people to decide what medical care they wish to have in the event they are unable to make those decisions themselves.

aerosolize: to disperse a substance through the air in such a way that it might be inhaled.

affected: term used to refer to the weaker side of the body after a stroke or injury; also called *involved*.

age-related macular degeneration (AMD): a condition in which the macula (part of the retina) gradually deteriorates, causing vision loss and problems such as the inability to recognize faces, drive, read, and write.

AIDS (acquired immunodeficiency syndrome): the final stage of HIV infection, in which infections, tumors, and central nervous system symptoms appear due to a weakened immune system that is unable to fight infection.

Alzheimer's disease (AD): a progressive, incurable disease that causes tangled nerve fibers and protein deposits to form in the brain, which eventually cause dementia.

ambulation: the act of moving or walking, with or without an assistive device.

ambulatory: capable of moving or walking.

Americans with Disabilities Act (ADA): a federal law that prohibits discrimination because of a disability.

amputation: the surgical removal of some or all of a body part.

amyotrophic lateral sclerosis (ALS): a progressive disease that causes muscle atrophy and eventually leads to death; also called *Lou Gehrig's disease*.

anaphylaxis: a dangerous reaction to an allergen that may cause swelling of the lips, tongue, and throat that can obstruct the airway.

anatomy: the structure of a body or body part.

anemia: a condition in which the blood has too few red blood cells to supply oxygen to body tissues.

angina: chest pain, pressure, or discomfort.

antimicrobial: an agent that destroys, resists, or prevents the development of pathogens.

anxiety: uneasiness, worry, or fear, often about a situation or condition.

apical pulse: the pulse located on the left side of the chest, just below the nipple.

apnea: the absence of breathing.

arthritis: a general term that refers to inflammation of the joints, causing stiffness, pain, and decreased mobility.

artifact: in an EKG, interference or distortion that appears on a tracing.

artificial airway: any tube inserted into the respiratory tract to maintain or promote breathing.

asexual: relating to emotional or romantic partners in a nonsexual way.

aspiration: the inhalation of food, fluid, or foreign material into the lungs.

assault: the use of words or actions to cause another person to feel fearful of being harmed.

assisted living facility: residence for people who do not need 24-hour skilled care, but do require some help with daily care.

asthma: a chronic inflammatory disease that makes it difficult to breathe and causes coughing and wheezing.

atherosclerosis: a hardening and narrowing of the blood vessels.

atrophy: the wasting away, decreasing in size, and weakening of muscles from lack of use.

augmented limb leads: in an EKG, the collective name for leads aVR, aVL, and aVF.

auscultation: the act of listening to sounds within the body using a stethoscope.

autoimmune illness: an illness in which the body's immune system attacks normal tissue in the body.

automated external defibrillator (AED): a device attached to a patient to analyze heart rhythm and deliver a shock, if needed, to restore a normal heart rhythm.

baseline: in relation to vital signs, an initial value that can be compared to future measurements.

battery: the intentional touching of another person without permission.

benign prostatic hyperplasia (BPH): a disorder that can occur in men as they age, in which the prostate becomes enlarged and causes problems with urination and/or emptying the bladder.

benign tumor: a tumor that is considered noncancerous.

bias: a judgmental response, which may be positive or negative, based on assumptions or personal beliefs.

bipolar disorder: a type of mental health disorder that causes a person to swing from periods of deep depression (a depressive episode) to periods of extreme activity (a manic episode).

bisexual: having physical, emotional, and/or romantic attraction for people of the same gender or a different gender.

bladder cancer: the rapid growth of abnormal cells in the bladder.

bladder scanning: placing a handheld ultrasound device (bladder scanner) on a patient's abdomen to measure the amount of urine in a patient's bladder.

bloodborne pathogens: microorganisms found in human blood that can cause infection and disease in humans.

Bloodborne Pathogens Standard: federal law that requires that healthcare facilities protect employees from bloodborne health hazards.

blood culture: a test for the presence of bacterial or fungal pathogens in the blood.

body mass index (BMI): a measurement found by dividing a person's weight in kilograms by the square of their height in meters; may be used as a screening tool for underweight or obesity.

body mechanics: the way the parts of the body work together when a person moves.

bone: rigid connective tissue that makes up the skeleton, protects organs, and allows the body to move.

bony prominence: area of the body where the bone lies close to the skin.

brachial pulse: the pulse located inside the elbow, about 1 to 1 1/2 inches above the elbow.

bradycardia: slow heart rate—under 60 beats per minute.

bradypnea: slow respirations.

breast cancer: the rapid growth of abnormal cells in one or both breasts.

bronchiectasis: a condition in which the bronchial tubes are abnormally enlarged, causing chronic coughing, thick sputum, recurrent pneumonia, and weight loss.

bronchitis: an irritation and inflammation of the lining of the bronchi.

cancer: general term to describe a disease in which abnormal cells grow in an uncontrolled way.

capillaries: tiny blood vessels that carry oxygen and nutrients to and remove carbon dioxide and wastes from cells throughout the body.

cardiac conduction system: the pathway of electrical impulses that controls the heart's pumping action.

cardiopulmonary resuscitation (CPR): medical procedures used when a person's heart or lungs have stopped working.

carotid pulse: the pulse located on the side of the neck, just below the jaw.

cataract: a condition in which cloudy spots develop in the lens of the eye, causing vision loss.

catheter: a thin tube inserted into the body to drain or inject fluids.

catheter-associated urinary tract infection (CAUTI): an infection that occurs in the urethra, bladder, ureter, or kidney when bacteria travels up a catheter.

causative agent: a pathogenic microorganism that causes disease.

cell: basic structural unit of the body that divides, develops, and dies, renewing tissues and organs.

cellulitis: a bacterial infection affecting the skin and soft tissue.

Centers for Disease Control and Prevention (CDC): a federal government agency that issues guidelines to protect and improve the health and safety of individuals and communities.

Centers for Medicare & Medicaid Services (CMS): a federal agency within the US Department of Health and Human Services that is responsible for Medicare and Medicaid, among many other responsibilities.

central nervous system (CNS): the part of the nervous system that is composed of the brain and spinal cord.

cerebrovascular accident (CVA): a condition that occurs when blood supply to a part of the brain is blocked or a blood vessel leaks or ruptures within the brain; also called *stroke*.

certified nurse-midwife (CNM): healthcare professional with graduate-level training in providing gynecological, prenatal, and postpartum care.

cervical cancer: the rapid growth of abnormal cells in the cervix.

chain of command: the line of authority within a facility.

chain of custody: documentation of the exact path an item (e.g., a blood specimen) takes from its origin to its destination; provides legal proof that the item is not changed or tampered with.

chain of infection: a way of describing how disease is transmitted from one human being to another.

chancres: open sores.

charting: documenting information and observations about patients.

chemical dependency: a disease related to substance use in which a person needs greater amounts of a drug to get the same effect and has symptoms when the drug is stopped (withdrawal).

chest tube: a hollow drainage tube that is inserted into the chest to drain air, blood or other fluid, or pus that has collected inside the pleural cavity.

Cheyne-Stokes: alternating periods of slow, irregular breathing and rapid, shallow respirations, along with periods of apnea.

chlamydia: a sexually transmitted infection that is caused by organisms introduced into the mucous membranes of the reproductive tract.

chronic obstructive pulmonary disease (COPD): a chronic, progressive, and incurable lung disease that causes difficulty breathing, weakness, and a high risk of lung infections.

chronic renal failure (CRF): a condition that occurs when the kidneys cannot eliminate certain waste products from the body; also called *chronic kidney failure.*

circadian rhythm: the 24-hour day-night cycle.

civil law: branch of law dealing with disputes between individuals.

clean: in health care, a condition in which an object has not been contaminated with pathogens.

clean-catch specimen: a urine specimen that does not include the first and last urine voided; also called *midstream specimen.*

Clinical and Laboratory Standards Institute (CLSI): a not-for-profit organization that develops standards of practice for medical testing.

Clinical Laboratory Improvement Amendments (CLIA): federal regulations regarding the staffing and operation of clinical laboratories.

closed fracture: a broken bone that does not break the skin.

***Clostridioides difficile* (*C. diff, C. difficile*):** a bacterium that is spread by spores in feces; it causes symptoms such as diarrhea and nausea and can lead to serious inflammation of the colon (colitis).

coagulation: the process of blood clotting.

code team: a team of healthcare workers who provide care in a medical emergency.

cognitive: related to thinking and learning.

cognitive behavioral therapy (CBT): a type of psychotherapy that is often used to treat anxiety disorders and depression and focuses on skills and solutions that a person can use to modify negative thinking and behavior patterns.

colorectal cancer: cancer of the gastrointestinal tract; also known as *colon cancer.*

colostomy: surgically created opening into the large intestine to allow stool to be expelled.

communication: the process of exchanging information with others by sending and receiving messages.

compassionate: being caring, concerned, considerate, empathetic, and understanding.

condom catheter: a type of urinary catheter that has an attachment on the end that fits onto the penis; also called an *external* or *Texas catheter.*

confidential: private.

congenital hypothyroidism: a form of hypothyroidism that affects infants and children that can stunt growth and development and cause intellectual deficits.

congestive heart failure (CHF): a condition in which the heart muscle is damaged and is no longer able to pump effectively; causes blood to back up in various parts of the body.

conscientious: guided by a sense of right and wrong; principled.

conscious: the state of being mentally alert and having awareness of surroundings, sensations, and thoughts.

constipation: the inability to eliminate stool, or the infrequent, difficult, and often painful elimination of hard, dry stool.

constrict: to narrow.

continuing education (CE): in health care, education that keeps healthcare workers up-to-date on changes that affect their jobs.

contracture: the permanent and often painful shortening of a muscle or tendon, usually due to a lack of activity.

controlled medication: a drug that is considered to have the potential for abuse, such as strong painkillers.

COVID-19 (coronavirus disease): a droplet and airborne disease transmitted through droplets and particles produced by an infected person; often characterized by respiratory symptoms and capable of progressing to severe symptoms, even death.

criminal law: branch of law dealing with offenses considered to harm all of society.

Crohn's disease: an inflammatory disease that can affect any part of the digestive tract, but most commonly affects the small intestine.

culture: a system of learned beliefs and behaviors practiced by a group of people.

cyanotic: having blue or gray skin color.

dangle: to sit up with the legs hanging over the side of the bed in order to regain balance and stabilize blood pressure.

debridement: a process of treating wounds that involves removing infected or necrotic tissue.

deep vein thrombosis (DVT): a condition in which a blood clot forms deep under the skin, usually in the legs.

dehydration: a serious condition resulting from an inadequate amount of fluid in the body.

delegation: transferring responsibility to a person for a specific task.

delusion: a persistent false belief.

dementia: a general term that refers to a serious, progressive loss of mental abilities such as thinking, remembering, reasoning, and communicating.

dentures: artificial teeth.

depression: a type of depressive disorder that causes pain, fatigue, apathy, sadness, irritability, anxiety, sleeplessness, and loss of appetite, as well as other symptoms; also called *major depressive disorder* or *clinical depression.*

developmental disabilities: disabilities that are present at birth or emerge during childhood, up to age 22, that restrict physical and/or mental ability.

diabetes: a condition in which the pancreas produces no insulin, too little insulin, or does not properly use insulin.

diabetic ketoacidosis (DKA): a complication of diabetes that is caused by having too little insulin in the body.

diabetic retinopathy: a complication of diabetes caused by damage to the retina; causes spots, blurred vision, and difficulty seeing well at night and may lead to blindness.

dialysis: an artificial means of removing the body's waste products when the kidneys are no longer able to function properly.

diarrhea: the frequent elimination of liquid or semiliquid feces.

diastole: phase when the heart relaxes or rests.

diastolic: the second measurement of blood pressure; phase when the heart relaxes or rests.

digestion: the process of preparing food physically and chemically so that it can be absorbed into the cells.

dilate: to widen.

direct contact: a way of transmitting pathogens through touching the infected person or their secretions.

dirty: in health care, a condition in which objects have been contaminated with pathogens.

disinfection: a process that destroys most, but not all, pathogens; it reduces the pathogen count to a level that is considered not infectious.

disposable: to be used only once and then discarded.

diversion: stealing medications prescribed for a patient for the purpose of personal use or sale to another person.

diversity: a term used to describe the variety found among people.

diverticulitis: a condition that occurs when diverticula in the colon become inflamed, causing fever, abdominal pain, tenderness, nausea, vomiting, and diarrhea.

diverticulosis: a condition in which small pouches called *diverticula* form in the colon.

doff: to remove.

don: to put on.

do not intubate (DNI): a type of advance directive indicating that the patient does not wish a breathing tube to be inserted to prolong life.

do not resuscitate (DNR): a type of advance directive indicating that the patient does not wish cardiopulmonary resuscitation (CPR) to be performed in the event of cardiac or respiratory arrest.

dorsiflexion: bending backward.

draw sheet: an extra sheet placed on top of the bottom sheet on a bed that is used for moving patients without causing shearing.

drug interaction: a situation in which a drug, vitamin, dietary supplement, herbal medication, food, beverage, or health condition affects how a drug works in a person's body.

durable power of attorney for health care: a type of advance directive designating a person other than the patient to make medical decisions if the person becomes ill or disabled.

dysphagia: difficulty swallowing.

dyspnea: difficulty breathing.

dysrhythmia: abnormal heart rhythm; also called *arrhythmia*.

edema: swelling caused by excess fluid in body tissues.

electrode: in health care, a pad that conducts electricity and is connected to the patient's body to conduct electrical signals from the body to a machine (e.g., an EKG machine) that interprets the signals.

electronic health record (EHR): an electronic version of a patient's medical record that can be shared between healthcare organizations.

electronic medical record (EMR): an electronic version of a patient's medical record that is used by a single healthcare facility.

elimination: the process of expelling wastes (made up of the waste products of food and fluids) that are not absorbed into the cells.

embolism: an obstruction of a blood vessel, usually by a blood clot.

emergency department (ED): department in a hospital that provides immediate medical care 24 hours a day, 7 days a week, for serious illnesses or injuries.

Emergency Medical Treatment and Labor Act (EMTALA): a federal law that requires hospitals to provide necessary emergency medical treatment to patients even if they cannot pay.

emesis: the act of vomiting, or ejecting stomach contents through the mouth and/or nose.

empathy: identifying with the feelings of others.

emphysema: a chronic disease of the lungs that usually results from cigarette smoking.

endometriosis: a condition that causes endometrial tissue to grow on the outer surface of the uterus.

enema: specific amount of water, with or without an additive, that is introduced into the colon to stimulate the elimination of stool.

engineering controls: features of medical devices that make their use less hazardous.

epilepsy: a brain disorder that results from a disruption in normal electrical impulses in the brain, which causes repeated seizures.

epistaxis: a nosebleed.

ergonomics: the science of designing equipment, areas, and work tasks to make them safer and to suit the worker's abilities.

ethanol: the intoxicating ingredient in alcoholic beverages.

ethics: the knowledge of right and wrong.

ethnicity: one aspect of a person's identity, often reflecting a combination of race, culture, nationality, language, and other factors.

eupnea: normal respirations.

expiration: the process of exhaling air out of the lungs.

exploitation: the act of taking advantage of a person for personal gain.

exposure control plan: a plan designed to eliminate or reduce employee exposure to infectious material.

extension: straightening a body part.

fasting: in medicine, the requirement to not eat or drink anything but water for a specified amount of time, usually 8–12 hours, before a test or procedure.

fecal impaction: hard stool that is stuck in the rectum and cannot be expelled.

fecal incontinence: the inability to control the bowels, leading to an involuntary passage of stool.

first aid: emergency care given immediately to an injured person by the first people to respond to an emergency.

flammable: easily ignited and capable of burning quickly.

flexion: bending a body part.

fluid balance: taking in and eliminating equal amounts of fluid.

fluid overload: a condition that occurs when the body cannot handle the amount of fluid consumed.

foot drop: a weakness of muscles in the feet and ankles that causes difficulty with the ability to flex the ankles and walk normally.

Fowler's: semisitting body position, in which a patient's head and shoulders are elevated 45 to 60 degrees.

fracture pan: a bedpan that is flatter than a regular bedpan.

fungus: a type of living organism that can sometimes cause infection; *Candida* is a common example.

gastroesophageal reflux disease (GERD): a chronic condition in which the liquid contents of the stomach back up into the esophagus.

gastrostomy: a surgically created opening into the stomach that allows insertion of a tube.

gauge: measurement of the size of a needle; higher gauge numbers correspond to thinner needles.

gay: having physical, emotional, and/or romantic attraction for people of the same gender.

gender identity: a deeply felt sense of one's gender.

generalized anxiety disorder (GAD): an anxiety disorder that is characterized by chronic anxiety and worry, even when there is no reason for concern.

Genetic Information Nondiscrimination Act (GINA): a federal law banning discrimination in employment and healthcare coverage based on genetic information.

genital herpes: an incurable type of sexually transmitted infection that is caused by herpes simplex viruses type 1 (HSV-1) or type 2 (HSV-2); causes painful sores on the genitals.

genital HPV infection: a sexually transmitted infection caused by human papillomavirus (HPV).

gestational diabetes: a type of diabetes that appears in pregnant women who have never had diabetes before but who have high glucose levels during pregnancy.

gland: an organ that produces and secretes chemicals called hormones.

glaucoma: a disease in which increased pressure inside the eye causes damage that often leads to vision loss and blindness.

glucose: natural sugar.

gonads: sex glands.

gonorrhea: a sexually transmitted infection caused by bacteria; if left untreated, it can cause blindness, joint infection, sterility, and pelvic inflammatory disease.

Graves' disease: an autoimmune disorder that often causes hyperthyroidism.

grief: deep distress or sorrow over a loss.

grooming: practices to care for oneself, such as caring for fingernails and hair.

hallucination: a false or distorted sensory perception.

hand hygiene: washing hands with soap and water or using an alcohol-based hand sanitizer.

Hashimoto's thyroiditis: an autoimmune disorder that often causes hypothyroidism.

hat: in health care, a plastic collection container that can be inserted into a toilet bowl to collect and measure urine or stool.

healthcare-associated infection (HAI): an infection acquired in a healthcare setting during the delivery of medical care.

Health Insurance Portability and Accountability Act (HIPAA): a federal law that requires health information be kept private and secure and that organizations take special steps to protect this information.

heartburn: a condition that results from a weakening of the sphincter muscle that joins the esophagus and the stomach and causes a burning sensation in the esophagus.

hematoma: injury caused by leaked blood beneath the skin.

hemorrhoid: an enlarged vein in the rectum or outside the anus that can cause rectal itching, burning, pain, and bleeding.

hepatitis: inflammation of the liver caused by certain viruses and other factors, such as alcohol abuse, some medications, and trauma.

HIV (human immunodeficiency virus): a virus that weakens the body's immune system so the body cannot effectively fight infections; eventually can cause AIDS.

holistic care: a type of care that involves caring for the whole person—including the person's physical, psychological, social, and spiritual needs.

home health care: health care that is provided in a person's home.

homeostasis: the condition in which all of the body's systems are balanced and are working together to maintain internal stability.

homophobia: prejudiced speech or actions toward LGBTQ people.

hormone: a chemical substance created by the body that controls a body function.

hospice care: holistic, compassionate, and person-centered care given to people who are dying and their families.

Hospital Consumer Assessment of Healthcare Providers and Systems (HCAHPS): a survey used to collect data about patients' experiences in hospitals.

hydrate: to absorb enough water or other fluid.

hydrocele: a condition in which fluid accumulates in the membrane around the testes.

hydrocephalus: abnormal accumulation of fluid in the head.

hygiene: practices that keep bodies clean and healthy.

hypertension (HTN): high blood pressure, regularly measuring 130/80 mm Hg or higher.

hyperthyroidism: a condition in which the thyroid produces too much thyroid hormone, causing body processes to speed up, resulting in rapid heartbeat, sweating, weight loss, and nervousness.

hypoglycemia: a complication of diabetes that can result from either too much insulin or too little food; also known as *insulin reaction*.

hypotension: low blood pressure, measuring 90/60 mm Hg or lower.

hypothyroidism: a condition in which the body lacks thyroid hormone, causing the body processes to slow down and resulting in fatigue, weight gain, constipation, and intolerance to cold.

hypoxia: inadequate (not enough) oxygen supply to the tissues of the body.

iatrogenic anemia: a type of anemia caused by removing too much of a patient's blood (e.g., by phlebotomy); especially common in infants and patients in intensive care units.

ileostomy: a surgically created opening into the end of the small intestine to allow stool to be expelled.

incident: an accident, problem, or unexpected event during the course of care that is not part of the normal routine in a healthcare facility.

incontinence: the inability to control the bladder or bowels.

indirect contact: a way of transmitting pathogens from touching an object contaminated by the infected person.

indwelling catheter: a type of urinary catheter that remains inside the bladder for a period of time; also called *Foley catheter*.

infection: the state resulting from pathogens invading the body and multiplying.

infection prevention: the set of methods practiced in healthcare facilities to prevent and control the spread of disease.

infectious: contagious.

inflammatory bowel disease (IBD): a condition in which the bowel is chronically inflamed.

influenza: a respiratory illness caused by a virus; common in the fall and winter months.

input: the fluid a person consumes; also called *intake*.

insomnia: the inability to fall asleep or remain asleep.

inspiration: the process of inhaling air into the lungs.

insulin: a hormone that works to move glucose from the blood and into the cells for energy for the body.

intake: the fluid a person consumes; also called *input*.

integument: a natural protective covering.

intensive care unit (ICU): unit in a hospital that provides care to patients who are critically ill and require constant skilled care.

intravenous therapy: the delivery of medication, nutrition, or fluids through a patient's vein; also called *IV therapy*.

intubation: the passage of a plastic tube through the mouth, nose, or opening in the neck and into the trachea.

involved: term used to refer to the weaker side of the body after a stroke or injury; also called *affected*.

irritable bowel syndrome (IBS): a condition that causes diarrhea, constipation, or both on a regular basis.

isolate: to keep something separate, or by itself.

jaundice: an excess of bilirubin in the blood.

joint: the place at which two bones meet.

Joint Commission: an independent, not-for-profit organization that evaluates and accredits healthcare organizations.

kidney stones: stones that form when urine crystallizes in the kidneys, which can block the kidneys and ureters, causing severe pain; also called *renal calculi*.

labor: the body's preparation for childbirth.

labor and delivery unit: unit in a hospital for patients who are giving birth.

latent TB infection (LTBI): a type of tuberculosis in which the person carries the disease but does not show symptoms and cannot infect others.

lateral: a body position in which a patient is lying on either side.

law: a rule set by the government to help people live peacefully together and to ensure order and safety.

lead: in an EKG, a "view" of the heart based on electrical activity measured by electrodes attached to the patient.

lesbian: a woman whose physical, emotional, and/or romantic attraction is for other women.

leukemia: a type of cancer in which the body's bone marrow produces defective white blood cells that are unable to fight disease.

liability: a legal term that means someone can be held responsible for harming someone else.

limb leads: in an EKG, the lead group made up of leads I, II, and III; also known as the *bipolar leads*.

living will: a document that outlines the medical care a person wants, or does not want, in case the person becomes unable to make those decisions.

localized infection: an infection that is limited to a specific location in the body and has local symptoms.

logrolling: moving a person as a unit without disturbing the alignment of the body.

long-term care (LTC): care given in long-term care facilities for people who need 24-hour skilled care.

lung cancer: the growth of abnormal cells or tumors in the lungs.

lupus: a chronic autoimmune disease in which the body attacks its own healthy tissues.

lymph: a clear yellowish fluid that carries disease-fighting cells called lymphocytes.

lymphedema: an abnormal buildup of lymph fluid in the body's tissues.

lymphoma: cancer of the lymphatic system; Hodgkin's and non-Hodgkin's lymphoma are two types.

major depressive disorder: a type of depressive disorder that causes pain, fatigue, apathy, sadness, irritability, anxiety, sleeplessness, and loss of appetite, as well as other symptoms; also called *depression* or *clinical depression*.

malaise: a general sense of feeling unwell.

malignant tumor: tumor that is cancerous.

mammogram: X-ray of the breast; regularly performed to screen for breast cancer.

mandated reporter: person who is legally required to report suspected or observed abuse or neglect because they have regular contact with vulnerable populations.

mastectomy: the surgical removal of all or part of the breast and sometimes other surrounding tissue.

Mayo stand: a portable stainless steel tray and holder often used to set up a sterile field.

mechanical ventilation: the use of a machine to inflate and deflate the lungs when a patient is unable to breathe on their own.

median cubital vein: well-anchored vein in the middle of the antecubital fossa; first priority site for venipuncture.

Medicaid: a medical assistance program for people who have a low income, as well as for people with disabilities.

medical asepsis: measures used to reduce and prevent the spread of pathogens.

medical/surgical unit: unit in a hospital for patients who are admitted for surgery, testing, observation, or treatment of an illness that does not require constant, intensive care.

Medicare: a federal health insurance program for people who are 65 or older, have certain disabilities or permanent kidney failure, or are ill and cannot work.

menopause: the end of menstruation; occurs when a woman has not had a menstrual period for 12 months.

mental health: the normal functioning of emotional and intellectual abilities.

mental health disorder: a disorder that affects a person's ability to function and often causes inappropriate behavior; confusion, disorientation, agitation, and anxiety are common symptoms.

metabolism: physical and chemical processes by which substances are broken down or transformed into energy or products for use by the body.

microorganism (MO): a living thing or organism that is so small that it can be seen only under a microscope; also called *microbe*.

miscarriage: the death of an embryo or fetus before it is mature enough to survive outside the womb.

mode of transmission: the method of describing how a pathogen travels.

mononucleosis: an illness caused by the Epstein-Barr virus (EBV); symptoms include extreme fatigue, sore throat, and fever.

MRSA (methicillin-resistant *Staphylococcus aureus*): bacteria (*Staphylococcus aureus*) that have developed resistance to the antibiotic methicillin.

mucous membranes: the membranes that line body cavities that open to the outside of the body, such as the linings of the mouth, nose, eyes, rectum, and genitals.

multidrug-resistant organisms (MDROs): microorganisms, mostly bacteria, that are resistant to one or more antimicrobial agents that are commonly used for treatment.

multidrug-resistant TB (MDR-TB): type of tuberculosis caused by an organism that is resistant to medication that is used to treat TB.

multiple myeloma: cancer of the plasma cells (type of white blood cells).

multiple sclerosis (MS): a progressive disease in which the myelin sheath breaks down over time; without this protective covering, nerves cannot send messages to and from the brain in a normal way, which causes problems with balance and walking, along with many other symptoms.

muscle: group of tissue that provides movement of body parts, protection of organs, and creation of heat.

muscular dystrophy (MD): a progressive, inherited disease that causes a gradual wasting away of muscle, weakness, and deformity.

myocardial infarction (MI): a condition that occurs when the heart muscle does not receive enough oxygen because blood flow to the heart is blocked; also called *heart attack.*

nasal cannula: an oxygen delivery device that consists of a piece of plastic tubing that fits around the face and 2 prongs that fit inside the nose.

nasogastric (NG) tube: a feeding tube that is inserted through the nose into the stomach.

neglect: the failure to provide needed care that results in physical, mental, or emotional harm to a person.

negligence: actions, or the failure to act or provide the proper care, resulting in unintended injury to a patient.

neuropathy: numbness, tingling, and pain in the feet and legs.

nitroglycerin: a medication that helps to relax the walls of the coronary arteries, allowing them to open and get more blood to the heart; comes in tablet, patch, or spray form.

nonintact skin: skin that is broken by abrasions, cuts, rashes, acne, pimples, lesions, surgical incisions, or boils.

nonspecific immunity: a type of immunity that protects the body from disease in general.

nonverbal communication: communication without words.

normal sinus rhythm (NSR): cardiac rhythm produced when the electrical system of the heart is functioning normally.

NPO: abbreviation for *nothing by mouth* from the Latin *nil per os*; medical order that means a patient should not have anything to eat or drink.

nutrient: a necessary substance that provides energy, promotes growth and health, and helps regulate metabolism.

nutrition: how the body uses food to maintain health.

objective information: information based on what a person sees, hears, touches, or smells; also called *signs.*

obsessive-compulsive disorder (OCD): a mental health disorder characterized by recurring intrusive behavior or thoughts that cause anxiety or stress.

obstructed airway: a condition in which something is blocking the tube through which air enters the lungs.

Occupational Safety and Health Administration (OSHA): a federal government agency that makes rules to protect workers from hazards on the job.

occupied bed: a bed made while a person is in the bed.

open fracture: a broken bone that penetrates the skin; also known as a *compound fracture.*

opposition: touching the thumb to any other finger.

oral care: care of the mouth, teeth, and gums.

order of draw: the standard sequence in which collection tubes are filled during a blood draw.

organ: a structural unit in the body that performs a specific function.

orthopnea: shortness of breath when lying down that is relieved by sitting up.

orthostatic hypotension: a sudden drop in blood pressure that occurs when a person stands or sits up.

orthotic device: a device applied externally that helps support and align a limb and improve its functioning; also called *orthosis.*

osteoarthritis: a common type of arthritis that usually affects the hips, knees, fingers, thumbs, and spine; also called *degenerative joint disease (DJD)* or *degenerative arthritis.*

osteoporosis: a condition in which bones become porous and brittle, causing them to break easily.

ostomy: surgical creation of an opening from an area inside the body to the outside.

output: fluid that is eliminated from the body through urine, feces, vomitus, perspiration, moisture that is exhaled in the air, and wound drainage.

oxygen therapy: the administration of oxygen to increase the supply of oxygen to a person's lungs.

palliative care: care that focuses on the comfort and dignity of a person who is very sick and/or dying, rather than on curing the person.

palpate: to touch body parts to feel structures beneath the skin.

panel: in phlebotomy, a group of tests either with related analytes or related to a particular condition or organ.

panic disorder: an anxiety disorder characterized by a person having regular panic attacks or living with chronic anxiety about having another attack.

pansexual: having physical, emotional, and/or romantic attraction for another person of any sex or gender identity.

paraplegia: the loss of function of the lower body and legs.

parenteral nutrition (PN): the intravenous infusion of nutrients administered directly into the bloodstream, bypassing the digestive system.

Parkinson's disease: a progressive, incurable disease that causes a section of the brain to degenerate, affecting muscle function and causing stooped posture, shuffling gait, pill-rolling, and tremors.

partial bath: a bath given on days when a complete bed bath, tub bath, or shower is not done; includes washing the face, hands, underarms, and perineum.

passive range of motion (PROM): exercises to put a joint through its full arc of motion that are performed by a healthcare worker, without the affected person's help.

pathogen: a microorganism capable of causing infection and disease.

Patient Self-Determination Act (PSDA): a federal law requiring that facilities provide patients with information about advance directives.

pediatric unit: unit in a hospital that provides care for children from birth through adolescence.

pediculosis: an infestation of lice.

peptic ulcer: raw sore in the stomach caused by excessive acid secretion that causes pain, belching, and vomiting; also called a *gastric ulcer.*

percutaneous endoscopic gastrostomy (PEG) tube: a feeding tube that is placed into the stomach through the abdominal wall.

perineal care: care of the genital and anal area.

perineum: the genital and anal area.

peripheral nervous system (PNS): a part of the nervous system made up of the nerves that extend throughout the body.

peripheral vascular disease (PVD): a disease in which the legs, feet, arms, or hands do not have enough blood circulation due to injury or to fatty deposits in the blood vessels that harden over time; causes cold legs, feet, arms, and hands, as well as pain, swelling, and ulcers of the legs and feet.

peristalsis: involuntary contractions that move food through the gastrointestinal system.

perseverating: repeating words, phrases, questions, or actions.

personal: relating to life outside one's job, such as family, friends, and home life.

personal protective equipment (PPE): equipment that helps protect employees from serious workplace injuries or illnesses resulting from contact with workplace hazards.

person-centered care: a type of care that places the emphasis on the person needing care and the person's individuality and capabilities.

phantom limb pain: pain in a limb (or extremity) that has been amputated.

phantom sensation: warmth, itching, or tingling from a body part that has been amputated.

phenylketonuria (PKU): a rare condition that can cause brain damage if left untreated; newborns are tested for this and other metabolic disorders.

phlegm: thick mucus from the respiratory passage.

phobia: an intense, irrational fear of or anxiety about an object, place, or situation.

Physician Orders for Life-Sustaining Treatment (POLST): a medical order that specifies the treatments a person wishes to receive when he is very ill; decisions are based on conversations between the patient and his healthcare providers.

physiological needs: needs that relate to the processes and activities that keep living things alive.

physiology: how a body or body system functions.

placenta: an organ that forms inside the uterus that supplies a fetus with oxygen and nutrients and removes wastes.

placental abruption: the sudden complete or partial separation of the placenta from the uterine wall.

placenta previa: a complication of pregnancy in which the placenta implants too low in the uterus, partially or completely covering the cervical outlet.

pneumonia: a bacterial, viral, or fungal infection that causes acute inflammation in lung tissue, causing fever, chills, cough, greenish sputum, and rapid pulse.

point-of-care test: a test that can be performed at the patient's bedside; fingerstick blood glucose testing is an example.

policy: a course of action that should be taken every time a certain situation occurs.

polydipsia: excessive thirst.

polyphagia: extreme hunger.

polyuria: frequent urination.

portable commode: a chair with a toilet seat and a removable container underneath; also called *bedside commode.*

portal of entry: any body opening on an uninfected person that allows pathogens to enter.

portal of exit: any body opening on an infected person that allows pathogens to leave.

positioning: the act of helping patients into positions that promote comfort and health.

postmortem care: care of the body after death.

postoperative: after surgery.

posttraumatic stress disorder (PTSD): a disorder caused by experiencing or witnessing a traumatic experience or series of events.

posture: the way a person holds and positions their body.

precordial leads: in an EKG, the unipolar lead group composed of leads V1, V2, V3, V4, V5, and V6; also known as the *chest leads.*

prediabetes: a condition that occurs when a person's blood glucose levels are above normal but not high enough for a diagnosis of type 2 diabetes.

preeclampsia: the sudden development of hypertension in pregnancy.

prenatal care: medical care provided during pregnancy.

preoperative: before surgery.

presbycusis: age-related hearing loss.

pressure injury: injury or wound that results from skin deterioration and shearing; also called *pressure ulcer, pressure sore, bed sore,* or *decubitus ulcer.*

pressure point: area of the body that bears much of the body's weight.

preterm birth: delivery of a baby before the 37th week of pregnancy.

procedure: a method, or way, of doing something.

professional: having to do with work or a job.

professionalism: the act of behaving properly when working.

pronation: turning downward.

prone: a body position in which a patient is lying on the stomach, or front side of the body.

prostate cancer: the rapid growth of abnormal cells in the prostate.

prosthesis: a device that replaces a body part that is missing or deformed because of an accident, injury, illness, or birth defect.

protected health information (PHI): a person's private health information, which includes name, address, telephone number, social security number, email address, and medical record number.

psoriasis: a condition that causes the body to create too many skin cells that die and build up, causing itchy and painful white or red scaly patches.

psychiatric unit: unit in a hospital for patients who need acute care related to mental health.

psychosocial needs: needs that involve social interaction, emotions, intellect, and spirituality.

psychotherapy: a method of treating mental health disorders that involves talking about one's problems with a mental health professional.

pulmonary embolism (PE): a blood clot or other blockage found in the lungs.

pulse oximeter: a noninvasive device that uses a light to determine the amount of oxygen in the blood.

puree: to blend or grind food into a thick paste of baby food consistency.

purulent drainage: yellow, green, brown, or white wound drainage that may have an odor and usually contains bacteria.

quadriplegia: the loss of function in the legs, trunk, and arms.

race: grouping of people based on physical characteristics shared by those with a common ancestry.

radial pulse: the pulse located on the inside of the wrist, where the radial artery runs just beneath the skin.

range of motion (ROM): exercises that put a particular joint through its full arc of motion.

renal cell cancer: the rapid growth of abnormal cells in the kidney.

renovascular hypertension: a condition in which a blockage of arteries in the kidneys causes high blood pressure.

reproduce: to create new human life.

requisition: a paper or electronic order for testing.

reservoir: a place where a pathogen lives and multiplies.

resistant: a state in which drugs no longer work to kill specific bacteria.

respiration: the process of inhaling air into the lungs (inspiration) and exhaling air out of the lungs (expiration).

restraint: a physical or chemical way to restrict voluntary movement or behavior.

rheumatoid arthritis (RA): a type of arthritis in which joints become red, swollen, and very painful, resulting in restricted movement and possible deformities.

***rigor mortis*:** the Latin term for the temporary condition after death in which the muscles in the body become stiff and rigid.

rotation: turning a joint.

route: the path that gets a drug into the patient's body.

routine urine specimen: a urine specimen that can be collected any time a patient voids.

Safety Data Sheet (SDS): document that details the ingredients, dangers, safe handling, storage, disposal procedures, and emergency response actions for chemicals in the workplace.

sanguineous drainage: bright red blood from a new cut.

scabies: a contagious skin infection caused by a tiny mite burrowing into the skin, where it lays eggs; causes intense itching and a skin rash that may look like thin burrow tracks.

schizophrenia: a type of psychotic disorder that causes problems with thinking, communication, and the ability to manage emotions, make decisions, and understand reality.

scope of practice: the roles, responsibilities, and procedures that are within the knowledge, training, and legal definition of a profession.

sedative: an agent or drug that helps calm and soothe a person and may cause sleep.

sentinel event: an unexpected occurrence that results in serious physical or psychological injury or death.

serosanguineous drainage: pink wound drainage that contains some red blood cells.

serous drainage: yellow or transparent wound drainage.

serum: the liquid portion of the blood that has been allowed to clot.

sexually transmitted infections (STIs): infections caused by sexual contact with infected people; signs and symptoms are not always apparent.

sexual orientation: a person's physical, emotional, and/or romantic attraction to another person.

sharps: needles or other sharp objects.

shearing: rubbing or friction that results from the skin moving one way and the bone underneath it remaining fixed or moving in the opposite direction.

shingles: a skin rash caused by the varicella-zoster virus (VZV) that causes pain, tingling, itching, and a rash of fluid-filled blisters.

shock: a condition that occurs when organs and tissues in the body do not receive an adequate blood supply.

sickle cell disease (SCD): an inherited blood condition in which unusual hemoglobin causes red blood cells to become deformed; these deformed cells can get stuck in blood vessels, causing pain and organ damage.

Sims': a body position in which a patient is lying on his left side with the upper knee flexed and raised toward the chest.

sinoatrial node: part of the cardiac conduction system of the heart, located in the upper part of the right atrium and acting as the primary pacemaker of the heart; also called the *SA node* or *sinus node*.

sitz bath: a warm soak of the perineal area to clean perineal wounds and reduce inflammation and pain.

slide board: a wooden board that helps transfer patients who are unable to bear weight on their legs; also called *transfer board.*

social anxiety disorder: an anxiety disorder in which a person has intense anxiety and extreme discomfort in social situations.

special diet: diet prescribed for certain illnesses, conditions, or food allergies; also called *therapeutic* or *modified diet.*

specific immunity: a type of immunity that protects the body against a particular disease that is invading the body at a given time.

specimen: a sample that is used for analysis in order to try to make a diagnosis.

sphygmomanometer: a device that measures blood pressure.

sputum: mucus coughed up from the lungs.

Standard Precautions: a method of infection prevention in which all blood and other body fluids, nonintact skin, and mucous membranes are treated as if they were infected.

stepdown unit: unit in a hospital for patients who no longer need intensive care but need more care than is given in the medical/surgical unit.

sterile field: a sterile area set up for a surgical procedure; everything within the sterile field must be sterilized and sterility must be maintained within this area.

sterilization: a cleaning measure used to decrease the spread of pathogens and disease by destroying all microorganisms, including those that form spores.

stethoscope: an instrument designed to listen to sounds within the body, such as the heart beating or air moving through the lungs.

stillbirth: death of a fetus from 20 weeks of pregnancy and beyond; may occur before or during delivery.

stoma: an artificial opening in the body.

straight: word to describe a person whose physical, emotional, and/or romantic attraction is for people of the opposite gender.

straight catheter: a type of urinary catheter that does not remain inside the person; it is removed immediately after urine is drained or collected.

subacute care unit: unit in a hospital for patients who no longer need the care given in the medical/surgical unit but who are not ready to go home.

subjective information: information that a person cannot or did not observe, but is based on something reported to the person that may or may not be true; also called *symptoms.*

substance use disorder (SUD): the repeated or uncontrolled use of legal or illegal substances in a way that is harmful to oneself or others.

sundowning: becoming restless and agitated in the late afternoon, evening, or night.

supination: turning upward.

supine: a body position in which a patient lies flat on his back.

surgical asepsis: the state of being completely free of all microorganisms; also called *sterile technique.*

surgical bed: a bed made to accept a patient who is returning to bed on a stretcher.

susceptible host: an uninfected person who could become sick.

sympathy: sharing in the feelings and difficulties of others.

syncope: loss of consciousness; also called *fainting.*

syphilis: a sexually transmitted infection caused by bacteria; causes open sores on the penis or inside the vagina, as well as headache, fever, weight loss, and muscle aches.

syringe: a barrel-shaped device with a plunger that is pulled to draw in fluid (e.g., blood).

systemic infection: an infection that travels through the bloodstream and is spread throughout the body, causing general symptoms.

systole: the phase where the heart is at work, contracting and pushing blood out of the left ventricle.

systolic: first measurement of blood pressure; phase when the heart is at work, contracting and pushing the blood out of the left ventricle.

tachycardia: rapid heart rate—over 100 beats per minute.

tachypnea: rapid respirations.

tactful: showing sensitivity and having a sense of what is appropriate when dealing with others.

TB disease: type of tuberculosis in which the person shows symptoms of the disease and can spread it to others.

telemetry: cardiac monitoring that sends information about the heart's rhythm and rate to a special monitoring room.

terminal illness: a disease or condition that will eventually cause death.

testicular cancer: the rapid growth of abnormal cells in one or both testicles.

tissues: groups of cells that perform similar functions.

tracheostomy: a surgically created opening through the neck into the trachea.

transfer belt: a belt made of canvas or other heavy material that is used to help people who are weak, unsteady, or uncoordinated to transfer or walk.

transient ischemic attack (TIA): a warning sign of a CVA/stroke resulting from a temporary lack of blood supply to the brain.

transmission: passage or transfer.

Transmission-Based Precautions: a method of infection prevention used when caring for persons who are infected or may be infected with certain infectious diseases.

trauma: severe injury due to accidents or acts of violence.

triage: the sorting of patients for care based on the urgency of their condition.

tuberculosis (TB): a highly contagious disease caused by a bacterium, *Mycobacterium tuberculosis,* that is carried on mucous droplets suspended in the air; causes fatigue, loss of appetite, slight fever, prolonged coughing, and shortness of breath.

tumor: a cluster of abnormally growing cells.

type 1 diabetes: a type of diabetes in which the pancreas produces no insulin or too little insulin; is usually diagnosed in children and young adults and will continue throughout a person's life.

type 2 diabetes: a common form of diabetes in which either the body does not produce enough insulin or the body fails to properly use insulin; typically develops after age 35 and is the milder form of diabetes.

ulceration: the process of eroding away.

ulcerative colitis: a chronic inflammatory disease of the large intestine that causes cramping, diarrhea, pain, rectal bleeding, loss of appetite, and weight loss.

unoccupied bed: a bed made while no person is in the bed.

ureterostomy: a surgically created opening from a ureter to the abdomen that allows urine to be eliminated.

urinary catheter: a catheter that is used to drain urine from the bladder.

urinary incontinence: the inability to control the bladder, which leads to an involuntary loss of urine.

urinary tract infection (UTI): a bacterial infection of the urethra, bladder, ureter, or kidney.

uterine fibroid: growth that occurs in or on the uterus and is almost always benign (non-cancerous).

vaginitis: an inflammation of the vagina that may be caused by bacteria, protozoa, or a fungus.

verbal communication: communication involving the use of spoken or written words or sounds.

vital signs: measurements—temperature, pulse, respirations, blood pressure— that monitor the functioning of the vital organs of the body.

VRE (vancomycin-resistant *Enterococcus*): bacteria (*enterococci*) that have developed resistance to the antibiotic vancomycin.

wound: a type of injury to the skin.

Yankauer suction catheter: a rigid, hollow tube with a bend that is used to perform suctioning.

Index